Handbook of Research on Environmental and Human Health Impacts of Plastic Pollution

Khursheed Ahmad Wani
Government Degree College Bijbehara, India

Lutfah Ariana
Indonesian Institute of Sciences, Indonesia

S.M. Zuber
Government Degree College Bijbehara, India

A volume in the Advances in Environmental Engineering and Green Technologies (AEEGT) Book Series

IGI Global
DISSEMINATOR OF KNOWLEDGE

Published in the United States of America by
IGI Global
Engineering Science Reference (an imprint of IGI Global)
701 E. Chocolate Avenue
Hershey PA, USA 17033
Tel: 717-533-8845
Fax: 717-533-8661
E-mail: cust@igi-global.com
Web site: http://www.igi-global.com

Library of Congress Cataloging-in-Publication Data

Names: Wani, Khursheed Ahmad, editor. | Ariana, Lutfah, editor. | Zuber, S. M., 1970- editor.
Title: Handbook of research on environmental and human health impacts of plastic pollution / Khursheed Ahmad Wani, Lutfah Ariana, and S.M. Zuber, editors.
Description: Hershey, PA : Engineering Science Reference, [2020] | Includes bibliographical references.
Identifiers: LCCN 2019001911| ISBN 9781522594529 (h/c) | ISBN 9781522594543 (eISBN)
Subjects: LCSH: Plastic scrap--Environmental aspects. | Plastics--Toxicology.
Classification: LCC TD427.P62 R57 2020 | DDC 363.738--dc23 LC record available at https://lccn.loc.gov/2019001911

This book is published in the IGI Global book series Advances in Environmental Engineering and Green Technologies (AEEGT) (ISSN: 2326-9162; eISSN: 2326-9170)

British Cataloguing in Publication Data
A Cataloguing in Publication record for this book is available from the British Library.

For electronic access to this publication, please contact: eresources@igi-global.com.

Advances in Environmental Engineering and Green Technologies (AEEGT) Book Series

Sang-Bing Tsai
University of Electronic Science and Technology of China Zhongshan Institute, China
Ming-Lang Tseng
Lunghwa University of Science and Technology, Taiwan
Yuchi Wang
University of Electronic Science and Technology of China Zhongshan Institute, China

ISSN:2326-9162
EISSN:2326-9170

Mission

Growing awareness and an increased focus on environmental issues such as climate change, energy use, and loss of non-renewable resources have brought about a greater need for research that provides potential solutions to these problems. Research in environmental science and engineering continues to play a vital role in uncovering new opportunities for a "green" future.

The **Advances in Environmental Engineering and Green Technologies (AEEGT)** book series is a mouthpiece for research in all aspects of environmental science, earth science, and green initiatives. This series supports the ongoing research in this field through publishing books that discuss topics within environmental engineering or that deal with the interdisciplinary field of green technologies.

Coverage

- Electric Vehicles
- Green Technology
- Renewable Energy
- Sustainable Communities
- Contaminated Site Remediation
- Air Quality
- Policies Involving Green Technologies and Environmental Engineering
- Green Transportation
- Radioactive Waste Treatment
- Cleantech

The Advances in Environmental Engineering and Green Technologies (AEEGT) Book Series (ISSN 2326-9162) is published by IGI Global, 701 E. Chocolate Avenue, Hershey, PA 17033-1240, USA, www.igi-global.com. This series is composed of titles available for purchase individually; each title is edited to be contextually exclusive from any other title within the series. For pricing and ordering information please visit http://www.igi-global.com/book-series/advances-environmental-engineering-green-technologies/73679. Postmaster: Send all address changes to above address.

Titles in this Series

For a list of additional titles in this series, please visit: www.igi-global.com/book-series

Advanced Design of Wastewater Treatment Plants Emerging Research and Opportunities
Athar Hussain (Ch. Brahm Prakash Government Engineering College, India) and Ayushman Bhattacharya (Ch. Brahm Prakash Government Engineering Colleg, India)
Engineering Science Reference • ©2019 • 350pp • H/C (ISBN: 9781522594413) • US $195.00

Advanced Multi-Criteria Decision Making for Addressing Complex Sustainability Issues
Prasenjit Chatterjee (MCKV Institute of Engineering, India) Morteza Yazdani (Universidad Loyola Andalucía, Spain) Shankar Chakraborty (Jadavpur University, India) Dilbagh Panchal (Dr. B. R. Ambedkar National Institute of Technology (NIT) Jalandhar, India) and Siddhartha Bhattacharyya (RCC Institute of Information Technology Kolkata, India)
Engineering Science Reference • ©2019 • 360pp • H/C (ISBN: 9781522585794) • US $195.00

Amelioration Technology for Soil Sustainability
Ashok K. Rathoure (Biohm Consultare Pvt Ltd, India)
Engineering Science Reference • ©2019 • 280pp • H/C (ISBN: 9781522579403) • US $185.00

Advanced Agro-Engineering Technologies for Rural Business Development
Valeriy Kharchenko (Federal Scientific Agroengineering Center VIM, Russia) and Pandian Vasant (Universiti Teknologi PETRONAS, Malaysia)
Engineering Science Reference • ©2019 • 484pp • H/C (ISBN: 9781522575733) • US $195.00

Spatial Planning in the Big Data Revolution
Angioletta Voghera (Politecnico di Torino, Italy) and Luigi La Riccia (Politecnico di Torino, Italy)
Engineering Science Reference • ©2019 • 359pp • H/C (ISBN: 9781522579274) • US $195.00

Global Initiatives for Waste Reduction and Cutting Food Loss
Aparna B. Gunjal (Asian Agri Food Consultancy Services Ltd, India) Meghmala S. Waghmode (Annasaheb Magar Mahavidyalaya, India) Neha N. Patil (Annasaheb Magar Mahavidyalaya, India) and Pankaj Bhatt (Dolphin (P.G) College of Biomedical and Natural Sciences Dehradun, India)
Engineering Science Reference • ©2019 • 328pp • H/C (ISBN: 9781522577065) • US $195.00

Green Public Procurement Strategies for Environmental Sustainability
Rajesh Kumar Shakya (The World Bank, USA)
Engineering Science Reference • ©2019 • 228pp • H/C (ISBN: 9781522570837) • US $185.00

IGI Global
DISSEMINATOR OF KNOWLEDGE

701 East Chocolate Avenue, Hershey, PA 17033, USA
Tel: 717-533-8845 x100 • Fax: 717-533-8661
E-Mail: cust@igi-global.com • www.igi-global.com

Editorial Advisory Board

List of Contributors

Table of Contents

Section 2
Plastics and Human Health

Detailed Table of Contents

pollution such as soil pollution, water pollution, and air pollution. Application of proper rules and regulations for the production and use of plastics can reduce the toxic effects of plastics on human health and the environment.

Plastic pollution is one of the prime and alarming issues in developing countries that has vast environmental and human health impacts which need to be addressed as a priority. Unfortunately, limited work has been done on the topic, especially on air and water pollution due to plastics in Pakistan. Informal solid waste management is being done by municipalities, which is not adequate, and the problem will increase with the upsurge in population and industrialization. There is a need to address the knowledge gap and improvements in the existing conditions to manage the issue of plastic pollution separately. In this chapter, causes; impacts of plastic pollution both on human and environmental health, plastic industries, and legislative context; and best practices to manage plastic pollution along with some important recommendations are discussed. It is expected the data presented may help the managers, environmental scientists, and policymakers to manage the problem of plastic pollution.

Rapid consumption of resources produces municipal solid wastes (MSW) in developing countries at the present time. MSW comprises the various kinds of waste present at different levels such as household products, industrial waste, biomedical waste, pesticides, sanitation residue, agriculture residue, building material waste, and so forth. The presence of solid waste in the water system is very hazardous and can cause severe health diseases in the human body such as dermatological disorder, respiratory infections, eye and blood infections, cholera, typhoid, tuberculosis, amoebic dysentery, anthrax, and so forth. Due to incineration of waste materials, the remaining ash is dumped into the water system so the amount of free oxygen in the water is diminished, which results in the death of fishes, beneficial bacteria, and worms, which play an important role in the fertility of the soil. This chapter reviews the challenges, methods, technologies, barriers, and opportunities associated with improving waste management worldwide.

Plastic pollution in the environment is currently receiving worldwide attention. Improper dumping of disused or abandoned plastic wastes leads to contamination of the environment. Contamination by bulk plastics and plastic debris is currently the one of the most serious problems in aquatic ecosystems.

Section 3
Plastic Waste Management

Foreword

Pollution in the form of solid, liquid, gas, heat, sound, or radioactivity effects our environment at a rate much quicker than it becomes harmless with major types as; air, water, noise, light and land pollution. Plastic pollution is a new edition to this with negative effects on the environment and wildlife and ultimately human health. The plastic was first invented in 1907 from a synthetic polymer made from phenol and formaldehyde. Today China contributes the highest share with over 25 percent of the global total, followed by Indonesia (10%), Philippines and Vietnam (6% each), Thailand, Egypt and Nigeria (3% each) and South Africa (2%). Plastics are the most affordable and easily available items at global level (Ritchie & Roser, 2018). About one trillion single-use plastic bags are used annually across the globe. That's nearly 2 million every minute. More than half a billion plastic straws are used every day around the world. More than 6.9 billion tons of plastics have become waste and a staggering 6.3 billion tons never made it to a recycling bin. No one knows how much unrecycled plastic waste exactly ends up in the ocean. In 1950, the world's population of 2.5 billion and they produced 1.5 million tons of plastic; in 2016, a global population of more than 7 billion people has produced over 320 million tons of plastic. This is set to double by 2034. Every day approximately 8 million pieces of plastic pollution find their way into our oceans (Jambeck et al., 2015).

Plastic waste is one of many types of wastes that take too long to decompose. Normally, plastic items can take up to 1000 years to decompose in landfills. But plastic bags we use in our everyday life take 10-1000 years to decompose, while plastic bottles can take 450 years or more. Different plastic pollution types are among our biggest environmental threats, hurting sea animals and making them sick. It is littering our oceans and threatening the lives of millions of marine animals because of this deadly environmental concern (Leblank, 2019).

More than 8 million tons of plastic annually end up in our oceans therefore more than hundred thousand activists from over 40 countries have taken a stand on plastic pollution. Estimates are that there will be half a kilogram of plastic for every 1.5 kg of fish in the ocean within next few years. The trash in our waters effects the smallest plankton to the biggest whales, some of the animals confuse plastic bags for food. World Wild Life fund is trying hard to be plastic-free by 2030 (UNEP & FAO, 2009).

Approximately 10-50 trillion microplastic particles weighing nearly 200.000 tonnes have been reported to keep floating in our oceans. Plastics also pollute without being littered through the release of its compounds. Burning of plastic releases poisonous chemicals, which when inhaled by living beings affect their health leading to respiratory diseases, lung cancer and others. The plastics contain toxic chemicals which can increase the chance of disease and affect reproduction in animals which may suffer for months or years before their death. Toxic chemicals accumulating in top predators can make these species unsafe to consume. The pollution of environment by chemicals leached from plastics into our surroundings is an area of concern. The toxic chemicals like bisphenol A are the most common types of plastic pollution and combined with plastic bags and food containers make up the majority of oceanic debris (Lebreton et al., 2017). Long term plastic polluting our waters has severe impacts on environment and economy. Seabirds, whales, sea turtles and other marine life are eating marine plastic and dying from choking, intestinal blockage and starvation. Approximately 700 marine species and according to some at least 100 million marine mammals are killed each year from plastic pollution. The non-biodegradable plastic when thrown on away reduces the soil fertitlity, chokes our ponds, rivers and oceans, and harms the sea life. The plastics circumnavigate the globe more than 4000 times and 100,000 of our marine life die annually from plastic entanglement and nearly 1 million sea birds die from plastic (Eriksen et al., 2014).

This volume titled *Handbook of Research on Environmental and Human Health Impacts of Plastic Pollution* edited by Khursheed Ahmad Wani, Lutfah Ariana, and S. M. Zuber from India and Indonesia is composed of three sections.

In Section 1 titled "Plastic Pollution and Environment" there are 11 contributions from India, Pakistan, and Indonesia. The topics include: plastic pollution and its effect on our environment; environmental and human health impacts of plastic waste; environmental and health implications of plastic pollution in Pakistan; environmental implications of incineration of municipal solid waste and ash disposal-a review; impact of plastic pollution on the aquatic ecosystems; marine plastic debris-distribution, abundance and impact on seafood; detrimental impact of plastics on agriculture-a threat to environment; plastic pollution and its remedies-an Indian scenario; plastic pollution and its impact on aquatic fauna; analysis of the recycling potential of medicinal plastic wastes: alternatives for treatment and disposal cost reduction of regulated medical waste.

Section 2 deals with "Plastics and Human Health". It is composed of seven chapters all from India discussing the topics like; association between urinary bisphenol A concentration and obesity prevalence in children and adolescents; bisphenol A and phthalates in the environment and their health effects; bisphenol A and phthalates exhibit similar toxicogenomics and health effects; exposure of phthalate to human health with special refernce to reproductive outcomes; environmental phthalate exposure in relation to reproductive outcomes and other health endpoints in humans; environmental phthalate exposure in relation to various health outcomes in humans; polyhydroxyalkanoates: an indispensable alternative.

The last section presents data on the "Plastic Waste Management". It has five chapters with titles from India, USA, and Malaysia; solid waste management and its impacts on environment; challenges and factors in plastic reutilization/recycling: a review, plastic pollution and its management in the age of globalization with special to India, biodegradation of plastic: an innovative solution to safe the human health and environment, framework proposition strategy for collection of returned products in reverse logistics environment.

The book emphasizes five Rs (i.e., recycle, reuse, reduce, remove, and refuse) for control of plastic pollution, stresses the need for education and outreach programs, strong laws and policies, and law enforcement for government and private institutions. They suggest that policy makers and advisers should sternly follow the steps like never throwing plastic bags on roads, carry nonplastic bags from home and use other items rather than plastics which can be reused. Microorganisms like bacteria, fungi and actinomycetes have developed a special strategy in order to use such materials as energy and carbon source. This needs to be developed further at a large scale. People should avoid using microbeads, replace plastics with jute or cotton bags, stop throwing plastic bags in rivers, cut down waste, carry reusable water bottles, avoid straws, reduce plastic waste to the minimum, follow reusable shopping and produce bags for markets, avoid using single-use plastics, avoid straws.

The book presents a wealth of information on plastic pollution and I must congratulatre the editorial team as well as the contributors for their excellent presentations.

Münir Öztürk
Islamic World Academy of Sciences, Turkey

Münir Öztürk *is Vice President of the Islamic World Academy of Sciences, Turkey.*

REFERENCES

Eriksen, M., Lebreton, L. C., Carson, H. S., Thiel, M., Moore, C. J., Borerro, J. C., ... Reisser, J. (2014). Plastic pollution in the world's oceans: More than 5 trillion plastic pieces weighing over 250,000 tons afloat at sea. *PLoS One*, *9*(12). doi:10.1371/journal.pone.0111913 PMID:25494041

Jambeck, J. R., Geyer, R., Wilcox, C., Siegler, T. R., Perryman, M., Andrady, A., ... Law, K. L. (2015). Plastic waste inputs from land into the ocean. *Science*, *347*(6223), 768–771. doi:10.1126cience.1260352 PMID:25678662

Leblank, R. (2019). *The Decomposition of Waste in Landfills: A Story of Time and Materials*. Available at: https://www.thebalancesmb.com/how-long-does-it-take-garbage-to-decompose-2878033

Lebreton, L. C., Van der Zwet, J., Damsteeg, J. W., Slat, B., Andrady, A., & Reisser, J. (2017). River plastic emissions to the world's oceans. *Nature Communications*, *8*(1), 15611. doi:10.1038/ncomms15611 PMID:28589961

Ritchie Hannah and Roser Max. (2018). *Plastic Pollution*. Avaılable at https://ourworldindata.org/plastic-pollution

UNEP & FAO. (2009). *Abandoned, lost or otherwise discarded fishing gear*. FAO Fisheries and Aquaculture Technical Paper No. 523, UNEP Regional Seas Reports and Studies No. 185. Available at: http://www.fao.org/docrep/011/i0620e/i0620e00.htm

Preface

Plastic usage in daily life has increased from 5 to 100 million tons per year since the 1950s due to their light-weight, non-corrosive nature, durability and cheap price. Plastic products consist mainly of polyethylene, polystyrene, polypropylene and polyvinyl chloride type plastics. The human society over the past century has enhanced the use of plastics in day to day life. Presently, there are more than 20 different major types of plastics used all over the globe and affect humans and the environment in one or the other way. Due to the non-biodegradability of these plastic substances, they have become an environmental nuisance and added extra burden to the already existing problem in the environment. It is obvious that plastics bring many societal benefits and offer future technological and medical advances. However, concerns about usage and disposal are diverse and include the accumulation of waste in landfills and in natural habitats, physical problems for wildlife resulting from ingestion or entanglement in plastic, the leaching of chemicals from plastic products and the potential for plastics to transfer chemicals to aquatic environment and humans. Monitoring the large quantity of debris in different ecosystems is important to establish rates of accumulation and the effectiveness of any remediation measures. The chapters included in this book have been received from different researchers across the globe have discussed the rising plastic pollution in the world and its impact on humanity and other ecosystems. The management strategies and policies have been also well discussed in the chapters.

We believe, these chapters included in the book are quite interesting and highly attractive to a student pursuing pre-research, research, and even masters and will be highly fruitful to NGO's and Industrialists.

Chapter 1 argues that the plastic pollution is treated as a dangerous and highly damaging phenomenon in marine environment and mostly hazardous to large marine mammals, amphibians, birds and people living in coastal areas of sea because plastic materials contain a number and verity kinds of chemicals, depending on the type of plastics and are mutagenic in nature. Finally, there are five R's named as Recycle, Reuse, Reduce, Remove and Refuse can control the plastic pollution from our environment.

Chapter 2 discusses the different concerns of plastics on the Environment and Human Health. The current understanding of the benefits and concerns surrounding the use of plastics and look to future priorities, challenges and opportunities are also explained. Plastics arise serious environment pollution such as soil pollution, water pollution, and air pollution.

Chapter 3 discusses the causes, impacts of plastic pollution both on human and environmental health, plastic industries and legislative context and best practices to manage plastic pollution along with some important recommendations are discussed. It is expected the data presented may help the managers, environmental scientist and policymakers to manage the problem of plastic pollution.

Chapter 4 reviews the challenges, methods, technologies, barriers, and opportunities associated with improving waste management worldwide. The presence of solid waste in the water system is very hazardous can cause severe health diseases in the human body such as dermatological disorder, respiratory infections, eye and blood infections, cholera, typhoid, tuberculosis, amoebic dysentery, and anthrax, and so forth.

Chapter 5 advocated that the abundance of plastics, combined with their small size and subsequent association with plankton in the water column, allows for direct ingestion by aquatic biota at different trophic levels.

Chapter 6 argues that we only have a limited understanding of marine plastic debris distribution, implication, fate, and behavior. Science is the key to getting the right alternative for processing debris. To prevent marine pollution successfully requires education and outreach programs, strong laws and policies, and law enforcement for government and private institutions.

Chapter 7 advocates that plastic is made-up non-biodegradable chemicals i.e. polyolefin, polyester, and polyurethanes. This can cause serious harm to the species that drink this water. Unlike natural organic material, they do not disintegrate with time and keep accumulating in the environment.

Chapter 8 discussed the harmful chemicals that get absorbed in the plastic debris, have a varied and harmful range of chronic effects like endocrine disorders. Therefore, it is high time for the government to take stringent steps to overcome the problems associated with plastic pollution. Policy makers and advisers should sternly follow the steps: never throw plastic bags on roads; always carry bags from home; and, use paper decorative items rather than of plastics as paper can be reused.

Chapter 9 describes that plastic pollution is the buildup of unwanted plastic products in the environment by its abundant and limitless use by the greedy human population in various ways. Plastics are usually made of chains of monomer units of ethylene and propylene linked together. Plastics are durable and resistant to degradation and tend to accumulate wherever disposed of. One more disaster this material causes is the release of toxic chemicals with time which affects the ecosystem badly where it is dumped. The same is the case with aquatic ecosystem because tons of plastic wastes are dumped into it in one way or the other.

The recycling issues like risk of transmitting infections, improper collection and separation, can be resolved by proper management, education and innovative waste collection, and disposal policies are explained in the tenth chapter.

The link between human health and environmental quality is made clearer; the commitment to safeguarding the natural environment is growing in major institutions as the health care industry is discussed in the eleventh chapter.

Chapter 12 argued that the adverse effects related to obesity include insulin resistance, adipocyte differentiation or aromatase-mediated transformation of androgen into estrogen. Apart from adipocyte hypertrophy and hyperplasia, bisphenol A has serious health risks particularly cardiovascular diseases, liver function abnormalities, alterations in the circulating thyroid hormone levels, association with diabetes, carcinogenic effect and its other aspects on health individually as well as in combination with other chemicals are worth mentioning.

Chapter 13 explains that plastics are also ubiquitous contaminants in the human body, wildlife, and the environment. BPA and PAEs have recently attracted the special attention of the scientific community, regulatory agencies and the general public due to their serious health concerns.

Chapter 14 explains Bisphenol A and phthalates are the most frequently detected organic pollutants found in our surroundings because of their regular use as plasticizers in daily use polymeric products are extensively studied.

The literature presented in Chapter 15 revealed that phthalate exposure has made alteration both to females and males, like reproductive alterations: including damaging the sperm quality, semen concentration and sperm DNA, breast cancer in females, AGD, endocrine disruption. Phthalate exposure has been shown to alter the behavior, which is an indication of nervous system damage. Phthalate exposure has been revealed to affect respiration. Phthalate after exposure has been found to get metabolized in various endpoints and their detection by various techniques has made an insight towards understanding the mechanism of phthalates toxicity.

The purpose of Chapter 16 is to review the environmental impact of phthalate exposure in relation to reproductive behavior and other health problems in humans. The primary exposure of Phthalates during fetal development stage results in a number of harmful effects in male offspring in humans, like abnormalities of the sperm-producing organs, abnormal development of penile, hypospadias, reduced anogenital distance as well as a risk for Prostate Cancer and cryptorchidism

The Chapter 17 on the hazards of phthalates would benefit the general population, academia, scientists, clinicians, environmentalists, and law or policymakers to decide upon whether usage of phthalates to be continued swiftly without sufficient deceleration or regulated by law or to be phased out from earth forever.

Chapter 18 is about the selections of suitable bacterial strains, inexpensive carbon sources, efficient fermentation, and recovery processes are also some aspects important aspects taken into consideration for the commercialization of PHA. PHA producers have been reported to reside at various ecological niches with few among them also produce some by-products like extracellular polymeric substances, rhamnolipids, and biohydrogen gas.

Chapter 19 discusses the advanced and new methods of disposal of solid waste such as pyrolysis, pulverization, incineration, and development of sanitary landfills, etc are used to solve the problem of managing solid waste.

Chapter 20 explores the plastic recycling methods and challenges during plastic recycling and deliberates more briefly how the government sector is working to clean most of the plastic waste from landfills to recycling over the next periods. In the last, this chapter highlights the plastic effects on the environment and how we can use them again through recycling.

Chapter 21 identifies the need to view globalization and its free flow of plastic commodities critically, so as to manage the menace of plastic pollution in India. Globalization as a process has undeniably been involved in ever-increasing mobility, of both men and material.

Chapter 22 advocated the importance of biodegradation of plastic products which is a rapidly growing field and offers a new dimension solution with novel properties in waste management areas. Microorganisms like bacteria, fungi, and actinomycetes have developed a special strategy in order to use such materials as energy and carbon source.

Chapter 23 argued that the importance of reverse logistics and product recovery is evident in various industries as well as in current UNESCO sustainable development goals. This includes plastics and recycling with the former "contributed" significantly towards environmental issues and the latter being one of the primary solutions.

Plastics offer substantial benefits for the future, but it is obvious that the approaches to production, use, and disposal are not sustainable and present concerns for aquatic life and human health. We have considerable knowledge about many of the environmental hazards, and information on human health effects is growing, but many concerns and uncertainties remain. There are solutions to control plastic pollution, but these can only be achieved by combined actions. There is a role for individuals, via appropriate use and disposal, particularly recycling; for industry by adopting green chemistry, material reduction and by designing products for reuse and/or end-of-life recyclability and for governments and policymakers by setting standards and targets, by defining appropriate product labelling to inform and incentivize change and by funding relevant academic research and technological developments.

Most of the chapters argue the abundance of all types of anthropogenic debris including data on plastics and/or plastic items is insufficient and needs further investigations at all fronts. In general, the abundance of debris on shorelines has been extensively monitored, in comparison to surveys from the open oceans or the seabed that need to be investigated. In addition to recording debris, there is a need to collect data on sources; for plastic debris, this should include discharges from rivers and sewers together with littering behavior.

The book will generate awareness towards the use of plastics and its impact on the environment, human health and other ecosystems. This publication will help the researchers to assess the negative impacts of plastic burden and they will start searching out different ways by involving biotechnological approaches to this menace. The literature included in this publication will help to reduce the burden of plastic pollution and will indirectly reduce the load of diseases caused due to plastic pollution on the planet earth.

Khursheed Ahmad Wani
Government Degree College Bijbehara, India

Lutfah Ariana
Indonesian Institute of Sciences, Indonesia

S. M. Zuber
Government Degree College Bijbehara, India

Acknowledgment

First and foremost, we would like to place on record our gratitude and sincere thanks to Almighty Allah[SWT] who always helped us surreptitiously while instilling passion of taking the stupendous jobs at hand. It is because of HIS divine intervention that we could finally complete this job in time.

We are at loss of words in extending heartfelt thanks to the anonymous learned reviewers who put every effort to make this project possible for us. We are thankful to the authorities at Govt. Degree College Bijbehara and Indonesian Institute of Sciences for providing facility of computers and internet during the course of editing. We are extremely thankful to Maria Rohde, Assistant Development Editor, IGI Global for being so kind to us during the editing of book.

To our parents, we are speechless! We can barely find the words to express all the wisdom, love and support you've given us. To our children: you were kind serene during the editing of the book. Our love for you has increased and we hope you will bear with us in future as well.

To rest of the family members, we do love you guys very much, collectively as well as, individually for different reasons. You all have always made us feel as if we are proud members, in spite of all our imperfections. Finally, our thanks are due to all the people who have supported us in completing and compiling this voluminous book directly or indirectly.

Khursheed Ahmad Wani
Government Degree College Bijbehara, India

Lutfah Ariana
Indonesian Institute of Sciences, Indonesia

S. M. Zuber
Government Degree College Bijbehara, India

Section 1
Plastic Pollution and the Environment

Chapter 1
Plastic Pollution and Its Effect on the Environment

Trinath Biswal
VSS University of Technology, India

Pravin Kumar Kar
Veer Surendra Sai University of Technology, India

ABSTRACT

Chlorinated plastics releases harmful chemicals and toxic substances into the surrounding soil, which can then seep into ground water or other surrounding surface water bodies in the form of a black thick liquid known as leachate causing sever water pollution. This water, if used as drinking water, causes serious harm to both plants and animals. Many advanced polymer composites used in various fields can leach into water forming hurdles. Plastic pollution is potentially poisonous to animals, which can then affect human food supplies. Plastic materials contain a number and variety of chemicals that are carcinogenic and mutagenic in nature. The five R's (recycle, reuse, reduce, remove, and refuse) can control the plastic pollution in our environment. This chapter explores plastic pollution and its effect on the environment.

INTRODUCTION

Plastic pollution may be defined as gathering of the various kinds of plastic materials, composites and Nano-composites of polymer on the surface of the earth, as well as in different surface water bodies such as rivers, sea and oceans, canals, some usable lakes, water reservoirs, dams, ponds etc. Now a day's plastic materials are utilized in different sectors on a large scale in different forms all over the world (Pavani et. al., 2014). The use of plastic materials are basically synthetic polymer or polymer composites and mostly the composition of some organic materials and some plastic materials may contain inorganic compounds and known as inorganic polymers. These are mainly derived from petrochemicals like alkenes and alkanes. While we discuss about the polymer or polymeric materials generally it means organic polymers because it is large in number and the number of inorganic polymers are quite less in number. Plastic materials are mainly classified as thermoplastics (polystyrene and polyvinyl chloride) and thermosetting polymers (poly-isoprene, Bakelite) on the basis of heat treatment. Apart from these

DOI: 10.4018/978-1-5225-9452-9.ch001

again polymeric materials are classified as biodegradable or non-biodegradable, engineering plastic materials, elastomers, fibers and plastics. Besides these there are several classifications of plastic materials. Plastic materials takes about 500-1000 years for its degradation but the actual time of degradation is not known to anyone. The monomer, initiators, catalyst, fillers, plasticizers, colouring materials used for the manufacture of plastic are highly poisonous and cause many dreadful diseases both in animals and human beings. If these waste plastic materials are not properly removed from the environment it may causes hazardous effect to our biological system.

Many vinyl monomers are carcinogenic in nature and its exposure for a long time causes cancer. (Elena - Diana et. al.2016, Plastic pollution Wikipedia) Plastic materials are light weight, durable, low cost and good looking, which is the cause of overuse of plastic materials in different sectors. The waste plastic materials such as bags, bottles, rejected electronic and electrical devices, toys, balls, packaging materials, home utensils, decorative materials etc., are used extensively in urban areas and therefore cause of clogging the water bodies mostly like canals, rivers, lakes and water pipelines particularly in the urban areas and this trend is increasing day by day (Annual *Review of Marine Science,* 9, 2017).

Many people throw their plastic bottles and polythene bags after limited use or even after a single use as this less expensive method of disposal. But these waste plastic materials finally reach in landfill sites, and are deposited in the form of layer over the land surface or soil in the surrounding area. Most of these are non-biodegradable in nature. Waste plastic materials are also dumped in landfill sites. The waste materials of plastic may interact with the water and soil and degraded partially into toxic chemical substances. If these toxic degraded polymeric materials infiltrated inside the surface of the earth and mixed with the groundwater aquifers, then it causes the change in quality if the ground water resulting ground water pollution.

It is estimated that globally about 70,000 tons of plastic waste materials finally reach sea or ocean (Moharam et. al., 2014). Sometimes the rejected unused fishing nets and some other synthetic plastic materials are eaten by both terrestrial and aquatic animals by mistake as food, and cause bioaccumulation inside their bodies. Ultimately this is the cause of death of these animals Due to accumulation of plastic waste it may causes breeding of mosquitoes and other harmful dangerous insects and it might cause several diseases to human beings and domestic animals. Not only terrestrial environment but the accumulation of plastic waste in ocean cause harm to marine biota along with marine plants (Grantham Institute Briefing Paper No. 19).

Large use of plastic materials also deteriorates the quality of the drinking water day by day because the plastic materials are made of toxic chemicals like vinyl chloride, Bisphenol-A, Styrene, Acrylonitrile, Methyl methacrylate etc. and these are undergoing partial degradation after many years. The Bisphenol-A sometimes damages our respiratory and reproductive system.

One of the methods to reduce plastic waste is controlled incineration, which is nothing but the combustion of plastic waste materials which releases huge amounts of toxic gases to the atmosphere. This leads to air pollution.

Many vagrant animals sometimes eat waste plastic materials because of inadequate disposal systems and improper management and carelessly thrown nearby the locality area leading to death of these animals (G. Scott, et. al.2007).

The deposited waste plastic materials are transferred from one place to another due to wind causing increase in the land littering. These waste plastic materials also get trapped by railings, plants and trees, long towers, huge buildings, etc. and any animal who comes nearby it might even get twisted and suffocated by it and ultimately resulting in death.

MAJOR PLASTIC MATERIALS USED BY US AND THEIR ENVIRONMENTAL IMPACTS

The word plastic is derived from the world 'Plasticos' which means fit for Moulding, i,e polymeric materials which is fit for moulding into desired shape and size are known as plastic materials otherwise it is known as polymeric materials. The plastic polymeric materials on the basis of heat treatment may be divided into two categories:

a. Thermoplastic materials
b. Thermosetting materials

These are a group of synthetic or natural organic materials that can be reshaped when soft and then again becomes hardened when cooled are known as thermoplastic materials but the plastic materials which is difficult to soften and cannot be reshaped and reused again are known as thermosetting materials .The polymeric materials includes a number of kinds of resins, polymers, cellulose derivatives, casein materials, elastomers and proteins, that are used in place of other materials such as glass, wood, and metals, in construction and decoration, for making many articles, as coatings, and, drawn into filaments, for weaving.

In chemistry, polymeric materials are considered as large molecules which are composed of small molecules of one kind or more than one kind forming a repeating unit called as structural repeating units and the small molecules are known as monomers which are basically made with carbon backbones. A polymer is simply a very large molecule or macromolecule made up of many smaller units joined together, generally end to end, to create a long chain. (Vipin Koushal et. al. 2014)

The first man-made plastic materials are made by Alexander Parkes and he demonstrated it publicly in 1862 at Great International Exhibition in London. The material, called parkesine, which is an organic material derived from cellulose, once on heating it can be moulded into articles of desired shape and retained its shape when cooled. Some plastic materials but not all, plastic products have a number – the resin identification code – moulded, formed or imprinted in or on the container, often on the bottom. This system of coding was developed in 1988 by the U.S.-based Society of the Plastics Industry to facilitate the recycling of post-consumer plastics. It is indeed, quite interesting to go through the fine lines (S F Wang et. al. 1987).

Polyethylene Terephthalate (PETE or PET)

PET is one of a most commonly used thermoplastic polymeric material in the world and is widely used in the textile industry by the trade name "polyester." It is a naturally transparent and semi-crystalline plastic widely used as a fiber for clothing, as an effective moisture barrier with wide applicability in bottling and packaging and also an engineering plastic when it is combined with other materials like glass fiber or carbon nanotubes to significantly increase the material's strength. PET is generally found to be colourless and a semi-solid material. This material is higher strength in comparison to its weight and also highly resistance to water, and it also shatterproof in naturei.e.it could not disrupt easily during processing and manufacturing and its wide availability as an economic and recyclable plastic.PET is very strong for its lightweight. It will not break or fracture and this makes it a great replacement for glass as a container. It is a naturally transparent polymeric material. It is generally used in soft drink, juice, water, beer, mouthwash, peanut butter, salad dressing, detergent, and cleaner containers.PET does not react with water or any food materials which is one of the reasons it is used for consumable packaging. Polyethylene terephthalate (PET) is a wonderful plastic for 3D printing and also widely available as sheet stock for CNC machine manufacturing (Xingyou Tian et. al. 2006)

Environmental Impact

- It was experimentally found that about 50 grams of the material (PET) required for fabrication of soft drinking bottle of about 2 L capacity and for the same purpose 2000 grams of glass is required.
- Since PET is light weight, therefore more and more number of its finished products are transported easily from manufacturing plat to the storage room resulting the reduction of fuel consumption. The use of less petroleum product as fuel may reduce the emission of potential greenhouse gases and also the gas responsible for smog formation.
- The containers made by PET materials have minimum impact on our environmental. Therefore, most of the soft drink containers and bottles are made from PET materials which contains less air and water borne waste (Ming-hui, XieQiQiao et. al 2011)

High-Density Polyethylene (HDPE)

Polyethylene is a widely used plastic material and classified mainly into two categories:

a. Low density polythene(LDPE)
b. High density polythene(HDPE)

The LDPE has high molecular weight and it can be recycled and reused easily from the waste but HDPE has low molecular weight more soft, flexible and widely used in our day to day life and can be used as packaging materials for milk, water bottles, juice packaging containers, bleaching materials, packaging materials and bottles for shampoo and detergent, can be used as garbage bags, and also liners of cereal box. LDPE is widely used as packaging materials generally for grocery products, dry cleaning, packaging of bread and frozen food, containers for honey mustard oil, soybean oil, palm oil and most of the food products. (H. Shaikh, A. Anis et. al.2016)

Environmental Impact

Both HDPE and LDPE have greater environmental impacts on air, water and land surfaces.

- The waste polythene materials after use carelessly finished to the land surface and its accumulation on the surface of the land resist infiltration of water inside the soil reducing the water absorption capacity and nutrient absorption capacity of the soil. The presence of polythene waste materials also increases the temperature of the soil and prevent the irradiation of sun light into the soil. The plants and crops are not properly grown in the soil where there is huge accumulation of polythene materials and the soil becomes unfit for agricultural use. It can present around 1000 years inside the soil and then slowly undergoes degradation. The roots of plants cannot be penetrated inside the soil for water, nutrient etc.

- Many small and large marine animals and also sea birds when take these waste polyethylene materials as food, these animals finally suffering painful injuries and finally death. Marine Plants and animals after death decomposes with that water bodies and caused marine water pollution and affect our marine projects, fishing and tourism. (Vince J. et. al. 2017)
- If the Polyethylene materials (Both LDPE &HDPE) subjected to incineration, then unpleasant gaseous products, soot, carbon particles, PM and aerosol products are emitted which mainly causes airborne diseases. The products obtained mostly Volatile Organic Compounds (VOCs) of alkanes and alkenes, aldehydes and dioxins.
- Plastic materials are ingested by animals persists within the digestive system and causes the decrease in rate of feeding stimuli. About 80 species of sea birds and mammals have been found to ingest plastic. These animals with the plastic bags in their stomachs face prolonged painful deaths (Alka Grover et. al. 2015)

Hence for a better lifestyle and creating sustainable environment massive awareness campaign should have made among enlightenment regarding the harmful effect of polyethylene products position to our environment.

Polyvinyl Chloride (PVC)

It is a widely used thermoplastic polymeric materials having vast applications and can be used in manufacturing toys, food packaging materials and containers, materials for packaging of shampoo, detergent powder, jam and jelly, cooking oil, medical cleaning container along with different household utensils. PVC is considered as one of the toxic material used by human being and in soil it undergoes slow degradation and leaches a very hazardous substance known as di- (2-ethylhexyl) phthalate or butyl benzyl phthalate depending upon its use. If it is used as softener and plasticiser its toxicity increases from usual value. Both the chemicals obtained during the time of degradation are the cause of disrupting endocrine gland representing the ejection of female hormone estrogen, and is the major cause of asthma and allergic specially for children. The chemicals di- (2-ethylhexyl) phthalate or butyl benzyl phthalate is also carcinogenic in nature and impacts negative effects on the impotent organs of our body such as liver, spleen, kidney, and affects bone formation and also body weight. In European countries the dangerous phthalates and its derivatives are totally banned for the manufacturing of plastic toys specially for children since 1999. Another group of toxic chemical known as dioxins which are produced during the manufacturing of chlorinated materials which includes PVC and other chlorinated plastic or polymeric materials and composites. Dioxin is found to be a common carcinogenic material for human beings and is the most powerful synthetic carcinogen ever verified in laboratory and toxic both for human beings and animals (Dorel Feldman et. al. 2014)

Environmental Impact

Within the lifecycle of PVC, a number of environmental hazards are observed. These are as follows

About 40% of the chlorine produced world wise is consumed by the manufacturing of PVC which is almost approximately 16 million tons. PVC is considered as the largest volume of the production of toxic organochlorine which is highly hazardous to our society, environment and ecological community. It sometimes enters our food chains and causes fatal to all kinds of living beings. The toxic hazardous organochlorine products generated as by-products during the manufacturing of chlorine gas and highly riches chlorine of hazardous solid waste are generated in the synthesis of the monomer of ethylene dichloride and **vinyl chloride.**

- The chemical mixture produced in the manufacturing of monomerethylene dichloride and vinyl chloride are extremely hazardous and persist within the environment for a longer period of time. These chlorinated chemical mixtures are the by-products during manufacturing of PVC. Since these chemical mixtures are highly persistent and non-biodegradable, therefore its toxicity effect is quite high and now a days considered as global pollutants. Almost all the living beings specially in industrial zones are affected by these chemical mixtures and suffers many health hazard problems.
- The chlorinated chemical substances bio-accumulated in the fatty tissue of plants and animals because of fat soluble properties and becomes fatal to them. Within the food chain and food web these chemical mixtures are transferred from one organism to another organism and finally becomes fatal to many organisms. Due to bioaccumulation the concentrations of these chlorinated substances gradually increases from lower species to high on the food chain and the toxicities increases. These chemical mixtures can easily crossover the placenta and concentrate in the breast milk of human beings and other mammals
- This polymeric materials containing chlorine is the cause of many harmful diseases mainly Cancer, disruption of the endocrine system, reproductive impairment, Impaired child development and birth defects, Neurotoxicity i,e it damages the brain function, and Immune system suppression (Comanita Eleana-Diana et. al.2015).

Polypropylene (PP)

This is a thermoplastic polymeric material and is considered as addition polymer and is formed by simple addition of the monomer propylene by free radical addition polymerization process. It can be used in a number of applications such as packaging of consumer products, different mechanical parts of plastic parts for various industries which mostly include automotive industry, textile industries and manufacturing of special devices like living hinges etc. This polymeric material is used in manufacturing of ketchup bottles, margarine tubes, medicine bottles, syrup bottles, straw, some opaque plastic containers including baby bottles and water bottles. It is generally used as a safer plastic material for manufacturing of bottles and other containers. Now a day's advance research is carried out to make this plastic material as safer and eco-friendly. The material polypropylene is mainly used in packaging industry and in this sector about 30% of the PP is utilized, the electrical and electronic equipment manufacturing industries uses nearly about 13% each i,e total of 26% . The industries manufacturing household utensils uses 10% and automotive industries uses 10% each of PP materials follows with about 5% of the market. Other applications whole together utilize the remaining of the global polypropylene consumption. It is a chemical resistant material and do not react easily with dilute acids and bases, therefore for manufacturing the container of liquids acids and bases PP material is the first choice. The container of cleaning agents, box of first-aid products, and some other materials polypropylene is also the first choice material. Although the plastic Polypropylene shows property of elasticity over a certain range of deflection like all other materials but it also has good plastic deformation property and can deform early in the process of deformation, this the reason for which it is generally considered a "tough" material. The term toughness may be defined as the ability of the material to deform plastically without rupture or breaking. This material retains its shape even after a lot of torsion, flexing and bending, this property of the material is valuable mainly for production of living hinge. It has a greater resistance to electricity and also much useful for manufacturing of electronic components.

Originally the polypropylene produced normally opaque in colour but it can be made transparent by addition of some suitable materials. It can be used for applications where there is some transfer of light is required or where it is of aesthetic value. If better transmissivity is desired for some applications, then plastic materials like Acrylic or Polycarbonate are generally better choices (Hisham A. Maddah et. al. 2016).

Environmental Impact

- The products of Polypropylene can easily undergo rupture if it is they are exposed to high temperatures during the manufacturing process and especially more breaking occurs when it is presented to a common mineral filler commonly termed as talc. It also produces allergic reaction to the workers exposed to the plastic polypropylene.
- This plastic material causes adverse effect to our endocrine system because it is the cause of genetic mutations and also sometimes tumours. It can damage our reproductive system and reduces the fertility capacity. It is the simulator of the female hormone oestrogen, resulting an overload of it in the woman's body and cause of problems with fertility and conceiving. Therefore, this plastic material is very much danger specially for women.

Polystyrene (PS)

This plastic material is generally amorphous, nonpolar and a good thermoplastic resin which is the cause of easy processing of this material. Hence this material can form readily a large number of semi-finished products such as foams, plastic sheets, films etc. It is considered to be as one of the largest volume of commodity plastic and comprises approximately about 7% of the total thermoplastic market of the world.

The plastic PS is a good non-conducting material and having excellent property of optical clarity due to the lack of crystallinity and possesses good chemical resistance property and resistance to dilute acids and alkalis and some other chemicals. It can easily have fabricated into a variety kinds of finished products. It is originally a viscous liquid above its glass transition temperature (Tg), therefore it can be easily moulded into articles of different shape and size. However, the material polystyrene has several disadvantages. It is always attacked by solvents, of hydrocarbon and has poor oxygen and UV resistance characteristics. It is not malleable but rather brittle in nature, i.e. it possesses poor impact strength because of the stiffness of the backbone of the polymer. Polystyrene is a polymer that is cheap and easy to process. It is the material of choice for many applications, including food-packing, optical, electronic, medical, and automotive parts. A large variety of products are formed in PS by injection moulding, including dining utensils, plastic cups, house wares, toys, CD cases, cosmetic containers, covers and fixtures. Medical applications include pipettes, Petri dishes and medicine containers. This plastic material is used in Styrofoam containers, egg cartons, disposable cups and bowls, food containers, plastic cutlery, and compact disc cases. On degradation it leaches styrene which is an endocrine disruptor impersonating the female hormone oestrogen, and thus has the capacity to cause reproductive and developmental problems.

Polystyrene is present generally in cigarette smoke, off chattering of construction materials, car exhaust gases and more possibly on drinking water. Styrene can migrate significantly from the containers of polystyrene into some other container specially where oily foods are cooked. Polystyrene is generally a non- biodegradable polymeric material and is more resistant to the process of photolysis. The major debris in ocean is waste polystyrene. This polymeric material is although recyclable but it is not recycled in many parts of our country due to high cost and other different reasons. The expandable polystyrene (EPS) creates a great problem due to its low density because these waste occupies relatively large amount of space in landfills sites (T. Maharanaa et. al.2007)

Environmental Impact

- Styrene as a probable human carcinogen which is the monomer for manufacturing polystyrene. It was reported that human and animal epidemiological testing result identified styrene as a risk factor for lymphomas and leukemias and possibly for pancreatic, kidney, and oesophageal cancers.
- Science polystyrene does not readily biodegrade, once it enters into the landfill site or anyway to the environment, including the ocean, it will persist within the environment for a very long time period and causes hazardous effect to both animals and human beings. (Martin B. 1991)
- On Long-term exposure of this materials by workers the brain and nervous system are badly affected and impacts adverse effects on red blood cells, liver, kidneys, and mainly stomach in animal studies

Polylactic Acid (PLA)

This polymeric material is a unique common plastic material in comparison to other polymers. It is mainly derived from the biomass products rather from the petroleum products and hence it is biodegrading in nature much quicker than traditional used plastic materials. Wallace Carothers first of all discovered this polymer in 1932 by continuous heating lactic acid in vacuum and continuously removing the condensed water. Initially only PLA of low density is produced by the ring-opening polymerization process taking lactide as raw material and later on high-density PLA was finally developed by using other techniques. PLA is an important polymeric material now a day because of its unique property of biodegradability. It is also a bioactive thermoplastic polymeric material mainly derived from renewable resources of our globe mainly from corn starch, roots of cassava, or starch and from sugarcane also.

It is mostly manufactured from the different renewable sources of our globe and is also compostable in nature by some bacteria. Hence the disposal of solid waste of PLA is not a problem to our society, which is the cause of more dependence on PLA than petroleum-based polymeric materials. Now a day PLA is the second most manufactured and consumed bioplastic material in the world in volume. It was found now a day that there is a variety of applications of PLA was observed and the most common applications are manufacturing of plastic films, plastic bottles, and biodegradable medical products such as screws, pins, rods, and plates which are expected to be biodegraded within six months to one year. Since PLA can shrink by action of heat therefore it is suitable for using for manufacturing of shrink wrap material. Another interesting applications of PLA is 3D printing because it can easily melt Since PLA has low glass transition temperature therefore it is not suitable to hold in hot form of liquid (Xuan Pang et.al. 2010).

Environmental Impact

- PLA is a proper substitute of plastic and is prepared from fermented plant starch mainly corn and now a day it becoming a proper alternative of traditional petroleum-based plastic materials. Due to biodegradability property it is used in many countries of the world mainly in China, South Africa, Uganda, Ireland etc. in which plastic bags are banned for grocery and vegetable packaging. The pollution of plastic in these countries are called "white pollution". PLAis now plays a great role as the alternative of plastic and not only replaces synthetic plastic in these countries but also throughout the whole world.
- During incineration of PLA no toxic fumes and gases are emitted but PLA is far from the solution of the problem of world's plastic waste and its adverse effect to society.
- PLA generally takes about 3 months for complete biodegradation into the gaseous products CO_2 and H_2O in a controlled composting environment. If no light and oxygen entering into the landfill sites or controlled composting environment, then it takes longer time for biodegradation.
- Another disadvantages of it that PLA is extracted from genetically modified corns but the future environment and human health of genetic modification are still largely unknown. (Donald Garlotta et. al. 2001)

Polycarbonate (PC)

It is a good transparent plastic material and is mainly applicable because of its high impact strength and load bearing capacity in comparison to other plastics materials. It is generally used in producing greenhouses where the materials having high transmissivity and strength both are required.

Due to its tendency to insulate high voltage material, Polycarbonate has over the period of time emerged as a much-liked material for the manufacture of electronic devices & appliances. Its high strength, impact resistance and transparency) also makes it a supreme material for different kinds of transparent structural applications. This is a naturally transparent amorphous thermoplastic polymeric materials and can be made commercially by adding different colours and it is available in the market in a variety of colours. The raw materials of polycarbonate are the cause of internal transmission of light nearly almost in the same capacity as glass. This polymeric material is used to produce a variety of advanced composite materials of high impact resistance, good transparency and mainly useful for manufacturing of bullet-proof glass. The major use of PC is manufacturing of plastic lenses, some medical devices, automotive components, protective gear, materials for greenhouses construction, digital disks such as CDs, DVDs and exterior decorative lighting fixtures.

Because of very good heat resistance capacity of this material it can also combined with the flame retardant materials without any significant degradation of the material. This polymeric material is considered as a good engineering plastic material because it specifically used as more capable and robust material such as in impact resistant "glass-like" surfaces. Polycarbonate is a valuable useful plastic material for the applications where transparency and high impact resistance is required. It is partially considered as an alternative to glass and natural UV filter which is the cause of using it as eyewear appliances. More recently Polycarbonate is used in a variety kind of applications across different industries. It was observed that there are certain kinds of polycarbonate are found to be toxic in contact with food because of the release of Bisphenol -A during hydrolysis i.e.it undergoes degradation when it is in contact with aqueous medium or water. The most commonly used polycarbonate is manufactured by using BPA and carbonyl chloride but the presence of BPA free polycarbonates marketable it particularly for applications involving containers and packaging materials of perishable food and water (K. A. Vijayalakshmi *et. al.*2011).**Environmental Impact:**

- It is more commonly used for manufacture of some smart materials such as CDs, DVDs, automotive parts and also the manufacture of baby bottles and some special kind of water bottles. Because of the presence of toxic bisphenol-A it is considered as an important carcinogen, hence many companies stopped using polycarbonate materials for manufacturing of products for human related applications.
- In the landfill site it is definitely a material of environmental alarming. It never biodegraded easily because it is obtained from petroleum products. The chemicals of this polymeric material slowly leach into the land surface causing significant damage to the environment. Since many of these chemicals produced from these polymers are consumed by marine organisms, fishes and other animals lot of damage and sometimes even on death was achieved.
- It is found that the unintentional dumping of this kind of plastic materials into seas and oceans may causes the death of mammals and birds by eating it. The use of CDs now increasing day by day and the volume of unused discarded CDs gradually increased in every year in worldwide which finally mixed with ocean water and becomes danger to marine biota and marine ecosystem, which is now a serious global pollution issue. Although now some specific methods are used to recycle CDs and DVDs, but these methods are not so effective novel method and its rate of pollution increased day by day (Altuwair IB et. al.2017).

Poly-Methyl Methacrylate (PMMA)

PMMA is commonly known as acrylic or acrylic glass and the trade name of this polymeric material is Crylux, Plexiglas, Acrylite, Lucite, and Perspex. This polymeric material belongs to thermoplastic type and is rigid and transparent material and is used as a perfect replacement of unbreakable glass. This polymeric material is considered as a perfect replacement for glass and many technical advantages than other transparent such as Polycarbonate, polystyrene etc. It is applied in various fields such as manufacturing of car windows of car and buses, smart phone cabinets and screens, aquariums. This kind of polymeric material is highly tough, therefore can be easily recycled and reshaped and found to be as a proper alternative of the high cost and less resilient glass.

It has refractive Index of 1.49 and also possess the property of high light transmittance. It was experimentally observed that a good quality of PMMA grades allows about 92% of light to pass through it, which is found to be more than any glass or plastic materials. Since this polymeric material can be easily reshaped and reused without losing the optical clarity of the material, therefore it is suitable for the use of many outdoor applications of high environmental stability. This polymer is highly tough, good durability and also a lightweight thermoplastic material. The density of this polymer ranges in between 1.17-1.20 g/cm3, which is almost half less than that of glass. It possesses excellent resistance to scratch as compared to other transparent polymeric materials like Polycarbonate but however it is less than glass. Because of low moisture and water absorption capacity the products obtained from this material has good dimensional and environmental stability.

This polymeric material possesses greater resistance to UV light and also good weathering resistance. Most of commercially available acrylic based polymeric materials are UV stabilized for good resistance to prolonged exposure to sunlight because its mechanical as well as optical properties fairly vary in these conditions, Hence, it is considered as suitable material for many outdoor applications projected for long-term exposure to open-air. Since PMMA is not affected by aqueous solutions of most of the laboratory chemicals, detergents, thinners, cleaners, dilute solution of inorganic acids, alkalis, and aliphatic hydrocarbons. But however this polymeric material cannot be recommended for use with chlorinated compounds, aromatic hydrocarbons, esters, or ketones.

PMMA is more commonly and widely used as construction materials such as window and door profiles, covering materials, panels, frontage design materials etc. This material facilitates the transmission of light and also has a good heat insulation capacity. Therefore, this material is considered as a good choice of construction of green houses. It can be used as to build aquariums and also marine canters.

The sheets made by PMMA are mainly used for designing of LED light bulbs and it maximizes the light emitting capacity if this bulb is used for house hold or other purposes. It is a good material for manufacturing lamps because of its transparency and better optical properties. The sheets of this material can be used for manufacturing windows of car and buses, windshields of motorcycle, interior and exterior panels of houses, fenders etc. The coloured form of acrylic sheets are used in indicator light covers of car and buses along with the interior light covers etc. This material can be utilized for manufacturing of windows of ships because of salt resistance properties and also used as aviation purposes.

Since this kind of materials possess outstanding optical clarity, very good light transmission along with scratch resistance properties it is extensively used in manufacturing of LCD and LED screens, laptop screens, smart phones display and all other electronic equipment displays. It can be used in the solar panels. Because of its excellent UV resistance and light transmission characteristics it has a property of allowing high energy conversion efficiencies and used as a better covering material.

The pure form of PMMA can be easily cleaned and for this reason it can be used for manufacturing of incubators, devices for drug testing, cabinets as storage container in hospitals and also in research labs. Because of the property of good bio-compatibility it is considered as a bio- active material and can be used infillings of dental cavity and bone cement. Since this material possess the exceptional properties like light transparency, good toughness and aesthetics, it can be used for manufacturing of chairs, tables, kitchen appliances, cabinets of many instruments, bowls, table mats etc. in any desired shape, size and colour in the finished form (Eshwar Pawar et. al.2016).

Environmental Impact

- On short term exposure MMA is harmful to invertebrates and fishes but it is not so harmful to algae. It is also not so harmful to aquatic organisms even on long-term exposure
- The persistence of MMA in the environment is very less because it is biodegrading normally in the sewage treatment plants and cannot be bind significantly to the soil or sediments due to its low water absorption coefficient. When it is released to the atmosphere within few days the photochemical degradation occurs. It is also not accumulated in the food chain and food web. Hence it has low bioaccumulation potential because of low octanal-water partition coefficient.
- PC is not suitable for human use and PMMA is the proper economical alternative polymeric material which replaces polycarbonate because of high tensile strength, flexural strength, good transparency to light, god polishability property and UV tolerance characteristics. This is more suitable

for human use because it does not contain the harmful toxic subunits of chemical bisphenol-A which is found in the polymeric material polycarbonate.

- It is mostly preferred because of its moderate properties, easy handling and processing, and low cost. Non-modified PMMA behaves in a brittle manner when under load, especially under an impact force, and is more prone to scratching than conventional inorganic glass, but modified PMMA is sometimes able to achieve high scratch and impact resistance (Kuo-Shen et. al. 2007).

Acetal (Polyoxymethyleneor POM)

The monomer molecule of this polymeric material contains alkopxy group as the functional group in which carbon is bonded with two alkoxy groups. This material was first of investigated by a German scientist Hermann Staudinger and he get the Nobel Prize in 1953 for his excellent discovery in chemistry. This material produced by Staudinger is thermally unstable and therefore not considered as commercially material. Then finally the POM of good stability homo-polymer was discovered by the scientist Dal Nagore.

This material possesses good tensile strength and high creep resistant properties for which the properties of this material is the bridge between most plastic materials and metals. This material has highly heat resistance capacity, abrasion resistance and resistance to water and chemicals. Because of low coefficient of friction and combined other essential characteristics this material is very useful for applications in manufacturing of gears and some other devices. Hence this polymeric material is useful material which possess following essential characteristics.

Stiffness is very high:

- Coefficient of friction is low
- High Hardness
- Abrasion resistance is also very high
- Good heat resistance characteristics
- Possess quite low water absorption properties
- Excellent electrical and dielectric properties
- Dimensional stability is much higher
- Better creep resistance even more than nylon
- Smoke emission is low and supports green environment.
- Gloss surface is much higher
- This material is crystalline in nature
- Liquid form is flammable and therefore possess dangerous property of fire hazard
- Less resistance to acids and bases
- The shrinkage rate is much higher than other polymeric materials
- Operating temperature range is also limited

It is an important engineering material and can be used indifferent practical fields. Applications for POM include high performance components such as gear and fasteners (screws, nuts, washers, spacers, etc.). This material is used in other applications such as bindings, yoyos, electronic, cigarettes, watch, ornaments, zippers, insulin pens, and metered dose inhalers. It is used in musical instruments for picks and instrument mouthpieces, in the food industry in applications like milk pumps and coffee spigots, and also as a solvent for perfumes and as a synthetic flavouring ingredient. (K. Mohan Babu et. al.2014)

Environmental Impact

- On heating or abraded mechanically Polyoxymethylene produces toxic formaldehyde. POM can also be broken down on heating, acids, alkalis, oxygen, abrasion, enzymes, and suitable high energy radiation. It is the only plastic material used in some artistic orthodontic brackets
- POM bracket generally melts at a temperature of about 178^{0}C, it starts degradation at a temperature of 250^{0}C and can completely converted into gaseous formaldehyde at higher temperature.
- Food and drug administration agency approved few of the grades of POM for milk pumps, coffee plugs, filter housings materials and food conveyors for manufacturing of aerosol cans, vehicle tanks. Hardware materials manufacture from it such as locks and key, handles, hinges etc. which are non-biodegradable in nature and causes environmental hazards (Alejandro Gallego-Schmid et. al 2016)

Nylon or Polyamide (PA)

- This polymeric material is found in variety of forms and can be used for a number of different kinds of applications including cloth manufacturing, as a reinforcing material in rubber like car and bus tires, utilized for manufacturing of rope and thread, and can be used for a number of injection moulded parts of different automobiles and in some mechanical equipments. It may be always used as an alternative of low strength metals in a number of applications such as manufacturing of car engines due to its high strength in comparison to other plastic materials, property of high temperature resilience, and chemical compatibility is also high.
- There are several kinds of poly amides used in verity of applications are as follows
  - Nylon 3, Nylon 6, Nylon 6 6, Nylon 6 10, Nylon8, Nylon10, Nylon11, Nylon 12 Nylon 6,12, Kevlar Nomex. The aliphatic polyamides are now-a days are manufactured in a very larger scale and considered as most important class of engineering thermoplastic materials. They are found to be amorphous or only moderately crystalline in nature when injection moulded, but the degree of crystallinity can be much increased for fiber and film applications by orientation via mechanical stretching. The two most important polyamides are Nylon 6,6) and Nylon 6 which has vast applications in different fields. Both have excellent mechanical properties including high tensile strength, high flexibility, good resilience, low creep and high impact strength (toughness)
- It was estimated that about 60%or more than that of it is produced are used in commercial fiber applications. This includes manufacturing of carpets, garments, seatbelts, upholstery, ropes and tire reinforcements. However, fabrics made from Nylon have less wrinkle resistance than cloth made from polyesters are costly. This is the reasons for which Nylon fibers are not more market applications than PET fibers all over the years.
- Fibers of Nylon and mineral powdered reinforced polyamide materials are widely used for different engineering and industrial applications. The without reinforced grades of materials have the operating temperature of BOUT 340 - 350 Whereas the glass and mineral reinforced grades have operating temperature of about 370 -390 K. Nylon of every kind is used in many industries and its

products are also sold in every market. For example, in the industry like automotive, nylon is used for making wire and cable jacket, cooling fans, intake to air, turbo air ducts, valves of different and also engine covers, reservoirs of brake and power steering, gears for the windshield wipers and speedometers. Polyamides of engineering materials arealso being used for power tool housings, vending for several machines, pumps and can be used for manufacturing of many electrical and electronic parts which includes electric switches, sockets, electric plugs and the devices for antenna-mounting.

- Although aromatic polyamides are much expensive but it possesses an excellent mechanical property. This material can be used as a challenging material and is applicable invarious industries. The industries utilize this material for manufacturing of ropes and cable materials, bulletproof Jackets and vests, tennis strings and composite of this material is used for hockey sticks. It is also being used for manufacturing of snowboards, enclosures of jet engine, friction parts of brake and transmission, gaskets (Partk K Vagholkar et. al.2016).

Environmental Impact

- During manufacturing of Nylon nitrous oxide is produced which is a potential greenhouse gas and about 300 times more powerful and dangerous than carbon dioxide. The manufacturing of polyester huge amounts of water is required for cooling and lubrication and it is a source of contamination.
- It is a synthetic fiber material and mainly derived from petrochemicals products and is a thermoplastic polymeric material. It is widely used in the fashion industry throughout the world. This material is an excellent and versatile material and is mostly used for manufacturing of stocks and parachutes, carpet materials, packaging materials and can be used for manufacturing of some car parts.
- For production of polyester almost about 70 billion barrels of oil are used in each year. Although more polyester materials are produced in comparison to Nylon in every year but the energy requirement is more for production of Nylon. The resin of Nylon utilizes almost about three times more energy than to produce cotton. By considering all these it is concluded that Nylon has great impotence and impact in day to day life of our society.
- Nylon manufacturing process cannot use natural dyes and it has also lower impact for chemical dyes during the process of production because in the process of colouring the fiber of Nylon causes substantial water pollution. Hence more is the nylon produced greater is its contribution towards the water contamination and causes increase in pollution load of water mainly in the developing countries of the world.
- All kinds of nylons are non-biodegradable in nature and these materials are persisting within the environment for a longer period. The two major sources of plastic pollution in the ocean world are mainly fishing nets made by nylon and synthetic textile fiber materials used during washing. Hence in the aquatic environment specially in marine environment nylonhas greater impact.
- The impact of nylon in the environment can be minimised by using recycled nylon for manufacturing of garments mainly swimwear and pantyhose. But if we can able to replace Nylon with suitable sustainable natural fibers it is better suited for our environment.

ABS (Acrylonitrile -Butadiene -Styrene)

The polymeric material ABS is prepared from three different kinds of monomers. The different proportion of monomers acrylonitrile, butadiene, and styrene in different compositions are used for manufacturing of amorphous blend. Each monomer of ABS has individual impact and separate function to ABS. The monomer acrylonitrile impacts chemical and thermal stability, butadiene is the cause of increase in toughness and impact strength whereas styrene provides a good finishing and nice looking to the plastic material ABS.

This polymeric material is very strong, resistance to corrosive, chemicals and also good resistance to physical impacts. Since this material is easily available and is of low melting temperature is can be easily fabricated by using the process of injection moulding or 3D printing.

This plastic material is a famous and popularly used material for manufacturing of basic items of our day to day life like keyboards of computer, kitchen appliances, imported toys, plastic guards, wall sockets, and the protective cases of power tools. Because of light weight this plastic material can be made easily into the desired shape and size by the process of injection moulding and is useful for manufacturing the products that needed for complex and accurate shaped, such as musical instruments, some automotive components, medical devices, protective headgear, golf club heads etc.

Not only it has good mechanical properties but also has good electrical insulation properties. The electrical properties of this polymeric material can evident easily at a wide range of frequencies, in an elevated temperature and also humid environments. Hence ABS is considered as a perfect material for electrical insulation specially the protective material for many electrical parts and mainly used for insulation of chips and cables.

The polymeric material ABS can have made very thin filament easily and therefore can be used as an appropriate material for 3D printers. Since this material can have operated at a very high temperature, shows good stability and durability even at high temperature also, therefore it is an appropriate material for 3D printing. Another advantages of it is that the Plastic appliances manufactured from ABS is glossy and shows opaque finish. For common 3D printing PLA may chose an alternative material.

Because of its durability and high resistance to heat most of the kitchen appliances and car panels are manufactured by using this material. Since this polymeric material shows an excellent physical and chemical properties, therefore it is selected as the best choice among the materials for manufacturing of plastic products. According to the data given by industry people the utilization of ABS is now going to increase from 4% to 5% annually. It is concluded that ABS has no replacement and it is a versatile plastic material for ever and anytime soon(Herman Alexander Bruson et. al.1942)

Environmental Impact

- Processing of ABS at an elevated temperature makes the material look nice with good finish and also better heat resistance property. If the material is processed at lower temperature, it shows high strength and also higher impact resistance.
- The major disadvantage of this material is that it is non-biodegradable in nature and not a renewable resource of material
- If this plastic material can have made an average diameter of less than 1 micrometre, then it can be used as colorant in some of the tattoo inks, Tattoo inks made of ABS are extremely vivid and toxic to our environment.

- At normal using condition and polymer processing conditions ABS decomposes and its exposure at the workplace causes carcinogenic effect to the workers. However, at elevated temperatures more than 400^0C ABS may decomposes into butadiene, acrylonitrile and styrene, all of these are highly carcinogenic in nature specially for human beings.
- The ultrafine particles of ABS produced during the process of 3D printing at lower temperatures is the cause of many air borne diseases and caused a number of adverse health hazard effect (Suraj Kumar Vishwakarma et. al. 2017).

Polyacrylonitrile (PAN)

It is commonly known as Creslan- 61 and is a semi -crystalline polymeric material having the general formula (C_3H_3N) n. It is a thermoplastic polymeric material but it does not melt easily under normal conditions and it degrades before melting. PAN has some unique properties such as light weight, good thermal stability, more strength and high modulus of elasticity, better stability to UV radiation, non-fusible in nature and also resistance to some of the chemical. These properties make it an essential plastic material for high end technology and textile applications.

- Since it has wool-like properties it can be used as a perfect material for textile applications.
- The production of fibers from these materials is done by either wet spinning process or dry spinning process.
- About 90% of the production of carbon fiber of the world is from PAN.
- Other different applications of PAN are as follows
- Used as Fiber material for reinforcement of cement
- Used for manufacturing of filtration membrane
- Used for preparation of some fabric materials and out-door applications
- The oxidized form of PAN used as fibers for thermal and acoustic insulation
- Used for manufacturing of anti-flame fibers
- Manufacture of hot air filtration
- The boiling point of Acrylonitrile was experimentally measured to be 77 ^{0}Cwhich is somewhat lower than other organic liquid. Because of this low boiling point acrylonitrile is sometimes considered as a volatile compound, which means that the liquid acrylonitrile molecules readily escape out into the gaseous phase and can evaporate. For this reason, it is a good idea to never leave a bottle of acrylonitrile open to the air because it will evaporate rather quickly (S K Nataraj et. al. 2012).

Environmental Impact

- The most common effects of PAN are mucosal irritation or injury or gastrointestinal tract irritation.
- It may cause irritation of our eye.
- It causes skin irritation and metabolized to cyanide and inhibits Cytochrome Oxidase resulting impairing of cellular respiration.

- It also causes irritation to the digestive tract. The toxicological characteristics of this material is not yet fully known. Metabolism may release cyanide, which causes headache, dizziness, weakness, collapse of our body, unconsciousness and may be possible death. Ingestion of this material may results the symptoms similar to that of the cyanide poisoning and it may be characterized by asphyxiation.
- It results irritation of our respiratory tract. Inhalation may result in symptoms similar to cyanide poisoning such as tachypnea, hyperpnea and dyspnea which is followed by rapid respiratory depression. Pulmonary edema may result because of the extensive use of PAN in our daily life.
- Since PAN is metabolized to cyanide, therefore it acts by inhibiting Cytochrome Oxidase causing impairing cellular respiration. Potential cancer hazard is mainly due to handling of this material (Ahamad Fausi Ismail et. al. 2008)

Styrene Acrylonitrile (SAN)

It is a hard rigid and transparent polymeric material. It can be easily coloured because the transmittance of this material in the visible range is more than 90%. It is also good thermal shock resistant and also resistance to chemicals. This polymeric material is rigid, transparent, tough, better resistant to oil and greases, resistance to cracking and crazing. It can be easily processed and better resistant to food stain. Science this material is a transparent material and resistance to fats, grease, oils, therefore it acts as a good cleaning agent and is very is an appropriate material for manufacturing kitchen appliances mainly mixing bowls, basins and refrigerator components. This material can be used for the outer casings of thermally insulated jugs, tableware, cutlery, coffee filters, designed jars and beakers and also manufacturing of storage containers for all kinds of foods. An additional application of this material is multi-trip tableware used for catering. This polymeric material can be made coloured easily and after colouring the appearance of this material is very attractive and nice looking. This is the cause of using this material for applications of many household and commercial purposes mainly manufacturing of toothbrushes, fittings of bathroom and packaging for cosmetic materials. Due to the property of hardness this material is used for different applications in office and industry in diversified way. It can be used as the outer covers of many appliances such as printers, calculators, instruments and lamps. In addition to that the other different applications of SAN are battery housings, winding cores, equipment of writing and drawing and cylindrical impellers for air-conditioners. SAN used in a number of applications in various fields mainly in lenses, automotive instrument lenses, dust covers, housewares, cups and glasses, handles of toothbrush, trays, some containers, industrial battery cases, knobs, switches, tractor components, automotive trim, some marine instruments, instrument panels, components of swimming pool (Yi jun Liao et.al. 2018).

Environmental Impact

- According to 1990s. EPA data about 10% of total generated municipal solid waste are only really recycled about 10% was subjected incinerated and around 80% was dumped into the landfill site areas but currently in many countries significant amount is it now recycled to avoid pollution load and about 20%of plastics is dumped into the landfill sites

- Very slowly SAN degrades in landfill sites within the soil and becomes a hazardous additive. These additive materials are mainly colorants, stabilizers and plasticizers and may contains toxic materials along with heavy metals like lead and cadmium. These toxic and hazardous pollutants leach slowly into the both surface and ground water and soil. According to the Current Survey Report there are at least 100 Mt of plastic in oceans posing which is a danger to marine life.
- The acrylonitrile generated from the containers of SAN can be easily migrated to the different parts of our environment in variable amounts and becomes toxic to environment. The International Agency for Research on Cancer (IARC) identified acrylonitrile as a Class 2B carcinogen. Therefore, the extensive use of SAN is the cause of increase in rate of cancer appearance in high dosage tests in male and female rats. It also causes of cancer diseases for human beings and other animals. (B D Gesner et. al. 1965)

Polyurethane (PUR and PU)

This polymeric material is consist of the organic units and is joined by carbamate i,e Urethane links. Most of the polyurethanes are mainly thermosetting polymers and it do not melt easily by action of heat but thermoplastic polyurethanes are also readily available. This plastic material can be synthesised by reaction of polyol with di-isocyanate or a polymeric isocyanate in the presence of a suitable catalysts and additives also. Since there is a wide range of di-isocyanates and polyols are available we may able to produce polyurethane in a broad range of spectrum which can meet the needs of different kinds of applications in different fields. Flexible polyurethane foam can be used as moderating agent in a variety of consumer and marketable products which includes bedding, furniture, automotive interiors, carpet underlay and packaging materials. This material is light weight, durable, supportive in nature and comfortable. The flexible polyurethane foam marketed about30% market cover of the entire North American and is used largely for bedding, furniture and in automotive industry. The rigid polyurethane and poly-isocyanate foams are considered as one of the world's most popular, energy-efficient and multipurpose insulating materials. These foams can expressively reduce the cost of energy when it is used as commercial and residential propose it becomes more efficient and also comfortable. These foams of PU are treated as effective insulating materials and mainly used in roof and wall insulation, insulated windows, doors and air barrier sealants. Polyurethanes materials can be used in the purpose of coatings, adhesives, sealants and elastomers and it also has wide range of commercial and industrial applications. Polyurethane coatings is the cause of increase in beauties and the lifespan of the product materials. Polyurethane adhesives has the advantages of strong bonding on the surface of product whereas the polyurethane sealants provide a tighter seal. This elastomeric material of Polyurethanes can be moulded into articles of any desired shape and size and is found to be lighter than metal. It also shows superior stress recovery characteristics and is resistant to many environmental factors.

The thermoplastic polyurethane (TPU) material possesses a good and useful physical property on combination with some other suitable materials and during processing applications. It shows high elastic property, flexible in nature and also excellent resistant to abrasion, impact and weather. TPUs can be made into coloured products or fabricated into a wide variety of products and their use can increase a product's overall durability. It mostly used in construction, automotive and footwear. Using injection moulding technique many useful products such as car bumpers, panels of electrical housing, computer parts and telecommunication equipment are prepared. The polyurethane products manufactured can exhibit good heat resistance, thermal insulation, dimensional stability and a high level of dynamic properties. Automotive, construction, appliance, furniture and recreation and sporting goods can be manufactured by using this type of technique. Binders of these kind of materials can be used to adhere several kinds of particles and fibers to each other. The major fields of using this material is the manufacturing of wood panels, rubber or elastomeric materials for flooring surfaces, sand casting material for the foundry industry. The major categories of application for polyurethane binder is for the manufacture of Oriented Strand Board (OSB). These prepared wood panels may be used as structural sheathing and flooring materials, manufactured housing, joists and beams and shop panels. Water mainly used as solvent for waterborne polyurethane dispersions (PUDs) .The material PUDs are widely used in industrial and commercial applications (Shoaib Suleman et. al. 2014).

Environmental Impact

- For environmental point of view this material can actively participate in fighting climate change in a number of ways. Since it is a good insulating material it can improve the energy efficiency of the buildings and also reduces the need for heating and cooling, results the lowering of carbon emissions. In vehicles this material not only do they ensure comfort and safety, but also cause of increase in fuel efficiency, because these materials are lighter than other alternative materials.
- Now a day the polyurethanes industry is continuously struggling to improve the life span of its manufactured products and becomes a more sustainable material. But now a day theschemes of recovery reduces the volume of polyurethane waste dumping into the landfill sites.It was estimated that more than 250,000 tons of polyurethane wastes from European countries are recycled and recovered in every year. Again another advantages of polyurethane waste is power generation in the process of incineration along with municipal solid waste and may decreases the requirement of fossil fuels of world.
- In the present day almost 45% of the fossil fuels are utilized for cooling and heating purposes of the interiors of buildings and individual homes. Although by the use of insulating materials, substantial amount of energy savings can be achieved but the result is a substantial reduction in CO_2 which is one of the major contributors to global warming effect.
- By using this material as an insulating material the energy efficiency achieved about 37% in the next ten years. Again by changing the design of manufactured products by the use of polyurethanes we can live a comfortable and energy-efficient life. This energy savings process substantially reduced the emission of greenhouse gases and also control the global warming effect. But however better cooling preserves more food which is another valuable technique to preserve our food resource.
- With the increase in production of numbers of vehicle they utilises polyurethane materials for light weighting purposes increases. Basically in the range density of 30to 50kg/m3, polyurethane foams used as a raw material to retain their strength and durability. The resulting weight loss of this material can yields substantial savings in fuel consumption and also emissions of carbon dioxide without compromising quality of the product (Paulina Parcheta et. al. 2017).

BIODEGRADABLE AND NON-BIODEGRADABLE PLASTIC

- Those plastic substances which can be easily decomposed or degraded by natural agents like water, oxygen, UV rays of the solar radiation, acid rains and different kinds of micro-organisms, etc. are generally called as biodegradable materials. It is a common observation that if some dead leaf or banana peel is thrown outside, these waste material is attacked by several bacteria's, fungi or sometimes small insects in a certain time period. The decomposition of these materials facilitated by the natural elements like oxygen, water, moisture, and heat and the plastic materials are broken down from complex organic forms to simpler sub units. These decomposed material partially mixes with the atmospheric air and partly returns back to the soil on land surface thus the nutrient content of soil again increases with various nutrients and minerals.
- Those materials which cannot undergoes biodegradation or decomposition into different simple materials by the help of bacteria and micro-organisms and returned to the soil by natural agents are called as non-biodegradable materials. These materials mainly composed of the plastic materials, metal scraps, aluminium cans plastic bottles and hazardous chemicals etc. These waste materials are practically resistant to biodegradation in natural processes and cannot be broken down even after thousands and thousands of years. Therefore, these waste materials rather than returning back to soil it contribute to solid waste which is very hazardous for the environment. The ever increasing load of non-biodegradable garbage is now a day an alarming issue in many countries all over the world.
- Hence the non-biodegradable waste cannot have returned back to the soil and persist within the environment as in the form of solid waste which contains very hazardous materials, chemicals along with metallic contaminates and become toxic to our environment. The\continuous increase in load of non-biodegradable garbage and rubbish materials is now a growing concern all over the globe and it is now the time for us to search eco-friendly alternative materials that can minimize the threat on aquatic life and also life on land surface.
- The biodegradable materials include food waste products of like vegetable and fruit peels, dead plants, leaves and dead body of animals, chicken waste, egg shells, paper materials, garden waste, agricultural waste etc. Non-biodegradable things consist of plastics, polystyrene, unused metals, plastic products, aluminium cans, toxic chemicals, paints, tyres, etc.
- The biodegradable materials on breaking produces simple organic matter and are aggregated in the soil and contributed a part of the carbon cycle of the atmosphere. On the other hand, non-biodegradable materials are resistant to the environmental factors and never decompose and mixed with the environment and a major part of the solid waste is contributed by non-biodegradable materials.

The biodegradable materials decompose within few days or months or even few hours while non-biodegradable waste materials may take thousands and thousands of years or may be never decomposed into simple products and remain in their original form as such (Dana Adamcova et. al. 2014).

TYPES OF BIODEGRADABLE PLASTICS

Definition: Biodegradable plastic materials are those that can be degraded by the microbial action and produces natural end products, like H_2O and CO_2, in an appropriate period of time. The time needed for complete decompose depends on the waste material, environmental conditions such as temperature and moisture, rain fall intensity and location of decomposition.

Biodegradable plastic materials can be classified into two categories:

- Bio -based Polyester Plastics
- Biomass Based Biodegradable Plastics
- Fossil fuel based plastic materials

Now in recent years' new types of plastic materials which are completely biodegradable in few days have been developed to protect our environment from plastic pollution.

Biobased Polyester Plastics

The bio -based plastic materials are mainly derived from plants are termed as bio- plastics that can be easily biodegraded and are made of two materials i,e biomass and polyesters derived from plants. There are mainly two types of bio -based polyesters: Polylactide acid (PLA) and polyhydroxyalkanoate (PHA).

Polyhydroxyalkanoate (PHA)

This material can be produced naturally by bacteria and it may be genetically modified organisms (GMO) plants. PHA is completely compostable in our natural environments mostly the microbe's rich environment, especially in microbe's rich soil. This material can automatically down by the microbes with the help of enzymes. The time necessary for biodegradation of this material depends on the concentration of microbes present in the soil. Within two months PHA undergoes complete decomposition or biodegradation and mixed with soil. The rate of biodegradation of this polymeric material is in marine environment is much less and it was found less than 50% of this material is decomposed even after six months.

Some items of some plastic materials are made entirely of PHA. The major disadvantages of it is the cost of production of this material is high, but it is can also be blended with starch or cellulose which can made it more economical and commercial. This is one of the advantage of PHA that its rate of decomposition is enhanced

Polylactide Acid (PLA)

It is a thermoplastic polymeric material which can be made through the process of fermentation of bacteria. This polymeric material is practically a long chain of lactic acid molecules bonded by covalent bonds. Since there are many inexpensive means for the production of lactic acid, these materials are only to be polymerized or may joined. Therefore, the products of PLA have less cost than PHA. But however, PLA is more brittle and its application is normally less than PHA.

- PLA cannot be easily composted because the temperature and level of water required are not suited in this environment.
- Normally 6 to 12 months are required for degradation of PLA in soil.
- But however in commercial facilities PLA degrades in one to six months.
- The end of the degraded products at the end are CO_2 & H_2O.
- The PLA degradation if carried out in landfill sites without oxygen, it produces CH_4 gas which is almost 20 times more damaging to the environment than CO_2.

Since PLA does not degrade rapidly in either soil or seawater; then it is littered arbitrarily and becomes a problem for environment.

BIOMASS BASED BIODEGRADABLE PLASTICS

This types of plastic materials are mostly manufactured from starch and cellulose which are mostly obtained from crop residues and wood. The two more commonly known biomass based biodegradable plastic materials are Cellulose acetate and starch.

Cellulose Acetate

Cellulose acetate is a synthetic material and is derived from cellulose and cellulosic materials which is mostly found in plants and trees. Cellulose is presently now used from cotton, wood, and crop waste. This material may be used for production of moulded solid plastics, cigarette filters, coatings, photographic-films and filters. Cellophane is a material of biodegradable film that produced from cellulose. Now advance research work is done to find out new advanced plastic films from waste crop products and wood materials which are water resistant and biodegradable in nature. About 70% of it is biodegradable after 18 months.

Starch

If starch is subjected to heat, water, and plasticizers a thermoplastic resin is produced and its strength can be improved on combination with filler materials and some other materials can be made by using it. Maize, wheat, potato, and cassava are the major sources of starch. This plastic material is used in packaging applications, bags, and agricultural mulch films, tableware, flower pots, and can also easily moulded to make packaging and consumer products. It is seen as an alternative for polystyrene (PS). Starch when added to bioplastic or conventional plastic materials it becomes more biodegradable

The composite material produced by using starch is either compostable or biodegradable. The compostable variants require 90 days to degrade in industrial facilities, whereas the biodegradable parts require about100 days for only46% to degrade and for complete degradation it requires more than two years.

FOSSIL FUEL BASED BIODEGRADABLE PLASTICS

There are a less number of fossil fuel based plastics are found all of these are biodegradable in nature. The most common among these are Polybutylene succinate (PBS), Polycaprolactone (PCL), Poly-butyrate adipate terephthalate (PBAT) and Polyvinyl alcohol (PVOH/PVA).

These are of the following categories:

- The polymeric material PBAT is synthesised from the derivatives of fossil fuel and is sometimes used in combination with starch. Now research work was continued to produce this polymeric material from renewable sources for environmental safety point of view. It is mostly used for manufacturing of garbage bags, wrapping films, disposable packaging materials and tableware such as cups, dishes etc. It is the not only biodegradable material which are also compostable.
- PCL is a synthetic polyester which can be used to synthesise compostable bags for medical application mainly sutures and fibers, as a surface coatings materials, adhesives for shoes and leather, and stiffeners for shoes and orthopaedic splints. This plastic material can be degraded by yeasts. More than 90% of films, and 40% of foam made of this material can be degraded within 15 days.
- PBS is an important polymeric resins synthesised from fossil fuels or can also be bio- based materials. It can be combined with other bio- based polymers or fibers like jute to improve its quality. It can be used for manufacturing of food packaging materials, service ware, agricultural mulch sheets, plant pots, hygiene products like diapers, and fishing nets.
- Poly vinyl alcohol is a resin that can be used to synthesise packaging films and it can replace both LDPE and HDPE from the market. The other important applications of PVOH are use in coatings and additives for paper and board production
- All these four fossil fuel based plastic materials are biodegrading with three months in industrial composting, in one year in backyard composting and in one to two years in normal soil or landfills areas.

NON-BIODEGRADABLE PLASTIC MATERIALS

The polymeric materials that are do not break down to a natural and environmentally safe condition in due time by bacteria are called as non-biodegradable polymers. Most of the plastic materials are non-biodegradable in nature and also widely used all over the world because of its low cost, light weight and durability. However, plastics can be made biodegradable with the addition of certain materials that breakdown the structure of the polymer.

The commonly used non-biodegradable plastic materials globally in our environment are as follows

- Polyethylene Terephthalate (PET or PETE)—Used as Plastic soft drink and water bottles, beer bottles, mouthwash bottles, peanut butter and salad dressing containers, openable film, openable pre-prepared food trays.
- High Density Polyethylene (HDPE)----Used as milk, water, juice, cosmetic, shampoo, dish and laundry detergent bottles; trash and retail bags, yogurt and margarine tubs, cereal box liners.

- Polyvinyl Chloride (PVC) ---Used as manufacturing of Toys, clear food and non-food packaging, shampoo bottles, medical tubing, wire and cable insulation, film and sheet; construction products such as pipes, fittings, siding, flooring, carpet backing, window frames.
- Low Density Polyethylene (LDPE)---Used as dry cleaning, bread, and frozen food bags; squeezable bottles (i.e., honey, mustard).
- Polypropylene (PP)—Used for manufacturing of Ketchup bottles, yogurt containers and margarine tubs, medicine bottles
- Polystyrene (PS)—Used for manufacturing of compact disc cases, foodservice applications, grocery store meat trays, egg cartons, aspirin bottles, cups, plates, cutler
- Other plastic materials like Nylon (PA) Acrylonitrile butadiene styrene (ABS) Polycarbonate (PC) Layered or multi-material mixed polymers---Used for making consumer products, bottles, plastic lumber (Martien van den Oever et.al.2017)

Environmental prospective and consequences of Bioplastic Materials:

Although bio-plastic materials have great potential to use and also many positive attributes, but it has almost equal number of disadvantages. Hence both sides are to be considered equally while considering its environmental impact in our society.

Prospective

- It reduces the consumption of fossil-fuels and faith on non-renewable resources of the environment.
- 65% less energy is required for its manufacturing process and generates less greenhouse gases than conventional plastic materials which is considered as a green synthesis method.
- Among these materials some are biodegradable and some are compostable in nature.
- Some of these plastic materials can be recycled along with conventional plastic materials.
- Some of these materials are non-toxic and safe for medical application and internal use and also for our environment.

Consequences

- Now a day many companies are begin to synthesise plastic materials from bioplastic even if its cost of manufacturing is much higher.
- Composting of these materials is easily possible only in industrial composting processes.
- Not all of these materials are recycled.
- Some of these materials can also interfere with or damage when plastic materials are recycled in standard procedure.
- All of these materials are not completely biodegradable in nature.
- In landfill sites some of these can release methane gas which is a potent greenhouse gas of the atmosphere.
- These materials are not appropriate for manufacturing of a number of products.
- The use of plant sugar and starch sources could have a negative impact on food prices.
- Bioplastic materials could not change the consumer behaviour regarding their use of plastic products (Abolfazl Jafari-Sales et. al. 2017).

Alternative Options to the Use Plastic that are Environmentally Friendly

1. **Bamboo Toothbrushes:** This is the product of natural plant species and can be easily biodegradable within few days only. So we have to switch to bamboo toothbrushes rather than the tooth brush made from conventional plastic materials. Toothbrush is a commonly used material mostly made from Nylon which is not completely biodegradable in nature.
2. **Stainless Steel or Glass Water Bottles:** The use of plastic bottles as drinking water is generally dangerous and toxic harmful because certain toxic chemicals enter into the drinking water and finally into your body. Hence the use of glass bottles and Stainless Steel bottles is more safe durable and it is also readily available in different designed forms in market.
3. **Eco-Friendly Tea and Coffee Mugs and Glasses**: We are using small and medium plastic mugs and glasses in different coffee stalls and tea stalls, which is a great contribution to garbage waste and increase the solid waste of our environment. But if eco-friendly cups are used instead of plastic cups, then it may decrease the pollution load of our environment.
4. **Use of Cloth Pads or Menstrual Cups:** In the conventional sanitary napkin generally more plastic materials are used. If we imagine the number of pads one woman will need to go through in one month, till she hits menopause. Then it is a huge contribution of plastic waste due to sanitary napkins and pads. The women in world wise uses the reusable cloth pads and menstrual cups which is recommended as a great alternative to conventional menstrual hygiene products.
5. **Cloth Diapers:** we are generally using plastic used diapers and its amount is very large and also a alarming frequency to environment. If we use reusable cloth diapers it is better for the baby's skin due to the lack of chemicals and easily biodegradable in landfill sites within few months.
6. **Reusable Shopping Bags:** The use of plastic bags is banned not only in our state and country but also throughout the world. People still using plastic bags specially for grocery and vegetable marketing and these are dumped in to garbage increasing solid waste volume and creates a problem. If we are used the reusable bags it can reduces the volume of generated solid waste. There are some bags which are made exclusively from vegetable products and is completely biodegradable in nature and is a better alternative to plastic bags.
7. **Compostable Garbage Bags:** The use of plastic garbage bag is due to no leakage of food waste and can hold quite a lot of stuff in it. But now a days biodegradable and compostable garbage bags are available in market which is a better alternative to plastic garbage bags
8. **Eco-Friendly Cutlery**: It is not always possible to use stainless steel spoons and forks, especially for an event, marriage or a picnic. In that case disposable cutlery is the only option you have is to pick those that can be friends of the environment. If we choose from wooden spoons and forks, leaf or bamboo plates and cups, and even edible cutlery It is better than throwing out an infinite number of plastic cutlery that will probably end up sticking around for a couple of centuries.
9. **Reusable Straws:** We are using plastic straws for drinking of fruit juice, cold drinks and other liquid drinks which are not biodegradable in nature. If we are using reused straw i,e the straw made of wood, steel, then the use of plastic straw is somewhat reduced. Now a day the straw of biomaterials is available in market which are completely biodegradable and compostable and is a good alternative to plastic straw.

CONCLUSION

Most of the plastic materials are found to be biologically non-degradable and not affected by any bacteria and micro-organisms. This is the main cause why the plastic garbage and waste generated today will last for longer period i,e thousand years and plays with our lives and also our environment. In such a situation, we have to think seriously about the production of plastic which seriously affecting our society and also its proper disposal. Now a day's marine plastic pollution is in world wise a serious environmental issue and it was expected that it may causes serious harm not only to the marine biota but also the whole environment. It was no doubt that the lesser the use of plastic on the earth, the lesser it will reach on the sea. Hence to reduce the plastic material in the ocean, we have to reduce its use globally. Since the marine water pollution is an extension of the whole earth's pollution, hence it is more dangerous than the earth's pollution for the world. Now in this situation the world has been transformed into a mountain of plastic waste and sea is affected by it. The indiscriminate use of polyethylene and other plastic material is much dangerous to selfish and other biota of marine ecosystem. Now in materialistic age we and our society should unaware about the danger of the use of polythene and other non-biodegradable plastic materials. The reusable bags should be developed and used instead of non-biodegradable plastic bags to reduce partly plastic pollution. If the use of non –biodegradable plastic is continued in the present rate, then a day comes when the whole world is covered with plastic materials and land surface becomes unusable for agriculture and other potential use and whole biological community will be demolished.

REFERENCES

Adamcova & Vaverkova. (2014). Biodegradable and non-biodegradable Plastic. *Polish J. of Environmental Studies, 23*(50), 1465-1474.

Ahamad Fausi Ismail, A. B. (2008). The effect of processing conditions on a polyacrylonitrile fiber produced using a solvent-free free coagulation process. *J of Material Science and Engineering A*, *485*(1-2), 251–257. doi:10.1016/j.msea.2007.08.060

Altuwair, I. B. (2017). *Environmental Performance Evaluation of Polycarbonates Production Processes. J. of Industrial Engineering & Management*, *6*(3), 2–11.

Bruson. (1942). Acrylonitrile -Butadiene –Styrene. *Journal of the American Chemical Society*, *64*(10), 2457–2461.

Chen, K.-S., & Hsu, R.-F. (2007). Evaluation of environmental effects on mechanical properties and characterization of creep behaviour of PMMA. *Zhongguo Gongcheng Xuekan*, *30*(2), 267–274. doi:10.1080/02533839.2007.9671253

Comanita, E.-D., Hlihor, R. M., Ghinea, C., & Gavrilescu, M. (2016). Occurrence of plastic waste in the environment: Ecological and health risks. *Environmental Engineering and Management Journal*, *15*(3), 675–685. doi:10.30638/eemj.2016.073

Eleana-Diana, C., & Rosca, M. (2015). Environmental impacts of polyvinyl chloride (PVC) production process. *Health and Bioengineering Conference*.

Feldman, D. (2014). Poly (vinyl chloride) Nanocomposites. *J. of Macromolecular Science Part-A, 51*(8), 659–667. doi:10.1080/10601325.2014.925265

Gallego-Schmid, A., Mendoza, J. M. F., Jeswani, H. K., & Azapagic, A. (2016). Life cycle environmental impacts of vacuum cleaners and the effects of European regulation. *The Science of the Total Environment, 559*, 192–203. doi:10.1016/j.scitotenv.2016.03.149 PMID:27060658

Garlotta, D. (2001). A Literature Review of Poly(Lactic Acid). *Journal of Polymers and the Environment, 9*(2), 63–84. doi:10.1023/A:1020200822435

Gesner, B. D. (1965). Environmental surface effects on ABS resins. *Journal of Applied Polymer Science, 9*(11), 3701–3706. doi:10.1002/app.1965.070091117

Grover, Gupta, Shivani, Kumari, & Khorana. (2015). Polythene and environment. *International Journal of Environmental Sciences, 5*(6), 1091-1104.

Hisham, A. (2016). Polypropylene as a Promising Plastic: A Review. *American Journal of Political Science, 6*(1), 1–11.

Hocking. (1991). *Relative merits of polystyrene foam and paper in hot drink cups: Implications for packaging*. Academic Press.

Jafari-Sales, Shahniani, & Bagherizadeh. (2017). Bioplastics and the Environment, Electronic. *Journal of Biology, 13*(3), 274–279.

Koushal, V., Sharma, R., Sharma, M., Sharma, R., & Sharma, V. (2014). Plastics: Issues Challenges and Remediation. *International Journal of Waste Resources, 4*(1), 2–6.

Liao, Wu, Zhu, & Yi. (n.d.). Synthesis and properties of novel styrene acrylonitrile/polypropylene blends with enhanced toughness. *Chemistry Central Journal.*

Maharanaa, T., Negia, Y. S., & Mohanty, B. (2007). Review Article: Recycling of Polystyrene. *Polymer-Plastics Technology and Engineering, 46*(7), 729–736. doi:10.1080/03602550701273963

Mohan Babu & Mettilda. (2014). Studies on Mechanical, Thermal, and Morphological Properties of Glass Fibre Reinforced Polyoxymethylene Nanocomposite. *Journal of Applied Chemistry.*

Nataraj, S. K., Yang, K. S., & Aminabhabi, T. M. (2012). Polyacrylonitrile-based nanofibers—A state-of-the-art review. *Progress in Polymer Science, 37*(3), 487–513. doi:10.1016/j.progpolymsci.2011.07.001

Pang, X., & Tang, Z. (2010). Polylactic acid (PLA): Research, development and industrialization. *Biotechnology Journal, 5*(11), 1125–1136. doi:10.1002/biot.201000135 PMID:21058315

Parcheta, P., & Datta, J. (2017). Environmental impact and industrial development of biorenewable resources for polyurethanes. *Critical Reviews in Environmental Science and Technology, 47*(20), 1986–2016. doi:10.1080/10643389.2017.1400861

Partk, K. (2016). Nylon (Chemistry, Properties and Uses). *International Journal of Scientific Research, 5*(9), 349–351.

Pavani & Rajeswari. (2014). Impact of plastics on environmental pollution. *Journal of Chemical and Pharmaceutical Sciences*, 87-93.

Pawar. (2016). A Review Article on Acrylic PMMA. *IOSR Journal of Mechanical and Civil Engineering, 13*(2), 1-4.

Plastics in the Marine Environment. (2017). *Annual Review of Marine Science, 9*, 205-229.

Riyad, Ali, & Maqtari. (2014). The Impact of Plastic Bags on the Environment: A field Survey of the City Of Sana'a And The Surrounding Areas, Yemen. *International Journal of Engineering Research and Reviews*, *2*(4), 61–69.

Scott, G. (2007). Plastic packaging and coastal pollution. *The International Journal of Environmental Studies*, *3*(4), 35–39.

Shaikh, H., Anis, A., Poulose, A. M., Alam, M., A-Otaibi, M. N., Alam, M. A., & Al-Zahrani, S. M. (2016). Studies on High Density Polyethylene Reinforced with Phosphate Ore Particles: Thermal, Rheological, Mechanical and Morphological Properties. *J of Polymer Plastic Technology and Engineering*, *55*(17), 1831–1841. doi:10.1080/03602559.2016.1171875

Suleman, Khan, Gull, Aleem, Shafiq, & Jamil. (2014). *A Comprehensive Short Review on Polyurethane Foam*. Academic Press.

The ocean plastic pollution challenge: Towards solutions in the UK. (n.d.). Grantham Institute.

Tian, X., Zhang, X., Liu, W., Zheng, J., Ruan, C., & Cui, P. (2006). Preparation and Properties of Poly (ethylene terephthalate)/Silica Nanocomposites. *Journal of Macromolecular Science, Part B: Physics*, *45*(4), 507–513. doi:10.1080/00222340600769782

van den Oever, Molenveld, van der Zee, & Bos. (2017). *Report No. 1722*. Wageningen Food & Biobased Research.

Vijayalakshmi, Mekala, Yoganand, & Pandiyaraj. (2011). Studies on Modification of Surface Properties in Polycarbonate (PC) Film Induced by DC Glow Discharge Plasma. *International Journal of Polymer Science*, 1-7.

Vince, J., & Hardesty, B. D. (2017). Plastic pollution challenges in marine and coastal environments: From local to global governance. *Restoration Ecology*, *25*(1), 123–128. doi:10.1111/rec.12388

Vishwakarma, S. K., Pandey, P., & Gupta, N. K. (2017). Characterization of ABS Material: A Review. *Journal of Research in Mechanical Engineering*, *3*(5), 13–16.

Wang, S. F., & Grosssman, S. J. (1987). Plastic materials for insulating applications. *Journal of Chemical Education*, *64*(1), 39–44. doi:10.1021/ed064p39

Xie & Qi. (2011). *Environmental impacts from PET packaging waste management using Life Cycle Assessment: A case study in China. International Symposium.*

Chapter 2
Plastic Waste Environmental and Human Health Impacts

Javid Manzoor
Jiwaji University Gwalior, India

Manoj Sharma
Jiwaji University Gwalior, India

Irfan Rashid Sofi
Jiwaji University Gwalior, India

Ashaq Ahmad Dar
Pondichery University, India

ABSTRACT

Plastics have become a vital asset for humanity. Plastics are known as synthetic materials produced from synthetic or semi-synthetic organic polymers derived from petro-based chemicals, able to displace traditional natural polymeric materials (wood, stone, ceramics, etc.). Plastics have malformed everyday life; usage is increasing, and annual production is likely to exceed 300 million tons by 2010. In this chapter, the authors blend current understanding of the benefits and concerns surrounding the use of plastics and look to future priorities, challenges, and opportunities. Plastics case serious environmental pollution such as soil pollution, water pollution, and air pollution. Application of proper rules and regulations for the production and use of plastics can reduce the toxic effects of plastics on human health and the environment.

INTRODUCTION

Plastic waste is a growing concern and the drivers behind it look set to continue. Although recently there has been a slight decrease in plastic production, this is unlikely to be maintained. Plastic is a highly useful material and its applications are expected to increase as more new products and plastics are developed to meet demands. The increased use and production of plastic in developing and merging countries is a

DOI: 10.4018/978-1-5225-9452-9.ch002

particular concern, as the sophistication of their waste management infrastructure may not be developing at an appropriate rate to deal with their increasing levels of plastic waste.

In the last 60 years, plastic has become a useful and versatile material with a wide range of applications. Its uses are likely to increase with ongoing developments in the plastic industry. In the future, plastic could help address some of the world's most pressing problems, such as climate change and food shortages. For example, plastics are used in the manufacture of rotors for wind turbines and tunnels made from polyethylene can help crops grow in otherwise unfavourable conditions. As demand for materials with certain qualities increases, the plastics industry will aim to supply them. Meanwhile, increasing plastic production and use in emerging economies looks set to continue, and waste management infrastructure will have to develop accordingly. Unfortunately, the properties of plastic that make it so valuable also make its disposal problematic, such as its durability, light weight and low cost. In many cases plastics are thrown away after one use, especially packaging and sheeting, but because they are durable, they persist in the environment. If plastic reaches the sea, its low density means it tends to remain on the surface.

Increasing attention has been paid to plastic waste by policymakers, scientists and the media and probably one of the most influential factors was the discovery of the Great Pacific Garbage Patch by Charles Moore in the late 1990s.This is a layer of rubbish floating between California and Hawaii that has been estimated to span about 3.43 million km^2 (the size of Europe). It is mostly plastic and contains everything from large abandoned fishing net to plastic bottles to tiny particles of plastic (or 'microplastics'). This type of mass in the seas can be known as 'plastic soup' and there are concerns that Europe hosts similar patches, in areas such as the Mediterranean and the North Sea. As such, marine litter and plastic waste is a priority on the EU policy agenda. Plastic is still a relatively new material, which means the problem of plastic waste has only recently been realized, as has knowledge about its environmental persistence (Barnes et al., 2009). Even more recent is the discovery of possible health and environmental effects, such as the impacts of the chemicals contained in plastics. The monitoring of plastic waste and research into its impacts are still in their infancy, but so far the implications are worrying.

INDIAN SCENARIO

Plastic waste is a major environmental and public health problem in Indian set up particularly in the urban areas (Tammemagi, 1999). Plastic shopping or carrier bags are one of the main sources of plastic waste in our country. Plastic bags of all sizes and colors dot the city's landscape due to the problems of misuse and overuse and littering in India. Besides this visual pollution, plastic bag wastes contribute to blockage of drains and gutters, are a threat to aquatic life when they find their way to water bodies, and can cause livestock deaths when the livestock consume them. Furthermore, when filled with rainwater, plastic bags become breeding grounds for mosquitoes, which cause malaria. We have become so accustomed to the ubiquitous presence of plastic that it is difficult to envision life when woods and metals were the primary materials used for consumer products. Plastic has become prevalent because it is inexpensive and it can be engineered with a wide range of properties. Plastics are strong but lightweight, resistant when degraded by chemicals, sunlight, and bacteria, and are thermally and electrically insulating. Plastics have become a critical material in the modern economy; the annual volume of plastics produced exceeds that volume of steel (Tammemagi,1999).The kind of recycling practiced in India is quite different from what is practiced in the rest of the world, in that state of the art technologies are not employed here. The starting point is the sorting of plastic waste (based on colour, transparency, hardness, density and opacity of the scrap). The sorted waste is then sent to the granulators to obtain granules using with the traditional mechanical and grinding techniques. The converters use these granules to make finished plastic products. The majority of such units (granulators and convertors) are often located in slums, and function single machine extruding units. Scrap storage is done in the backyards, and washing is done in open drums. These activities are often termed as backyard recycling. The technologies used in these industries are also old and local Narayan, (2001). Of the types of plastics recycled in India, PVC (polyvinyl chloride) accounts for 45%, LDPE (low density polyethylene) for 25%, HDPE (high density polyethylene) for 20%, PP (polypropylene) for 7.6% and other polymers such as PS (polystyrene) for 2.4% Shah, (2001). This recycling is usually results in the down cycling of plastics into lower-quality products that have higher and more 4 leachable levels of toxic additives Chaturvedi, (2002). During recycling, the plastic scrap is cleaned to remove the dirt and foreign matter adhering to it. The waste water generated used for this purpose is finally disposed of into open drains. This wastewater has high pollution load in terms of BOD, COD, and TSS (Narayan, 2001).The final stage in the life cycle of plastics is disposal. In India, there are three common ways of getting rid off plastics - by dumping them in landfills, by burning them in incinerators or by littering them. In the case of littering, plastic wastes fail to reach landfills or incinerators. It is the improper way of disposing plastics and is identified as the cause of manifold ecological problems. Incineration of plastic wastes also significantly reduces the volume of waste requiring disposal Begum, (2010). It is believed that the volume reduction brought about by incineration ranges from 80 to 95%. But the burning of these chlorine-containing substances releases toxic heavy metals and emits noxious gasses like dioxins and furans. The latter two are two of the most toxic and poisonous substances on earth and can cause a variety of health

EFFECTS OF PLASTIC ON HUMAN HEALTH

Human health risks from plastics can stem from their monomeric building blocks (e.g., Bisphenol A), their additives (e.g., plasticizers) or from a combination of the two (e.g., antimicrobial polycarbonate) (Rahman & Brazel 2004). There are several toxic materials which are secreted by plastics. Among them, we concentrate on plastics components and additives of principal concern such as Bisphenol A and phthalates. Bisphenol A (BPA) is best known as the monomeric building block of polycarbonate plastics. It was first synthesized in 1891 and used frequently as an additive to other plastics such as polyvinyl chloride (PVC) (Dodds & Lawson1936). The yearly yield of BPA in the worldwide was 2.2 million metric tons in 2003. A sizable part of this mass comes into contact with nourishment. Since the polymerization of BPA abandons a few monomers unbound, BPA atoms can be discharged from refreshment and nourishment holders into beverage and sustenance after some time. The draining procedure is quickened by continued washing of holders and while putting away in the acidic or fundamental things that separate the polymer. Accordingly, reusable water bottles, infant bottles, and the inward linings of nourishment jars, all made by utilizing BPA, are known to filter the questionable monomer into sustenance after some time, especially at raised temperatures (Raloff 1999; Kang et al. 2003). Studies have indicated that food and drinks stored in such containers including those ubiquitous clear water bottles hanging from just about every hiker's backpack can contain a trace amount of Bisphenol A (BPA) that may interfere with the body's natural hormonal messaging system. Food and inhalation are considered the main source of exposure to BPA in the human body (Wilson et al.2007). The BPA is considered to be a hormone because it is the mimics of reproductive hormones 'estrogen'. As found in various studies, BPA has been associated with a number of health problems such as ovarian chromosomal damage, decreased sperm production, rapid puberty, rapid changes in immune system, type-2diabetes, cardiovascular disorder, obesity etc. Some studies have also claimed that BPA increases the risk of breast cancer, prostate cancer, pains, metabolic disorders, etc. BPA in women and impaired health, including obesity, endometrial hyperplasia, recurrent miscarriages, sterility, and polycystic ovarian syndrome(Warner et al. 2002; Rayner et al. 2004; Eskenazi et al. 2007).Levels of unconjugated BPA in human blood and tissues are in the range of 0.1 to 10 µg/L in the human body and is assessed in blood serum and urine (Ikezuki et al. 2002; Schonfelder et al.2002). BPA is controlled by catalyst connected insusceptible sorbent test (ELISA). Geometric methods for every day admission of BPA assessed from urinary dimensions are higher for guys than females (53.8 versus 41 ng/kg/day) and higher in youngsters and teenagers (64.6 and 71 ng/kg/day, individually) than in grown-ups, whose presentation levels decline with age from 52.9 ng/kg/day in 20– 39-year olds to 33.5 ng/kg/day in seniors 60 years and more established (Lakind and Naiman 2008). Raised introduction of ladies of childbearing age and of youngsters are of specific concern as a result of known windows of defenselessness to BPA that put the creating hatchling and kids at raised hazard, contrasted with grown-ups uncovered with indistinguishable dimensions of the contaminant (Vandenberg et al. 2009).In its determination of a reference dose for humans, the U.S. EPA arrived at a value of 50 µg per kg per day by applying a safety factor, to account for extrapolation from animals to humans, variability in the human population, and extrapolation from subchronic to chronic exposures (Welshons et al. 2003). This reference dose for BPA was calculated on the basis of the lowest observable adverse effect level (LOAL) as adverse responses were found even at the lowest dose tested (Vandenberg et al. 2009).Today's concerns about BPA are driven primarily by low-dose effects observed in human populations, and by the recognition that biologically active levels of BPA detectable in human blood are within or above the range of concentrations demonstrated in vitro to cause changes in the function of human tissues (Vom & Hughes2005). Phthalates are a diverse group of compounds that represent diesters of phthalic acid, a compound also known as 1, 2-benzenedicarboxylic acid produced in large quantities since the1930s. The properties of phthalates are dependent on the length and branching of the dialkyl or alkyl/aryl side chains, i.e., the alcohol moiety of the ester. Di (2-ethylhexyl) phthalate (DEHP), produced at annual quantities of 2 million tons and widely used in medical devices. Important routes of human exposure to phthalates include, most notably, medical exposures caused by direct release of phthalates into the human body, e.g., through dialysis, blood transfusions, and extracorporeal membrane oxygenation (ECMO); ingestion of contaminated materials, including contaminated food, house dust etc. (Sathyanarayana 2008; Kamrin2009; Meeker et al. 2009). Thalates usually work to increase plastic flexibility or flexibility. Here is an example of adding some plastic such as polyvinyl chloride (PVC) thalates. Thales like BPA has hormonal imbalances, which also cause them to disrupt hormones normal and daily work. Both BPA and thalates can enterthe body of the newborn through pregnancy and through fetal and breast feeding, they will be able to harm them. However, it is important to remember that, Thales is a little less damaging to human than the BPA. So all kinds of plastic containers have harmful BPAand thalates.

The harmful effects of plastic on aquatic life are devastating, and accelerating. The impacts of plastic waste on our health and the environment are only just becoming apparent. Most of our knowledge is around plastic waste in the marine environment, although there is research that indicates that plastic waste in landfill and in badly managed recycling systems could be having an impact, mainly from the chemicals contained in plastic. Ingestion of plastic occurs more frequently than entanglement. The MFSD has recognized ingestion of waste as a marker for checking natural status. Ingestion of plastic waste has been reported in various species. For certain species, practically all people contain ingested plastic Ryan at al., (2009), including ocean flying creatures, fish, turtles, mussels and warm blooded animals. Obviously unique species ingest diverse sorts and sizes of plastic flotsam and jetsam. Numerous creatures botch plastic waste for prey, for instance, fish can mistake plastic pellets for tiny fish, flying creatures may confuse bits of plastic with cuttlefish or other prey (Derraik, 2002, Gregory, 2009). There are a few synthetic substances inside plastic material itself that have been added to give it certain properties, for example, Bisphenol A, phthalates and fire retardants. These all have known negative effects on human and animal health, mainly affecting the endocrine system. There are also toxic monomers, which have been linked to cancer and reproductive problems. The actual role of plastic waste in causing these health impacts is uncertain. This is partly because it is not clear what level of exposure is caused by plastic waste, and partly because the mechanisms by which the chemicals from plastic may have an impact on humans and animals are not fully established. The most likely pathway is through ingestion, after which chemicals could bioaccumulate up the food chain, meaning that those at the top could be exposed to greater levels of chemicals Science for Environment Policy (2011).Plastic waste also has the ability to attract contaminants, such as persistent organic pollutants (POPs). Plastic could potentially transport these chemicals to otherwise clean environments and, when ingested by wildlife, plastic could cause the transfer of chemicals into the organism's system. However, in some conditions plastic could potentially act as a sink for contaminants, making them less available to wildlife, particularly if they are buried on the seafloor. With their large surface area-to-volume ratio, micro plastics may have the capacity to make chemicals more available to wildlife and the environment in comparison to larger sized plastics. However, once ingested, micro plastics may pass through the digestive system more quickly than larger plastics, potentially providing less opportunity for chemicals to be absorbed into the circulatory system Science for Environment Policy (2011). Unfortunately, the properties of plastic that make it so valuable also make its disposal problematic, such as its durability, light weight and low cost. In many cases plastics are thrown away after one use, especially packaging and sheeting, but because they are durable, they persist in the environment. If plastic reaches the sea, its low density means it tends to remain on the surface. Most types of plastic are not biodegradable. Some plastics are designed to be biodegradable and can be broken down in a controlled environment, such as landfill, but it is uncertain if this will occur under other conditions, especially in oceans where the temperature is colder Schuler, (2008). Even if plastic does eventually biodegrade, it will temporarily break into smaller fragments, which then produce so-called 'microplastics'. These have a specific and significant set of impacts. The harmful effects of chemicals additives in plastics are also pronounced in newborns via mothers exposed to these toxins during their pregnancy. The second vulnerable groups are young children exposed directly to these chemicals. Since many of these chemicals (BPA and phthalates) can cross the placenta, resulting in growth retardation and neurological harm. There are also evidences to suggest hormonal derangements and cancers in children Zaman, (2010).

Impact on Environment

Plastic is one of the major toxic pollutants of present time. Being composed of toxic chemicals and most importantly a non biodegradable substance, plastic pollutes earth and leads to air pollution and water pollution. This also mixes with food chain effecting Environment Humans and animals. There is no safe way to dispose plastic waste and waste causes serious damage to environment during its production process, during its usage and during its disposal process. Harmful synthetic concoctions discharge amid assembling process is another huge wellspring of the negative natural effect of plastics. An entire host of cancer-causing, neurotoxic, and hormone-problematic synthetic concoctions are standard fixings and waste results of plastic generation, and they unavoidably discover their way into our nature through water, land, and air contamination. A portion of the significant mixes incorporate vinyl chloride (in PVC), dioxins (in PVC), benzene (in polystyrene), phthalates and different plasticizers (in PVC and others), formaldehyde, and bisphenol-An, or BPA (in polycarbonate). Huge numbers of these are relentless natural contaminations (POPs) probably the most harming poisons on earth, inferable from a mix of their steadiness in the earth and their elevated amounts of harmfulness; in any case, their unmitigated discharge into the earth influences all earthbound and oceanic existence with which they come into contact. It is in the use phase that the benefits of plastics in durability and effectiveness are most evident. Though most plastics are benign in their intended use form, many release toxic gases in their in-place curing(such as spray foam) or by virtue of their formulation (as with PVC additives off-gassing during their use phase). Occupational exposure during installation, such as inhalation of dust while cutting plastic pipe or off-gassing vapors of curing products, is also a great concern for human health and the environment. The disposal of plastics—the "grave" phase, is one of the least recognized and most highly problematic areas of plastic's ecological impact. Ironically, one of plastic's most desirable traits-its durability and resistance to decomposition-is also the source of one of its greatest liabilities when it comes to the disposal of plastics. Natural organisms have a very difficult time breaking down the synthetic chemical bonds in plastic, creating the tremendous problem of the material's persistence. A very small amount of total plastic production (less than10%) is effectively recycled; the remaining plastic is sent to landfills, where it is destined to remain entombed in limbo for hundreds of thousands of years, or to incinerators, where its toxic compounds are spewed throughout the atmosphere to be accumulated in biotic forms throughout the surrounding ecosystems. Unfortunately, because of plastic's low density, it frequently migrates "downstream," blowing out of landfills and off garbage barges. In 1997, Captain Charles Moore discovered widespread plastic garbage contamination area, called a gyre, in the North Pacific Ocean. By 2005, the estimated area of contamination expanded to 10 million square miles. 90% of this garbage was determined to be plastic, and 80% was originally sourced from land, such as construction waste. It has been reported that there are six similar gyres across the planet's oceans, each laden with plastic refuse.

CONCLUSION

Toxicity of plastic is a problem in nature on a universal scale, from the individual level to the level of populations. The chapter reveals that the negative consequences of plastic on human health and environment as a result of exposure to toxic chemicals used in the production of plastics. Peoples use unconsciously plastics without knowing its toxicity. The toxic effect of plastics on human health and environment is very much evident by the most of the reviews. The government, law implementing agencies and health authorities of the country should take more steps and pay attention to sustainable production, use, and disposal of plastics. Phthalates of high concern should be banned and implemented, primary in consumer products or product in contact with children. Bisphenols should be banned from use in materials that come into contact with food and beverages and children and in the long term in other consumer products like thermal cash receipt. Every company must take their responsibility in terms of the decline of unnecessary plastic consumption.

REFERENCES

Andrady, A. (2003). An environmental primer. In A. Andrady (Ed.), *Plastics and theenvironment* (pp. 3–76). Hoboken, NJ: Wiley Interscience. doi:10.1002/0471721557

Andrady, AL & Neal MA (2009). Applications and societal benefitsof plastics. *Phil. Trans. R. Soc. B, 364*, 1977–1984. doi:10.1098/rstb.2008.0304

APME. (2006). *An Analysis of Plastics Production, Demand and Recovery in Europe*. APME.

Barnes, D. K. A., Galgani, F., Thompson, R. C., & Barlaz, M. (2009). Accumulation and fragmentation of plastic debris in global environments. *Philosophical Transactions of the Royal Society of London. Series B, Biological Sciences, 364*(1526), 1985–1998. doi:10.1098/rstb.2008.0205 PMID:19528051

Barnes, D. K. A., Galgani, F., Thompson, R. C., & Barlaz, M. (2009). Accumulation and fragmentation of plastic debris in global environments. *Philosophical Transactions of the Royal Society of London. Series B, Biological Sciences, 364*(1526), 1985–1998. doi:10.1098/rstb.2008.0205 PMID:19528051

Begum, Z. (2010). *Plastics and environment. Dissemination Paper for the Ministryof Environment and Forest*. Government of India.

Biello & David. (2011). Are Biodegradeable Plastics Doing More Harm Than Good? *Scientific American*.

Chaturvedi, B. (2002). *The source of this information is a press release of NoPlastics in the Environment (Nope) Imports Versus Surplus: A Glut of Plasticsin India Today*. Chintan Environmental Organization.

Derraik, J. G. B. (2002). The pollution of the marine environment by plastic debris: Areview. *Marine Pollution Bulletin, 44*(9), 842–852. doi:10.1016/S0025-326X(02)00220-5 PMID:12405208

Dodds, E. C., & Lawson, W. (1936). Synthetic estrogenic agents without the phenantthrene nucleus. *Nature, 137*(3476), 996. doi:10.1038/137996a0

Eskenazi, B., Warner, M., Samuels, S., Young, J., & Gerthoux, P. M. (2007). Serum dioxin concentrations and risk of uterine leiomyomain the Seveso Women's Health Study. *American Journal of Epidemiology, 166*, 79–87. doi:10.1093/aje/kwm048

Gregory, M. R. (2009). Environmental implications of plastic debris in marinesettings-entanglement ingestion smothering hangers-on hitch-hiking and alieninvasions. *Philosophical Transactions of the Royal Society of London. Series B, Biological Sciences, 364*(1526), 2013–2025. doi:10.1098/rstb.2008.0265 PMID:19528053

Halden, R. U. (2010). Plastics and health risks. *Annual Review of Public Health, 31*(1), 179–194. doi:10.1146/annurev.publhealth.012809.103714 PMID:20070188

Ikezuki, Y., Tsutsumi, O., Takai, Y., Kamei, Y., & Taketani, Y. (2002). Determination of bisphenol a concentrations in human biologicalfluids reveals significant early prenatal exposure. *Human Reproduction (Oxford, England), 17*(11), 2839–2841. doi:10.1093/humrep/17.11.2839 PMID:12407035

Kamrin, M. A. (2009). Phthalate risks, phthalate regulation, and public health: A review. *J. Toxicol. Environ. Health B, 12*(2), 157–174. doi:10.1080/10937400902729226 PMID:19235623

Kang, J. H., Kito, K., & Kondo, F. (2003). Factors influencing the migration of bisphenol A from cans. *Journal of Food Protection, 66*(8), 1444–1447. doi:10.4315/0362-028X-66.8.1444 PMID:12929833

Lakind, J. S., & Naiman, D. Q. (2008). Bisphenol A (BPA) daily intakesin the United States: Estimates from the 2003–2004 NHANES urinary BPA data. *Journal of Exposure Science & Environmental Epidemiology, 18*(6), 608–615. doi:10.1038/jes.2008.20 PMID:18414515

Meeker, J.D., Sathyanarayana, S., & Swan, S.H. (2009). Phthalates andother additives in plastics: human exposure and associated healthoutcomes. *Phil. Trans. R. Soc. B, 364*, 2097–2113. doi:10.1098/rstb.2008.0268

Narayan, P. (2001). *Analyzing Plastic Waste Management in India: Case study of Polybags and PET bottles published by IIIEE*. Lund University Sweden.

Plastics Europe. (2008). The compelling facts about Plastics 2007: An analysis of plastics production, demand and recovery for 2007 in Europe. Brussels, Belgium: Plastics Europe.

Rahman, M., & Brazel, C. S. (2004). The plasticizer market: An assessment of traditional plasticizers and research trends to meet new challenges. *Progress in Polymer Science, 29*(12), 1223–1248. doi:10.1016/j.progpolymsci.2004.10.001

Raloff, J. (1999). Food for thought: What's coming out of baby's bottle? *Sci. News Online, 156*, 1–4.

Rayner, J. L., Wood, C., & Fenton, S. E. (2004). Exposure parameters necessary for delayed puberty and mammary gland development in Long-Evans rats exposed in utero to atrazine. *Toxicology and Applied Pharmacology, 195*(1), 23–34. doi:10.1016/j.taap.2003.11.005 PMID:14962502

Rudel, R.A., Dodson, R.E., Newton, E., Zota, A.R., & Brody, J.G. (2008). Correlations between urinary phthalate metabolites and phthalates, estrogenic compounds 4-butyl phenol and o-phenyl phenol, and some pesticides in home indoor air and house dust. *Epidemiology, 19*, S332.

Ryan, P.G., Moore, C.J., Franeker, J.A., & Moloney, C.L. (2009). Monitoring the abundanceof plastic debris in the marine environment. *Philos Trans R Soc Lond BBiol Sci B, 364*, 1999-2012.

Sathyanarayana, S. (2008). Phthalates and children's health. *Current Problems in Pediatric and Adolescent Health Care, 38*(2), 34–49. doi:10.1016/j.cppeds.2007.11.001 PMID:18237855

Schonfelder, G., Wittfoht, W., Hopp, H., Talsness, C. E., Paul, M., & Chahoud, I. (2002). Parent bisphenol A accumulation in the human maternal-fetal-placental unit. *Environmental Health Perspectives, 110*(11), 703–707. doi:10.1289/ehp.021100703 PMID:12417499

Schuler, K. (2008). *Smart Plastics Guide: Healthier Food Uses of Plastics*. Minneapolis, MN: Academic Press.

Science for Environment Policy. (2011). *Plastic Waste: Ecological and HumanHealth Impacts*. In-depth Reports.

Shah, P. (2001). *The Plastic Devil: Ecological Menace*. Academic Press.

Tammemagi, H. Y. (1999). *The Waste Crisis: Landfills Incinerators and the Searchfor a Sustainable Future*. Oxford University Press.

Vandenberg, L. N., Maffini, M. V., Sonnenschein, C., Rubin, B. S., & Soto, A. M. (2009). Bisphenol-A and the great divide: A review of controversies in the field of endocrine disruption. *Endocrine Reviews*, *30*(1), 75–95. doi:10.1210/er.2008-0021 PMID:19074586

Vom Saal, F. S., & Hughes, C. (2005). an extensive new literature concerning low-dose effecs of bisphenol A shows the need for a newrisk assessment. *Environmental Health Perspectives*, *113*(8), 926–933. doi:10.1289/ehp.7713 PMID:16079060

Wagner, M., & Oehlmann, J. (2009). Endocrine disruptors in bottledmineral water: total estrogenic burden and migration from plasticbottles. *Environ. Sci. Pollut. Res*, *16*, 278–286. -009-0107-7 doi:10.100711356

Warner, M., Eskenazi, B., Mocarelli, P., Gerthoux, P. M., Samuels, S., Needham, L., ... Brambilla, P. (2002). Serum dioxin concentrations and breast cancer risk in the Seveso Women's Health Study. *Environmental Health Perspectives*, *110*(7), 625–628. doi:10.1289/ehp.02110625 PMID:12117637

Welshons, W. V., Thayer, K. A., Judy, B. M., Taylor, J. A., Curran, E. M., & Vom Saal, F. S. (2003). large effects from small exposures. I. Mechanisms for endocrine-disrupting chemicals with estrogenic activity. *Environmental Health Perspectives*, *111*(8), 994–1006. doi:10.1289/ehp.5494 PMID:12826473

Wilson, N. K., Chuang, J. C., Morgan, M. K., Lordo, R. A., & Sheldon, L. S. (2007). An observational study of the potential exposures of preschool children to pentachlorophenol, bisphenol-A, and nonylphenol at home and daycare. *Environmental Research*, *103*(1), 9–20. doi:10.1016/j.envres.2006.04.006 PMID:16750524

Yarsley, V. E., & Couzens, E. G. (1945). *Plastics*. Middlesex, UK: Penguin Books Limited.

Zaman, T. (2010). *The Prevalence and Environmental Impact of Single Use Plastic Products*. Academic Press.

Chapter 3
Environmental and Health Implications of Plastic Pollution:
A Pakistan Perspective

Toqeer Ahmed
COMSATS University Islamabad, Pakistan

Hassaan Fayyaz Khan Sipra
COMSATS University Islamabad, Pakistan

ABSTRACT

Plastic pollution is one of the prime and alarming issues in developing countries that has vast environmental and human health impacts which need to be addressed as a priority. Unfortunately, limited work has been done on the topic, especially on air and water pollution due to plastics in Pakistan. Informal solid waste management is being done by municipalities, which is not adequate, and the problem will increase with the upsurge in population and industrialization. There is a need to address the knowledge gap and improvements in the existing conditions to manage the issue of plastic pollution separately. In this chapter, causes; impacts of plastic pollution both on human and environmental health, plastic industries, and legislative context; and best practices to manage plastic pollution along with some important recommendations are discussed. It is expected the data presented may help the managers, environmental scientists, and policymakers to manage the problem of plastic pollution.

INTRODUCTION

Plastics reached large-scale production and consumption beginning in 1950 (Geyer, Jambeck, & Law, 2017), and the global lack of coordination on waste management and recycling has led to plastic waste accumulation, with effects on health and environment (Raynaud, 2014). Given that plastic is made to not degrade (Hopewell, Dvorak, & Kosior, 2009), plastic can be considered a sign of the Age of the Anthropocene (Zalasiewicz, et al., 2016). In order to better manage plastic waste, the principles of sustainable development and circular economy must be applied on production and consumption resource loops (Stahel, 2016).

DOI: 10.4018/978-1-5225-9452-9.ch003

Such a transformation of production and consumption systems is considerably challenging because of a lack of data on plastic waste. However, estimates point towards mismanagement at the production and consumption levels in terms of the state of plastic waste today. In terms of production, 8.3 billion metric tons of virgin plastic were produced between 1950 and 2015, of which 6.3billion metric tons was converted into plastic waste – with 79% reaching end of life in a landfill or the environment (Geyer, Jambeck, & Law, 2017).

It is unsurprising that the demand for plastic and its subsequent conversion to plastic waste is rising rapidly, since it is linked to rising living standards. As countries urbanize and economic growth occurs, production and consumption patterns change; waste generation and waste composition change as well. Higher living standards means more plastics enter the waste stream (Hoornweg & Bhada-Tata, 2012), and where mismanaged, they accumulate as plastic pollution. Better plastic waste management strategies (namely recovery and recycling) need to be instituted as urbanization continues. Its impacts on human health and our surrounding environment need to be studied closely to ensure that sound policies can be made to address plastic pollution.

Data on plastic pollution is limited, making its study difficult. There are also inherent biases and knowledge gaps within the global assessment of plastic pollution, with the focus being on ocean and freshwater plastic pollution. The most recent review effort of scientific literature on the global scale finds 87% of studies focus on marine plastic pollution, while 13% of studies focus on freshwater plastic pollution (Figure 1); marine based papers have a growth rate five times higher than that of freshwater based pollution papers (Blettler, Abrial, Khan, Sivri, & Espinola, 2018).Water based studies on plastic pollution are given extreme importance when trying to understand the local, regional and global plastic flows, since the majority of mismanaged plastic waste ends up in river systems and eventually flushes out to the oceans (Tibbetts, 2015). The United Nations Environment Programme estimates the costs of plastic pollution to be at $13 billion in terms of environmental damage to marine ecosystems (Raynaud, 2014).

Figure 1. Freshwater and marine plastic pollution studies globally (Blettler, Abrial, Khan, Sivri, & Espinola, 2018)

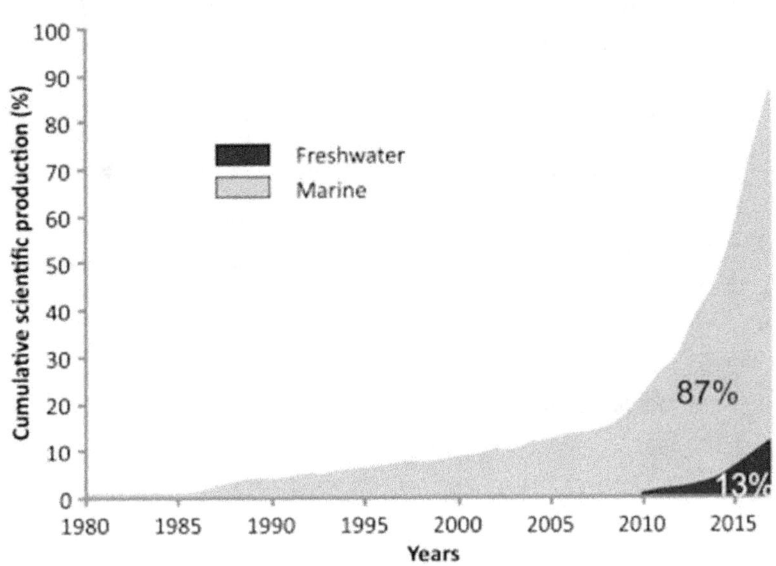

Another review of plastic wastes including bottles, bags and microscopic fibers and beads found that more than a quarter of all of marine plastic pollution comes from only 10 major rivers – eight in Asia, and two in Africa. Of particular note is the Indus River, situated in Pakistan, which contributes the second largest amount of plastic pollution to the global ocean circulation system (Schmidt, Krauth, & Wagner, 2017). Per a 2010 estimate where Pakistan was ranked number 15 in an index of mismanaged plastic waste, in a classification that found 83% of marine debris comes from just 20 countries, with Pakistan contributing 1.5% (Jambeck, et al., 2015).

At its core then, plastic pollution is a waste management issue for Pakistan. Its impacts on environment and health are largely unexplored. In an analysis of the Web of Knowledge (Figure 2), using key terms related to plastic pollution (management, recycling, air pollution, water pollution, soil pollution and health impacts) within selected Asian countries found that a total of 489 studies were published in peer-reviewed journals on the topic from 1975 to 2018. The Chinese contribution to plastic pollution research was the highest at 59%, while Pakistan had among the lowest contributions at 3%, only 17 publications. The major focus in Pakistan was on management (9 publications), followed by recycling (5 publications), health impacts (2 publications) and soil pollution (1 publication). No publications on air and water pollution due to plastics were found in Pakistan.

CAUSES / SOURCES OF PLASTIC POLLUTION

Waste tends to increase and change its characteristic as a result of economic growth, rising populations and urbanization (Chen, 2018). Although most developing countries primarily produce organic waste, economic growth and affluence are resulting in changes to most countries' waste characteristics, leading to increases in plastic, paper and other high valuable recycling materials in the waste supply chain (Medina, 2010). It can be classified as pollution when the waste is not properly managed, leading to unwanted impacts on human health and the environment. As the world moves towards more consumerist

Figure 2. Analysis of web of knowledge for plastic pollution peer-reviewed publications in selected Asian countries (based on data available on Web of Knowledge in Dec. 2018)

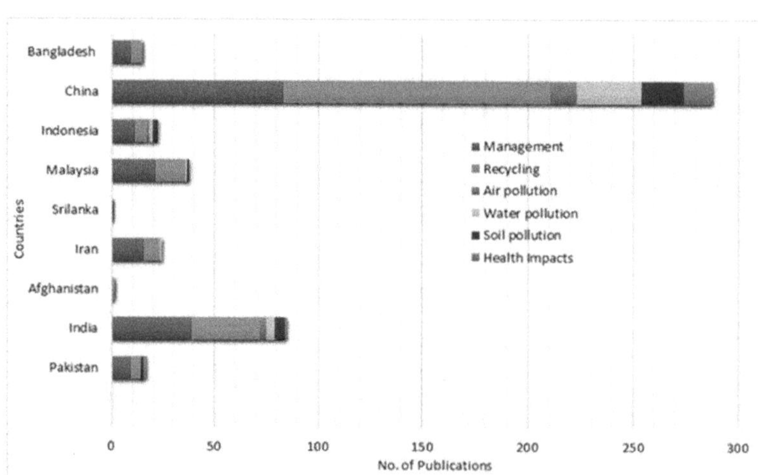

pathways due to rising living standard, societies need to come to terms with the reality that out of sight should not mean out of mind, in a world of plastics proliferation (Boetzkes, 2016).

Plastics present a problem for waste management due to two reasons: they are cheap, and they are easy to use (Ni, Lu, Mo, & Zeng, 2016). This quality means that plastics tend to largely come in the form of single-use plastics – the largest contributors to the pollution problem; their cheap and easy to use nature have allowed them to ramp up both production and consumption without the systematic presence of waste management. A global review found that single-use plastics contributed 60%-95% of marine plastic pollution, contending that interventions to reduce their production and consumption may well solve many of the problems associated with plastic pollution (Schnurr, et al., 2018). Many developing countries are facing the challenges of plastic pollution since their waste management systems are not on par with their increasing waste generation rates and changing waste characteristics (Hopewell, Dvorak, & Kosior, 2009). With global waste generation rates expected to increase by 70% in 2050, the budgets for municipal waste management systems need to increase as a proportion of waste generation in order to be effective (The World Bank, 2018).

Most developing countries continue to rely on informal waste management systems in the absence of municipal waste management due to budget constraints (Wilson, Costas, & Cheeseman, Role of informal sector recycling in waste management in developing countries, 2006). The informal system provides a valuable service to their societies where governments are unable to perform basic municipal functions, but they operate in an environment of lax or nonexistent regulations, open to exploitation and health impacts (Aparacana, 2017). Due to the lack of communication and data with regard to informal waste management, it is difficult to determine the recycling rate for plastics in most developing countries. However, it can be assumed that due to the high organic content in the waste of most developing countries, the overall contribution of high valuable recyclables such as plastics is small (Velis, 2017). Developing world cities are generally only able to achieve collection efficiency of 50%-80%(Wilson, Costas, & Cheeseman, Role of informal sector recycling in waste management in developing countries, 2006), with open dumping and burning presenting as the major pollution issue that is rarely considered in many developing countries (Wiedinmyer, Yokelson, & Gullett, 2014).

Burning of plastic in open fields and dumpsites release a variety of toxic gases, including, polybrominated diphenyl ethers (Ni, Lu, Mo, & Zeng, 2016), polychlorinated biphenyls, mercury and dioxins, which have severe health impacts to land, air and water (Verma, Vinoda, Papireddy, & Gowda, 2016). Within the context of Pakistan, a baseline study conducted in Lahore found that burning of such wastes presented low to moderate risk to the local population through different exposure mechanisms (Hafeez, et al., 2016).

Another major risk has begun to present itself in terms of plastics burning and recycling. It relates to the import of electronic waste into developing countries, particularly India and Pakistan – among the largest importers of electronic waste globally due to lax development and enforcement of customs regulations (Iqbal, et al., 2015). Although plastics are among the top contributors to composition and revenue from the dismantling and recycling processes associated with electronic waste, their extraction is needlessly difficult due to a lack of foresight by producers into design-for-environment/recycling (Cucchiella, D'Adamo, Koh, & Rosa, 2015). Specifically within the Pakistan context, it has been observed that plastics are often burned during the electronic waste recycling processes (Imran, Haydar, Kim, Awam, & Bhatti, 2017), causing numerous ailments associated with heart disease, respiratory and central nervous system issues (Cucchiella, D'Adamo, Koh, & Rosa, 2015).

PLASTICS POLLUTION STATUS IN PAKISTAN

Globally, plastic waste management began to be seriously considered and implemented approximately 30 years ago, once its impacts on human health and environment started being studied (Lam, et al., 2018). Today, as the world's population and affluence increases, rapid urbanization in developing countries is resulting in unsustainable pressures on cities in terms of waste management, particularly plastics and electronic waste (Vergara & Tchobanoglous, 2012). Pakistan, being a highly populous, rapidly urbanizing developing country (Pakistan Bureau of Statistics, 2017), faces many challenges with regard to municipal waste management. The country is struggling with implementation of regulatory mechanisms to strengthen waste management institutions, raise waste collection efficiency, formalize recycling processes, and build awareness of waste generation (Masood & Barlow, Framework for integration of informal waste management sector with the formal sector in Pakistan, 2013) to furnish a circular economy.

Pakistan is a South Asian country with a population of 207.7 million persons, an annual growth rate of 2.4% and 36.4% urbanization (Pakistan Bureau of Statistics, 2017). It is the fifth largest country in the world by population (United States Census Bureau, 2018), with a growing youth base; 64% of its population under the age of 29 (Najam & Bari, 2017).Already the country's largest city, Karachi is expected to become the third largest city in the world by 2030, per Euro Monitor International, a global market research firm (Baloch, 2018). Its waste generation rates vary across its cities (Table 1), with a national average of 0.6 kg/capita/day (Korai, Mahar, & Uqaili, 2017).

The ten largest cities of Pakistan are all over one million in population, and rapidly expanding (Pakistan Bureau of Statistics, 2017). The growing and urbanizing population is apparent in the country's waste composition. In a waste composition study conducted in 1996, Pakistan generated 3% plastic waste. By comparison, the United Kingdom and the United States had a share of 7% and 8% of plastic in their waste, respectively (Mahar, et al., 2007). It is important to set a population benchmark as well – the 1998 Census counted 132.4 million persons. Given a 2017 population of 207.8 million (Pakistan Bureau of Statistics, 2017), as compiled for the United Nations Environment Programme, Pakistan's municipal solid waste composition found that 9% of the country's waste is plastic (International Trade

Table 1. Waste generation rates and tons of waste per day across Pakistan cities (Pakistan Bureau of Statistics, 2015)

City Name	Waste Generation Rate	Tons of Waste/Day
Karachi	0.49	12,000
Hyderabad	0.212	300
Peshawar	0.629	781
Bannu	0.68	68
Quetta	0.56	1,250
Sibi	1.276	46
Faisalabad	0.50	1,759
Lahore	0.56	5,000
Bahawalpur	0.50	398

Administration, 2018). Nonetheless, waste characterization studies across the various cities of Pakistan are sorely needed to determine the amount of plastic waste.

It is difficult to conduct such studies, given the level of informal waste collection that takes place within Pakistani cities (Masood & Barlow, Framework for integration of informal waste management sector with the formal sector in Pakistan, 2013). Data for Lahore's dumpsites, operated under the municipal administration, is available; approximately 10% of the total waste is plastics, vastly low density polyethylene (Sadef, et al., 2016). In developing countries, the amount of high value waste secured at dumpsites and landfills, is much lower than the original waste amount. Recycling rates through the informal waste sector can vary between 20%-50%, with up to half in the form of clean, source segregated materials from households and businesses (Wilson, Araba, Chinwah, & Cheeseman, 2009). In Lahore, the recycling rate is estimated to be 27% (Masood & Barlow, Framework for integration of informal waste management sector with the formal sector in Pakistan, 2013), mostly made of high value recyclables such as plastic and paper (Batool, Chaudhry, & Majeed, Economic potential of recycling business in Lahore, Pakistan, 2008). This recycling operates outside the bounds of the formal waste management system. Such activities allow for a significant reduction in the burden on municipal collection, transport and disposal services/sites (Medina, 2010).

With regard to the informal waste sector, one of the common complaints by the various municipal waste management companies of the Punjab province is that waste pickers collect, reuse and improperly dispose of hospital waste. In Lahore, the 72% of hospital waste was plastics, against an infectious waste rate of 15% to 25% (Javed, Majeed, Farhan, & Nadeem, 2016). In Gujranwala, 25.8% was infectious, and 13.4% was plastic among the general waste (Ali, Wang, & Chaudhry, 2015). In Faisalabad hospitals, 14% infectious waste was found (Hameed, Riaz, Nassar u Minallah, & Munawar, 2017). In a review of such studies, it was noted that hospital staff do not follow the Hospital Waste Management Rules 2005, with multiple gaps identified in storage, transportation and disposal, allowing for greater access by informal waste pickers (Zeeshan, et al., 2018), who are reported to not use personal protection equipment, even when faced with infectious waste.(Masood & Barlow, 2014). Beyond safety equipment, informal waste pickers also have not been immunization to many of the infectious diseases they are exposed to during their collection and recycling efforts (Ali M., Wang, Chaudhry, & Geng, 2017).

In Pakistan, major plastic pollutants contain plastic bags, straws, beverages and chemicals empty plastic bottles and their caps cause environmental pollution. Karachi also deserves special attention from a plastic waste perspective in Pakistan since it is on the coast, in a country where 88% of plastic waste is mismanaged (Tibbetts, 2015). In a global review of freshwater plastic pollution (Figure 3), no data was present for Pakistan's freshwater plastic pollution (Blettler, Abrial, Khan, Sivri, & Espinola, 2018), although other Asia countries, such as China, Vietnam and India, have conducted such research. In a 2014 study, marine debris along the Karachi coast was characterized. It was found that 49.4% of the debris was plastic, across four locations (Qari & Shaffat, 2015). In a regional study of nine countries on microplastic fibers, Pakistan (Karachi coast) had the third highest amount (12 fibers/25 gram sand sample) of microplastic fibers, behind only Bangladesh (12.3) and India (13) (Balasubramaniam & Phillott, 2016).

Environmental and Health Implications of Plastic Pollution in Pakistan

The mismanagement of plastic waste in Pakistan is of high environmental concern, leading to freshwater (Tibbetts, 2015) and marine plastic pollution (Ivar do Sul & Costa, 2014). Since plastic does not degrade, through weathering processes it only becomes smaller, under it is microplastic. Microplastic is easily

Figure 3. Number of freshwater plastic pollution studies globally. Note that Pakistan has no such studies conducted (Blettler, Abrial, Khan, Sivri, & Espinola, 2018)

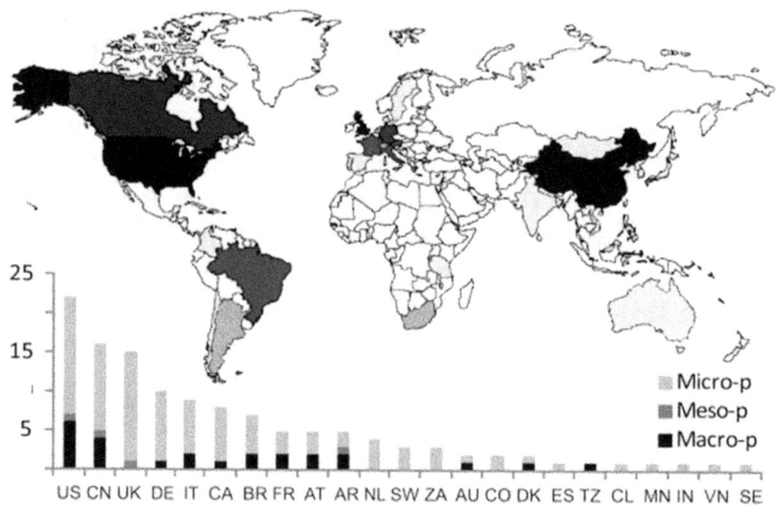

ingested by aquatic biota, particularly filter feeders like mollusks and oysters. Once ingested, it enters the food chain and impacts both on aquatic life and human beings as final consumer (Ogunola, Onada, & Falaye, 2018). More dedicated research on actual exposure and impacts on ingestion of microplastics is still needed. It is clear, however, that chemical additives to microplastics adsorb pollutants and metals to their surface, which are absorbed by the animal and human digestive systems. The bio-magnification of the microplastic due to increasing trophic levels have yet to be fully comprehended, but are likely to have an impact on gene expression, may result in cell death and be held responsible for immune-toxicological responses (Seltenrich, 2015).While the effects of microplastics are still being studied, macroplastics are also wreaking havoc on aquatic life, either through digestive issues after ingestion, or via entanglement (Derraik, 2002). Similarly, plastic dumped on the land, reduce land fertility and cause serious damage to the environment (Khan, Nawaz, Usama, & Ashraf, 2015).

One of the primary additives in plastics manufacturing is Bisphenol A (BPA) (Vandenberg, Hauser, Marcus, Olea, & Welshons, 2007), an endocrine disrupting chemical known for causing molecular changes in oestrogen levels (Leonardi, et al., 2017), impacting animals and humans at various stages of development (Table 2). The manufacturing use of BPA is prolific; it is used in many consumer-grade plastic products, such as food and beverage containers, in dental sealants and in the production of heat resistant papers (Galloway, et al., 2018). Concern over the carcinogenic potential of BPA has been thoroughly examined, and the US Environment Protection Agency noted that BPA leaching of 1 million pounds occurs annually, with over 90% of tested humans showing detectable levels of the chemical in their bloodstream, highlighting the risk of breast and prostate tumor development (Seachrist, et al., 2016).

Although many countries have adopted regulations to reduce the use of BPA in plastics manufacturing, no such regulations exist in Pakistan, despite research work on the matter having been conducted locally (Taskeen, Qualitative and Quantitative Analysis of Bisphenol-A in Foods and Beverages Stored in Plastic Containers and Wraps in Pakistan, 2012). BPA has been noted to have significantly contaminated the Indus River and its Sindh tributaries (Shaikh, Memon, Bhanger, & Nizamani, 2014), and its discharge at trace levels in milk packaging raise a specific concern for infants and young children(Taskeen

Table 2. BPA Impacts in Animals when exposed to Low-dose (Adopted from (Huang, 2012)

Dose (µg/kg/day)	BPA Effects (measured in studies of animals)	References
2	"Increased prostate weight 30%"	Nagel et al., 1997
1	Long-term adverse reproductive and carcinogenic effects	Newbold et al., 2009
0.025	"Changes in breast tissue that predispose cells to hormones and carcinogens"	Muñoz-de-Toro et al., 2005
0.025	"Permanent changes to genital tract"	Markey et al., 2005
2	"Lower bodyweight, increase of anogenital distance in both genders, signs of early puberty and longer estrus."	Honma et al., 2002
10	"Prostate cells more sensitive to hormones and cancer"	Ho et al., 2006
2.5	"Breast cells predisposed to cancer"	Murray et al., 2007
2.4	"Decline in testicular testosterone"	Akingbemi et al., 2004
10	"Decreased maternal behaviors"	Palanza et al., 2002
50	Adverse neurological effects occur in non-human primates	Leranth et al., 2008
30	"Reversed the normal sex differences in brain structure and behavior"	Kubo et al., 2003
50	Disrupts ovarian development	Adewale et al., 2009

& Naeem, 2009). It has also been linked to chronic diseases, such as obesity, diabetes, liver disease (Lang, Galloway, & Scarlett, 2008), cardiovascular disorders and sexual dysfunction (Li, et al., 2009), through a variety of exposure sources, including contaminated food from plastic containers. Although, the US, Canada, European Union have put limits on the amount of BPA, none of the limits established are above the 1 µg/kg of body weight/day recommended daily intake amount limit (Rezg, El-Fazaa, Gharbi, & Mornagui, 2014).

With the cross cutting health effects of BPA, some 40 countries have adopted policies to regulate and restrict its use, particularly with regard to food container safety for infants and young children (Duraisamy & Shrinithivihahshini, 2017). The need of the hour for Pakistan is to also adopt such measures against the use of BPA in plastics to offset its exposure to the public.

Beyond BPA, a most serious concern observed in developing countries is the use of ordinary plastic bags for the consumption of processed and/or cooked food items can lead to serious health issues, such as hypertension and diabetes in infants and young children (Reese, 2012). Further, the use of microwaves to warm food in plastic containers can cause as leaching of plastic particles that lead to testicular cancer (Richiardi, et al., 2004).

Other than BPA, phthalates and polybrominated diphenyl ether are important regarding health which comes under regulations. Expanding on the health impacts of plastic (Figure 4), burning in open dumps and containers has lasting damaging effects on human health, particularly causing thyroid imbalance, cancer and neurodevelopment toxicity (Siddiqi, Laessig, & Reed, 2003).Burning releases toxic gases like mercury, furans, polychlorinated biphenyls and dioxins into the environment. Polyvinyl chloride burning releases harmful halogens and pollutes air, resulting in climate change. Other increased risks with burning of plastics include asthma, nausea, skin problems, heart related issues and effects on nervous system (Verma, Vinoda, Papireddy, & Gowda, 2016), as well as financial effects and losses(Singh & Sharma, 2016). In a country like Pakistan, where open burning of plastic waste continues to occur

Figure 4. Impact of plastics on human health (Adapted from Proshad et al., 2018)

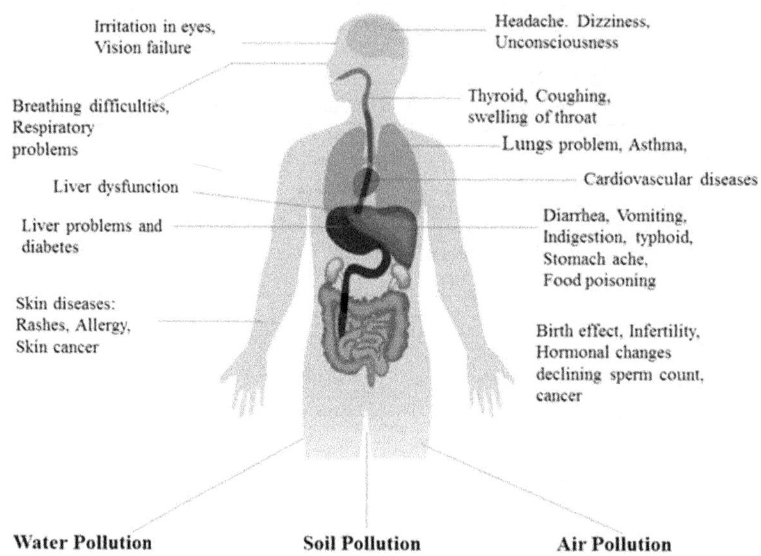

despite bans suggests that a more sustainable, poverty alleviating solution for the management of plastic waste is urgently needed (Wiedinmyer, Yokelson, & Gullett, 2014). Specific focus should be on the waste pickers' health; due to their nature of work and close proximity to the waste, they are more prone to diseases. Adoption of safe strategies and local government provision of facilities is necessary to assist them in their day-to-day activities and with their ailments (Black, et al., 2019). Multiple impacts have been reported against short- and long-term exposure to people and children working in plastic industries, such as issues in the development of nervous system in children, cancer and genetic susceptibility to other diseases (Sarigiannis, 2017). Other health effects include irritation to eyes, liver dysfunctions, birth effects, dizziness, cardiovascular impacts, genotoxic and gastrointestinal issues (Proshad, et al., 2018).

PLASTIC INDUSTRY AND LEGISLATIVE CONTEXT

Within the perspective of Pakistan's growing plastics industry, it is clear that Pakistan must take policy decisions on the production, use and disposal of plastics locally. The plastic industry of Pakistan is growing at an unprecedented rate of 15% per annum, on average (Khan Z. A., 2018).Approximately 8,000 small-scale plastic production units, on average producing 250-500 kilograms of plastics, end up producing 55 billion plastic bags per year, according to the Ministry of Climate Change of Pakistan (Khan A., Pakistan uses 55 billion shopping bags every year, 2018).

Further, Pakistan is dependent on the import of plastic materials for production of mainly packaging materials. Little data is available on the import and production of plastics in Pakistan, with none found within available scientific literature of the past decade, highlighting a major research gap within the country. However, support from the government for plastics industry in Pakistan is strong. In recent developments, the State Bank of Pakistan noted that local manufacturers were importing large amounts of plastic waste for the purpose of recycling without the implementation of any standards, which violates several trade conventions. The report also highlighted the need for better disposal and management systems for plastic uptake to reduce the overall burden of virgin plastics import, citing the principle of circular economy and resource efficiency (M/s Corporate Partners, 2010).

Plastics data is unavailable in Pakistan due to a lack of policy development and enforcement. Therefore, to resolve the health and environmental impacts of plastics, the legislative apparatus of Pakistan must be understood. The Constitution of 1973 provides certain inalienable protections/fundamental rights to the people of Pakistan; of relevance to the country's waste management scenario is Article 38e, which seeks to ensure that the State is responsible for the provision of the basic necessities of life: specifically mentioning food, clothing, housing, education and medical relief. Specifically, protecting natural resources and citizens from environmental pollution was included in the Concurrent Legislative List of Schedule IV (National Assembly of Pakistan, 2012), providing legislative authority to the federal and provincial legislatures to enact protections against environmental pollution (Alam, 2010).

In the landmark 1994 case Zia v. WAPDA (the Water and Power Regulatory Authority) (Supreme Court of Pakistan, 1994), the Supreme Court of Pakistan struck down WAPDA's plans for construction of an electric grid station, citing health concerns and expanding upon the definition of basic necessities to life to include a clean and healthy environment, free of pollution (IUCN, 2005). With this decision, a link between environmental pollution and human health was established within the Pakistan legislative context. The newly established precedent for extending fundamental rights led to the approval of the Pakistan Environment Protection Act in 1997 by the National Assembly and Senate (Senate of Pakistan, 1997). The act lay the groundwork for the need to prevent and control pollution and promote sustainable development.

The Act provided final authority for overseeing and guiding the process of environmental protection to the Pakistan Environmental Protection Council. The Council along with sub-functionaries, the Pakistan Environmental Protection Agency and Provincial Environmental Protection Agencies were to enforce the Act and its protections. Namely, the requirement was the development of comprehensive national environmental policies, the development of a national conservation strategy, the development and enforcement of the National Environmental Quality Standards, provision of guidelines for conservation and integration of sustainable development (Senate of Pakistan, 1997). However, with the 18th Constitutional Amendment in 2010, the Concurrent Legislative List of Schedule IV (Alam, 2010) was excluded from the federal legislature and became the sole responsibility of the provinces (Khan, Chaudhry, Ahmad, Saif, & Mehmood, 2018).

Pakistani legislation is taking its first steps towards addressing the proliferation plastics, particularly single-use plastics, by replacing them with biodegradable plastics. The Punjab government has already banned the use of plastics under thickness of 30 microns (Government of the Punjab, 2004), and Cabinet approval was received in Sindh for a phase-wise ban on plastic bags (Mansoor, 2018). Major outlets have begun providing cloth bags and charging for the plastic bags, while others have begun offering biodegradable plastic bags. Further, the Khyber Pakhtunkhwa province has declared that only oxo-biodegradable bags can be manufactured, sold and distributed (Ali M., 2017). Biodegradability requires another component that is missing from the Pakistani perspective – disposal conditions (Lacy & Rutqvist, 2015). To date, Pakistan only has one sanitary landfill that is capable of handling biodegradable matter in plastic form, Lakhodair Landfill in Lahore. Without the appropriate disposal conditions biodegradable bags release methane, a greenhouse gas, at the rate of 14.18 Gg per year (Zuberi & Ali, 2015).

PLASTICS, PAKISTAN, AND SUSTAINABLE DEVELOPMENT AGENDA

Plastic pollution must be reduced if sustainable development is to be achieved in Pakistan. Several of the UN Sustainable Development Goals, to which Pakistan is a signatory, are directly impacted by plastic pollution. Production and consumption (Goal 12) have an important role to play in reducing plastic pollution, in order to ensure that the health (Goal 3) and environmental impacts to land and sea (Goals 14-15) do not continue to place an exorbitant cost on society (ten Brink, et al., 2018).

With reference to sustainable production and consumption, there is a need for engaging the circular economy approach to maintain resource loops of the already present plastic within production and consumption cycles (Stahel, 2016) – in essence, people must practice recovery and recycling globally, while plastic production is on the rise, post-consumption recovery and recycling programs are laggard (Gourmelon, 2015). Investments in waste management capacity alongside societal awareness programs can improve recovery and recycling, as long as municipal authorities ensure convenience and quality assurance (Khan, Ahmed, & Najmi, 2019).

At the production level, the integration of design-for-environment is crucial to reducing plastics or for finding less impactful alternatives. Lifecycle assessment, eco-indicators and other similar impact assessment tools are necessary for realizing a world where plastics are used in a sustainable manner (Lewis, Gertsakis, Grant, Morelli, & Sweatman, 2017). Of particular concern is the single largest user of plastics – packaging, which accounted for roughly 40% of all plastic use in 2015 (Groh, et al., 2019). Despite global calls for reduction in plastics, the plastics industry in Pakistan continues to grow and be incentivized (M/s Corporate Partners, 2010). It is noteworthy that the plastics and packaging industry has grown at an accelerated rate of 15% per annum, contributing 1.7% to the national GDP (The News International, 2016). Against this backdrop, the use of circular economy and design-for-environment tools is not yet apparent in Pakistan (Umer & Abid, 2017).

In conjunction with production, on the consumer front, greater awareness is required regarding the role of plastics in the current global pollution scenario. Production strongly correlates to consumption, and the reduction in production or promotion of plastics re-use raises the level of awareness among consumer of plastic use, hazards and waste (Ragaert, Delva, & Van Geem, 2017). Till now in Pakistan, the reduction, reuse and recycling of plastic waste is limited to the informal waste sector, which is driven by monetary gains. However, consumers (specifically households) that engage in recycling tend to have a higher awareness of the negative impacts of plastics, and are driven by more than just the monetary gains associated with plastics recycling (Abbasi & Sheikh, 2016).

Given the interplay between production and consumption, the role of regulation becomes extremely important in combating plastic pollution. Common approaches for disposal of solid waste especially plastic waste includes landfilling, dumping, incineration and recycling. These approaches generally lead to greenhouse gas emissions, health impacts for formal and informal waste management labor forces (Sadef, et al., 2016), environmental degradation and public health issues (McKay, 2017). Further, the inequity of the global production and consumption scenarios is that the most economically disadvantaged groups suffer the greatest burden of plastic use (Han, 2017). Within this context, implementation of rules and regulation relating to waste management and plastics can help Pakistan in managing plastic pollution and reducing the impacts on human health and the environment (Masood & Barlow, 2013). Efforts to ban single use plastics can only go so far without also guiding the plastic industry's growth towards biodegradable alternatives (Ali M., 2017). Introducing biodegradable plastics without establishing sanitary landfills and bio-gasification plants in an economic and environmentally friendly way will not curtail the plastic pollution problem that now faces Pakistan (Batool & Chaudhry, 2008). Further, transparent implementation and enforcement of policies is needed, particularly with regard to recycling through the imposition of fines/fees for waste management, and eco-labeling to foment behavioral changes in reduction and reuse of plastics (Ogunola, Onada, & Falaye, 2018). Different companies and mega malls have already introduced biodegradable plastic bags and some NGOs have raised voice to use alternate to plastic bags.

CONCLUSION

Plastic pollution is one of the big challenges in the years and has vast impacts both on human and environmental health. There is dire need to change the mind of the society and raise awareness for reducing the impacts. In Pakistan, there is a need to consider alternatives to plastic manufacture, use and disposal. A mix of evidence-based policy approaches, technology transfer and public awareness need to be employed to implement effective waste management, with a focus on plastic use reduction, its recovery, recycling and incineration.

The legislative framework for plastic waste is now present in Pakistan, with bans of plastic bags and a requirement for biodegradability. After the 18th Amendment of the Pakistani Constitution and the subsequent devolution of the subject of environment to the provincial levels, this is occurring in a disparate manner. It is, therefore, recommended that a national level policy be devised to align and monitor the various sub-national policies. The advantage of doing so would be increased resource allocation towards capacity development of municipal waste management through federally distributed provincial budgets. Accomplishing this requires a focus on management of processes, inter-departmental coordination and good governance that targets better control of plastic pollution.

The various municipal governments of Pakistan must look towards resolving the hurdles of planning to develop large-scale waste-to-energy plants, given the high calorific value of plastic, and need for energy capacity in the country (Khan et al., 2015; Al-Salem, 2019). Further, a focus on the waste supply chain is paramount to the deployment of sorting, resource recovery, bio-gasification, composting and landfilling (Batool and Chuadhry, 2009). Such activities require the development of standards and protocols, particularly at hospitals, for informal waste pickers and sanitary workers (Rasheed et al., 2001). The occupational risks and health hazards of labor dealing with management of plastic waste and those in the plastic industries must also be ensured.

Finally, an enabling environment that incentivizes private sector to offer alternatives to plastic must be a legislative measure with specific targets for major plastic producers. Data collection and tagging of production by plastic type can provide decision-makers with a sense of the scope of the program. By enabling the private sector to offer alternatives, consumer behavior can be changed, but it will also require public awareness in local languages to the impacts of plastic on health and environment to cause a paradigm shift in the demand for plastics and move towards acceptance of recycling.

ACKNOWLEDGMENT

The authors gratefully the facilities of CCRD, CUI, Islamabad used for writing this chapter.

REFERENCES

Abbasi, M. N., & Sheikh, N. A. (2016). Attitudes and Motivations towards Plastics Recycling: A Multi-tier Supply Chain Approach. *Pakistan Journal of Social Sciences, 36*(2), 705-722. Retrieved from https://www.bzu.edu.pk/PJSS/Vol36No22016/PJSS-Vol36-No2-10.pdf

Alam, R. (2010, July 02). *Environment and the 18th Amendment.* Retrieved from The Express Tribune: https://tribune.com.pk/story/25273/environment-and-the-18th-amendment/

Ali, M. (2017, June 22). *Manufacture, use of non-biodegradable plastic products banned.* Retrieved from https://www.dawn.com/news/1341056

Ali, M., Wang, W., & Chaudhry, N. (2015). Management of wastes from hospitals: A case study of Pakistan. *Waste Management and Research, 34*(1), 87-90.

Ali, M., Wang, W., Chaudhry, N., & Geng, Y. (2017). Hospital waste management in developing countries: A mini review. *Waste Management and Research, 35*(6), 581-592.

Aparacana, S. (2017). Approaches to formalization of the informal waste sector into municipal solid waste management systems in low- and middle-income countries: Review of barriers and success factors. *Waste Management (New York, N.Y.), 61*, 593–607. doi:10.1016/j.wasman.2016.12.028 PMID:28038906

Balasubramaniam, M., & Phillott, A. D. (2016, January). Preliminary Observations of Microplastics from Beaches in the Indian Ocean. *Indian Ocean Turtle Newsletter,* (23), 13-16. Retrieved from https://www.iotn.org/wp-content/uploads/2017/05/IOTN-23.pdf#page=15

Baloch, F. (2018, November 6). *Karachi to become the world's third most populated city by 2030.* Retrieved from Samaa News: https://www.samaa.tv/news/2018/11/karachi-to-become-the-worlds-third-most-populated-city-by-2030/

Batool, S. A., & Chaudhry, M. N. (2008). The impact of municipal solid waste treatment methods on greenhouse gas emissions in Lahore, Pakistan. *Waste Management (New York, N.Y.), 29*(1), 63–69. doi:10.1016/j.wasman.2008.01.013 PMID:18387288

Batool, S. A., Chaudhry, N., & Majeed, K. (2008). Economic potential of recycling business in Lahore, Pakistan. *Waste Management (New York, N.Y.), 28*(2), 294–298. doi:10.1016/j.wasman.2006.12.007 PMID:17475469

Black, M., Karki, J., Lee, A. C., Makai, P., Barai, Y. R., Kritsotakis, E. I., ... Heckmann, A. F. (2019). The health risks of informal waste workers in the Kathmandu Valley: A cross-sectional survey. *Public Health, 166*, 10–18. doi:10.1016/j.puhe.2018.09.026 PMID:30419409

Blettler, M. C., Abrial, E., Khan, F. R., Sivri, N., & Espinola, L. A. (2018). Freshwater plastic pollution: Recognizing research biases and identifying knowledge gaps. *Water Research, 143*, 416–424. doi:10.1016/j.watres.2018.06.015 PMID:29986250

Boetzkes, A. (2016). Plastic, Oil Culture, and the Ethics of Waste. In C. Mauch (Ed.), *Out of Sight, Out of Mind: The Politics and Culture of Waste* (pp. 51–58). Berlin, Germany: Federal Ministry of Education and Research, Germany. Retrieved from http://www.environmentandsociety.org/sites/default/files/2016_i1.pdf

Chen, Y.-C. (2018). Effects of urbanization on municipal solid waste composition. *Waste Management (New York, N.Y.)*, *79*, 828–836. doi:10.1016/j.wasman.2018.04.017 PMID:30078496

Cucchiella, F., D'Adamo, I., Koh, S. C., & Rosa, P. (2015). Recycling of WEEEs: An economic assessment of present and future e-waste streams. *Renewable & Sustainable Energy Reviews*, *51*, 263–272. doi:10.1016/j.rser.2015.06.010

Derraik, J. G. (2002). The pollution of the marine environment by plastic debris: A review. *Marine Pollution Bulletin*, *44*(9), 842–852. doi:10.1016/S0025-326X(02)00220-5 PMID:12405208

Duraisamy, M., & Shrinithivihahshini, N. D. (2017). Need for regulatory policies in India, on the use of bisphenol A in food contact plastic containers. *Current Science, 113*(5), 861-868. Retrieved from https://web.a.ebscohost.com/abstract?direct=true&profile=ehost&scope=site&authtype=crawler&jrnl=00113891&AN=125124518&h=oIMQUSRyn1d%2b6Xbkfq8CFnbQ0hlJEVdR7NYqWIh58E0eHLEL6FDlS1DjZhW3EVKknYFr2yO1apriRXga4GTrSQ%3d%3d&crl=c&resultNs=AdminWebAuth&resultLocal=

Galloway, T. S., Baglin, N., Lee, B. P., Kocur, A. L., Shepherd, M. H., Steele, A. M., & Harries, L. W. (2018). An engaged research study to assess the effect of a 'real-world' dietary intervention on urinary bisphenol A (BPA) levels in teenagers. *BMJ Open*, *8*(2), e018742. doi:10.1136/bmjopen-2017-018742 PMID:29431133

Geyer, R., Jambeck, J. R., & Law, K. L. (2017). Production, use, and fate of all plastics ever made. *Science Advances*, *3*(7), e1700782. doi:10.1126ciadv.1700782 PMID:28776036

Gourmelon, G. (2015, January 27). *Global Plastic Production Rises, Recycling Lags.* Retrieved from World Watch Institute: http://worldwatch.net/sites/default/files/vital_signs_trend_plastic_full_pdf.pdf

Government of the Punjab. (2004, May 18). *The Punjab Polythene Bag Rules 2004.* Retrieved from Environment Protection Department Punjab: https://epd.punjab.gov.pk/system/files/The_Punjab_Polythene_Bag_Rules_2004.pdf

Groh, K. J., Backhaus, T., Carney-Almorth, B., Geueke, B., Inostroza, P. A., Lennquist, A., ... Muncke, J. (2019). Overview of known plastic packaging-associated chemicals and their hazards. *The Science of the Total Environment*, *651*(Part 2), 3253–3268. doi:10.1016/j.scitotenv.2018.10.015 PMID:30463173

Hafeez, S., Mahmood, A., Syed, J. H., Li, J., Ali, U., Malik, R. N., & Zhang, G. (2016). Waste dumping sites as a potential source of POPs and associated health risks in perspective of current waste management practices in Lahore city, Pakistan. *The Science of the Total Environment*, *562*, 953–961. doi:10.1016/j.scitotenv.2016.01.120 PMID:27153484

Hahladakis, J. N., & Aljabri, H. M. (2019). Delineating the plastic waste status in the State of Qatar: Potential opportunities, recovery and recycling routes. *The Science of the Total Environment*, *653*, 294–299. doi:10.1016/j.scitotenv.2018.10.390 PMID:30412874

Hameed, K., Riaz, O., Nassar u Minallah, M., & Munawar, H. (2017). Types of Hospital Waste and Waste Generation Rate in Different Hospitals of Faisalabad City, Pakistan. *Journal of Basic & Applied Scienes*, *13*, 386-391. Retrieved from http://lifescienceglobal.com/pms/index.php/jbas/article/view/4777/2709

Han, H. (2017). Environmental Injustice in the Production and Disposal of Plastics. *The Undergraduate Sociological Journal of Boston College,* (8), 47-53. Retrieved from https://pdfs.semanticscholar.org/751d/3f07b908ed69303c03797b0f2a4b45fba521.pdf#page=47

Hoornweg, D., & Bhada-Tata, P. (2012). *What a Waste: A Global Review of Solid Waste Management*. Washington, DC: The World Bank. Retrieved from https://openknowledge.worldbank.org/handle/10986/17388

Hopewell, J., Dvorak, R., & Kosior, E. (2009). Plastics recycling: Challenges and opportunities. *Philosophical Transactions of the Royal Society of London. Series B, Biological Sciences*, *364*(1526), 2115–2126. doi:10.1098/rstb.2008.0311 PMID:19528059

Huang, Y. W., Wong, C. K. C., Zheng, J. S., Bouwman, H., Barra, R., Wahlström, B., ... Wong, M. H. (2012). Bisphenol A (BPA) in China: A review of sources, environmental levels, and potential human health impacts. *Environment International*, *42*, 91–99. doi:10.1016/j.envint.2011.04.010 PMID:21596439

Imran, M., Haydar, S., Kim, J., Awam, M. R., & Bhatti, A. A. (2017). E-waste flows, resource recovery and improvement of legal framework in Pakistan. *Resources, Conservation and Recycling*, *125*, 131–138. doi:10.1016/j.resconrec.2017.06.015

International Trade Administration. (2018, September 8). *Pakistan - Waste Management*. Retrieved from https://www.export.gov/article?id=Pakistan-Waste-Management

Iqbal, M., Breivik, K., Syed, J. H., Malik, R. N., Li, J., Zhang, G., & Jones, K. C. (2015). Emerging issue of e-waste in Pakistan: A review of status, research needs and data gaps. *Environmental Pollution*, *207*, 308–318. doi:10.1016/j.envpol.2015.09.002 PMID:26433180

IUCN. (2005). *Environmental Law in Pakistan: Governing Natural Resources and the Process and Instituitions that Affect Them.* Karachi: IUCN, Environmental Law Programme. Retrieved from https://portals.iucn.org/library/sites/library/files/documents/ELC-016-1.pdf

Ivar do Sul, J. A., & Costa, M. F. (2014). The present and future of microplastic pollution in the marine environment. *Environmental Pollution*, *185*, 352–364. doi:10.1016/j.envpol.2013.10.036 PMID:24275078

Jambeck, J. R., Geyer, R., Wilcox, C., Siegler, T. R., Perryman, M., Andrady, A., . . . Law, K. L. (2015). Plastic waste inputs from land into the ocean. *Science Magazine*. Retrieved from http://wedocs.unep.org/bitstream/handle/20.500.11822/17969/Plastic_waste_inputs_from_land_into_the_ocean.pdf?sequence=1&isAllowed=y

Javed, N., Majeed, K., Farhan, K., & Nadeem, K. (2016). *Healthcare Waste Treatment and Disposal Lahore*. Lahore: The Urban Unit.

Khan, A. (2018). *Pakistan uses 55 billion shopping bags every year*. Retrieved from The Nation: https://nation.com.pk/17-Dec-2018/pakistan-uses-55-billion-shopping-bags-every-year

Khan, A., Nawaz, K., Usama, M., & Ashraf, Z. (2015). Feasibility Study of Municipal Plastic Waste for Power Generation in Lahore City, Pakistan. *Journal of Chemical Engineering & Process Technology*, *229*(6). doi:10.4172/2157-7048.1000229

Khan, M., Chaudhry, M. N., Ahmad, S. R., Saif, S., & Mehmood, A. (2018). Challenges to EIA consultants whilst dealing with stakeholders in Punjab, Pakistan. *Environmental Impact Assessment Review, 73*, 201–209. doi:10.1016/j.eiar.2018.09.001

Khan, Z. A. (2018, March 19). *Hazardous plastic scraps imports continue unabated in Pakistan*. Retrieved from https://www.dawn.com/news/1396102

Korai, M. S., Mahar, R. B., & Uqaili, M. A. (2017). The feasibility of municipal solid waste for energy generation and its existing management practices in Pakistan. *Renewable & Sustainable Energy Reviews, 72*, 338–353. doi:10.1016/j.rser.2017.01.051

Lacy, P., & Rutqvist, J. (2015). *Waste to Wealth: The Circular Economy Advantage*. New York: Palgrave Macmillan. Retrieved from https://books.google.com.pk/books?hl=en&lr=&id=DmKkCgAAQBAJ&oi=fnd&pg=PP1&dq=plastic+pollution+circular+economy+pakistan&ots=7WOHBD1Rc5&sig=sR30Noypse-sYRhuHTQFtA2bk74#v=onepage&q&f=false

Lam, S.-S., Ramanathan, S., Carbery, M., Gray, K., Vanka, K. S., Maurin, C., ... Palanisami, T. (2018). A Comprehensive Analysis of Plastics and Microplastic Legislation Worldwide. *Water, Air, and Soil Pollution*, 229–345. doi:10.100711270-018-4002-z

Lang, I. A., Galloway, T. S., & Scarlett, A. (2008). Association of Urinary Bisphenol A Concentration With Medical Disorders and Laboratory Abnormalities in Adults. *Journal of the American Medical Association, 300*(11), 1303–1310. doi:10.1001/jama.300.11.1303 PMID:18799442

Leonardi, A., Cofini, M., Rigante, D., Lucchetti, L., Cipolla, C., Penta, L., & Esposito, S. (2017). The Effect of Bisphenol A on Puberty: A Critical Review of the Medical Literature. *International Journal of Environmental Research and Public Health, 14*(9), 1044. doi:10.3390/ijerph14091044 PMID:28891963

Lewis, H., Gertsakis, J., Grant, T., Morelli, N., & Sweatman, A. (2017). *Design + Envrionment: A Global Guide to Designing Greener Goods*. London: Routledge. Retrieved from https://www.taylorfrancis.com/books/9781351282208

Li, D., Zhou, Z., Qing, D., He, Y., Wu, T., Miao, M., ... Yuan, W. (2009). Occupational exposure to bisphenol-A (BPA) and the risk of self-reported male sexual dysfunction. *Journal of Human Reproduction, 25*(2), 519–527. doi:10.1093/humrep/dep381

Mahar, A., Malik, R. N., Qadir, A., Ahmed, T., Khan, Z., & Khan, M. A. (2007). Review and Analysis of Current Solid Waste Management Situation. In *Proceedings of the International Conference on Sustainable Solid Waste Management* (pp. 33-41). Chennai: Academic Press. Retrieved from http://citeseerx.ist.psu.edu/viewdoc/download?doi=10.1.1.529.3759&rep=rep1&type=pdf

Mansoor, H. (2018, November 11). *Cabinet approves phase-wise ban on plastic bags across Sindh*. Retrieved from https://www.dawn.com/news/1444812

Masood, M., & Barlow, C. Y. (2013). Framework for integration of informal waste management sector with the formal sector in Pakistan. *Waste Management & Research, 31*(10), 93–105. doi:10.1177/0734242X13499811 PMID:23999020

Masood, M., & Barlow, C. Y. (2014). Informal waste sector in Lahore: Role & Motivation. *Second Pakistan Urban Forum*. Retrieved from https://www.researchgate.net/publication/273950122_Informal_waste_sector_in_Lahore_Role_Motivation

McKay, J. (2017). *A Healthier Planet. Defence Journal, 20(12)*, 41–42. Retrieved from https://search.proquest.com/openview/4905f31a8aacd1a842962bdd2ea2bed3/1?pq-origsite=gscholar&cbl=616545

Medina, M. (2010). *Solid wastes, poverty and the environment in developing country cities: Challenges and opportunities*. Helsinki: The United Nations University World Institute for Development Economics Research. Retrieved from https://www.econstor.eu/bitstream/10419/54107/1/63649439X.pdf

Najam, A., & Bari, F. (2017). *Pakistan National Human Development Report 2017*. Islamabad: United Nations Development Programme. Retrieved from http://www.pk.undp.org/content/dam/pakistan/docs/HDR/PK-NHDR.pdf

National Assembly of Pakistan. (2012, February 28). *The Constitution of the Islamic Republic of Pakistan*. Retrieved from National Assembly of Pakistan: http://na.gov.pk/uploads/documents/1333523681_951.pdf

Ni, H.-G., Lu, S.-Y., Mo, T., & Zeng, H. (2016). Brominated flame retardant emissions from the open burning of five plastic wastes and implications for environmental exposure in China. *Environmental Pollution, 214*, 70–76. doi:10.1016/j.envpol.2016.03.049 PMID:27064612

Ogunola, O. S., Onada, O. A., & Falaye, A. E. (2018). Mitigation measures to avert the impacts of plastics and microplasticsin the marine environment (a review). *Environmental Science and Pollution Research International, 25*(12). doi:10.100711356-018-1499-z PMID:29470754

Pakistan Bureau of Statistics. (2015). *Compendium on Environment Statistics 2015*. Islamabad: Bueau of Statistics, Government of Pakistan. Retrieved from http://www.pbs.gov.pk/sites/default/files//crops_and_climates/compendium_environment/compendium_environment_2015.pdf

Pakistan Bureau of Statistics. (2017). *Provisional Summary Results of 6th Population and Housing Census-2017*. Retrieved from Pakistan Bureau of Statistics, Government of Pakistan: http://www.pbs.gov.pk/content/provisional-summary-results-6th-population-and-housing-census-2017-0

Partners, C. (2010). *Plastic Products*. Islamabad: State Bank of Pakistan; Retrieved from http://www.sbp.org.pk/departments/ihfd/Sub-Segment%20Booklets/Plastic%20Products.pdf

Proshad, R., Kormoker, T., Islam, M. S., Haque, M. A., Rahman, M. M., & Mithu, M. M. (2018). Toxic effects of plastic on human health and environment: A consequences of health risk assessment in Bangladesh. *International Journal of Health, 6*(1), 1–5. doi:10.14419/ijh.v6i1.8655

Qari, R., & Shaffat, M. (2015). Distribution and Abundance of Marine Debris Along the Coast of Karachi (Arabian Sea), Pakistan. *Pakistan Journal of Scientific and Industrial Research, Series B: Biological Sciences, 58*(2), 98-103. Retrieved from https://www.researchgate.net/profile/Rashida_Qari2/publication/314261050_Distribution_and_Abundance_of_Marine_Debris_Along_the_Coast_of_Karachi_Arabian_Sea_Pakistan/links/58be93c6aca272b9b1805b77/Distribution-and-Abundance-of-Marine-Debris-Along-the-Coast

Ragaert, K., Delva, L., & Van Geem, K. (2017). Mechanical and chemical recycling of solid plastic waste. *Waste Management (New York, N.Y.), 69*, 24–58. doi:10.1016/j.wasman.2017.07.044 PMID:28823699

Raynaud, J. (2014). *Valuing Plastics: The Business Case for Measuring, Managing and Disclosing Plastic Use in the Consumer Goods Industry.* UNEP. Retrieved from http://wedocs.unep.org/bitstream/handle/20.500.11822/9238/-Valuing%20plastic%3a%20the%20business%20case%20for%20measuring%2c%20managing%20and%20disclosing%20plastic%20use%20in%20the%20consumer%20goods%20industry-2014Valuing%20plasticsF.pdf?sequence=8&isAl

Reese, A. (2012, September 26). *Eating hot food in plastic containers can lead to serious health problems - Doctor.* Retrieved from https://www.modernghana.com/lifestyle/3733/eating-hot-food-in-plastic-containers-can-lead-to-serious-he.html

Rezg, R., El-Fazaa, S., Gharbi, N., & Mornagui, B. (2014). Bisphenol A and human chronic diseases: Current evidences, possible mechanisms, and future perspectives. *Environment International, 64*, 83–90. doi:10.1016/j.envint.2013.12.007 PMID:24382480

Richiardi, L., Bellocco, R., Adami, H.-O., Torrang, A., Barlow, L., Hakulinen, T., . . . Akre, O. (2004). Testicular Cancer Incidence in Eight Northern European Countries: Secular and Recent Trends. *Cancer Epidemiology, Biomarkers & Prevention, 13*(12), 2157-2166. Retrieved from http://cebp.aacrjournals.org/content/13/12/2157.full-text.pdf

Sadef, Y., Nizami, A. S., Batool, S. A., Chaudary, M. N., Ouda, O. K., Asam, Z. Z., ... Demirbas, A. (2016). Waste-to-energy and recycling value for developing integrated solid waste management plan in Lahore. *Energy Sources. Part B, Economics, Planning, and Policy, 11*(7), 569–579. doi:10.1080/15567249.2015.1052595

Sarigiannis, D. A. (2017). Assessing the impact of hazardous waste on children's health: The exposome paradigm. *Environmental Research, 158*, 531–541. doi:10.1016/j.envres.2017.06.031 PMID:28711809

Schmidt, C., Krauth, T., & Wagner, S. (2017). Export of Plastic Debris by Rivers into the Sea. *Environmental Science & Technology, 51*(21), 12246–12253. doi:10.1021/acs.est.7b02368 PMID:29019247

Schnurr, R. E., Alboiu, V., Chaudhary, M., Corbett, R. A., Quanz, M. E., Sankar, K., ... Walker, T. R. (2018). Reducing marine pollution from single-use plastics (SUPs): A review. *Marine Pollution Bulletin, 137*, 157–171. doi:10.1016/j.marpolbul.2018.10.001 PMID:30503422

Seachrist, D. D., Bonk, K. W., Ho, S.-M., Prins, G. S., Soto, A. M., & Keri, R. A. (2016). A review of the carcinogenic potential of bisphenol A. *Reproductive Toxicology (Elmsford, N.Y.), 59*, 167–182. doi:10.1016/j.reprotox.2015.09.006 PMID:26493093

Seltenrich, N. (2015). New Link in the Food Chain? Marine Plastic Pollution and Seafood Safety. *Environmental Health Perspectives, 123*(2), A34-A41.

Senate of Pakistan. (1997). *Act,1997.* Retrieved from ELAW: https://www.elaw.org/system/files/Law-PEPA-1997.pdf

Shaikh, H., Memon, N., Bhanger, M. I., & Nizamani, S. M. (2014). GC/MS Based Non-target Screening of Organic Contaminants in River Indus and its Tributaries in Sindh (Pakistan). *Pakistan Journal of Analytical & Environmental Chemistry, 15*(1), 24. Retrieved from http://pjaec.pk/index.php/pjaec/article/view/210

Siddiqi, M. A., Laessig, R. H., & Reed, K. D. (2003). Polybrominated Diphenyl Ethers (PBDEs): New Pollutants-Old Diseases. *Clinical Medicine & Research, 1*(4), 281–290. doi:10.3121/cmr.1.4.281 PMID:15931321

Singh, P., & Sharma, V. P. (2016). Integrated Plastic Waste Management: Environmental and Improved Health Approaches. *Procedia Environmental Sciences, 35*, 692–700. doi:10.1016/j.proenv.2016.07.068

Stahel, W. R. (2016, March 23). The circular economy. *Nature International Weekly Journal of Science, 531*, 435–438. doi:10.1038/531435a PMID:27008952

Supreme Court of Pakistan. (1994). *Zia v. WAPDA, PLD 1994 Supreme Court 693*. Islamabad: Supreme Court of Pakistan. Retrieved from https://www.elaw.org/pk.shehla.zia.1994

Taskeen, A. (2012). *Qualitative and Quantitative Analysis of Bisphenol-A in Foods and Beverages Stored in Plastic Containers and Wraps in Pakistan*. Lahore: Department of Chemistry, Lahore College for Women University. Retrieved from http://prr.hec.gov.pk/jspui/bitstream/123456789/504/1/1734S.pdf

Taskeen, A., & Naeem, I. (2009). Bisphenol A Toxicity in Milk: A Review. *Nature and Science, 7*(8), 83-85. Retrieved from http://www.sciencepub.net/nature/0708/10_0981_Bisphenol_ns0708.pdf

ten Brink, P., Schweitzer, J.-P., Watkins, E., Janssens, C., De Smet, M., Leslie, H., & Galgani, F. (2018). Circular economy measures to keep plastics and their value in the economy, avoid waste and reduce marine litter. *Economics*. Retrieved from https://archimer.ifremer.fr/doc/00419/53002/53950.pdf

The News International. (2016, August 21). *Packaging industry enjoys 15 percent annual growth*. Retrieved from https://www.thenews.com.pk/print/143977-Packaging-industry-enjoys-15-percent-annual-growth

The World Bank. (2018a). *Solid Waste Management*. Washington DC: The World Bank. Retrieved from http://www.worldbank.org/en/topic/urbandevelopment/brief/solid-waste-management

The World Bank. (2018b). *Urban population (% of total)*. Retrieved from The World Bank Group: https://data.worldbank.org/indicator/SP.URB.TOTL.IN.ZS

Tibbetts, J. H. (2015). Managing Marine Plastic Pollution: Policy Initiatives to Address Wayward Waste. *Environmental Health Perspectives, 123*(4), A90-A93.

Umer, M., & Abid, M. (2017). Economic Practices in Plastic Industry from Raw Material to Waste in Pakistan: A Case Study. *Asian Journal of Water, Environment and Pollution, 14*(2), 81-90. Retrieved from https://content.iospress.com/articles/asian-journal-of-water-environment-and-pollution/ajw170018

United States Census Bureau. (2018, December 28). *Current Population*. Retrieved from https://www.census.gov/popclock/print.php?component=counter

Vandenberg, L. N., Hauser, R., Marcus, M., Olea, N., & Welshons, W. V. (2007). Human exposure to bisphenol A (BPA). *Reproductive Toxicology (Elmsford, N.Y.)*, *24*(2), 139–177. doi:10.1016/j.reprotox.2007.07.010 PMID:17825522

Velis, C. (2017). Waste pickers in Global South: Informal recycling sector in a circular economy era. *Waste Management & Research, 35*(4), 329-331.

Vergara, S. E., & Tchobanoglous, G. (2012). Municipal Solid Waste and the Environment: A Global Perspective. *Annual Review of Environment and Resources*, *37*(1), 277–309. doi:10.1146/annurev-environ-050511-122532

Verma, R., Vinoda, K. S., Papireddy, M., & Gowda, A. N. (2016). Toxic Polluntants from Plasti Waste - A Review. *Procedia Environmental Sciences*, *35*, 701–708. doi:10.1016/j.proenv.2016.07.069

Wiedinmyer, C., Yokelson, R. J., & Gullett, B. K. (2014). Global Emissions of Trace Gases, Particulate Matter, and Hazardous Air Pollutants from Open Burning of Domestic Waste. *Environmental Science & Technology*, *48*(16), 9523–9530. doi:10.1021/es502250z PMID:25019173

Wilson, D. C., Araba, A. O., Chinwah, K., & Cheeseman, C. R. (2009). Building recycling rates through the informal sector. *Waste Management (New York, N.Y.)*, *29*(2), 629–635. doi:10.1016/j.wasman.2008.06.016 PMID:18701272

Wilson, D. C., Costas, V., & Cheeseman, C. (2006). Role of informal sector recycling in waste management in developing countries. *Habitat International*, *30*(4), 797–808. doi:10.1016/j.habitatint.2005.09.005

Zalasiewicz, J., Waters, C. N., Ivar do Sul, J. A., Corcoran, P. L., Barnosky, A. D., Cearreta, A., ... Yonan, Y. (2016). The geological cycle of plastics and their use as a stratigraphic indicator of the Anthropocene. *Anthropocene*, *13*, 4–17. doi:10.1016/j.ancene.2016.01.002

Zeeshan, M. F., Al Ibad, A., Aziz, A., Subhani, A., Shah, A., & Khan, T. (2018). Practice and enforcement of national Hospital Waste Management 2005 rules in Pakistan. *Eastern Mediterranean Health Journal, 24*(5), 443+. doi:10.26719/2018.24.5.443

Zuberi, M. J., & Ali, S. F. (2015). Greenhouse effect reduction by recovering energy from waste landfills in Pakistan. *Renewable & Sustainable Energy Reviews*, *44*, 117–131. doi:10.1016/j.rser.2014.12.028

ADDITIONAL READING

Barnes, S. J. (2019). Understanding Plastics Pollution: The Role of Economic Development and Technological Research. *Environmental Pollution*, *249*, 812–821. doi:10.1016/j.envpol.2019.03.108 PMID:30953943

Bonefeld-Jorgensen, E. C., Long, M., Hofmeister, M. V., & Vinggaard, A. M. (2007). Endocrine-disrupting potential of bisphenol A, bisphenol A dimethacrylate, 4-n-nonylphenol, and 4-n-octylphenol in vitro: New data and a brief review. *Environmental Health Perspectives*, *115*(Suppl. 1), 69–76. doi:10.1289/ehp.9368 PMID:18174953

Chae, Y., & Youn-Joo, A. (2018). Current Research Trends on Plastic Pollution and Ecological Impacts on the Soil Ecosystem: A Review. *Environmental Pollution*, *240*, 387–395. doi:10.1016/j.envpol.2018.05.008 PMID:29753246

Duty, S. M., Singh, N. P., Silva, M. J., Barr, D. B., Brock, J. W., Ryan, L., ... Hauser, R. (2003). The relationship between environmental exposures to phthalates and DNA damage in human sperm using the neutral comet assay. *Environmental Health Perspectives*, *111*(9), 1164–1169. doi:10.1289/ehp.5756 PMID:12842768

Halden, R. U. (2010). Plastics and health risks. *Annual Review of Public Health*, *31*(1), 179–194. doi:10.1146/annurev.publhealth.012809.103714 PMID:20070188

Hassan, S. (2019). Plastics: A brief review of its disasters and degradation techniques. *Science Proceedings Series*, *1*(2), 100–102. doi:10.31580ps.v1i2.698

Liboiron, M. (2016). Redefining pollution and action: The matter of plastics. *Journal of Material Culture*, *21*(1), 87–110. doi:10.1177/1359183515622966

North, E. J., & Halden, R. U. (2013). Plastics and environmental health: The road ahead. *Reviews on Environmental Health*, *28*(1), 1–8. doi:10.1515/reveh-2012-0030 PMID:23337043

Tibbetts, J. H. (2015). Managing Marine Plastic Pollution: Policy Initiatives to Address Wayward Waste. *Environmental Health Perspectives*, *123*(4). doi:10.1289/ehp.123-A90 PMID:25830293

KEY TERMS AND DEFINITIONS

Anthropocene: The time period in which human influence was dominant on environment.

Bio-Gasification: A process of converting biomass into biogas.

Biodegradability: Conversion of organic substances into simple substances by the microbial enzymes.

Carcinogenic: Cancer-causing agent.

Genotoxic: Toxic èffects on genes.

Hepatic Dysfunctions: disturbances in liver functioning that may lead to life threatening liver failure.

Ingestion: The process of taking in food or any other substance but here it means plastic material.

Microplastic Fibers: Microscopic size of the plastic threads, have a size less than 5mm which have more dangerous potential as compared to large size plastics.

Neurological Effects: Effects on human brain, spinal cord and other nerve cells.

Plastic: A synthetic material prepared by human that can be easily shaped or molded.

Chapter 4
Review Environmental Implications of Incineration of Municipal Solid Waste and Ash Disposal

Sapna
Banasthali Vidyapith, India

Sapna Raghav
Banasthali Vidyapith, India

Dinesh Kumar
https://orcid.org/0000-0001-5488-951X
Central University of Gujarat, India

ABSTRACT

Rapid consumption of resources produces municipal solid wastes (MSW) in developing countries at the present time. MSW comprises the various kinds of waste present at different levels such as household products, industrial waste, biomedical waste, pesticides, sanitation residue, agriculture residue, building material waste, and so forth. The presence of solid waste in the water system is very hazardous and can cause severe health diseases in the human body such as dermatological disorder, respiratory infections, eye and blood infections, cholera, typhoid, tuberculosis, amoebic dysentery, anthrax, and so forth. Due to incineration of waste materials, the remaining ash is dumped into the water system so the amount of free oxygen in the water is diminished, which results in the death of fishes, beneficial bacteria, and worms, which play an important role in the fertility of the soil. This chapter reviews the challenges, methods, technologies, barriers, and opportunities associated with improving waste management worldwide.

DOI: 10.4018/978-1-5225-9452-9.ch004

INTRODUCTION

Currently, the global production of MSW is remarkably high. The production of MSW was about 1.3 billion tons in 2012 only, and it has been predicted that it may be increased up to 2.2 billion tons by 2025 (Hoornweg & Bhada-Tata, 2012). The main constituents of MSW are paper, food, metals, textiles, and glass and the amount of these constituents depends on the practices of different cultures, policies and legislation related to the management of wastes, and on the major economic sectors of various regions (Burnley, 2007; Liu, Liu, &Li, 2006;Wu, Wang, Chai, Takahashi, &Shimaoka, 2016). The basic step of the life cycle of MSW and its management is the incineration with energy recovery which reduces its mass and volume by 70 and 90%, respectively. Hence, the incineration of MSW is the best and cost-effective method for waste treatment, which also saves landfill space area. About 70% of the total mass of MSW is lost in the form of flue gas and only a small amount left as residue in the air pollution control (APC) systems (Brunner & Rechberger, 2015). The significant components of the flue gases are NOx, HCl, CO, furans (polychlorinated dibenzofurans (PCDF)), dioxins –(polychlorinated dibenzo-p-dioxins (PCDD)), and so forth. Waste management especially industrial and municipal is a global problem which is continuously increasing. The European Union (EU)has imposed regulation, and it is allowed only a restricted amount of waste to go to landfill. Due to the strict regulation of the atmospheric emissions, various incinerator plants have been closed in the past few years, and near future, all incinerator plants must obey new standards established in a recent European Commission draft directive. The world has long-lasting alternative solutions to tackle the waste disaster. The primary alternative solutions are the implementation of waste prevention strategies, waste recycling, reuse, and so forth. Despite the said solution, there is another solution which is also in trend like construction or plans to build new incinerators to provide a 'quick fix' solution to the waste calamity. Incinerators are supposed to be more favorable because it is expected that they can reduce the waste up to one-tenth of the original volume, and as a crux, the volume of waste for the landfill sites will also reduce. However, the construction of incinerators is contentious due to their potential impacts on the environment and human health and the economic point of view because they discharge several toxic chemicals into the troposphere and release ashes and other solid waste residues. The Philippine is the only country which has taken a serious step at a government level due to the strong public opposition to incinerators and passed the resolution of "Clean Air Act of 1999". The "Clean Air Act of 1999" of the Philippine has barred the incineration of medical, municipal and hazardous wastes. Waste reduction, reuse, and recycling are being promoted while non-burn technologies are recommended for waste that needs some form of treatment. Some governments of the EU have been promoting the creation of extra incinerators. This report is commenced to draw the attention of the scientific community on incinerator discharges and their effects on human being. The effect appears in those who live near the incinerators and in those who work in this type of installations. These impacts are adverse for the respiratory system, cancer (among both children and adults), heart disease increased allergies, immune system effects, and congenital abnormalities. It has been found that cancer is caused due to older incinerators rather than a modern one. Though, the modern incinerators (operational from the last few years) have also related to the antagonistic effect on health. Despite the reduction of some chemicals in mass discharges, they are still releasing several toxic chemicals and other residues like fly ash and bottom ash into the environment. Mostly, the health implications due to the incinerators are not related to the specific contaminant, and the finding related to a health issue is limited. It is difficult to forecast the health impact of incinerators either new or updated one. These health-related issues show that there is a crucial requirement for the complete shutdown of incineration and the execution of sound waste management policies based on waste prevention, reuse, and recycling.

INCINERATION

Incineration is a process for the degradation of MSW having solid waste, by complete combustion in controlled conditions. It leashes to the recovery of energy and demolition of toxic wastes, likewise hospitals waste. The solid waste incinerates at the temperature range of 980 -2000 °C. The most important feature of the incineration process is the combustible waste reduces its original volume up to 80–90%. In some newly designed incinerators, are maintained at a high temperature to produce a molten material, it can be probable to decrease the original volume up to 5% or even less (Jha, Sondhi & Pansare, 2003; Peavey, Donald, & Gorge, 1985; Jha, Sondhi, & Pansare 2003). Inappropriately, in the Indian cities, as it is not very much experienced. This might be due to the high moisture content, high inert content (30–50%), organic material, and low calorific value content in MSW (Kansal, 2002; Joardar, 2000; Sudhire, Muraleedharan, & Srinivasan 1996; Chakrabarti, 1995). Some incineration plants are as,

1. Timarpur place in New Delhi first large-scale MSW incineration plant was established with a capacity of 300 ton per day, and its manufacturing cost is Rs. 250 million.
2. BARC in Mumbai for burning of paper waste and many more small incinerators plastic have been established for burning of hospital waste.

It is a common misconception that things simply disappear when they are burned. Matter cannot be destroyed - it merely changes its form. This can be exemplified by looking at the fate of some substances in wastes which are burned in MSW incinerators. The incinerators are fed with mixed waste which releases streams of hazardous materials, i.e., chlorinated organic chemicals and heavy metals on burning. These heavy metals present in the incinerator stack emitted in the form of stack gases or adhered with tiny particles and they are also available in the remaining ashes and other residues. The burning of chlorinated wastes, like PVC, produce new chlorinated chemicals, viz. highly toxic dioxins, and it releases in stack gases, ashes, and other residues. Incinerators are not the solution to the problems of toxic constituents of wastes. They make it more complicated by converting these toxic constituents into more toxic. Mostly are persistent, toxic and bio-accumulative. These properties make them possibly the most challenging chemicals for natural systems. Some emitted chemicals are carcinogenic, and few of them are endocrine disruptors. While, others like nitrogen dioxide (NO_2), sulfur dioxide (SO_2) and fine particulate matter, cause an antagonistic effect on the respiratory system. There is a delusion that the weight and volume both reduce during incineration of waste. It is frequently mentioned that the volume of garbage reduces by about 90% during incineration, but the actual figure is close to 45% only. While the weight of waste is supposed to be reduced about one-third on incineration. Though, this refers only to ashes and negates while other incinerator emissions in the form of gases that increased the output in weight. In sum, if the mass of all the outputs including the incinerator to the gaseous outputs are added together, the output surpasses the input(Allsopp, Costner, &Johnston,2010).

The rapid urbanization, industrialization and the current lifestyle of human being have significantly increased the quantity of MSW in recent decades. In New Zealand, the MSW sent to landfills have rubble (16%), organics (28%), treated timber (11%), non-recyclable plastics (8%), non-recyclable cardboards

(7%), glass (2%), rubber tires (2%), hazardous materials (15%) sanitary items (3%), and other solids (10%). More than 2.4 million tons of solid wastes were disposed to municipal landfill sites in New Zealand in 2012 only, and their main sources were commercial, domestic, institutional and industrial waste sources. Globally, the major portion of non-organic solid waste presents in MSW is treated timber, non-recyclable plastics, tires, sanitary items (i.e., nappies), and non-recyclable cardboards. These materials are untreatable before their disposal and on treatment by biological and thermal processes cause an antagonistic environmental effect. The plastic waste stream that covers almost 20% volume in landfill sites, mainly contains polypropylene, polyethylene, and polyethylene terephthalate. Rubber tires which cover larger landfill space degrade in a long time due to their high embodied energy. It provides space for insects and other vermin which spread diseases.

According to recent data that 10% of waste in Auckland is sanitary items in which nappies are the major component, and it may increase in the future. Methane emissions, as well as its leaching to groundwater, may be dangerous for human health. The bulky and non-recyclable cardboards viz. pizza boxes and disposable coffee cups when sent to landfills, it covers larger space, and they produce methane and other greenhouse gases. The effective processing and disposal of the increasing amount of MSW area challenging task. Exhausting natural resources and increasing environmental restrictions encourage the development of appropriate waste management tactics (Chalmin&Gaillochet, 2009). Landfilling is the most common waste management technique in the world. Butits expenses are increasing continuously because it covers a large landfill area because of the large volumes of waste while resource recovery is also very less.

Additionally, landfilled waste releases leachate, toxins, and greenhouse gas emissions. Besides the landfilling technique, other waste management techniques are also being used, i.e. biological and thermal processing techniques. In biological processing technique, aerobic or anaerobic decomposition of organic compounds present in solid waste is done with the help of microbes. It is expensive and time-consuming, and it needs a large area also. Some materials, mainly plastics require pre-treatment before biological degradation (Eckenfelder & O'Connor, 2013).Thermal processing technique needs several additional techniques like gasification, incineration, and pyrolysis, which include high-temperature degradation of materials. However, this technique can also be used for the treatment of several non-hazardous wastes, which emits carcinogenic volatile organics and greenhouse gases (Lu, Namioka, &Yoshikawa, 2011). Moreover, it also needs a pre-treatment step, i.e., drying of waste, which is costly and a highly energy-intensive process.

SPECIFIC TOXICANTS

Heavy Metals

The production of many heavy metals due to consequences of MSW incineration(Carlsson, 1986). Incinerated MSW produces many toxic elements as pollutants. Their high toxicity includes many toxicants like fine ash or suspended particulates. **Tables 1** and **2** show level of elements found in bottom ash, suspended particulates, and fly ash produced during the MSW incineration. The incineration of MSW and its secondary pollutants affected the environment seasonal cycle as well as the economic status of the country.

Table 1. Heavy metal concentration in MSW, bottom ash, fly as hand suspended particulates

Element	Concentration (μg/g unless % indicated)			
	MSW	Bottom ssh	Fly ash	Suspended particulates
Antimony	20		139–760	610–12000
Aluminium (%)	0.54–1.17	2.6 – 14.2	9.0 – 14.2	0.58 – 4.8
Arsenic			9.4 –74	81 – 510
Barium	47– 47	80 – 9000	1600– 3600	40 – 1700
Beryllium	< 2			
Bismuth	< 15–30			
Carbon (%)		1.0–28.7	1.7–7.4	1.8 – 2.2
Calcium (%)	0.59–1.65	3.6–11.2	3.3–8.6	0.66 – 5.3
Cadmium	4.22	3.8–442	< 1–477	520 –2100
Chlorine (%)		0.2–1.0	0.12–1.12	9.29
Cobalt	< 3–5		25–54	3.8–28
Chromium	22–96		730 - 1900	122–1800
Cupper	79–877	630–4281	69 - 2000	122–1800
Fluorine	140–200	130–250	1500 - 3100	990–6800
Iron (%)	0.10–0.35	2.1–32	2.4 – 8.7	0.17–1.8
Mercury	1–4.4	0.03–3.5	0.09 – 25	20–2000
Magnesium	0.09–0.21	0.04–0.86	0.5–2.1	0.31–2.8
Manganese	0.005–0.02	0.08–39	0.20–0.85	0.03–0.57
Nitrogen		0–0.35		
Potassium	0.09–0.19	0.42–2.41		
Sodium	0.18–0.74	2.3–14.2	1.12–1.94	5.1–9.8
Silver	< 3–7		52–220	84–2000
Nickel	9–90	110–210	38.6–960	65–440
Phosphorus (%)		0.04–0.83		
Sulfur (%)		0.27–1.0	1.9–3.6	0.001–0.01
Strontium	11–35		110–220	
Selenium			1.4–13	7.0–122
Silicon (%)		4.7–9.4		
Tin (%)	<0.002–0.004	0.01 – 0.1	0.12 – 0.26	0.4–1.51
Titanium (%)	0.14–0.31	0.04 – 0.90	2.5 – 4.2	0.13–1.29
Thallium				150
Vanadium			110 – 166	6–60
Zinc (%)	0.02–0.25	0.35–3.61	0.08–2.6	4.7–24

The elements like aluminum, titanium, iron, copper, zinc, and lead are found in the slag of MSW incineration in large amount, while cadmium, lead, antimony, selenium, and tin are found in the vapor-

Table 2. The composition of bottom ash from a municipal incinerator

Component	% dry wt.
Iron: cans, wire, miscellaneous	28.2
Metals (non-ferrous)	1.4
Stones, bricks	1.0
Ceramics	0.9
Carbon (as charcoal, carbonized paper)	8.3
Partially burned organics	0.7
Ash	15.4
Glass	44.1

ized combustion products or combustion zone due to their volatile nature, these combustion products are condensed in fine particles in the atmosphere as suspended particulates(Greenberg, Zoller, & Gordon, 1978; Brunner, & Ernst, 1986).As these particles are very small, hence have a large surface area, so they are more reactive and toxic(Wadge & Hutton, 1986). Aluminum, calcium, and titanium are found in the clay particles, dust, and dirt. Iron, lead, zinc, magnesium, molybdenum, chromium, copper, and barium are significantly found in magazine paper (Campbell, 1976). PVC polymer is responsible for chlorine production in MSW. Its incineration releases hydrochloric acid which enhances the corrosion of incinerator components. The chlorides of arsenic, cadmium, nickel, lead, antimony, and zinc are volatile, which increase the concentration of suspended particulates and fly ash. The chlorides of aluminum and iron are also volatile, but they do not find in fly ash. The aluminosilicates of these elements lead to the melting of material instead of vaporization. The evaporation of few elements may be higher if they are disseminated inflammable material like additives to plastics, consequently evaporated at least for a short time as the material burns the emission of toxic elements and magnitude of vaporization affected by several factors. The garbage having higher the calorific value and higher vaporization will emit like copper, zinc, lead, and cadmium.

Mercury is one of the most toxic and volatile elements of MSW. About80% of the MSW contains mercury in the gas phase. The oxidized form of mercury halides is present in MSW. The major source of mercury content in MSW is mercury batteries. Other than mercury silver, cadmium, lithium, manganese, nickel, lead, and zinc are also present in these batteries(Takizawa, Sasaki, Muto, & Karino, 1984). Incineration of MSW yields much higher concentrations of cadmium and lead in fly ash and far greater emission of arsenic cadmium, chloride, and lead. The concentration of such elements in MSW, bottom ash, fly ash and suspended particulates are given Table 1.

Plastic Waste

Plastics are being used as the main constituent of various products and in their production processes like textiles, packaging, and construction. The use of plastic products worldwide increases the plastic pollution in the environment from the last few decades. The accumulation of plastic waste in the atmosphere causes severe problems from flora to fauna. About 80% of the marine residues having plastic products which are coming from the environment land-based, i.e. beach waste. As plastic waste reaches to the marines, they are degraded into smaller pieces. Plastics are long chains of polymeric materials that originated from organic or inorganic materials. The polyethylene polymer (PEP) is one of the utmost utilized in human-made or synthetic polymers. PEP is being used in many applications in their different forms, likewise high-density polyethylene (HDPE) with 12.1% production and low-density polyethylene (LDPE) 17.5% production in the European plastic production. In the marine waste, about 79% PE presents HDPE and LDPE have densities, lower than water (1 g/cm^3). Hence, they can be easily transported by wind to the nearby marine or coastal environment. As the plastic waste subjected to UV-radiation, the fragmentation of waste increases due to the rise in surface temperature of the water. The buoyancy of plastic waste enhances ocean driven transport(Ivar do Sul and Costa, 2014).

The plastic waste in the oceans affects the marine species; about hundreds of marine species are broadly affected including the higher trophic level to lower trophic level. In higher trophic level turtles, crabs, fish, and whale while in lower trophic level, zooplankton. These marine animals consume macro and meso plastics, which accumulated in their bodies. This plastic impacts to flora and fauna (Herzke et al., 2016). The plastic particles less than 5 mm are termed microplastic(MPs). The plastic waste in marine fragmented into the MPs waste; thereby plastic waste is concerning issue for marine life(Andrady, 2011).

Potential Toxicological Pathways of Plastic

Plastics materials are contemplated as an inert. The plastic waste harms the animals by long-term oral administration, the small microplastics (MPs) deposition such as PVC granules, affects the embolization of small vessels. The microplastic surface charge, shape, and size affect the toxicity of particles during the in vivo of tissues and cells (Nel, Xia, Madler, Li, 2006).The bio-persistence might lead to a set of biological responses such as oxidative stress, apoptosis, necrosis, inflammation, and genotoxicity; these are the physical effects of it. If these circumstances are continued, a range of consequences can arise such as carcinogenesis, fibrosis, and tissue damage. The Chemical effects begin by the composition of it, such as leaching of free ions or chemical, untreated monomers units, and hydrophobic organic residue contaminants desorption. These are common precedence contaminants with well-known health effects on humans. Cellular uptake of MPs would permit endogenous or adhered pollutants in the cellular entry (Khan, Syberg, Shashoua, Bury, 2015).

The inhalation acquaintance studies have earlier confirmed that inflammation and oxidative stress presents the best example for the particle toxicity. The oxidative stress due to challenge with NPs including quartz, titanium oxide NPs, and particulate matter outcomes in intestinal fibrosis and airway inflammation. This type of toxicity mechanism also observed due to MPs and nanoplastics, might be due to its small size and hence the large surface area, which provide higher functional sites(Gewert, Plassmann, MacLeod, 2015).

Gastrointestinal Tract (GIT) and Airway Surface

In the GIT, the normal cellular effect of MPs will increase possibly due to adjuvant activity, which is the enrichment of present immune response to surface-adsorbed biomolecules (Powell, Faria, Thomas-McKay, Pele, 2010). When macrophages were presented with antigens and toxins conjugated to their soluble equivalents. Additionally, titanium oxide NPs have been exposed to increase the inflammatory response of marginal cells to the endotoxin lipopolysaccharide. This can also improve by incorporating bridging between the biomolecule and adsorption of luminal protein by enrichment of cell culture medium with Ca, it acts as cation and provides bridging potential (Ashwood, Thompson, Powell, 2007).

Hydrophobicity, charge, (Evans, Ashwood, Warley, Berisha, Thompson, Powell, 2002) shape, and surface morphology (surface pits and cracks) of the particle will influence the extent of this. The corona impacts not only on particle uptake but its toxicity also (Lundqvist, Stigler, Elia, Lynch, Cedervall, Dawson, 2008).

Nevertheless, the expansion of coronas on environmental MPs is largely unaware by researchers. The zeta potential of PS NPs (193.8–344.5 nm) was accompanying with parameters indicative of acute pulmonary inflammation. (Lundqvist, Stigler, Elia, Lynch, Cedervall, Dawson, 2016) Cationic PS NPs (NH_2attachment) displayed more toxicity lung epithelial cells and macrophages (Xia, Kovochich, Liong, Zink, Nel, 2008). The surface charge of MPs has been allied with the destruction of the cellular membrane and destabilization of membrane potential.

METHODS TO REDUCE THE MSW

The treatment and disposal methods for MSW are shown in Fig. 1, and two first innovative ways to waste disposal being accepted worldwide are composting and waste-to-energy (WTE).

To discard MSW, many WTE projects have been sanctioned test and examine MSW, and they are showing positive results especially in developed countries (Lal, 1996; Khan, 1994). Various methods have been used to dispose of MSW; some of them are discussed below.

Landfill

In metropolitan cities, unrestrained, open, and weakly managed discarding of MSW is normally experienced, which is responsible for degrading the environment. About 90% of MSW is directly disposed to the open area in towns and cities. This dumping in the open environment increases the heavy metal contamination in the air.

Figure 1. Flow chart of degradation steps of MSW

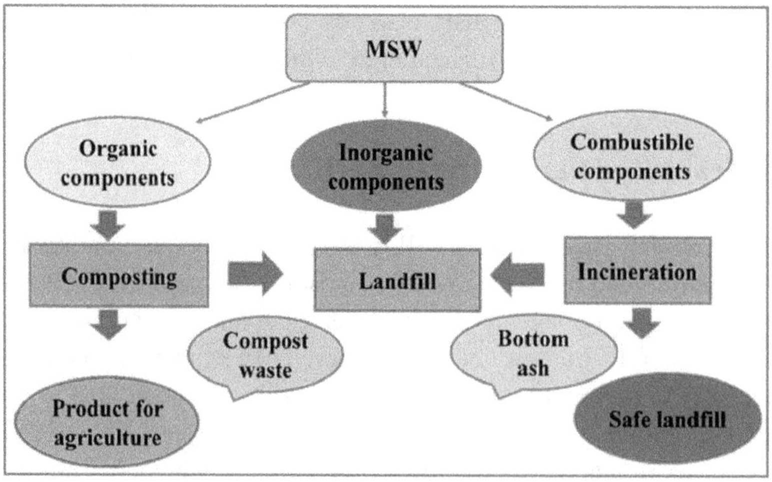

Vermicomposting

Vermicomposting includes maintenance of organic waste through the combined action of aerobic microorganisms and earthworms. Primarily, microbial disintegration of biodegradable waste ensues through extracellular enzymatic activity; then the enzymatically degraded waste feed up by earthworms. It consumes the degraded waste up to five times their body weight per day. The ingested food of earthworm is further disintegrated into the gut, subsequently in the reduction of the particle. The worm cast is a granular, odorless, and fine product; this reduced product used as a biofertilizer. Mumbai, Hyderabad, Faridabad, and Bangalore have been utilized this technique (Sannigrahi & Chakrabortty, 2002; Bezboruah & Bhargava, 2003)In gasification technology; the solid MSW decomposed in the absence of oxygen environment. It has usually been used to produce fuel gas, which would be stored and utilized. Some gasifiers have been utilized for burning of biomass such as sawmill dust waste, forest waste, and agriculture-residues (Dogru, Beltran, Mitra, Erdem, Park, and E.S., 2019).They have also been utilized for the treatment of MSW after drying. In India, two different gasifiers have been designed.

1. NERIFIER gasification unit at Nohar, Hanungarh, Rajasthan by Narvreet Energy Research and Information (NERI) for the ablaze of sawmill dust, agriculture, and forest wastes.
2. TERI gasification unit installed at Gaul Pahari campus, New Delhi by Tata Energy Research Institute (TERI)(CPCB, 2004).

About 25% of the fuel gas has been produced by using this technique, which is further utilized for the system support of the process. About 50–150 kg of MSW per hour treated in the plant and its efficiency is approximately 70–80%.

Anaerobic Digestion

The MSW of organic waste is obscured into the bottomless pits in moderately anaerobic circumstances, the anaerobic microorganisms degrade the waste and release of CO_2 and CH_4, and the left residue is good manure. Its digestion is very slow than aerobic composting. Aerobic digestion occurs naturally in landfills. Nevertheless, thermophilic digestion is an ultrafast method for waste degradation and biomethanation, so it has been commercialized. Anaerobic digestion leads to energy recovery through biogas generation. The biogas produces from the anaerobic digestion, and it has been used as fuels. It is evaluated that by organized anaerobic digestion methods, one tone of waste produces 2–4 times much methane in three weeks as compared landfills in 6–7 years (Ahsan, 1999). The Indian government is trying to utilize industrial, municipal, and agriculture waste for producing biomethanation. There are various schemes for biomethanation of the yard, MSW, and vegetable market wastes for some cities (Bhide & Shekdar, 1998). It has been estimated that in all circumstances where space is vacant, composting is the healthier and good option, because it avoids the load on municipalities for transport and collection of MSW and then decreases the burden on the landfills.

Pyrolysis

This method has been using across the globe due to its high efficiency and good eco-friendly performance. It is utilized for the conversion of biomass via thermal technology (Agarwal, 2014). It offers the prospect for the conversion of municipal solid wastes comprises scrap tires, non-recyclable plastics, agricultural residues, etc. into clean energy. It provides a significant way of conversion of urban wastes into usable products which further can be effectively utilized to produce heat, electricity, and chemicals. Generally, in municipal waste pyrolysis process, the carbon-rich organic material is heated in a non-reactive atmosphere. Pyrolysis is a kind of thermal degradation of organic materials in the absence of oxygen. In the waste streams, thermal decomposition of organic components begins from 350 to 550°C and reaches up to 700-800°C in the absence of oxygen. Pyrolysis of municipal wastes initiates with separation of glass, mechanical preparation, and inert materials and metals before processing the remaining waste in a pyrolysis reactor (Perrot & Subiantoro, (2018). During the pyrolysis usually used reactors are rotary hearth furnaces, rotary kilns, and fluidized bed furnaces. External heat source necessitates maintaining the high temperature in the reactors. This method can be implied at a smaller scale.

Consequently it reduces transport and handling costs and makes the method to be very efficient and cheaper. Its products have high calorific value as a gas like a synthesis gas or syngas and as a biofuel like bio-oil or pyrolysis oil, as solid residue like char. It depends on the final temperature of pyrolysis. When the temperature range below than 450 ^{0}C and slow heating rate than mainly MSW pyrolysis yields solid residues. The gases will be produced at a heating rate, and the temperature range reaches up to 800 ^{0}C and more than that. The range of temperature between 450 and 800^{0}C with relatively high heating rates, the formation of the main product is a liquid fuel commonly identified as bio-oil.

Partial Oxidation

Direct combustion and the incineration of the MSW in the water system as well as on the surface of the ground causing hazardous effects on plant and the animal life. Generally, various polymers present in MSW. Plastic polymers contain a high calorific value. When the MSW direct goes in combustion state without partial oxidation, it releases the very noxious substance to the environment. These noxious substances including toxic gases such as NOx, sulfur oxides, hydrocarbons, and dioxins. Before the combustion, MSW should be undergone to a partial oxidation process to reduce the toxic effect of noxious substances. This is performed by using oxygen and steam. It could be generated the mixture of hydrocarbons and synthesis gas like CO and H_2. The formation of side product quantity and quality is dependent on the type of polymer used. Yamamoto and coworkers introduced a new type of waste gasification and smelting system to the development of steelmaking and iron-making technologies to produce a dioxin-free and high-calorie purified gas. As a result of two-stage pyrolysis and partial oxidation process, 60-70% of the hydrogen production efficiency has been reported from polymer waste. Co-gasification of biomass with polymer waste the production of hydrogen increases while the CO content reduced. The production of bulk chemicals, such as acetic acid, from polyolefins via oxidation using NO and/or O_2, is also possible (Yamamoto, Isaka, Sato, Matsukura, & Ishida 2000.

Hydrothermal Carbonization (HTC)

HTC is the advanced thermal conversion method that sterilizes the MSW. It is mostly used for the inspection of some restricted number of feedstocks like some pure substances along with more complex biomass like wood. It converts the feedstocks into nanostructure form. A few studies are available which have been used the carbonization or HTC method for the treatment of complex waste streams. This method can be optimized as considering the environmental effects because carbonization of complex wastes and chemicals, and physical and thermal properties of the produced hydrochar. Results from batch carbonization experiments indicate 49-75% of the initially present carbon is retained within the char, while 20-37% and 2-11% of the carbon is transferred to the liquid and gas phases, respectively. The dehydration and decarboxylation occur during carbonization the produced hydrochar. Process energetics suggest that feedstock carbonization is exothermic (Fiori, Bassoa, Castelloa,& Baratierib2014).

Mechanical Recycling

In this method, reprocess the used plastic into the manufacturing of new similar kind of product. In primary and secondary recycling of plastic waste, homogeneous waste plastics are converted into products with nearly same or less performance level than the original product. A lot of efforts had taken in the 1970s by polymer technologists to turn waste plastics materials into the usable materials. The practical assessment found the less mechanical as well as minimal durability in the polymer polyblends than the virgin polymers which reprocessed by the mixed contaminated plastics present in the MSW(Scott, 2000). The mechanical recycling of plastic wastes seems to be a greener approach except fora few limitations like less strength and durability. Its re-processing operation is very cost efficient as it required high energy for cleaning, transportation, sorting, and processing in addition to the additives used to provide a serviceable product (Mantia, 2000).

Further recycling of household waste plastics materials is predominantly difficult because household waste consists of a mixture of various types of contaminated plastic and biological residues. Therefore, an urgent need to be introduced the specific technology to sort plastics automatically. Some of the techniques have been used for a similar process such as infrared and near-infrared spectroscopy, X-ray fluorescence, flotation, and electrostatics. Though, the practicability and economic viability of these processes not so recognizable, in industrial application (Panda, Singh, & Mishra (2010).The enterprise vision makes tremendous efforts to elaborate the superior processing equipment which helps in the conversion of mixed plastics wastes of concrete as well as wood substitutes into the preparation of benches, boat docks, fenceposts, etc. While by doing this causing creates lots of serious questions for the polymer technologist whether it is eco-friendly or not at a certain level. Although they have been achieved the success in the limited areas like the formation of plastics-based underground chambers, concrete roads by utilization of mixed plastics wastes, this application is suitable in much more extent there is no long-term deterioration due to exposure to the weather. The main limitation of this procedure is it can't be continued at large scale due to less availability of the mixed plastic polymers including stiff plastic and concrete or less stability of the bare polymer blends (Bonhomme, Cuer, Delort, Lemaire, Sancelme,& Scott(2003). Therefore, in polymer chemistry utilization of the compatibilizers attains considerable attention to enhance the stability of the immiscible blend of a polymer. It is the solid phase dispersant substance which provides stability and upgrades of the mechanical performance of mixed plastics polyblends. Other than this it also increases the yield properties of blend generally not achieved in either single pure component. The overall compatibilization process is an expensive and energy-intensive procedure which cannot be acceptable for domestic mixed plastics wastes. Although mechanical recycling widely employed, it is not apparent suitable method when the quality of secondary production and ecological aspects are considered.

INNOVATIVE METHODS

Drying Methods for MSW

Dryers act as exterior heat as well as internal energy sources utilized in the organic waste decomposition (Velis Longhurst, Drew, Smith, & Pollard 2009). Mostly dryers have been employed concerning wide application environmental engineering purposes, for instance, refuse-derived fuel (RDF) drying, dewatering sludge and MSW drying for fuel and reduced disposal at landfills. The most communal involved drying methods have been utilized crosswise the world to optimize MSW quality like biodrying, stabilization, solar drying, and thermal drying.

Biodrying

Biodrying method has been gaining much attention in many countries in Europe together with Poland, Italy, Germany, Greece, United Kingdom, Spain, Romania (Yuan, Zhang & Li 2017; Sugni, Calcaterra, & Adani 2005; Debicka, Zygadlo, & Latosinska 2013) and in some parts of Asia as well as India, Malaysia, China (Tom, Haridas, & Pawels 2016; Ab Jalil, Basri, Ahmad Basri, & Abushammala 2015). Several studies have explored the drying process, at the various labs, pilot scales, and industrial scale. The researchers have shown intense concern toward the solid wastes like mixed or separated MSW, organic wastes and other wastes comes and agricultural sectors from municipal sectors. It is an eco-friendly method that reproduced heat by natural aerobic bioconversion of some organic matter to dry the waste (Robles-Martinez, Silva-Rodriguez, Espinosa-Solares, Pina-Guzman, Calixto-Mosqueda, Colomer-Mendoza, & Duran-Paramo 2012). The main aim of the drying process is employed internal energy by organic waste decomposition. Generally, microorganisms tangled in the breakdown of organic matters. Some of the bacteria and fungi involved in the degradation including actinomycetes and celluloses degraders. In the total amount of organic degradation, the mixing of inoculating materials at the different times also show various effects on the degradation rate of total organics and the performance of water removal and water content reduction (Zhang, He, Yu, &Shao 2009)(Anilkumar, Sukumaran &Vincent,2015). The temperature range in between 40 to 70°C is enough with a proper aeration system inside the reactor for the good growth of the microorganisms to degrade organic parts of MSW. Other than this it acts greenhouse dryer is also utilized through striking of solar-energy directly on the product present inside the reactor. The greenhouse process provides the mainly two outcome results one is the metabolic heat generation by natural aerobic bioconversion of the organic matter, and Second is solar energy accumulated as heat inside the greenhouse that will increase the air temperature. In the drying method process, in comparison to the outdoor condition inside the greenhouse with temperature, relative humidity also higher.

Biostabilization

This method comprises the increase biological decomposition of organic matter, contributes the diminished MSW in weight and volume ratio, and reduce the environmental contaminations as landfill gas and leachate. The similar metabolism of microbial has been reported to that of biodrying. It is more time consuming than biodrying. Other than the degradation application these materials could be considered as agricultural drives and might be stored safely in a landfill whereas bio-dried materials showed utility as an energy source like fuel (He, Shao, Zhang, & Shao 2009).

Solar Drying

The substitute for the use of traditional drying replaced by utilization of solar dryers. Many agriculture residues are accumulated in an open area, and they degrade in along period. It is used to overcome the limitation of open-air drying. Other than MSW solar drying is used in the drying of plant leaves and other residual waste like plastic. The solar collectors have been utilized for the recycling of waste. They generate a lot of heat from solar energy to melt the plastic to transform the plastic into the 3D printing filament on a small scale (Wrya, Joseph, Carroll, Paul & Embery 2018). The main constituents of organic fertilizer are nitrogen, phosphorus, and potassium, and they generate from the olive mill wastewater by the treatment of the solar drying process. The wastewater from the mill was collected in a chamber where solar energy died the sewer, and inside swine manure also used as the bulking agent. They found that the mean evaporation rate was 5.2 kg $H_2O/m^2/d$ for a drying period of six months. (Galliou, Markakis, Fountoulakis, Nikolaidis, & Manios 2018).

Thermal Drying

Thermal drying treatment is an efficient method for the treatment of sewage sludge, which is filled with the biodegradable as well as nonbiodegradable debris. Nowadays, researchers have been tried to modify the thermal drying of sewage sludge by introducing electromagnetic induction heating. During electromagnetic induction heating (EMI) it has been observed that shrinkage and cracking of sludge rapidly occur, and a huge amount of moisture disappears. At higher working voltage a significant weight reduction of sludge is reported. To prevent the release of volatile organic compounds, a lower working voltage (200–350 V) is recommended during EMI drying process. At working voltage, 200 V sample EMI-P-C1 and EMI-N-D1 shows the difference in the reduction of moisture content at time intervals. 25 g of sludge sample EMI-P-C1 reduced the moisture content from 84 to 19.60% within 18 min, and 300 g of sludge sample EMI-N-D1 reduced the moisture content from 84 to 17% during 30 min (Xue, Wang, Hu, Zhou, Liu, Hou, & Li (2018). Avelar et al. demonstrated the utilization of eucalyptus chips and bark as a bulking agent for the thermal drying of sludge. These bulking agents increase the pores in the biosludge mass. The mixing of 25% eucalyptus raised the moisture evaporation as well as total final solid content (Avelar, Ribeiro, Rezende, Silva, Carneiro, & Martins2018).

Applications of MSW in Agriculture

Direct supply of MSW in water as well agriculture system causing a toxic effect on soil and grown crop. But after the implication of various degrading method, it converts into the usable form and further can be utilized in the field of agriculture. Over the period MSW turns into compost form which is very useful to produce the crop. The MSW compost is the kind of soil conditioner and acts as a fertilizer. The loading of soil with metals can result in increased metal content in crops.

In some cases, metals and excess nutrients can move through the soil profile into groundwater. A large concentration of salt has been reported in the MSW compost which may prevent the plant growth and can destruct the soil structure. Compost quality should be examined before bringing in utilization in the agriculture field. The quality of MSW can be determined based on several parameters including feedstock source, composting facility design, composting procedure, and proportions used, and length of maturation. With all differences in between MSW composts, when it is applied to the different types of field soils, and it shows further variations in the plant growth (Hargreaves, Adl, & Warman 2008).

Ash Disposal

Major portions of ash are generated as a by-product in the process of incineration of MSW. Generally, ash consists of 1–30% by wet weight and 5–15% by volume of the wet MSW, which depends upon the nature of the incineration plant. As a result of incineration two types of ashes are produced; One is bottom ash and second is fly ash. In overall MSW ash around 75–80% bottom ash. The major ratio of around 90% consists of grate or fly ash. The bottom ash appearances to porous, grayish, silty sand with gravel, and comprises some extent of unburnt organic material and chunks. The metal glass, ferrous and nonferrous metals, ceramics, and minerals are the main constituent of the grate ash stream (Siddique 2010).

USAGE OF FLY ASH IN CONCRETE

In the concrete mixture, and is utilized as a fine aggregate, and Rashid & Frantz 1992 stated that the fly ash produces from the MSW as bottom ash and fly ash. Both ashes can be used in the formation of cement. Single sand is not enough to produce concrete. In past fly ash releases into the atmosphere and cause air pollution. But nowadays researchers focus on developing the reactor and technologies which captured this and use for further applications. Generally, fly ash is produced from coal combustion. Another classification of MSW flies ash known as pulverized fuel ash. Role of fly ash in the formation of various products including concrete, cement production, glass and glass–ceramics, road surface, embankment, and soil stabilization.

Agriculture

Fly ash mainly comprises the various major useful content which enhances the fertility of soil like silicon, iron, magnesium, sodium, calcium, and aluminum. It improves the physical property of soil. Due to the presence of major useful constituents, it acts as good fertilizer and promotes plant growth. This is a controversial subject here questions of toxicity raise; therefore, this must be carefully addressed, additionally since plants belong to the first trophic level of the food chain. With the excellent constituent as nutrient the tendency of another toxic ion like copper, zinc, mercury, nickel, lead and so forth. Therefore, possibilities of mobility of the metals in the soil and the causing contamination of surface and ground waters. These nutrients enhance the yield of the crop.

Salinity

The accumulation of salt concentration on to the surface of the soil as the result of the addition of fly ash on to the surface of the soil. Many soluble salts present in the ash and these cause the stress in plants. The tolerance level of salination of each plant is varied from the species to species. Based on the tolerance level, it is classified into further categories which can be moderately sensitive or moderately tolerant. A few reports have declared the with the increasing salinity crop productivity reduced with several plants (Ferreira, 2003). Phytotoxicity has been observed in plants due to the presence of high salinity (Giordano, Behel, Lawrence, Soileau, & Bradford 1983). Some artificial zeolite has been reported in the literature which synthesized from coal fly ash with NaOH by using hydrothermal treatment (Querol, Alastuey, Lopez-Soler, Plana, Andres, Juan, & Ruiz 1997). The thought implies the coal fly ash for the artificial synthesis zeolite is built based on the similar chemical composition of both the materials. They contain a higher amount of aluminosilicate glass and showed a high specific surface. MSW fly ash also contains minerals like Al_2O_3 and SiO_2 and a high specific surface which play the major role in the synthesis of zeolite materials. These kinds of chemical composition seem in less amount in MSW fly ash rather than coal fly ash. Yang and coworkers demonstrated the synthesis of zeolite-like materials obtained from MSW fly ash via hydrothermal alkaline processing, very similar to that reported for coal fly ash (Yang & Yang 1998). They conclude the although zeolites quality is lower than that of commercially available adsorbents such as natural zeolite and activated carbon synthesized zeolite is environmentally safe to use, according to the toxicity characteristic leaching procedure (TLCP) extraction procedure.

FUTURE SCOPE

The review of the literature shows that significant efforts have been made on the degradation of MSW by several useful methods. However, all discussed methods are widely used for MSW with ash disposal. But it possesses some subsequent limitations which should be solved shortly. The should have to mark scale up, economically viable, eco-friendly, and easy in operation.

The pyrolysis technique considered as significant for the cycling of the plastic waste present in the MSW. So, there is a need to design the pyrolysis reactor for a plastic constituent of MSW waste which applicable at small-scaled as middle-scaled production.

It needs to improve the pyrolysis and recycling of waste polyvinyl chloride and optimize operational conditions of pyrolysis for waste plastics to subside the production including PCBs and dioxins and as highly noxious toxin substances.

Among all degradation methods in India composting and landfilling techniques proved to be the best approach is for the dumping of MSW. But incineration is the least favorable method for the dispose of MSW because it generated highly toxic metal and the other hazardous substance in the atmosphere which creates pollution in the environment.

In the anaerobic digestion of MSW, a massive amount of energy produced which can be utilized for domestic purposes.

Microturbine technology should be implied at the site of landfilling of MSW which is capable of generating the electricity.

CONCLUSION

Among all kind of pollutions, incineration of MSW deteriorates every aspect of the life of the environment like a water system, mountains, soil system, plant system, etc. Direct combustion has been done due to lack of awareness and not enough amount of facilities provides for the collection of waste material. Most metropolitan cities have current situation suffering from insufficient waste infrastructure, waste dumping, and unceremonious sector. There is an urgent need for campaigns about how to manage the waste at the individual level and save the environment. Only government policies did not work to clean the environment people have to change their attitude towards waste management. At the community level awareness program should be organized to minimize the waste in domestic works. Until basic needs like proper landfill areas, collection waste, sorting of waste, primary degradation method of requirements are met, India will continue to suffer from environmental pollution.

ACKNOWLEDGMENT

We gratefully acknowledge support from the Ministry of Science and Technology and Department of Science and Technology, Government of India under the scheme of Establishment of Women Technology Park, for providing the necessary financial support to carry out this study vide letter No, F. No SEED/WTP/063/2014.

REFERENCES

Ab Jalil, N., Basri, H., Basri, N. A., & Abushammala, M. F. (2015). The Potential of Biodrying as Pretreatment for municipal solid waste in Malaysia. *Journal of Advanced Review on Scientific Research*, *7*, 5–13.

Ahsan, N. (1999). Solid waste management plan for Indian megacities. *Indian Journal of Environmental Protection*, *19*, 90–95.

Allsopp, M., Costner, P., & Johnston, P. (2001). Incineration and human health. *Environmental Science and Pollution Research International*, *8*(2), 141–145. doi:10.1007/BF02987308 PMID:11400640

Andrady, A. L. (2011). Microplastics in the marine environment. *Marine Pollution Bulletin*, *62*(8), 1596–1605. doi:10.1016/j.marpolbul.2011.05.030 PMID:21742351

Anilkumar, A., Sukamaran, D., & Vincent, S. G. T. (2015). Effect of municipal solid waste leachate on groundwater quality of Thiruvananthapuram District, Kerala, India. *Applied Ecology and Environmental Sciences*, *3*, 151–157.

Ashwood, P., Thompson, R. P., & Powell, J. J. (2007). Fine particles that adsorb lipopolysaccharide via bridging calcium cations may mimic bacterial pathogenicity towards cells. *Experimental Biology and Medicine (Maywood, N.J.)*, *232*, 107–117. PMID:17202591

Avelar, N. V., Ribeiro, B. C., Rezende, A. A. P., Silva, C. M., Carneiro, A. D. C. O., & Martins, M. A. (2018). Thermal drying of industrial sludge using forced aeration. *Environmental Technology*, 1–11. doi:10.1080/09593330.2018.1470679 PMID:29701122

Bezboruah, A. N., & Bhargava, D. S. (2003). Vermicomposting of municipal solid waste from a campus. *Indian Journal of Environmental Protection*, *23*, 1120–1136.

Bhide, A. D., & Shekdar, A. V. (1998). Solid waste management in Indian urban centers. *International Solid Waste Association Times*, *1*, 26–28.

Bonhomme, S., Cuer, A., Delort, A. M., Lemaire, J., Sancelme, M., & Scott, G. (2003). Environmental biodegradation of polyethylene. *Polymer Degradation & Stability*, *81*(3), 441–452. doi:10.1016/S0141-3910(03)00129-0

Brunner, P. H., & Ernst, W. R. (1986). Alternative methods for the analysis of municipal solid waste. *Waste Management & Research*, *4*(1), 147–160. doi:10.1177/0734242X8600400116

Brunner, P. H., & Rechberger, H. (2015). Waste to energy – key element for sustainable waste management. *Waste Management*, 373–12.

Burnley, S. J. (2007). The use of chemical composition data in waste management planning –a case study. *Waste Management (New York, N.Y.)*, *27*(3), 327–336. doi:10.1016/j.wasman.2005.12.020 PMID:16647255

Carlsson, K. (1986). Heavy metals from "energy from waste" plants– comparison of gas cleaning systems. *Waste Management & Research*, *4*(1), 15–20. doi:10.1177/0734242X8600400103

Chakrabarty, P., Srivastava, V. K., & Chakrabarti, S. N. (1995). Solid waste disposal and the environment– a review. *Indian Journal of Environmental Protection*, *15*, 39–43.

Colomer-Mendoza, F. J., Robles-Martinez, F., Herrera-Prats, L., Gallardo-Izquierdo, A., & Bovea, M. D. (2012). Biodrying as a biological process to diminish moisture in gardening and harvest wastes. *Environment, Development and Sustainability*, *14*(6), 1013–1026. doi:10.100710668-012-9369-1

Debicka, M., Zygadlo, M., & Latosinska, J. (2013). Investigations of bio– drying process of municipal solid waste. *Ecological Chemistry and Engineering A*, *20*, 1–28.

Desforges, J. P. W., Galbraith, M., & Ross, P. S. (2015). Ingestion of microplastics by zooplankton in the Northeast Pacific Ocean. *Archives of Environmental Contamination and Toxicology*, *69*(3), 320–330. doi:10.100700244-015-0172-5 PMID:26066061

do Sul, J. A. I., & Costa, M. F. (2014). The present and future of microplastic pollution in the marine environment. *Environmental Pollution*, *185*, 352–364. doi:10.1016/j.envpol.2013.10.036 PMID:24275078

Eckenfelder, W. W., & O'Connor, D. J. (2013). Biological waste treatment. Elsevier.

Evans, S. M., Ashwood, P., Warley, A., Berisha, F., Thompson, R. P. H., & Powell, J. J. (2002). The role of dietary microparticles and calcium in apoptosis and interleukin-1β release of intestinal macrophages. *Gastroenterology*, *123*(5), 1543–1553. doi:10.1053/gast.2002.36554 PMID:12404229

Fiori, L., Bassoa, D., Castelloa, D., & Baratierib, M. (2014). Hydrothermal carbonization of biomass: Design of a batch reactor and preliminary experimental results. *Chemical Engineering Transactions*, *37*, 55–60.

Galliou, F., Markakis, N., Fountoulakis, M. S., Nikolaidis, N., & Manios, T. (2018). Production of organic fertilizer from olive mill wastewater by combining solar greenhouse drying and composting. *Waste Management (New York, N.Y.), 75*, 305–311. doi:10.1016/j.wasman.2018.01.020 PMID:29366800

Gewert, B; Plassmann, M. M., & MacLeod, M. (2015). Pathways for degradation of plastic polymers floating in the marine environment. *Environmental Science Processes Impacts, 17*, 1095-1513.

Giordano, P. M., Behel, A. D., Lawrence, J. E., Soileau, J. M., & Bradford, B. N. (1983). Mobility in soil and plant availability of metals derived from incinerated municipal refuse. *Environmental Science & Technology, 17*(4), 193–198. doi:10.1021/es00110a003 PMID:22304633

Greenberg, R. R., Zoller, W. H., & Gordon, G. E. (1978). Composition and size distributions of particles released in refuse incineration. *Environmental Science & Technology, 12*(5), 566–573. doi:10.1021/es60141a011

Hargreaves, J. C., Adl, M. S., & Warman, P. R. (2008). A review of the use of composted municipal solid waste in agriculture. *Agriculture, Ecosystems & Environment, 123*(1-3), 1–14. doi:10.1016/j.agee.2007.07.004

Herzke, D., Anker-Nilssen, T., Nost, T. H., Gotsch, A., Christensen-Dalsgaard, S., Langset, M., ... Koelmans, A. A. (2016). Negligible impact of ingested microplastics on tissue concentrations of persistent organic pollutants in northern fulmars off coastal Norway. *Environmental Science & Technology, 50*(4), 1924–1933. doi:10.1021/acs.est.5b04663 PMID:26694206

Hoornweg, D., & Bhada-Tata, P. (2012). What a Waste: a Global Review of Solid Waste Management. *Urban Development Series Knowledge Papers*, 151–198.

Jha, M. K., Sondhi, O. A. K., & Pansare, M. (2003). Solid waste management – a case study. *Indian Journal of Environmental Protection, 23*, 1153–1160.

Joardar, S. D. (2000). Urban residential solid waste management in India. *Public Works Management & Policy, 4*(4), 319–330. doi:10.1177/1087724X0044006

Kansal, A. (2002). Solid waste management strategies for India. *Indian Journal of Environmental Protection, 22*, 444–448.

Khan, F. R., Syberg, K., Shashoua, Y., & Bury, N. R. (2015). Influence of polyethylene microplastic beads on the uptake and localization of silver in zebrafish (*Danio rerio*). *Environmental Pollution, 206*, 73–79. doi:10.1016/j.envpol.2015.06.009 PMID:26142753

Khan, R. R. (1994). Environmental management of municipal solid wastes. *Indian Journal of Environmental Protection, 14*, 26–30.

Lal, A. K. (1996). Environmental status of Delhi. *Indian Journal of Environmental Protection, 16*, 1–11.

Liu, Z., Liu, Z., & Li, X. (2006). Status and prospect of the application of municipal solid waste incineration in China. *Applied Thermal Engineering, 26*(11-12), 1193–1197. doi:10.1016/j.applthermaleng.2005.07.036

Lu, L., Namioka, T., & Yoshikawa, K. (2011). Effects of hydrothermal treatment on characteristics and combustion behaviors of municipal solid wastes. *Applied Energy*, *8*(11), 3659–3664. doi:10.1016/j.apenergy.2011.04.022

Lundqvist, M., Stigler, J., Elia, G., Lynch, I., Cedervall, T., & Dawson, K. A. (2008). Nanoparticle size and surface properties determine the protein corona with possible implications for biological impacts. *Proceedings of the National Academy of Sciences of the United States of America*, *105*(38), 14265–14270. doi:10.1073/pnas.0805135105 PMID:18809927

Mahar, R. B., Yue, D., Liu, J., Zhang, Y., & Nie, Y. (2009). Biological pretreatment of municipal solid waste prior to landfilling. *Global NEST Journal*, *11*, 510–517.

Mantia, P. L. (2002). *Handbook of plastics recycling*. Francesco.

Ministry for the Environment. (2006). *Product stewardship case study for end– of– life tyres*. Author.

Ministry for the Environment. (2012). Quantity of solid waste sent to landfill indicator update. *Info*, 654.

Mohammed, M., Ozbay, I., Karademir, A., & Isleyen, M. (2017). Pre– treatment and utilization of food waste as energy source by bio– drying process. *Energy Procedia*, *128*, 100–107. doi:10.1016/j.egypro.2017.09.021

Nel, A. (2006, February 3). Toxic Potential of Materials at the Nanolevel. *Science*, *311*(5761), 622–627. doi:10.1126cience.1114397

Nel, A., Xia, T., Madler, L., Li, N. (2006). *Toxic Potential of Materials at the Nanolevel*. Academic Press.

Panda, A. K., Singh, R. K., & Mishra, D. K. (2010). Thermolysis of waste plastics to liquid fuel: A suitable method for plastic waste management and manufacture of value added products—A world prospective. *Renewable & Sustainable Energy Reviews*, *14*(1), 233–248. doi:10.1016/j.rser.2009.07.005

Peavey, H. S., Donald, R. R., & Gorge, G. (1985). *Environmental Engineering*. Singapore: McGraw–Hill Book Co.

Perrot, J. F., & Subiantoro, A. (2018). Municipal waste management strategy review and waste– to–energy potentials in New Zealand. *Sustainability*, *10*(9), 1–12. doi:10.3390u10093114 PMID:30607262

Powell, J. J., Faria, N., Thomas-McKay, E., & Pele, L. C. (2010). Origin and fate of dietary nanoparticles and microparticles in the gastrointestinal tract. *Journal of Autoimmunity*, *34*(3), 226–233. doi:10.1016/j.jaut.2009.11.006 PMID:20096538

Querol, X., Alastuey, A., López-Soler, A., Plana, F., Andrés, J. M., Juan, R., ... Ruiz, C. R. (1997). A fast method for recycling fly ash: Microwave– assisted zeolite synthesis. *Environmental Science & Technology*, *31*(9), 2527–2533. doi:10.1021/es960937t

Rashid, R. A., & Frantz, G. C. (1992). MSW incinerator ash as aggregate in concrete and masonry. *Journal of Materials in Civil Engineering*, *4*(4), 353–368. doi:10.1061/(ASCE)0899-1561(1992)4:4(353)

Robles-Martínez, F. (2012). Biodrying under greenhouse conditions as pretreatment for horticultural waste. *Journal of Environmental Protection*, *3*(04), 298–303. doi:10.4236/jep.2012.34038

Sannigrahi, A. K., & Chakrabortty, S. (2002). Beneficial management of organic wastes by vermi composting. *Indian Journal of Environmental Protection*, *22*, 405–408.

Scott, G. (2000). 'Green'polymers. *Polymer Degradation & Stability*, *68*(1), 1–7. doi:10.1016/S0141-3910(99)00182-2

Siddique, R. (2010). Utilization of municipal solid waste (MSW) ash in cement and mortar. *Resources, Conservation and Recycling*, *54*(12), 1037–1047. doi:10.1016/j.resconrec.2010.05.002

Sudhire, V., Muraleedharan, V. R., &Srinivasan, G. (1996). Integrated solid waste management in urban India: a critical operational research framework. *Journal of Socio-Economic Planning Science, 30*, 163–181.

Sugni, M., Calcaterra, E., & Adani, F. (2005). Biostabilization–biodrying of municipal solid waste by inverting air– flow. *Bioresource Technology*, *96*(12), 1331–1337. doi:10.1016/j.biortech.2004.11.016 PMID:15792579

Tom, A. P., Haridas, A., & Pawels, R. (2016). Biodrying process efficiency: – significance of reactor matrix height. *Procedia Technology*, *25*, 130–137. doi:10.1016/j.protcy.2016.08.240

Urban, R. M., Jacobs, J. J., Tomlinson, M. J., Gavrilovic, J., Black, J., & Peoc'H, M. (2000, April). Dissemination of wear particles to the liver, spleen, and abdominal lymph nodes of patients with hip or knee replacement. *J. Bone. Joint. Surg.*, *82*(4), 457–457. doi:10.2106/00004623-200004000-00002 PMID:10761937

Velis, C. A., Longhurst, P. J., Drew, G. H., Smith, R., & Pollard, S. J. (2009). Biodrying for mechanical–biological treatment of wastes: A review of process science and engineering. *Bioresource Technology*, *100*(11), 2747–2761. doi:10.1016/j.biortech.2008.12.026 PMID:19216072

Wadge, A., & Hutton, M. (1986). The uptake of cadmium, lead and selenium by barley and cabbage grown on soils amended with refuse incinerator fly ash. *Plant and Soil*, *96*(3), 407–412. doi:10.1007/BF02375144

Wrya, M., Joseph, R. C., & Paul, D. E. (2018). Using Solar Thermal Collectors for Plastic Recycling in Additive Manufacturing. *UKH Journal of Science and Engineering*.

Wu, B., Wang, D., Chai, X., Takahashi, F., & Shimaoka, T. (2016). Characterization of chlorine and heavy metals for the potential recycling of bottom ash from municipal solid waste incinerators as cement additives. *Frontiers of Environmental Science & Engineering*, *10*(4), 1–8. doi:10.100711783-016-0847-9

Xia, T., Kovochich, M., Liong, M., Zink, J. I., & Nel, A. E. (2008). Cationic polystyrene nanosphere toxicity depends on cell-specific endocytic and mitochondrial injury pathways. *ACS Nano*, *2*(1), 85–96. doi:10.1021/nn700256c PMID:19206551

Xue, Y., Wang, C., Hu, Z., Zhou, Y., Liu, G., Hou, H., ... Li, J. (2018). Thermal treatment on sewage sludge by electromagnetic induction heating: Methodology and drying characterization. *Waste Management (New York, N.Y.)*, *78*, 917–928. doi:10.1016/j.wasman.2018.07.009

Yamamoto, T., Isaka, K., Sato, H., Matsukura, Y., & Ishida, H. (2000). Gasification and smelting system using oxygen blowing for municipal waste. *ISIJ International*, *40*(3), 260–265. doi:10.2355/isijinternational.40.260

Yang, G. C., & Yang, T. Y. (1998). Synthesis of zeolites from municipal incinerator fly ash. *Journal of Hazardous Materials*, *62*(1), 75–89. doi:10.1016/S0304-3894(98)00163-0

Zhang, D. Q., He, P. J., Yu, L. Z., & Shao, L. M. (2009). Effect of inoculation time on the bio– drying performance of combined hydrolytic–aerobic process. *Bioresource Technology*, *100*(3), 1087–1093. doi:10.1016/j.biortech.2008.07.059 PMID:18835776

KEY TERMS AND DEFINITIONS

Biomethanation: Here the microbes are involved in the degradation of organic waste under the anaerobic condition and produce the biogas. So, it helps in reduction of consumption of fossil fuel and emission of CO_2 gas.

Carbonization: It the method in which conversion takes place of organic waste like plants and animals into the carbon through destructive distillation.

Incineration: In this method municipal waste degraded by giving higher thermal condition and recover the energy, so this is the waste to energy generating technology .technology.

Landfill: It is the isolated place where the municipal waste buried and seems to be most oldest technique for the waste treatment.

MSW: It is the commonly waste refers to the garbage which found in the society in the form of food waste, cleaning waste, medical waste, etc.

Pyrolysis: It is the method in which decompose the organic waste at elevated temperature in inert gas atmospheric condition.

Chapter 5
Plastic Pollution and the Ecological Impact on the Aquatic Ecosystem

Irfan Rashid Sofi
Jiwaji University, India

Javid Manzoor
Jiwaji University, India

Rayees Ahmad Bhat
Government Adarsh Science College, India

Rafiya Munvar
Jiwaji University, India

ABSTRACT

Plastic pollution in the environment is currently receiving worldwide attention. Improper dumping of disused or abandoned plastic wastes leads to contamination of the environment. Contamination by bulk plastics and plastic debris is currently the one of the most serious problems in aquatic ecosystems. In particular, small-scale plastic debris such as microplastics and nanoplastics has become a leading contributor to the pollution of marine and freshwater ecosystems. Over 300 million tons of plastic is produced annually, and around 75% of all marine litter is plastic. Plastic litter is widespread in aquatic ecosystems and comes from a variety of sources. The abundance of plastics, combined with their small size and subsequent association with plankton in the water column, allows for direct ingestion by aquatic biota at different trophic levels.

INTRODUCTION

Plastics are ubiquitous materials and find applications in all parts of our life and economy. They are lightweight (energy saving) and low cost, and exhibit unique and versatile properties. They find use in agriculture, aviation, railways, telecommunication, building construction, electrical, electronics,

DOI: 10.4018/978-1-5225-9452-9.ch005

medicine and health, automotive, packaging, thermal insulation, household, furniture, toys, and others. The usage of plastic packaging's and products has increased multifold in the last one decade due to its low price and convenience. However, general public is not aware of its impact on the human and environment on littering or dumping. In India, approximately 12 million tonnes plastic products are consumed every year (2012), which is expected to rise further. It is also known that about 50 to 60% of its consumption is converted into waste. Main usage of plastics is in the form of carry bags, packaging films, wrappingmaterials, fluid containers, clothing, toys, household applications, industrial products, engineering applications, building materials, etc. It is true that conventional (petro-based) plastic waste is non-biodegradable and remains on landscape for several years polluting the environment. It is also well established that all types of plastic wastes cannot be recycled and therefore, it gets accumulated in open drains, low-lying areas, river banks, coastal areas, sea beaches, etc. Further, recycling of a virgin plastic product can be done 3 to 4 times only by mixing with virgin plastics granules. Therefore, after every recycling, its tensile strength and quality of plastic product gets deteriorated. Besides, recycled plastic materials are more harmful to the health and environment than the virgin products due to mixing of color, additives, stabilizers, flame retardants, etc.

By 2014 the top three global producers of plastics were China, Europe and North America at 26%, 20% and 19%, respectively.337 Five countries accounted for 63.9% of the total European demand for plastics: Germany (24.9%), Italy (14.3%), France (9.6%), the United Kingdom (7.7%) and Spain (7.4%).337 The plastics in most demand worldwide were polyethylene and polypropylene, and the packaging industry was by far the biggest consumer of these materials. By 2015 the worldwide consumption of plastic materials was almost 300 million tonnes.

The presence of small plastic pieces in the oceans was first noted by scientists in the early1970s (Carpenter et al., 1972). Since that time, many scientists have studied the potential problems associated with what we now term "microplastics." Microplastic debris in aquatic ecosystems is currently considered one of the most important global pollution problems of our time.

The majority of synthetic plastics polluting the aquatic environment include polyethyleneterephthalate (PET), low- and high-density polyethylene (PE), polypropylene (PP), polyvinyl chloride (PVC), and polystyrene (PS). Microplastics are categorized as primary or secondary and then further classified as fragments, pellets, fibers, film, or foam for further study. The term "microplastic" generally refers to plastic particles that are<5 mm, with the term "nanoplastic" being used to describe a plastic particle that is<1 μm in at least one of its dimensions (da Costa et al., 2016).

Primary microplastics are those plastic particles intentionally manufactured in sizes<5 mm for use in personal care products or industrial applications, such as blasting scrubbers. Plastic microbeads have become common components in consumer products such as toothpastes, body washes, and facial cleansers. As such, they frequently flush into municipal wastewater treatment facilities (Fendall and Sewell, 2009). While wastewater treatment processes remove much of this material, a certain portion bypasses the treatment process to be discharged into the aquatic environment (Carr et al., 2016;Talvitie et al., 2015). Mason et al. (2016a) estimate that an average of 13 billion microbeads is released each day into waterways of the United States alone.

Secondary microplastics are the degraded fragments of larger plastic debris that have made their way into the environment. In the environment, plastic items degrade through photo-oxidative pathways (Singh and Sharma, 2008) that make the plastic brittle enough to break into pieces that become increasingly smaller over time. The formation of secondary microplastics from plastic debris depends upon a number of exposure factors including ultraviolet exposure, oxygen concentrations, temperature, mechanical forces, biofouling, and the size and shape of the debris pieces (Andrady, 2011). In a recent study, Weinstein et al.(2016) demonstrated that microplastic production from strips of polyethylene, polypropylene, and polystyrene placed in an open estuary can begin in as little as 8 weeks, producing both fragments and fibers.

It has even been shown that isopod crustaceans (*Sphaeroma quoianum*) can add secondary microplastic fragments to marine waters by boring into polystyrene floats under docks (Davidson, 2012). Other contributors to microplastic pollution are plastic fibers. Plastic fibers come fromthe degradation of larger debris (Weinstein et al., 2016), from the breakdown of geotextile liners (Wiewel and Lamoree, 2016), or from household washing of synthetic textiles (Napper and Thompson, 2016). In the case of synthetic textiles, microplastic fibers are discharged in wash water and then, like microbeads, make their way into municipal wastewater treatment facilities where some fibers are ultimately released at the outfall (Browne et al., 2011). Agricultural application of sewage sludge also serves as an additional source of microplastic fiber pollution through runoff into the watershed (Zubris and Richards, 2005).

PREVALENCE OF MICROPLASTICS IN WATER AND SEDIMENT

There are many published studies that measure the presence of microplastic pollutants in water and sediments around the world and the result of these analyses vary in specific numbers, all agree that microplastics have become a problem of great concern because of the enormous volume of these materials in the world's oceans, lakes, and rivers. The global nature of the predicament is further evident in the fact that microplastics have even been found in the atmospheric fallout (Dris et al., 2016), arctic waters and sea ice (Tekman et al., 2017), the waters of remote lakes (Zhang et al., 2016), and the guts of organisms collected from deep-sea sediments (Taylor et al., 2016). The ubiquitous presence of these materials leads to many questions related to how these particles affect aquatic organisms at individual and population levels.

THE CONCERN OVER MICROPLASTICS IN THE AQUATIC ENVIRONMENT

In aquatic ecosystems, microplastics can be found in the sediments, floating on the surface, and suspended throughout the water column, thus leading to numerous pathways of potential problems for aquatic organisms and populations. The plastics themselves cause direct physical or nutritional problems when ingested, and these problems may be exacerbated by the presence of plasticizers in the particles themselves or by the presence of other toxic pollutants that have adhered to the surface. There are also some indications that microplastics can affect primary producers at the base of aquatic food webs. The abundance of microplastics, combined with their small size and close proximity to plankton in the water column, allows for direct ingestion by aquatic biota at different trophic levels. Microplastic ingestion by marine and estuarine organisms has been noted by many scientists over the years and from locations all over the world. It has been reported by many researchers that microplastic is ingested by a long list of marine organisms, including fish, seabirds, marine mammals, and a host of marine/estuarine invertebrates. While microplastic pollution in freshwater systems has drawn less attention than marine systems, as we know that freshwater organisms are also exposed and that they also ingest microplastic pollutants.

MICROPLASTICS AS PART OF AN AQUATIC ORGANISM'S DIET AND ITS IMPACT ON SOME AQUATIC BIODIVERSITY

While many studies have reported microplastic ingestion by fish (Bellas et al., 2016; and also it has been reported that physical damage happens to the fish (Peda et al., 2016). Tadpoles of Xenopustropicalis were shown to accumulate and eliminate polystyrene microspheres with no negative effects (Hu et al., 2016). Likewise, there have also been a number of investigations on invertebrates where ingestion was observed, but no negative effects were reported. While ingestion did occur, there was no indication of translocation into the tissues and no indication of physical harm. Imhof and Laforsch (2016) found that microplastic exposure caused no morphological changes or developmental effects in mud snails (Potampoyrgusantipodarum) after exposing to irregular shaped microplastic particles in their food. Kaposi et al. (2014) reported that the ingestion of microspheres by the larvae of sea urchins (*Tripneustes gratilla*) caused no measurable dose-dependent effects. On the other hand, there are numerous publications showing physical effects to some lower-trophic-level aquatic species. The initial concerns related to the direct ingestion of nanosized and microplastic particles include physical damage to feeding structures or digestive organs, accumulation within organisms, and translocation of the particles from the digestive tract to other tissues.

SEALS AND SEA OTTERS

It is entirely possible for higher organisms to be exposed to microplastics and contaminants purely as a result of their diet. Indeed, it has been suggested that the exposure of seals to POPs is primarily via ingestion of contaminated food sources, such as fish, and not as a result of their contact with the aquatic environment. For example, in a study which examined the faeces of Antarctic fur seals on Macquarie Island, Australia, it was revealed that microplastics were present in the faeces and 93% of the microplastics were composed of polyethylene. Considering that the main diet of these fur seals was mesopelagic fish, such as lantern fish, it is likely that the fish consumed the microplastics, after which they were then consumed by the seals, as opposed to the seals directly consuming the microplastics.

In a study2010 which analysed samples of blubber taken from various grey seal pups in the Farne Islands, United Kingdom between 1998 and 2000, polybrominateddiphenyl ethers (PBDEs), Polychlorinated biphenyls (PCBs) and organochloride pesticides (DDE and DDT) were found in the blubber. These persistent organic pollutants (POPs) are passed from mother to pup in the womb and via milk following birth. However, upon maturation, dietary habits, such as the ingestion of fish, become the predominant exposure route to these pollutants.

While there are no reports thus far of sea otters ingesting plastics, it is expected that sea otter populations in the North Pacific will suffer increasingly detrimental effects from anthropogenic pollution of the aquatic environment. Populations in California in the United States have exhibited the highest effects from pollutants, suffering infectious diseases and increased morbidity and thus have been deemed as threatened by the United States Endangered Species Act.18

WHALES

There have been several documented incidences of many species of whale ingesting plastic litter, such as the killer whale, the beaked whale and the sperm whale. Furthermore, a dead sperm whale recovered from the Mediterranean Sea was ascertained to have died as a result of a ruptured stomach, which contained 7.6 kg of plastic material. However, microplastics were directly identified for the first time in a cetacean species during a study of True's beaked whale carcasses discovered on the North and West coasts of Ireland. In the carcass examined, the average size of the microplastics was reported to be 2.16 mm while the greatest accumulation of microplastics (38%) was in the whale's main stomach. Furthermore, the main type of plastic recovered overall was rayon, which comprised 53% of the recovered microplastics. This was significantly higher than other types of plastic and the next most abundant, polyester at 16%. However, as the largest filter feeder in the ocean, baleen whales (such as the blue whale) were expected to be exposed to large quantities of microplastics on a daily

FISH

Microplastics are ingested by fish, and the consumption of microplastics by fish can interfere with biological processes, such as the inhibition of gastrointestinal function, as well as causing blockages and inducing feeding impairment.

ENVIRONMENTAL POSITIVES AND NEGATIVES OF PLASTIC

The production of plastics has an associated greenhouse gas footprint, and the "per functional unit" footprint may be less than that of alternatives. However, this is highly dependent on how the impacts of the production are distributed across a product's life cycle. The use of plastics has undeniable benefits for humanity and the utility of these materials is reflected in both the speed at which they were adopted and the vast range of applications in which they are now used. Their positive characteristics include the fact that they are lightweight, easily moldable, as tough or flexible as desired, easy to color, transparent, water resistant, and cheap to produce. The variety of ways in which these characteristics provide benefits are broad; however, the focus here is on environmental implications. Perhaps counter-intuitively, the use of plastic has been linked to improved environmental outcomes in certain applications, due to both their properties and resource efficiency. A joint report by the American Chemical Council and Trucost calculates that there would be greater environmental consequences (up to a 3.8 times increase for consumer goods) if plastic materials were replaced with alternative materials (e.g., wood, glass, metal) (Trucost 2013). This would mainly be due to the large increase in the volume and weight of materials that would be associated with using the alternatives. A good example of this is the replacement of metal with plastic for many vehicle parts, which reduces the weight of the vehicle and thus reduces fuel usage for transport (Andrary 2009).

While the use phase of plastics can lead to environmental benefits, the major environmental burden associated with plastics is in their end-of-life (EOL) phase. This has been neglected in many studies because the burden is difficult to quantify through a conventional life-cycle assessment (Anderson, 2016). One of the major issues is plastic accumulation, which occurs due to the durability of plastics in landfill and the environment (and the large amount of waste which is mismanaged) (Bergmann, 2016). The impacts of accumulation can be separated into two separate issues relating to plastics in landfills and plastics as litter in the ocean. These will require different approaches to alleviate and are explored further in the sections below.

ACCUMULATION IN THE OCEANS

The quantity of plastics in the marine environment is substantial but the exact amount and relative proportions of different plastic types in the ocean remain largely unknown. This is due to a lack of reliable information on the sources, originating sectors, and users (UNEP 2016). However, recently Jambeck and Geyer attempted to model the inputs of plastic waste to the marine environments for 192 coastal countries, considering plastic waste mismanagement and direct litter. Their results for the distribution of plastic waste that is produced and mismanaged, by country. Population size and quality of waste management systems determine which countries contribute the greatest portion of plastics to marine litter, with over 50% of the plastic waste entering the oceans predicted to originate in just five Southeast Asian countries (Jambeck and Geyer 2016).Even their most conservative estimates predicted an input of 100 million tons of plastic waste to the oceans over the 15-year time period 2010-25, or around 1.5%-4.1% of total plastic production entering the ocean per year. This input is predicted to increase by an order of magnitude by 2025 and by 2050 there are reports that the oceans could contain more plastics than fish, by weight. When discussing plastic accumulation in the oceans, there are two main groups of plastics referred to: macroplastics (which are solid articles such as bags, packaging, cigarette lighters, etc.) and microplastics. Microplastics are microscopic fragments of plastic debris and result from either direct release of small plastic particles (plastic pellets andpowders), or the fragmentation of larger items (under conditions of UV, heat, and physical action in the environment (Andrady 2009), or through everyday usage such as clothes washing (Browne 2011, Hartlin 2016). Their presence has been documented from the poles to the equator (Thompson 2015). Whilst Jambeck et al. (2015) considered macroplastics, in regard to microplastics, it is estimated that in the United States alone 100 tons of microplastics directly enter the oceans annually, mainly through wastewater streams. At least similar volumes would be expected from other developed nations.

Although, the measured volume may appear to be small compared to the scale of annual plastic flows. Microplastics have the potential to be a significant issue as they affect animals (such as fish) that are otherwise relatively unaffected by large plastic items and can accumulate up the food chain (Thompson 2015). In regard to the types of products most likely to enter the oceans, typically 40% to 80% of marine waste items are plastic, and these items are often light-weight, single use, and can be linked to the food industry (Barnes 2009).The plastics most commonly associated with litter include the main polymer types as well as cellulose acetate, which, although having low production levels, is used in cigarette filters that probably enter the oceans due to their abundance and small size. This highlights the fact that light-weight, single-use materials need to be the targets when attempting to address ocean litter. The main entry points for these plastics are wastewater discharge points, rivers, and coastal areas. Other sources of marine plastics such as new agricultural products (e.g., polymer encapsulation for slow release fertilizers) have been identified; however, their contribution to the problem is currently unknown.

MARINE DEBRIS AND PLASTIC IN THE ENVIRONMENT

One of the most alarming concerns for the environment is the growing amount of plastic and other trash in the world's oceans and lakes. Trash is sometimes illegally or accidentally dumped directly into the ocean, such as from ships and offshore platforms, but more often is carried by rivers and streams, washed overland by stormwater runoff or via raw sewage overspills, or blown in by wind. Many developing countries cannot afford wide-scale trash pickup and safe landfilling, and instead, they resort to open dumping. Improper handling of waste occurs in all countries, however, and is a global problem. Millions of tons of plastics and other marine debris in the ocean get concentrated in giant gyres that swirl in circular patterns created by winds and the Coriolis effect from the rotation of the earth. One such gyre or giant vortex that accumulates trash is called the Great Pacific Garbage Patch. It stretches from California to Japan in the gyre of the North Pacific Subtropical Convergence Zone. There are presently five major garbage patches that are located in the North Pacific, South Pacific, North Atlantic, South Atlantic, and Indian Oceans.

The marine debris will move in and out of these gyres, but the sea floors accumulate more garbage below the middle of these gyres than elsewhere. Natural materials such as cotton can biodegrade rapidly, but plastics can take possibly hundreds of years to completely break down. Sunlight and physical stressors can break down plastic trash such as water bottles into pieces of plastic. Birds and fish mistakenly ingest the plastic as food. In the most concentrated parts of these gyres, there is more plastic than biomass. Pieces of plastic debris also adsorb other pollutants in the ocean, such as PCBs. Thus, when an organism ingests the plastic, it is also ingesting contaminants that have collected on the plastic. Plastics may themselves contain toxins such as bisphenol A (an endocrine-disrupting chemical), phthalates, or vinyl chloride, depending on the type of plastic. The most persistent and bioaccumulating of chemicals will be transferred throughout the food chain. Humans should be very concerned because it is probable if not likely that all fish contain some measure of these chemicals. When pieces of plastic break down into particles of less than 1 mm in diameter, they are called microplastics. In addition to the microplastics created from the decomposition of trash, microplastics enter the environment from sewage discharges carrying personal care products. Tiny microplastic beads make good facial scrubs and have been used in various cosmetics and toothpastes. But now the growing concern and awareness that marine biota including zooplanktons ingest microplastics has led to a federal ban of microplastics in personal care products in the United States, starting in 2017.

INGESTION OF CONTAMINATED MICROPLASTICS

The ingestion of contaminated microplastics by aquatic organisms provides a viable route for the transfer of toxic chemicals into the tissues of the organism, in which microplastics act as a vector for the transport of sorbed contaminants and chemical additives into organisms. While the investigation of such phenomena and the mechanisms by which this occurs is very much in its infancy, there has been a significant garnering of evidence thus far. Certainly, microplastics can pick up waterborne chemical contaminants during their time spent in polluted waters and can concentrate these contaminants up to 1 million times greater than the surrounding water.

However, the formation of a definitive link between the ingestion of contaminated microplastics and the body condition of pelagic fish is still in its infancy and requires further research. Indeed, it has been suggested that contaminated microplastics may not contribute significantly to the bioaccumulation of contaminants and that the levels of microplastics shown to have adverse effects on organisms in the laboratory are higher than microplastic concentrations measured in subtidal sediments, and similar to the maximum concentrations measured in beach sediments. Furthermore, based on the utilization of model analyses, it has been suggested that the bioaccumulation of persistent organic pollutants (POPs) from the ingestion of contaminated plastics by organisms may be small due to the absence of a gradient between POPs and the fatty tissues of the aquatic organisms, and that some mechanism of removing POPs may take place.

However, many models do not take into account the role of gut surfactants in the desorption of these contaminants, especially at different temperatures and pH. For example, in simulated physiological conditions, the desorption of several common pollutants in the aquatic environment from contaminated polyethylene microplastics (phenanthrene, DEHP, PFOA and DDT) was faster when gut surfactant was present and was further increased at elevated temperatures typically present in warm-blooded aquatic species. Furthermore, the desorption of contaminants from microplastics in the conditions typically found in the gut may be up to 30 times greater than in the conditions typically found in seawater. Consequently, pollutants desorbed from ingested microplastics become freely available to diffuse into the tissues of the organisms. Indeed, the concentration of a chemical pollutants in an organism has been noted to increase, the greater the ability of that pollutant to dissolve in fats, lipids and oils (lipophilicity). Since many POPs are lipophilic, they tend bioaccumulate and readily distribute throughout the food web, ranging from small planktonic species to large air-breathers, such as whales. Ultimately, the vast majority of researchers concede that drastic worldwide action must be taken since many aquatic regions have high levels of pollutants and global concentrations of microplastics in the aquatic environment are increasing.

SOURCES OF NANOPARTICLES IN THE AQUATIC ENVIRONMENT

Nanoplastics in the aquatic system are derived from primary and secondary particles. Primary particles are intentionally manufactured to a fixed size whereas secondary particles arise from fragmentation of larger matter. Industrial operations and human activities contribute to the distribution of secondary particles, that is, plastic litter in freshwater and marine ecosystems. Human-originating sources include solid waste disposal from land and individual vessels at sea and coastal landfill operations (Pruter, 1987). Furthermore, accidental loss or spillage of plastics during transportation and manufacturing practices in the plastics industry also contribute to the accumulation of secondary particles in aquatic environments (Derraik, 2002; Mato et al., 2001). Microplastic and nanoplastic particles used in consumer products from pharmaceutical and cosmetic industries (Lorenz et al., 2011) can reach the environment via wastewater or during consumer use (Sharma and Chatterjee, 2017). Most microplastics are removed in the wastewater treatment plants (Carr et al., 2016); however, not all particles are removed, and the plants may constitute to a considerable source of microplastics (Talvitie et al., 2017). Ecologically induced processes, such as tsunamis and storms, may also partially contribute to the widespread of plastic particles (Zettler et al., 2013). It has been argued that the increase in the amount of primary particles in the aquatic environment is caused by the recent expansion in the manufacturing and use of nanoparticles (Biswas and Wu, 2005) and engineered nanoparticles released into the atmosphere inevitably end up in the aquatic environment or in soil (Nowack and Bucheli, 2007; Ryan et al., 2009;). Nanoplastic particles produced from research and medical applications can also contribute as a source for nanoplastics in the environment. However, a more pronounced amount can arise from cosmetic consumer products that can, for example, enter the aquatic environment through the wastewater or during use. However, how small particles can escape through the wastewater plants is not known since most studies in wastewater plants do not detect particles with a size smaller than20 µm (Carr et al., 2016).

Biodegradable plastics are plastics that can be broken down into water, carbon monoxide, and some biomaterials from microorganisms, such as fungi and bacteria. Some plastics are made from biomaterials or materials made from biological and renewable resources such as grains, corn, potatoes, beet sugar, sugar cane, or vegetable oils, but many biodegradable plastics are made from oil (PlasticsEurope, 2015). Nonetheless, most plastics are thermoplastics which means that they can be remelted into the liquid phase, and this type is generally considered non biodegradable (Plastics Europe, 2015). The degree of biodegradability depends on the properties of the polymer and those of the biological environment. When a product is defined as biodegradable, it is considered to be biodegradable under specific conditions, such as when an industrial composter reaches a temperature of 70°C(UNEP, 2015). However, this is not the case in aquatic environments where the temperature, UV exposure and microbial colonizations are different to the preceding conditions (Moore, 2008).

In 2010, O'Brine and Thompson studied the degradation of four different plastic carrier bags in the marine environment—two oxo-biodegradable polyethylene (PE) bags, one biodegradable bag of polyester, and one standard PE bag produced from 33% of recycled materials. After 4 weeks of exposure, they saw the formation of biofilms on the samples and a decrease in tensile strength. Moreover, after 24 weeks, the compostable polyester was no longer detectable, whereas 98% of the other plastic remained intact even after 40 weeks. Another study, made by Lambert and Wagner (2016), investigated the degradation of 1cm pieces of polystyrene (PS) disposable coffee cup lids and found an increase in the number of nanoparticles over time. In other words, larger plastics were degraded into nano sized particles. The pieces were placed in a weathering chamber for 24h together with 20mL demineralized water at 30°C and exposed to both visible and ultraviolet radiation. According to nanoparticle tracking analysis (NTA), the remaining plastic pieces had decreased in particle size and had unquantifiable weights during the experiment.

REFERENCES

Anderson, J. C., Park, B. J., & Palace, V. P. (2016). Microplastics in aquatic environments: Implications for Canadian ecosystems. *Environmental Pollution*, *218*, 269–280. doi:10.1016/j.envpol.2016.06.074 PMID:27431693

Andrady, A. L. (2011). Microplastics in the marine environment. *Marine Pollution Bulletin*, *62*(8), 1596–1605. doi:10.1016/j.marpolbul.2011.05.030 PMID:21742351

Andrady, A. L. (2015). Persistence of plastic litter in the oceans. In *Marine anthropogenic litter* (pp. 57–72). Cham: Springer. doi:10.1007/978-3-319-16510-3_3

Andrady, A. L., & Neal, M. A. (2009). Applications and societal benefits of plastics. *Philosophical Transactions of the Royal Society of London. Series B, Biological Sciences*, *364*(1526), 1977–1984. doi:10.1098/rstb.2008.0304 PMID:19528050

Barnes, D. K., Galgani, F., Thompson, R. C., & Barlaz, M. (2009). Accumulation and fragmentation of plastic debris in global environments. *Philosophical Transactions of the Royal Society of London. Series B, Biological Sciences*, *364*(1526), 1985–1998. doi:10.1098/rstb.2008.0205 PMID:19528051

Bellas, J., Martínez-Armental, J., Martínez-Cámara, A., Besada, V., & Martínez-Gómez, C. (2016). Ingestion of microplastics by demersal fish from the Spanish Atlantic and Mediterranean coasts. *Marine Pollution Bulletin*, *109*(1), 55–60. doi:10.1016/j.marpolbul.2016.06.026 PMID:27289284

Bergmann, M., Sandhop, N., Schewe, I., & D'Hert, D. (2016). Observations of floating anthropogenic litter in the Barents Sea and Fram Strait, Arctic. *Polar Biology*, *39*(3), 553–560. doi:10.100700300-015-1795-8

Biswas, P., & Wu, C. Y. (2005). Nanoparticles and the environment. *Journal of the Air & Waste Management Association*, *55*(6), 708–746. doi:10.1080/10473289.2005.10464656 PMID:16022411

Browne, M. A., Crump, P., Niven, S. J., Teuten, E., Tonkin, A., Galloway, T., & Thompson, R. (2011). Accumulation of microplastic on shorelines woldwide: Sources and sinks. *Environmental Science & Technology*, *45*(21), 9175–9179. doi:10.1021/es201811s PMID:21894925

Carpenter, E. J., & Smith, K. L. (1972). Plastics on the Sargasso Sea surface. *Science*, *175*(4027), 1240–1241. doi:10.1126cience.175.4027.1240 PMID:5061243

Carr, S. A., Liu, J., & Tesoro, A. G. (2016). Transport and fate of microplastic particles in wastewater treatment plants. *Water Research*, *91*, 174–182. doi:10.1016/j.watres.2016.01.002 PMID:26795302

da Costa, J. P., Santos, P. S., Duarte, A. C., & Rocha-Santos, T. (2016). (Nano) plastics in the environment–sources, fates and effects. *The Science of the Total Environment*, *566*, 15–26. doi:10.1016/j.scitotenv.2016.05.041 PMID:27213666

Davidson, T. M. (2012). Boring crustaceans damage polystyrene floats under docks polluting marine waters with microplastic. *Marine Pollution Bulletin*, *64*(9), 1821–1828. doi:10.1016/j.marpolbul.2012.06.005 PMID:22763283

Derraik, J. G. (2002). The pollution of the marine environment by plastic debris: A review. *Marine Pollution Bulletin*, *44*(9), 842–852. doi:10.1016/S0025-326X(02)00220-5 PMID:12405208

Dris, R., Gasperi, J., Saad, M., Mirande, C., & Tassin, B. (2016). Synthetic fibers in atmospheric fallout: A source of microplastics in the environment? *Marine Pollution Bulletin*, *104*(1-2), 290–293. doi:10.1016/j.marpolbul.2016.01.006 PMID:26787549

Fendall, L. S., & Sewell, M. A. (2009). Contributing to marine pollution by washing your face: Microplastics in facial cleansers. *Marine Pollution Bulletin*, *58*(8), 1225–1228. doi:10.1016/j.marpolbul.2009.04.025 PMID:19481226

Hartline, N. L., Bruce, N. J., Karba, S. N., Ruff, E. O., Sonar, S. U., & Holden, P. A. (2016). Microfiber masses recovered from conventional machine washing of new or aged garments. *Environmental Science & Technology*, *50*(21), 11532–11538. doi:10.1021/acs.est.6b03045 PMID:27689236

Hu, L., Su, L., Xue, Y., Mu, J., Zhu, J., Xu, J., & Shi, H. (2016). Uptake, accumulation and elimination of polystyrene microspheres in tadpoles of Xenopustropicalis. *Chemosphere*, *164*, 611–617. doi:10.1016/j.chemosphere.2016.09.002 PMID:27635643

Imhof, H. K., & Laforsch, C. (2016). Hazardous or not–Are adult and juvenile individuals of Potamopyrgusantipodarum affected by non-buoyant microplastic particles? *Environmental Pollution*, *218*, 383–391. doi:10.1016/j.envpol.2016.07.017 PMID:27431695

Jambeck, J. R., Geyer, R., Wilcox, C., Siegler, T. R., Perryman, M., Andrady, A., ... Law, K. L. (2015). Plastic waste inputs from land into the ocean. *Science*, *347*(6223), 768–771. doi:10.1126cience.1260352 PMID:25678662

Kaposi, K. L., Mos, B., Kelaher, B. P., & Dworjanyn, S. A. (2014). Ingestion of microplastic has limited impact on a marine larva. *Environmental Science & Technology*, *48*(3), 1638–1645. doi:10.1021/es404295e PMID:24341789

Lambert, S., & Wagner, M. (2016). Characterisation of nanoplastics during the degradation of polystyrene. *Chemosphere*, *145*, 265–268. doi:10.1016/j.chemosphere.2015.11.078 PMID:26688263

Lorenz, C., Von Goetz, N., Scheringer, M., Wormuth, M., & Hungerbühler, K. (2011). Potential exposure of German consumers to engineered nanoparticles in cosmetics and personal care products. *Nanotoxicology*, *5*(1), 12–29. doi:10.3109/17435390.2010.484554 PMID:21417685

Mason, S. A., Kammin, L., Eriksen, M., Aleid, G., Wilson, S., Box, C., ... Riley, A. (2016). Pelagic plastic pollution within the surface waters of Lake Michigan, USA. *Journal of Great Lakes Research*, *42*(4), 753–759. doi:10.1016/j.jglr.2016.05.009

Mato, Y., Isobe, T., Takada, H., Kanehiro, H., Ohtake, C., & Kaminuma, T. (2001). Plastic resin pellets as a transport medium for toxic chemicals in the marine environment. *Environmental Science & Technology*, *35*(2), 318–324. doi:10.1021/es0010498 PMID:11347604

Moore, C. J. (2008). Synthetic polymers in the marine environment: A rapidly increasing, long-term threat. *Environmental Research*, *108*(2), 131–139. doi:10.1016/j.envres.2008.07.025 PMID:18949831

Napper, I. E., & Thompson, R. C. (2016). Release of synthetic microplastic plastic fibres from domestic washing machines: Effects of fabric type and washing conditions. *Marine Pollution Bulletin*, *112*(1-2), 39–45. doi:10.1016/j.marpolbul.2016.09.025 PMID:27686821

Nowack, B., & Bucheli, T. D. (2007). Occurrence, behavior and effects of nanoparticles in the environment. *Environmental Pollution*, *150*(1), 5–22. doi:10.1016/j.envpol.2007.06.006 PMID:17658673

O'Brine, T., & Thompson, R. C. (2010). Degradation of plastic carrier bags in the marine environment. *Marine Pollution Bulletin*, *60*(12), 2279–2283. doi:10.1016/j.marpolbul.2010.08.005 PMID:20961585

Pedà, C., Caccamo, L., Fossi, M. C., Gai, F., Andaloro, F., Genovese, L., ... Maricchiolo, G. (2016). Intestinal alterations in European sea bass Dicentrarchuslabrax (Linnaeus, 1758) exposed to microplastics: Preliminary results. *Environmental Pollution*, *212*, 251–256. doi:10.1016/j.envpol.2016.01.083 PMID:26851981

Plastics Europe. (2015). *Plastics—The Facts 2014/2015 an Analysis of European Plastics Production, Demand and Waste Data. In Plastics Europe* (p. 34). Brussels: Association of Plastic Manufactures.

Pruter, A. T. (1987). Sources, quantities and distribution of persistent plastics in the marine environment. *Marine Pollution Bulletin*, *18*(6), 305–310. doi:10.1016/S0025-326X(87)80016-4

Ryan, P. G., Moore, C. J., van Franeker, J. A., & Moloney, C. L. (2009). Monitoring the abundance of plastic debris in the marine environment. *Philosophical Transactions of the Royal Society of London. Series B, Biological Sciences*, *364*(1526), 1999–2012. doi:10.1098/rstb.2008.0207 PMID:19528052

Sharma, S., & Chatterjee, S. (2017). Microplastic pollution, a threat to marine ecosystem and human health: A short review. *Environmental Science and Pollution Research International*, *24*(27), 21530–21547. doi:10.100711356-017-9910-8 PMID:28815367

Singh, B., & Sharma, N. (2008). Mechanistic implications of plastic degradation. *Polymer Degradation & Stability*, *93*(3), 561–584. doi:10.1016/j.polymdegradstab.2007.11.008

Talvitie, J., Heinonen, M., Pääkkönen, J. P., Vahtera, E., Mikola, A., Setälä, O., & Vahala, R. (2015). Do wastewater treatment plants act as a potential point source of microplastics? Preliminary study in the coastal Gulf of Finland, Baltic Sea. *Water Science and Technology*. PMID:26524440

Talvitie, J., Mikola, A., Setälä, O., Heinonen, M., & Koistinen, A. (2017). How well is microlitter purified from wastewater?–A detailed study on the stepwise removal of microlitter in a tertiary level wastewater treatment plant. *Water Research*, *109*, 164–172. doi:10.1016/j.watres.2016.11.046 PMID:27883921

Taylor, M. L., Gwinnett, C., Robinson, L. F., & Woodall, L. C. (2016). Plastic microfibre ingestion by deep-sea organisms. *Scientific Reports*, *6*(1), 33997. doi:10.1038rep33997 PMID:27687574

Tekman, M. B., Krumpen, T., & Bergmann, M. (2017). Marine litter on deep Arctic seafloor continues to increase and spreads to the North at the HAUSGARTEN observatory. *Deep-sea Research. Part I, Oceanographic Research Papers*, *120*, 88–99. doi:10.1016/j.dsr.2016.12.011

Thompson, R. C. (2015). Microplastics in the marine environment: Sources, consequences and solutions. In *Marine anthropogenic litter* (pp. 185–200). Cham: Springer. doi:10.1007/978-3-319-16510-3_7

UNEP. (2015). *Biodegradable Plastics and Marine Litter.Misconceptions, concerns and impacts on marine environments.* UNEP.

Weinstein, J. E., Crocker, B. K., & Gray, A. D. (2016). From macroplastic to microplastic: Degradation of high-density polyethylene, polypropylene, and polystyrene in a salt marsh habitat. *Environmental Toxicology and Chemistry*, *35*(7), 1632–1640. doi:10.1002/etc.3432 PMID:26992845

Wiewel, B. V., & Lamoree, M. (2016). Geotextile composition, application and ecotoxicology—A review. *Journal of Hazardous Materials*, *317*, 640–655. doi:10.1016/j.jhazmat.2016.04.060 PMID:27283344

Woods, L., & Bakshi, B. R. (2014). Reusable vs. disposable cups revisited: Guidance in life cycle comparisons addressing scenario, model, and parameter uncertainties for the US consumer. *The International Journal of Life Cycle Assessment*, *19*(4), 931–940. doi:10.100711367-013-0697-7

Zettler, E. R., Mincer, T. J., & Amaral-Zettler, L. A. (2013). Life in the "plastisphere": Microbial communities on plastic marine debris. *Environmental Science & Technology*, *47*(13), 7137–7146. doi:10.1021/es401288x PMID:23745679

Zhang, K., Su, J., Xiong, X., Wu, X., Wu, C., & Liu, J. (2016). Microplastic pollution of lakeshore sediments from remote lakes in Tibet plateau, China. *Environmental Pollution*, *219*, 450–455. doi:10.1016/j.envpol.2016.05.048 PMID:27238763

Zubris, K. A. V., & Richards, B. K. (2005). Synthetic fibers as an indicator of land application of sludge. *Environmental Pollution*, *138*(2), 201–211. doi:10.1016/j.envpol.2005.04.013 PMID:15967553

ADDITIONAL READING

Barlow, C. Y., & Morgan, D. C. (2013). Polymer film packaging for food: An environmental assessment. *Resources, Conservation and Recycling*, *78*, 74–80. doi:10.1016/j.resconrec.2013.07.003

Eriksen, M., Lebreton, L. C., Carson, H. S., Thiel, M., Moore, C. J., Borerro, J. C., ... Reisser, J. (2014). Plastic pollution in the world's oceans: More than 5 trillion plastic pieces weighing over 250,000 tons afloat at sea. *PLoS One*, *9*(12), 111913. doi:10.1371/journal.pone.0111913 PMID:25494041

Moore, C. J. (2008). Synthetic polymers in the marine environment: A rapidly increasing, long-term threat. *Environmental Research*, *108*(2), 131–139. doi:10.1016/j.envres.2008.07.025 PMID:18949831

Thompson, R. C., Moore, C. J., VomSaal, F. S., & Swan, S. H. (2009). Plastics, the environment and human health: Current consensus and future trends. *Philosophical Transactions of the Royal Society of London. Series B, Biological Sciences*, *364*(1526), 2153–2166. doi:10.1098/rstb.2009.0053 PMID:19528062

Tolinksi, M. (2011). *Plastics and Sustainability: Towards a Peaceful Co-existence Between Bio-based and Fossil Fuel-based Plastics*. Scrivener.

Van Sebille, E., England, M. H., & Froyland, G. (2012). Origin, dynamics and evolution of ocean garbage patches from observed surface drifters. *Environmental Research Letters*, *7*(4), 044040. doi:10.1088/1748-9326/7/4/044040

KEY TERMS AND DEFINITIONS

Effects of Plastic on Land: Chlorinated plastic can release harmful chemicals into the surrounding soil, which can then seep into groundwater or other surrounding water sources and also the ecosystem of the world. This can cause serious harm to the species that drink the water.

Macrodebris: Plastic debris is categorized as macrodebris when it is larger than 20 mm. These include items such as plastic grocery bags. Macrodebris are often found in ocean waters, and can have a serious impact on the native organisms. Fishing nets have been prime pollutants. Even after they have been abandoned, they continue to trap marine organisms and other plastic debris. Eventually, these abandoned nets become too difficult to remove from the water because they become too heavy, having grown in weight up to 6 tons.

Marine Debris: The term marine debris encompasses more than plastic, including metals (derelict vessels, dumped vehicles, beverage containers), glass (light bulbs, beverage containers, older fishing floats), and other materials (rubber, textiles, lumber). Plastic certainly makes up the majority of floating litter, but in some areas the debris on the ocean floor may contain sizeable amounts of those other denser types.

Microdebris: Microdebrisare plastic pieces between 2 mm and 5 mm in size. Plastic debris that starts off as meso- or macrodebris can become microdebris through degradation and collisions that break it down into smaller pieces. Microdebris is more commonly referred to as nurdles. They often end up in ocean waters through rivers and streams. Microdebris that come from cleaning and cosmetic products are also referred to as scrubbers. Because microdebris and scrubbers are so small in size, filter-feeding organisms often consume them.

Persistent Organic Pollutants: It was estimated that global production of plastics is approximately 250 mt/yr. Their abundance has been found to transport persistent organic pollutants, also known as POPs. These pollutants have been linked to an increased distribution of algae associated with red tides.

Plastic: Plastic is versatile, lightweight, flexible, moisture resistant, strong, and relatively inexpensive. Those are the attractive qualities that lead us, around the world, to such a voracious appetite and over-consumption of plastic goods. However, durable and very slow to degrade, plastic materials that are used in the production of so many products all, ultimately, become waste with staying power.

Chapter 6
Marine Plastic Debris:
Distribution, Abundance, and Impact on Our Seafood

Muhammad Reza Cordova
https://orcid.org/0000-0002-4756-9646
Indonesian Institute of Sciences, Indonesia

ABSTRACT

Marine pollution due to littering from anthropogenic activities is a serious global environmental problem—the main reason accumulation of debris in the environment, including in the ocean. There is a significant hazard coming from plastic debris. Besides entanglement and ingestion, marine plastics debris has more complex problems and can release additional and by-product chemical substances. If we keep producing and not doing anything, a recent study said by 2050 there would be three times more plastic than fish in the ocean. We only have a limited understanding of marine plastic debris distribution, implication, fate, and behavior. Science is the key to getting the right alternative for processing debris. To prevent marine pollution successfully requires education and outreach programs, strong laws and policies, and law enforcement for government and private institutions. This chapter explores marine plastic debris.

INTRODUCTION

Plastic is a material that is successfully made by humans. Plastic materials are durable, reliable, lightweight, and has versatility; made this material come to provide many serve a wide range of products, including packaging, building and construction, transportation, electronics and energy, agriculture, healthcare, sport,and leisure. As a result of these properties, plastics production reach 348 million tons (Rosevelt, Los Huertos, Garza, & Nevins, 2013a) withannual production reached78 million tons(Foin et al., 2014). This trend continuously uplifting about 4% per year (Rosevelt et al., 2013a) and by 2050, plastic production expected quadruple (Jovanović, 2017). However, from this massive plastics production due to litter mismanagement andillegally dumping,only 40% ofplastics litter going to landfilled and32% of plastic material trash leaks out to the environment (Foin et al., 2014), including to the ocean. Jambeck

DOI: 10.4018/978-1-5225-9452-9.ch006

et al.(2015), Thompson (2006) and Van Cauwenberghe et al. (2015)estimate 10% of plastic litter will be end up into the sea.The fast increment in worldwide plastic creation has expanded the number of plastic materials in marine frameworks, which as a rule has balanced the increases made by diminishing misfortunes of mechanical pellets and dumping of ship-produced litter.In 2025, plastic material in the ocean estimated to be 250 million metric tons (Jovanović, 2017). Plastic litter that leaks out, made plastic continuously increase over recent years in aquatic ecosystems worldwide, including the ocean, sea surface, shoreline,andseafloor.Plastic litter was seen as an aesthetic problem and has been ignored for a long time, but recent decades shows the presence of this litter gives negative impact to marine animals (Boerger, Lattin, Moore, & Moore, 2010; Carrasco, Harvey, & Saravia, 2009; F. Galgani, Hanke, Werner, & De Vrees, 2013; C. J. Moore, Moore, Leecaster, & Weisberg, 2001). Marine plastic litter already causes $ 13 billion in global financial damage every year (Vigiak, Ribolzi, Pierret, Sengtaheuanghoung, & Valentin, 2008). The cost of cleaning up plastic litter operations is requires very high costs, National Oceanic and Atmospheric Administration (2012)explain to clean 1% area of north plastic would need $ 489 million for the year. From these high numbers, it can be said that plastic is too expensive to be trash.

Enormous plastic litter in the aquatic environment worldwide, especially to the ocean, as the case may be new and big challenges, beside climate change and ocean acidification in human history. On 2050, plastic expected to exceed ocean fish stock by mass ratio (Foin et al., 2014; Jovanović, 2017). Whereas, ocean fish stock could disappear on 2048 (Worm et al., 2006). The majority of plastic litters entering the sea came from diffuse (Figure 1), land-based sources which are harder to control. Land-based activities contribute 80% of all pollution in seas and oceans, and the rest comes from ocean activities (Law, 2017). Eunomia Research & Consulting (2016) explain there is different area of plastics accumulation in the marine ecosystem. Average global concentration of plastic litter in the beaches is highest at 2,000 kg/km^2; in the seafloor is 70 kg/km^2, and in the sea surface is less than 1 kg/km^2(Law, 2017).

Plastic after entering the aquatic environment can be degraded by UV thermal oxidation, mechanic processes, or bacterial process up to the microscopic size(Andrady, 2011; Wagner et al., 2014). This plastic waste with the micrometers size has been known as microplastics. Besides commonly-used

Figure 1. The fate of land and sea-based plastics litter (Law, 2017)

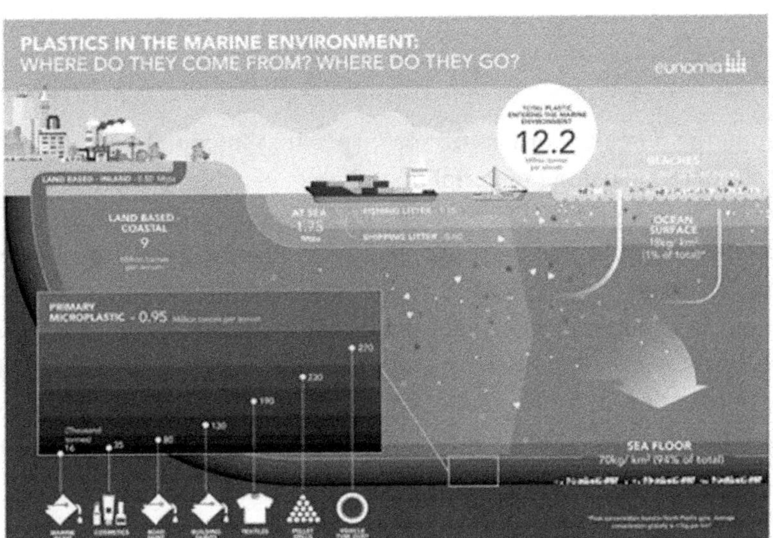

plastic, microplastic sources may come from industrial pellets and microbeads contained in cosmetic or fabric(Browne et al., 2011; Fendall & Sewell, 2009).According to previous studies, microplastic can be found in the coastal area, coral reefs area, mangrove ecosystem, water column, and in the sediment of the sea bottom(Abayomi et al., 2017; Claessens, Meester, Landuyt, Clerck, & Janssen, 2011; Cordova, Hadi, & Prayudha, 2018; Cordova & Wahyudi, 2016; Mohamed Nor & Obbard, 2014; C. J. Moore, Moore, Weisberg, Lattin, & Zellers, 2002; Lisbeth Van Cauwenberghe, Vanreusel, Mees, & Janssen, 2013). With small size, microplastics will increase plastic bioavailability for marine organisms and possible to enter the natural food chain. Some laboratory studies showed that detritivores organism (e.g., Amphipods), deposit feeders (e.g., lugworm), filter feeders (e.g., barnacles and bivalves) or deposit and suspension feeders (e.g., sea cucumber and Copepods) consumes microplastic(Graham & Thompson, 2009; Thompson et al., 2004). (Micro) Plastic consumption will irritate the digestive system(Betts, 2008) and furthermore, it will cause other severe problems since the consumed plastic may adsorp organic pollutant (Teuten et al., 2009). Microplastic consumption by marine organisms may happen because they identified the microplastic as edible foods(Jovanović, 2017; L. Van Cauwenberghe, Claessens, Vandegehuchte, & Janssen, 2014).

However, the effect of the plastic particle to the aquatic ecosystem, particularly to the ocean is still unclear. The research regarding the ingestion of smaller size plastics by marine organism the matter has since been consistently expanding (Jovanović, 2017).Microplastics will degrade to a smaller size, to nano-plastics(Gigault, Pedrono, Maxit, & Ter Halle, 2016; Lambert, Sinclair, Bradley, & Boxall, 2013; Lambert & Wagner, 2016; O'Brine & Thompson, 2010)or smaller, as pico-particles. This smaller plastic particles have more significantthreat because, smaller particles able to penetrate cellular and biological tissue, accumulate and can affect metabolism and life behavior(Cedervall, Hansson, Lard, Frohm, & Linse, 2012; Kashiwada, 2006; Mattsson et al., 2016, 2015; Mattsson, Hansson, Linse, Malmendal, & Cedervall, 2014; Mattsson et al., 2017; Von Moos, Burkhardt-Holm, & Köhler, 2012; Wegner, Besseling, Foekema, Kamermans, & Koelmans, 2012). The threat of plastic litter, from big size to smallest size, in the marine ecosystem, has been ignored since it was first discovered, and it is time to getting the right alternative, such as a science, for prevent and processing plastics litter before it is going to the environment.

DEFINITION

Plastics derives from the Greek word“πλαστός” (plastos) meaning molded or shaped, andthe word“πλαστικός” (plastikos), meaning material that pliable, capable to molded or shaped (BPF, 2016; Crawford & Quinn, 2017; WARKENTIN, SODHI, ESPIE, & POOLE, 2005; Yin, Zhang, & Wang, 2004a). Plastic isa synthetic organic polymer with an additive chemical that can improve the materials(da Costa, Santos, Duarte, & Rocha-Santos, 2016). Additional material that added to plastics includeplasticizers, colorants, stabilizers coupling agents, antioxidant, UV absorber, lubricant, flame retardants and organic preservative(Jovanović, 2017).Plastic material typically derived from petrochemicals with two main processes, polymerization, and polycondensation. These procedures need a specific catalyst and additional material, to create specific structure and properties based on used monomer.

History of Plastic

Organic compound plastic (perkesine)were introduced at 1862 by Alexander Parkes. However,perkesine was not a commercial success(PLASTICS, 2012). At 1869, John Wesley Hyatt develops the first synthetic polymer (Yin et al., 2004a). In 1907 Leo Baekeland invented Bakelite, the first fully synthetic plastic. Hermann Staudinger at 1920 discovered polymers. From this product invented until 1945, early "plastic materials" production increased. Innovation for the polymer such as polyethylene (in 1933), nylon (in 1939), expanded polystyrene (in 1941), and in 1950 polyesterwas discovered(BPF, 2016; Crawford & Quinn, 2017; PLASTICS, 2012; Yin et al., 2004a). More plastic material was developed after a world war,and plastic industry started to produce consumer product after 1950.Due to innovative applications, strength and design flexibility, plastic production increase more than 20x from 1964 to today(Foin et al., 2014).

Thermoplastic and Thermosetting

Plastics classified by chemical structure and product design.Based on the characteristic, plastics can categorized into thermoplastic and thermoset(Do, Boonmongkon, Paek, & Guadamuz, 2017). A thermoplastic is a polymer material that moldable or flexible on a specific temperature(Rosevelt et al., 2013a), for examples polyethylene, polypropylene, polyamides, polycarbonate, polystyrene, polyethylene terephthalate, and polyvinyl-chloride. A thermosetting plastic is a polymer substance that has permanent form after the hardening process at a particular temperature(Rosevelt et al., 2013a), such as acrylic resins, polyurethane, epoxy resins, vinyl ester, silicone, and unsaturated polyester.Thermosetting plastics have a stable covalent bond between polymer chain and have a three-dimensional bond crosslink network that suited to high and decomposition temperature(Dodiuk & Goodman, 2013). Those bond lead thermosetting plastics stronger than thermoplastic.

Plastic Size Range

Plastics, although not yet having a nomenclature, are divided by size according to the agreement of the international research community, namely the size of mega, macro, meso, micro and nano (Figure 2, GESAMP, 2015). Megaplastic is plastic with a size of more than 1 m. Macroplastic with a size between less than 1 m to more than 2.5 cm. Mesoplastic sizes range from 2.5 cm to 1 mm. Microplastic includes plastic with a size between 1 mm to 1 μm, but many categorize the size from less than 5 mm to 1 μm. Microplastic defined as a plastic size less than 5 mm which provides a different threat to the larger size of plastic. Nanoplastic is plastic with a size of less than 1 μm.

Plastic Density in Marine Environment

The position of materials in the water column depends on the density. The density of an object in the waters determines the vertical position of the depth of the object in the water column. Materials that have a lower density will float in the water column while materials that have higher densities than the water density will sink to the bottom of the water or are above the surface of the water column. In general, plastics have a lower density when compared to seawater (1.27 kg/m³). Plastic density has a range of 0.9 - 1.39 kg/m³(Kershaw, 2015; Meier, 2009). Plastic density and examples of plastic objects found in the marine environment can be seen in Table 1.

Figure 2. Plastic size range (right) in coastal and marine ecosystems and their comparison with living creatures (left) (GESAMP Joint Group of Experts on the Scientific Aspects of Marine Environmental Protection, 2015)

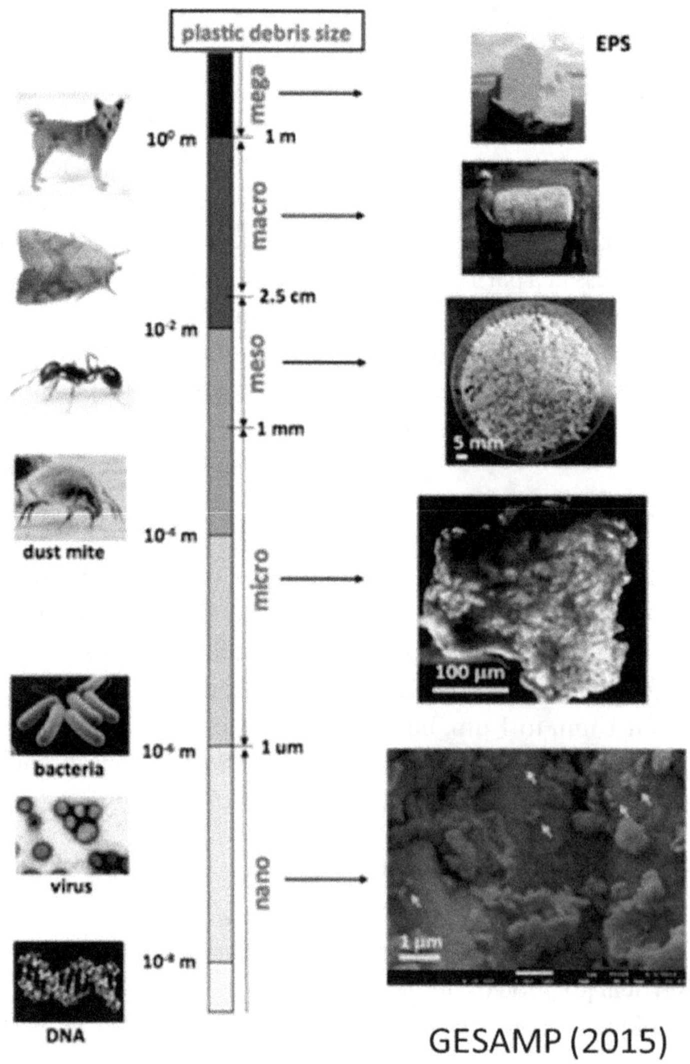

Table 1. Plastic density and examples of plastic objects found in the marine environment

Material	Density (kg/m³)	Examples of plastic objects found in the marine environment
ABS	1,052	pipe, automatic bumper
Acetal (Delrin)	1,356	gear wheels, eyeglasses
Acrylic	1,163	roof windows, lenses and screens
Neoprene	1,384	flashings and automotive fan belts
Polyamide (Nylon)	1,100	fishing net and food packaging
Polycarbonate	1,190	electronic applications, construction industry and data storage
LDPE (Low-Density Polyethylene)	913	various containers, dispensing bottles, and plastic bags
HDPE (High-Density Polyethylene)	941	plastic bottles, geomembranes and plastic lumber
Polyethylene terephtalate	1,34 – 1,39	packaging foods and beverages
Polyester	>1,35	conveyor belts, safety belts, coated fabrics, and various clothing
Polypropylene	913	various packaging, automotive industry, and textiles
Polystyrene (expanded)	1,01 – 1,05	cool boxes dan cups
PVC (Polyvinyl chloride)	1,467	pipe
Polytetrafluoroethylene (Teflon)	2,159	wiring and cookware

PLASTIC PROBLEM

Plastics Litter in Marine Environment

The issue of plastic litter in the all oceans regime has pulled scientific community concern. Perception of the plastic litter threats to aquatic ecosystems started the 1960s (Figure 3) and relatively increases every year (Ryan, 2015). The fate of plastic litter in the ocean (amount, sources, transport, and ingestion) were still the main study, then followed by management, policy and regulation of marine plastic litter (Fig 3). Started from the 2000s, there was also growing recognition regarding microplastics (and plastic particles smaller than microplastic) including the potential consequences on the health of marine ecosystems.By 2025, United Nation Development Programme (2016)have a target from Sustainable Development Goal 14 (SDGs) to reduce and prevent pollution to the ocean significantly, mainly marine debris.

Figure 3. Increasing record of plastic litter research from 1960s to today (Ryan, 2015)

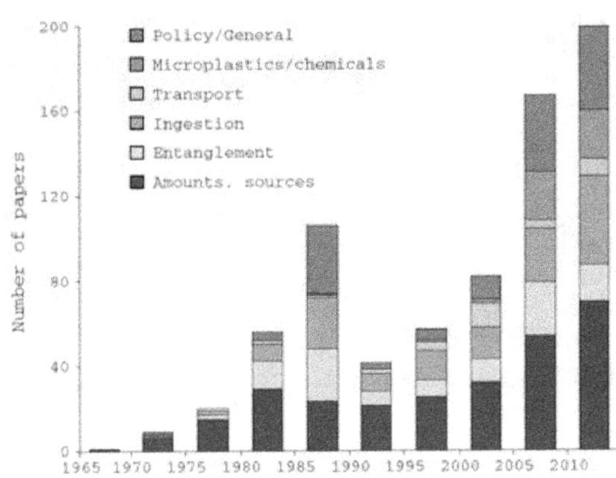

Interpretation of the composition and structure of marine plastic litter provides information that can investigate its origins. The sources of marine litter, including plastics material, dominated from land, as unprotected landfill from domestic and industry litter (Jambeck et al., 2015; Jang, Kim, Seong, Chung, & Yoon, 2014); or by river run-off (Díaz-Torres, Ortega-Ortiz, Silva-Iñiguez, Nene-Preciado, & Orozco, 2017; Jang et al., 2014; Laurent C.M. Lebreton et al., 2017; Sadri & Thompson, 2014); or extreme event, such as Tsunami-Driven Debris (Nistor, Goseberg, & Stolle, 2017; Shafiei, Melville, Beskhyroun, & Shamseldin, 2014). About 20% marine litter sources comes from ocean activity, such as shipping, fishing, and aquaculture (François Galgani, Hanke, & Maes, 2015). Marine litter comprises fundamentally of plastics (Derraik, 2002; Eriksen et al., 2014; Lisbeth Van Cauwenberghe, Claessens, Vandegehuchte, Mees, & Janssen, 2013). The predominance of plastic litter in the marine environment, due to persistence and durability of plastics. Inappropriate handled plastic litter make a significant environmental threat. Plastic ability generates that this material remains in the marine environment for a lifetime and potentially drifted by wind and water. Plastic litter can accumulate in the shoreline or sea surface far from the sources area. UNEP (2016)describe the allocation of plastic litter in the ocean spread the most on open ocean water (39%), thenon the coastline and the sea floor (33.8%) and accumulated on coastal ocean waters (26.8%).

Multiple types of research have been carried out to estimate the trajectories of floating marine plastic litter globally. Plastic litter could travel long distance following ocean currents.A massive cluster of floating plastic litter is formed in the center of five gyres by converging Ekman currents (Dohan & Maximenko, 2010), it is also identified as "plastic trash vortex" or "the plastic garbage patch" (Figure 4). Based on surface trawl data, Cozar et al. (2014) expected a global total of 10,000-40,000 tonnes of plastic floats in the ocean. Eriksen et al. (2014) investigates, from surface trawls and visual surveys, that more than 5 trillion plastic pieces with weight of 268,000 tonnes are drifting at sea.Calculation of the mass distribution of floating plastic litter in the five gyres (Eriksen et al., 2014) can be seen in Figure 5.

Plastic litter from anthropogenic activity estimated accumulated in the beach. A numerical model prognosticated that sea-based and land-based litter as a source for litter in the beach, 28% and 40% respectively (L. C.M. Lebreton, Greer, & Borrero, 2012). Beach litter studies have been conducted globally for better judgment the characters of marine debris. Some research studies related to the accumulation and the percentage of plastic waste on the beach can be seen in the Table 2.

Figure 4. A huge of plastic trash vortex in five gyres (NOWPAP MERRAC, 2017)

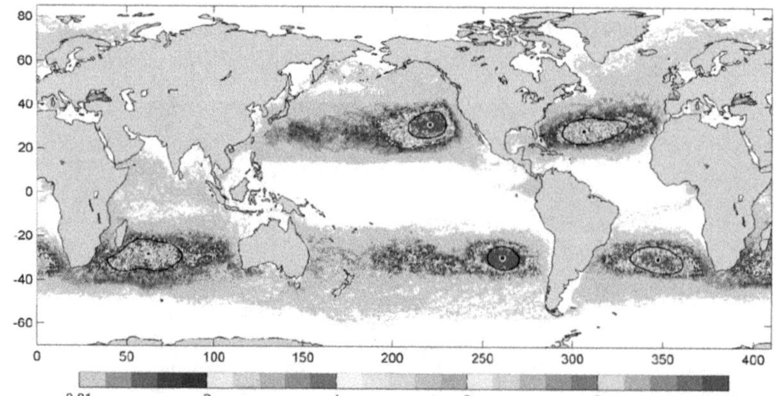

Figure 5.Estimation of the weight distribution of floating plastic litter in the five gyres(modified after Eriksen et al., 2014)

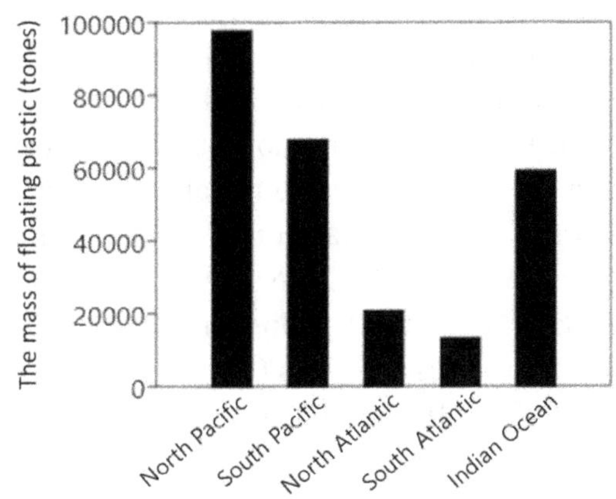

Table 2. Density and percentage of plastic in some beach region

Region	Density (m^{-2}) Average (range)	Plastic (%)	References
11 beaches of Northern Oman	na (0.43–6.01)	61.8	(Claereboudt, 2004)
Portuguese coastline	185.1 (28.6-392.85)	na	(Martins & Sobral, 2011)
Bootless Bay, Papua New Guinea	15.3 (1.2–78.3)	89	(Smith, 2012)
Recreational beaches in Mumbai, India	68.83 (12–960)	na	(Jayasiri, Purushothaman, & Vennila, 2013)
Monterey Bay, United State of America	1 (0.03-17.1)	68	(Rosevelt, Los Huertos, Garza, & Nevins, 2013b)
Kaosiung, Taiwan	0.9 (na)	78.7	(Liu, Wang, & Chen, 2013)
Turkish Western Black Sea Coast	0.88 (0.008–5.06)	91	(Topçu, Tonay, Dede, Öztürk, & Öztürk, 2013)
Marina beach, Chennai, India	1.37 (na)	44.8	(Kumar et al., 2016)
18 Indonesian beaches	1.71 (0.29-5.86)	36-38	(RCO-LIPI, 2018)

na: not available

The position of the plastic naturally will be on the surface of the water. With the value of plastic density on seawater density and ignoring buoyancy, it can conclude that polyethylene, polypropylene and some types of polystyrene plastic will float in seawater. In freshwater, polyethylene and polypropylene will float in the water column by ignoring buoyancy in all types of plastic (Kershaw, 2015). Litter from land which eventually accumulates on the seafloor comes from the river, mostly in the rainy season (Jang et al., 2014). In addition to waste, the river is also a source of organic and inorganic waste materials, because of which plastic waste material is "attached" by materials and organism. This event is termed fouling. Plastic also has uniqueness properties, such as 'sponge' as a medium for organic material, POPs (persistent organic pollutant) and heavy metal adsorption from/to the waters that causes changes in density (Bakir, Rowland, & Thompson, 2014; Holmes, Turner, & Thompson, 2014). Besides, microorganism communities can form a biofilm layer on plastic which increases the density of the plastic(Lobelle & Cunliffe, 2011; Rummel, Jahnke, Gorokhova, Kühnel, & Schmitt-Jansen, 2017; Webb, Crawford, Sawabe, & Ivanova, 2009). With adsorption of that material, plastic density will increase and cause that composite material going down towards the bottom.The existence of a strong current makes the plastic litter material carried away from the source when the slow current makes the plastic litter material (with fouling material) accumulate to the seafloor (F. Galgani et al., 2000; François Galgani et al., 2015).

In shallow water seabed (<200m), the study was done with trawl sampling, scuba, research submarine and remotely operated vehicles (Abu-Hilal & Al-Najjar, 2009; Booth et al., 2007; F. Galgani et al., 2000; Watters, Yoklavich, Love, & Schroeder, 2010).In aquaculture and fishing area, waste in seafloor dominated by plastic materials from fisheries activities (Lee, Cho, & Jeong, 2006). Recent studies(Abu-Hilal & Al-Najjar, 2009; Booth et al., 2007; F. Galgani et al., 2000; Watters et al., 2010) highlight plastic litter density in the shallow water seabed from 0 to 6 items.m^{-2}, dominated by abandoned fishing gear (60-90%). Abandoned fishing gear may persist in the seabed in a long time(Gilman, 2016; Ortega & Dorrance, 2011),not only cause severe damage to the seabed ecosystem, such as to coral reefs and benthic organism (Chiappone, Dienes, Swanson, & Miller, 2005; Mirenda & Beukelman, 1987; Uhrin, Matthews, & Lewis, 2014), but also disrupt marine tourism activities, as troubling propeller.

Plastic wastes also found in the deep-sea realm. Plastic litter found on the seafloor of all seas and oceans, with a different amount. The study of litter on the seabed, especially on the deep-sea floor is still low, and most use bottom trawls. This condition happened because of the high cost of conducting the study. This plastic phenomenon found in four oceans, namely Arctic, Atlantic, Indian, and Pacific (Barnes, Galgani, Thompson, & Barlaz, 2009; Bergmann & Klages, 2012; Woodall, Robinson, Rogers, Narayanaswamy, & Paterson, 2015). Public development, fishing, tourism activity and transshipment are anthropogenic activities that contribute to waste on the seabed. This fact also found on the South Java Deep Sea Expedition, from more than 30 stations, only five to six station found without plastics litter; one of the new species found hidden in discarded clothes (Boh, 2018).

Plastic including smaller size, such as microplastic, will be heading to the seabed so-called "marine snow" would be considered as a portion of food by sea-bottom-living organisms(Goldberg, 1997). Marine snow has widely known as the component in a biogeochemical vector of the biological pump, especially for its role in the downward export of organic matter(Turner, 2015). However, as suggested by(Goldberg, 1997; Lisbeth Van Cauwenberghe, Vanreusel, et al., 2013), the marine snow may become a vector for a microplastic downward pump. Furthermore, it widely known that the formation of marine snow is not merely composed of organic materials (e.g., fecal pellets, phytodetritus or transparent exopolymer/ TEP), but inorganic materials or others (M. Graham, MacIntyre, & Alldredge, 1999; U. Passow, Ziervogel, Asper, & Diercks, 2012; Uta Passow, De La Rocha, Fairfield, & Schmidt, 2014). Plastic from the surface to the bottom of the ocean water to a depth of >2000 m, within a few days a year, depending on the currents in the ocean(Lisbeth Van Cauwenberghe, Vanreusel, et al., 2013). Microplastic will reach the seabed and covered with sand and mud(Ivar Do Sul & Costa, 2014).

Entanglement and Ingestion of Plastic Litter in Marine Organism

As a major global concern, plastic litter has consequences to the organism, including human as an end consumer(UNEP, 2011). However, for other marine organism investigation of plastic entanglement still not done clearly.Entanglement and ingestion of plastic on the marine organism, give an impact to over 46,000 individuals and 663 species, that can reduce survival rate (Mazur & Hitchcock, 2001).Entanglement majority caused by abandoned or derelict fishing gear or ghost fishing, ropes, plastic bags, or discarded clothes(Francois Galgani, Pham, Claro, & Consoli, 2018; E. Moore et al., 2009; Raum-Suryan, Jemison, & Pitcher, 2009; Rodríguez, Bécares, Rodríguez, & Arcos, 2013; Stelfox, Hudgins, & Sweet, 2016).Kühn et al. (2015) found a high percentage of marine organism entangled by plastic, for example 100% species of sea turtle, 67% species of seals, 31% species of whales, and 36% species of seabirds(Ryan, 2018). Moreover, ghost fishing gear entangled more than 5400 individuals from 40 different species of elasmobranchs, reptiles and, marine mammals(Stelfox et al., 2016).The negative impact of plastic entanglement on the marine organism is interfere breathing, lowered appetite, reduce movement and escape from the predator, caused wound and injury, skin infection, amputation, and non-direct mortality(Barreiros & Guerreiro, 2014; Barreiros & Raykov, 2014; Kühn et al., 2015; Laist, 1997; E. Moore et al., 2009; Orós, Torrent, Calabuig, & Déniz, 2005; Program, 2014; Wabnitz & Nichols, 2010). Although not immediately perceptible, plastic litter entanglement can have a severe consequence on naturally born populations of marine organism (Kühn et al., 2015).

Ingestion of plastic often caused by misidentification plastic litter materials as food(Laist, 1997). Compared with entanglement case, plastic ingestion phenomenon is difficult to detect(Kühn et al., 2015), even though whereas these events have a more severe impact, such as can affect fitness and reproductive pattern(McCauley & Bjorndal, 1999).The presence of 5.9kg, more than 1,100 pieces, plastic material in the stomach of 9.5m sperm whales stranded in Wakatobi, Indonesia(Associated Press in Jakarta, 2018), could be one of the causes of the whale's death.In sea turtle, ingestion of plastic can cause decreasing growth rates with the result that poor health or mortality because plastic can directly cause intestinal injury, may block absorption of food essence and dietary dilution(Bjorndal, Bolten, & Lagueux, 1994; Nelms et al., 2016).In fish, ingestion of tiny plastic (nanoparticle size plastic) can cause behavioral disorders, because plastic can enter the blood-to-brain barrier to the brain and disrupting brain function(Mattsson et al., 2017).Ingestion of microscopic size plastic (microplastic) in oyster preventing allocation and energy uptake, which resulted in inefficient offspring performance (Sussarellu et al., 2016). A recent study found that 74% of investigated species northeastern Atlantic recorded ingesting plastic(O'Hanlon, James, Masden, & Bond, 2017). Seabird with high levels of ingested plastic showed weakened body fitness and increased contaminant load (Lavers, Bond, & Hutton, 2014).This condition is worrying, considering seabirds are a sentinelorganism for the marine environment.

Ingestion of microplastics in organisms is found from primary and secondary consumers such as zooxanthellae, rotifers, echinoderms, annelid worms,shellfish (moluscs and crustaceans) and fish as consumer and top predator intermediates(de Sá, Oliveira, Ribeiro, Rocha, & Futter, 2018). de Sá, Oliveira, Ribeiro, Rocha, & Futter (2018)added that the study of the impact of microplastics was mostly carried out on fish and shellfish with a total percentage of 84% from 130 studies. Considering the three marine organisms as a seafood, they can be a source of microplastics contaminants from marine environments to humans(Bouwmeester, Hollman, & Peters, 2015). Microplastics uptake on aquatic organisms that become seafood from local fish market can be seen in Table 3. Microplastics which enters the human digestive tract through seafood may occur gastrointestinal lymphatics uptake. Translocation of inert particulate

Table 3. Microplastics level from commercial shellfish and fish

Common name	Scientific name	Microplastics level (mean ± SD)	Sources	Reference
Asian hard clam	*Meretrixlusoria*	9.22	China	Li et al.(2015)
Mediterranean mussel	*Mytilusgalloprovincialis*	4.33 ± 2.62	China	Li et al.(2015)
Yesso scallop	*Patinopectenyessoensis*	57.17 ± 17.34	China	Li et al.(2015)
Manila clam	*Ruditapesphilippinarum*	5.72 ± 2.86	China	Li et al.(2015)
Anadara gray	*Scapharcasubcrenata*	45 ± 14.98	China	Li et al.(2015)
Chinese razor clam	*Sinonovaculaconstricta*	14.33 ± 2.21	China	Li et al.(2015)
Ark clam	*Tegillarcagranosa*	5.33 ± 2.21	China	Li et al.(2015)
Pacific oyster	*Crassostreagigas*	0.6 ± 0.9	California, USA	Rochman et al. (2015)
Pacific oyster	*Crassostreagigas*	0.47 ± 0.16 * particles/g individual	Brittany, France	Van Cauwenberghe & Janssen (2014)
Jacksmelt	*Atherinopsiscaliforniensis*	1.6 ± 3.7	California, USA	Rochman et al. (2015)
Pacific anchovy	*Engraulismordax*	0.3 ± 0.5	California, USA	Rochman et al. (2015)
Yellowtail Rockfish	*Sebastes flavidus*	0.3 ± 0.6	California, USA	Rochman et al. (2015)
Striped bass	*Moronesaxatilis*	0.9 ± 1.2	California, USA	Rochman et al. (2015)
Chinook salmon	*Oncorhynchustshawytscha*	0.25 ± 0.5	California, USA	Rochman et al. (2015)
Blue rockfish	*Sebastes mystinus*	0.2 ± 0.4	California, USA	Rochman et al. (2015)
Pacific sanddab	*Citharichthyssordidus*	1 ± 1.2	California, USA	Rochman et al. (2015)
Lingcod	*Ophiodon elongatus*	0.1 ± 0.3	California, USA	Rochman et al. (2015)
Indian mackerel	*Rastrelligerkanagurta*	1 ± 1.1	Eastern Indonesia	Rochman et al. (2015)
Shortfin scad	*Decapterusmacrosoma*	2.5 ± 6.3	Eastern Indonesia	Rochman et al. (2015)
Silver-stripe round herring	*Spratelloidesgracilis*	1.1 ± 1.7	Eastern Indonesia	Rochman et al. (2015)
Rabbitfish	*Siganus argenteus*	0.5 ± 0.7	Eastern Indonesia	Rochman et al. (2015)
Rabbitfish	*Siganuscanaliculatus*	0.3 ± 0.6	Eastern Indonesia	Rochman et al. (2015)
Jewfish	*Argyrosomusregius*	0.80 ± 0.8	Portuguese Coast	Neves, Sobral, Ferreira, & Pereira (2015)
Atlantic pomfret	*Bramabrama*	0.67 ± 1.2	Portuguese Coast	Neves, Sobral, Ferreira, & Pereira (2015)
Large-eyed Dentex	*Dentexmacrophthalmus*	1	Portuguese Coast	Neves, Sobral, Ferreira, & Pereira (2015)
Angler	*Lophiuspiscatorius*	0.5	Portuguese Coast	Neves, Sobral, Ferreira, & Pereira (2015)
European hake	*Merlucciusmerluccius*	0.40 ± 0.89	Portuguese Coast	Neves, Sobral, Ferreira, & Pereira (2015)
Striped red mullet	*Mullussurmuletus*	1.66 ± 0.57	Portuguese Coast	Neves, Sobral, Ferreira, & Pereira (2015)
Starry Skate	*Raja asterias*	0.57 ± 0.79	Portuguese Coast	Neves, Sobral, Ferreira, & Pereira (2015)
Small-spotted catshark	*Scyliorhinuscanicula*	0.67 ± 0.58	Portuguese Coast	Neves, Sobral, Ferreira, & Pereira (2015)

matter, including plastics, will occur in microparticles with a size less than 150 µm (Hussain, Jaitley, & Florence, 2001). Currently, research associated with the influence of microplastics in seafood on human health is still insufficient. This information is needed as the foundation of the plastics risk assessment. Understanding the processes of fate and the possible effect of microplastics in human health become one of the studies that need to be prioritized.

Plastic Litter Material as Releaser and Medium of Toxic Pollutant

In addition to physically disrupting, plastic ingested by a marine organism has more complex problems due to the content of substances added or produced during plastic production, and other pollutants that "attached" to the plastic litter (Hahladakis, Velis, Weber, Iacovidou, & Purnell, 2018; Lithner, Larsson, & Dave, 2011; Mato et al., 2001; Rochman, Hoh, Kurobe, & Teh, 2013; Teuten et al., 2009; vom Saal & Hughes, 2005). Rochman (2015) declared the plastic litter that was in the aquatic environment to be 'cocktail of chemicals' (Figure 6). Plastic litter material not only can release toxic chemical ingredients and by-product but also can be a medium to sorb contaminant and released later (Rochman, 2015). In this case, plastic litter can be a source and be a sink for a pollutant.Lithner et al. (2011)stated some plastics polymers are a combination of dangerous monomers such as polyurethane (PUR) foam, polyvinyl chloride (PVC), polycarbonate (PC) and high-impact polystyrene (HIPS). besides, because of the complexity of the polymerization, the residue from the monomer or additive ingredients, such as phthalates, brominated flame retardants, bisphenol A, and formaldehyde, can be released because it is not bound to the polymer matrix (Lithner et al., 2011; Lithner, Nordensvan, & Dave, 2012).The hazardous materials from plastic acutely toxic to aquatic life considered carcinogenic, mutagenic or interfere reproduction (Lithner et al., 2011, 2012).

The hazardous potential of plastic litter as pollutant transporter can occur globally because ocean current can transport far from the sources (Engler, 2012; Martinez, Maamaatuaiahutapu, & Taillandier, 2009; Maximenko, Hafner, & Niiler, 2012; Pearce, Jackson, & Cresswell, 2018), furthermore, there is a higher probability of releasing pollutant from plastic litter in the pristine remote area (Hirai et al., 2011).Toxicant can also be released from the plastic on the stomach marine organism which ingests plastic. The accumulation due to ingestion of litter that can release pollutants will cause further impacts. Beside plastic can be dangerous as described earlier, releasing pollutant can become bioavailable to marine life. Bioavailable is a pollutant entering the circulation of metabolism in living organisms and can have an active toxic effect. This means there is a possibility for marine organisms to be affected by the toxic pollutant associated with plastic debris. Bioavailable in living organism means toxic pollutant can interfere with the performance of the metabolic system, disrupting endocrine, and carcinogenic and

Figure 6. The "cocktail of contaminants" correlated with marine plastic litter (Rochman, 2015).

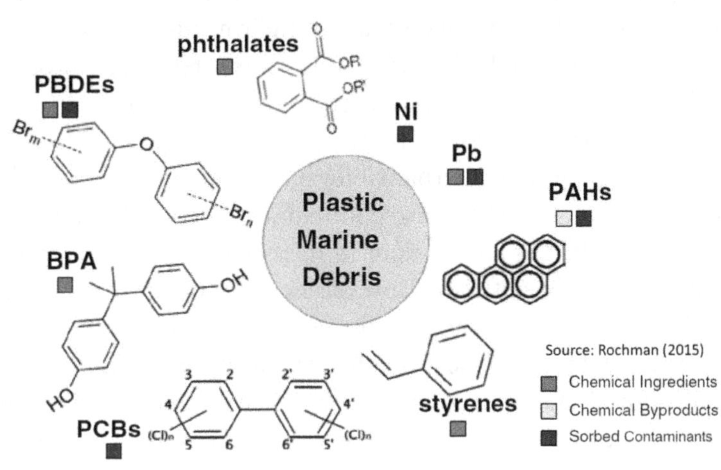

mutagenic (Gallo et al., 2018; Porte et al., 2006; Teuten et al., 2009; Varotto et al., 2013; vom Saal & Hughes, 2005).There is an indication plastic enter food chains and trophic transfer of plastic from prey to top predators(Carbery, O'Connor, & Palanisami, 2018; Farrell & Nelson, 2013; Lusher, 2015; Nelms et al., 2016). This possibility raised when plastic has a smaller size(Chae, Kim, Kim, & An, 2018; Rummel et al., 2017; Wright, Thompson, & Galloway, 2013). However, the plastic implications in the food chain have not been further understood (Thompson, Moore, Saal, & Swan, 2009);it only understood it implies bioaccumulation and biomagnification (Lusher, 2015). High dosage and smaller size of plastic easily transferred through the food chain(Chae et al., 2018; Welden, Abylkhani, & Howarth, 2018). However, still few studies track the fate of plastics and "attached" pollutant through a complex marine food web (including to humans), that can identify the real level of risk and the implication for human health(Carbery et al., 2018; da Costa et al., 2016; Sheavly & Register, 2007; Thompson et al., 2009). We recommend that theme as a future research question.

Mitigating Plastic Litter Problem

To prevent the plastic litter problem in the ocean, a necessary management approach that involves all stakeholders needs to be done. The management approach is generally carried out with a triple helix concept consisting of Academics and Universities, Industry, and Government. Academia and industry provide environment-friendly products. Governments provide the regulatory framework and the financial support for the definition and implementation of innovation strategies and policies. Yawson (2009) added one protagonist, civil society who not only applies knowledge and demands for innovation, in this case in combating marine plastic debris, not only products and services but also becomes an active part of the innovation system. The concept with four implementing elements is known as the Quadruple Helix Constellation.

Quadruple Helix has a concept; government formulates policies and financing and supporting advisory service(Carayannis, Barth, & Campbell, 2012; Carayannis & Campbell, 2011). All government-developed regulation must support the combating of marine plastic debris by including all stakeholders involved from the Quadruple Helix, both in each country and regionally and globally. Academia in this case research institutions and universities to conduct research and development, as incubators and spin-offs from industry and education providers for civil society(Miller, McAdam, & McAdam, 2018). The industry as entrepreneurial venturing and product and service development to environment-friendly products. Civil society is innovation users who give information about their needs and experiences. The civil society has a role as a collaboration platform, legitimating link, competence and process development of the industry(Arnkil et al., 2010). Civil society is also carrying individual and structural perspective(Arnkil et al., 2010; Carayannis et al., 2012; Yawson, 2009).

Science is the key to getting the right alternative for processing plastic litters. The problem of plastic pollution in the world oceans has attracted global community concern. The author suggests adapting the Quadruple Helix model to combating plastic litter in the ocean. Academics work with the Industry to design products that minimize the use of disposable plastics, plastic that can be used repeatedly and high durability and plastics that can and, in the end, can always be recycled. Regulations set by the government protects all these products, and the use of the product get approval from civil society. Academics become a platform for providing appropriate environmental education to civil society by involving industry and government supporting advisory services. The waste management process, especially plastic is carried

Figure 7. The Quadruple Helix Concept to combating marine plastic litter (modified after Lindberg, Lindgren, & Packendorff, 2014)

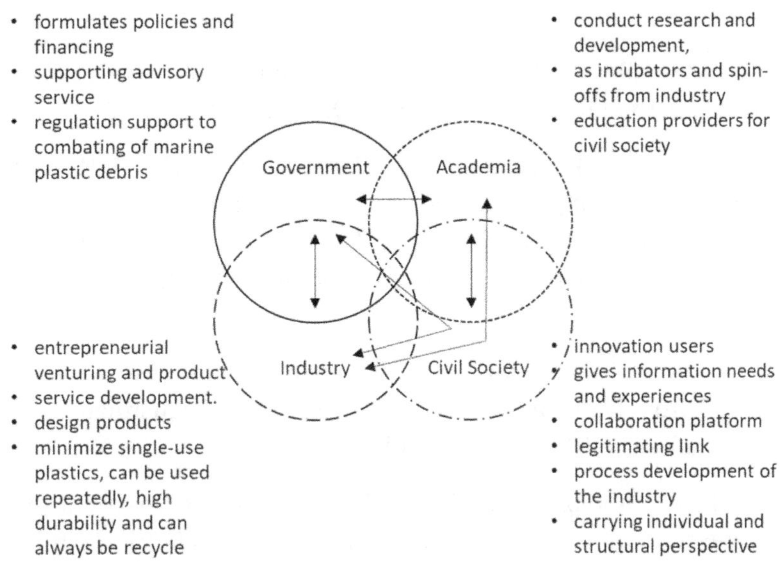

out through recognized waste management involving competent industries, implementation of appropriate regulations and supervision of the community and academics.

CONCLUSION

Plastic pollution problem in the oceans has attracted community concern. Plastic as relatively new materials has invaded ocean areas, not only accumulating close to anthropogenic activity area but also including pristine areas. Ocean spread open ocean water, on the coastline, the sea floor and on coastal waters. Entanglement and ingestion of plastic on the marine organism can reduce survival rate. Plastic litter has more complex problems due to the content of substances added or produced during plastic production, and other pollutants that "attached" to the plastic litter. There is a lack of study to track the fate of plastics and "attached" pollutant through a complex marine food web and the implication for human health. To combating marine pollution successfully, mainly marine plastic debris, we recommend applying the Quadruple Helix Concept, integrate implementation of education and outreach programs, strong laws and policies, and law enforcement for government and private institutions.

REFERENCES

Abayomi, O. A., Range, P., Al-Ghouti, M. A., Obbard, J. P., Almeer, S. H., & Ben-Hamadou, R. (2017). Microplastics in coastal environments of the Arabian Gulf. *Marine Pollution Bulletin, 124*(1), 181–188. doi:10.1016/j.marpolbul.2017.07.011 PMID:28739102

Abu-Hilal, A., & Al-Najjar, T. (2009). Marine litter in coral reef areas along the Jordan Gulf of Aqaba, Red Sea. *Journal of Environmental Management*, *90*(2), 1043–1049. doi:10.1016/j.jenvman.2008.03.014 PMID:18490098

Andrady, A. L. (2011). Microplastics in the marine environment. *Marine Pollution Bulletin*, *62*(8), 1596–1605. doi:10.1016/j.marpolbul.2011.05.030 PMID:21742351

Arnkil, R. A., Jarvensivu, A., Korski, P., Piirainen, T., Järvensivu, A., Koski, P., & Piirainen, T. (2010). *Exploring Quadruple Helix: Outlining user-oriented innovation models.* Tampere: The CLIQ. Retrieved from http://tampub.uta.fi/bitstream/handle/10024/65758/978-951-44-8209-0.pdf?sequenc%0Ahttp://www.arnkildialogues.com/files/testataan.kotisivukone.com/julkaisut/exploring_quadruple_helix-2010-1.pdf

Associated Press in Jakarta. (2018). *Indonesia: dead whale had 1,000 pieces of plastic in stomach*. Retrieved November 27, 2018, from The Guardian website: https://www.theguardian.com/environment/2018/nov/20/indonesia-dead-whale-had-1000-pieces-of-plastic-in-stomach

Bakir, A., Rowland, S. J., & Thompson, R. C. (2014). Transport of persistent organic pollutants by microplastics in estuarine conditions. *Estuarine, Coastal and Shelf Science*, *140*, 14–21. doi:10.1016/j.ecss.2014.01.004

Barnes, D. K. A., Galgani, F., Thompson, R. C., & Barlaz, M. (2009). Accumulation and fragmentation of plastic debris in global environments. *Philosophical Transactions of the Royal Society of London. Series B, Biological Sciences*, *364*(1526), 1985–1998. doi:10.1098/rstb.2008.0205 PMID:19528051

Barreiros, J. P., & Guerreiro, O. (2014). Notes on a plastic debris collar on a juvenile Pagellus acarne (Perciformes : Sparidae) from Terceira Island, Azores, NE Atlantic. *Bothalia Journal*, *44*(4), 42–45.

Barreiros, J. P., & Raykov, V. S. (2014). Lethal lesions and amputation caused by plastic debris and fishing gear on the loggerhead turtle Caretta caretta (Linnaeus, 1758). Three case reports from Terceira Island, Azores (NE Atlantic). *Marine Pollution Bulletin*, *86*(1–2), 518–522. doi:10.1016/j.marpolbul.2014.07.020 PMID:25066455

Bergmann, M., & Klages, M. (2012). Increase of litter at the Arctic deep-sea observatory HAUSGARTEN. *Marine Pollution Bulletin*, *64*(12), 2734–2741. doi:10.1016/j.marpolbul.2012.09.018 PMID:23083926

Betts, K. (2008). Why small plastic particles may pose a big problem in the oceans. *Environmental Science & Technology*, *42*(24), 8996. doi:10.1021/es802970v PMID:19174862

Bjorndal, K. A., Bolten, A. B., & Lagueux, C. J. (1994). Ingestion of marine debris by juvenile sea turtles in coastal Florida habitats. *Marine Pollution Bulletin*, *28*(3), 154–158. doi:10.1016/0025-326X(94)90391-3

Boerger, C. M., Lattin, G. L., Moore, S. L., & Moore, C. J. (2010). Plastic ingestion by planktivorous fishes in the North Pacific Central Gyre. *Marine Pollution Bulletin*, *60*(12), 2275–2278. doi:10.1016/j.marpolbul.2010.08.007 PMID:21067782

Boh, S. (2018). *Singapore-Indonesia deep-sea expedition team discovers over a dozen species new to science.* Retrieved May 29, 2018, from The Straits Times website: https://www.straitstimes.com/singapore/singapore-indonesia-deep-sea-expedition-team-discover-over-a-dozen-species-new-to-science

Booth, C. H., Christianson, A. D., Lawrence, J. M., Pham, L. D., Lashley, J. C., & Drymiotis, F. R. (2007). Ytterbium divalency and lattice disorder in near-zero thermal expansion YbGaGe. *Physical Review B: Condensed Matter and Materials Physics*, *75*(1), 401–407. doi:10.1103/PhysRevB.75.012301

Bouwmeester, H., Hollman, P. C. H., & Peters, R. J. B. (2015). Potential Health Impact of Environmentally Released Micro- and Nanoplastics in the Human Food Production Chain: Experiences from Nanotoxicology. *Environmental Science & Technology*, *49*(15), 8932–8947. doi:10.1021/acs.est.5b01090 PMID:26130306

BPF. (2016). *A History of Plastics*. Retrieved from British Plastic Federation website: http://www.bpf.co.uk/plastipedia/plastics_history/default.aspx

Brine, T., & Thompson, R. C. (2010). Degradation of plastic carrier bags in the marine environment. *Marine Pollution Bulletin*, *60*(12), 2279–2283. doi:10.1016/j.marpolbul.2010.08.005

Browne, M. A., Crump, P., Niven, S. J., Teuten, E., Tonkin, A., Galloway, T., & Thompson, R. (2011). Accumulation of microplastic on shorelines woldwide: Sources and sinks. *Environmental Science & Technology*, *45*(21), 9175–9179. doi:10.1021/es201811s PMID:21894925

Carayannis, E. G., Barth, T. D., & Campbell, D. F. (2012). The Quintuple Helix innovation model: global warming as a challenge and driver for innovation. *Journal of Innovation and Entrepreneurship*. doi:10.1186/2192-5372-1-2

Carayannis, E. G., & Campbell, D. F. J. (2011). Open Innovation Diplomacy and a 21st Century Fractal Research, Education and Innovation (FREIE) Ecosystem: Building on the Quadruple and Quintuple Helix Innovation Concepts and the "Mode 3" Knowledge Production System. *Journal of the Knowledge Economy*, *2*(3), 327–372. doi:10.100713132-011-0058-3

Carbery, M., O'Connor, W., & Palanisami, T. (2018). Trophic transfer of microplastics and mixed contaminants in the marine food web and implications for human health. *Environment International*, *115*, 400–409. doi:10.1016/j.envint.2018.03.007 PMID:29653694

Carrasco, P. A., Harvey, M. B., & Saravia, A. M. (2009). The rare andean pitviper rhinocerophis jonathani (Serpentes: Viperidae: Crotalinae): Redescription with comments on its systematics and biogeography. *Zootaxa*, *364*(2283), 1–15. doi:10.1098/rstb.2008.0265

Cedervall, T., Hansson, L. A., Lard, M., Frohm, B., & Linse, S. (2012). Food chain transport of nanoparticles affects behaviour and fat metabolism in fish. *PLoS One*, *7*(2), e32254. doi:10.1371/journal.pone.0032254 PMID:22384193

Chae, Y., Kim, D., Kim, S. W., & An, Y. J. (2018). Trophic transfer and individual impact of nano-sized polystyrene in a four-species freshwater food chain. *Scientific Reports*, *8*(1), 284. doi:10.103841598-017-18849-y PMID:29321604

Chiappone, M., Dienes, H., Swanson, D. W., & Miller, S. L. (2005). Impacts of lost fishing gear on coral reef sessile invertebrates in the Florida Keys National Marine Sanctuary. *Biological Conservation*, *121*(2), 221–230. doi:10.1016/j.biocon.2004.04.023

Claereboudt, M. R. (2004). Shore litter along sandy beaches of the Gulf of Oman. *Marine Pollution Bulletin*, *49*(9–10), 770–777. doi:10.1016/j.marpolbul.2004.06.004 PMID:15530520

Claessens, M., De Meester, S., Van Landuyt, L., De Clerck, K., & Janssen, C. R. (2011). Occurrence and distribution of microplastics in marine sediments along the Belgian coast. *Marine Pollution Bulletin*, *62*(10), 2199–2204. doi:10.1016/j.marpolbul.2011.06.030 PMID:21802098

Cordova, M. R., Hadi, T. A., & Prayudha, B. (2018). Occurrence and abundance of microplastics in coral reef sediment : A case study in Sekotong, Lombok-Indonesia. *Advances in Environmental Sciences Bioflux*, *10*(1), 23–29. doi:10.5281/zenodo.1297719

Cordova, M. R., & Wahyudi, A. J. (2016). Microplastic in the Deep-Sea Sediment of Southwestern Sumatran Waters. *Marine Research in Indonesia*, *41*(1), 27. doi:10.14203/mri.v41i1.99

Cozar, A., Echevarria, F., Gonzalez-Gordillo, J. I., Irigoien, X., Ubeda, B., Hernandez-Leon, S., … Duarte, C. M. (2014). Plastic debris in the open ocean. *Proceedings of the National Academy of Sciences*, *111*(28), 10239–10244. 10.1073/pnas.1314705111

Crawford, C. B., & Quinn, B. (2017). The contemporary history of plastics. In Microplastic Pollutants (pp. 19–37). Academic Press. doi:10.1016/B978-0-12-809406-8.00002-5

da Costa, J. P., Santos, P. S. M., Duarte, A. C., & Rocha-Santos, T. (2016). (Nano)plastics in the environment - Sources, fates and effects. *The Science of the Total Environment*, *566–567*, 15–26. doi:10.1016/j.scitotenv.2016.05.041 PMID:27213666

de Sá, L. C., Oliveira, M., Ribeiro, F., Rocha, T. L., & Futter, M. N. (2018). Studies of the effects of microplastics on aquatic organisms: What do we know and where should we focus our efforts in the future? *The Science of the Total Environment*, *645*, 1029–1039. doi:10.1016/j.scitotenv.2018.07.207 PMID:30248828

Derraik, J. G. B. (2002). The pollution of the marine environment by plastic debris: A review. *Marine Pollution Bulletin*, *44*(9), 842–852. doi:10.1016/S0025-326X(02)00220-5 PMID:12405208

Díaz-Torres, E. R., Ortega-Ortiz, C. D., Silva-Iñiguez, L., Nene-Preciado, A., & Orozco, E. T. (2017). Floating Marine Debris in waters of the Mexican Central Pacific. *Marine Pollution Bulletin*, *115*(1–2), 225–232. doi:10.1016/j.marpolbul.2016.11.065 PMID:27974156

Do, L. A. T., Boonmongkon, P., Paek, S. C., & Guadamuz, T. E. (2017). *'Hu Hong' (bad thing): parental perceptions of teenagers' sexuality in urban Vietnam*. doi:10.118612889-017-4133-y

Dodiuk, H., & Goodman, S. H. (2013). Handbook of Thermoset Plastics. In Handbook of Thermoset Plastics. doi:10.1016/C2011-0-09694-1

Dohan, K., & Maximenko, N. (2010). Monitoring Ocean Currents with Satellite Sensors. *Oceanography (Washington, D.C.)*, *23*(4), 94–103. doi:10.5670/oceanog.2010.08

Engler, R. E. (2012). The complex interaction between marine debris and toxic chemicals in the ocean. *Environmental Science & Technology*, *46*(22), 12302–12315. doi:10.1021/es3027105 PMID:23088563

Eriksen, M., Lebreton, L. C. M., Carson, H. S., Thiel, M., Moore, C. J., Borerro, J. C., ... Reisser, J. (2014). Plastic Pollution in the World's Oceans: More than 5 Trillion Plastic Pieces Weighing over 250,000 Tons Afloat at Sea. *PLoS One*, *9*(12), e111913. doi:10.1371/journal.pone.0111913 PMID:25494041

Farrell, P., & Nelson, K. (2013). Trophic level transfer of microplastic: Mytilus edulis (L.) to Carcinus maenas (L.). *Environmental Pollution*, *177*, 1–3. doi:10.1016/j.envpol.2013.01.046 PMID:23434827

Fendall, L. S., & Sewell, M. A. (2009). Contributing to marine pollution by washing your face: Microplastics in facial cleansers. *Marine Pollution Bulletin*, *58*(8), 1225–1228. doi:10.1016/j.marpolbul.2009.04.025 PMID:19481226

Foin, N., Lee, R. D., Torii, R., Guitierrez-Chico, J. L., Mattesini, A., Nijjer, S., ... Wong, P. (2014). Impact of stent strut design in metallic stents and biodegradable scaffolds. *International Journal of Cardiology*, *177*(3), 800–808. doi:10.1016/j.ijcard.2014.09.143 PMID:25449502

Galgani, F., Hanke, G., & Maes, T. (2015). Global distribution, composition and abundance of marine litter. In Marine Anthropogenic Litter (pp. 29–56). doi:10.1007/978-3-319-16510-3_2

Galgani, F., Hanke, G., Werner, S., & De Vrees, L. (2013). Marine litter within the European Marine Strategy Framework Directive. *ICES Journal of Marine Science*, *70*(6), 1055–1064. doi:10.1093/icesjms/fst122

Galgani, F., Leaute, J. P., Moguedet, P., Souplet, A., Verin, Y., Carpentier, A., ... Nerisson, P. (2000). Litter on the sea floor along European coasts. *Marine Pollution Bulletin*, *40*(6), 516–527. doi:10.1016/S0025-326X(99)00234-9

Galgani, F., Pham, C. K., Claro, F., & Consoli, P. (2018). Marine animal forests as useful indicators of entanglement by marine litter. *Marine Pollution Bulletin*, *135*, 735–738. doi:10.1016/j.marpolbul.2018.08.004 PMID:30301092

Gallo, F., Fossi, C., Weber, R., Santillo, D., Sousa, J., Ingram, I., ... Romano, D. (2018). Marine litter plastics and microplastics and their toxic chemicals components: The need for urgent preventive measures. *Environmental Sciences Europe*, *30*(1), 13. doi:10.118612302-018-0139-z PMID:29721401

GESAMP Joint Group of Experts on the Scientific Aspects of Marine Environmental Protection. (2015). Sources, fate and effects of microplastics in the marine environment: A global assessment. *Reports and Studies GESAMP*, *90*, 96. doi:10.13140/RG.2.1.3803.7925

Gigault, J., Pedrono, B., Maxit, B., & Ter Halle, A. (2016). Marine plastic litter: The unanalyzed nanofraction. *Environmental Science. Nano*, *3*(2), 346–350. doi:10.1039/C6EN00008H

Gilman, E. (2016). Abandoned, lost and discarded gillnets and trammel nets. Methods to estimate ghost fishing mortality, and the status of regional monitoring and management. In E. Gilman, F. Chopin, P. Suuronen, & B. Kuemlangan (Eds.), *FAO Fisheries Technical Paper* (Vol. 600). Retrieved from www.fao.org/3/a-i5051e.pdf

Goldberg, E. D. (1997). Plasticizing the seafloor: An overview. *Environmental Technology (United Kingdom)*, *18*(2), 195–201. doi:10.1080/09593331808616527

Graham, E. R., & Thompson, J. T. (2009). Deposit- and suspension-feeding sea cucumbers (Echinodermata) ingest plastic fragments. *Journal of Experimental Marine Biology and Ecology*, *368*(1), 22–29. doi:10.1016/j.jembe.2008.09.007

Graham, M., Mac, W., Intyre, S., & Alldredge, A. L. (1999). Diel variations of marine snow concentration in surface waters and implications for particle flux in the sea. *Deep-sea Research. Part I, Oceanographic Research Papers*, *47*(3), 367–395. doi:10.1016/S0967-0637(99)00063-1

Hahladakis, J. N., Velis, C. A., Weber, R., Iacovidou, E., & Purnell, P. (2018). An overview of chemical additives present in plastics: Migration, release, fate and environmental impact during their use, disposal and recycling. *Journal of Hazardous Materials*, *344*, 179–199. doi:10.1016/j.jhazmat.2017.10.014 PMID:29035713

Hirai, H., Takada, H., Ogata, Y., Yamashita, R., Mizukawa, K., Saha, M., ... Ward, M. W. (2011). Organic micropollutants in marine plastics debris from the open ocean and remote and urban beaches. *Marine Pollution Bulletin*, *62*(8), 1683–1692. doi:10.1016/j.marpolbul.2011.06.004 PMID:21719036

Hoegh-Guldberg, O., Cai, R., Poloczanska, E. S., Brewer, P. G., Sundby, S., Hilmi, K., ... Jung, S. (2015). The ocean. *Climate Change 2014: Impacts, Adaptation and Vulnerability: Part B: Regional Aspects. Working Group II Contribution to the Fifth Assessment Report of the Intergovernmental Panel on Climate Change*, *347*(6223), 1655–1734. doi:10.1017/CBO9781107415386.010

Holmes, L. A., Turner, A., & Thompson, R. C. (2014). Interactions between trace metals and plastic production pellets under estuarine conditions. *Marine Chemistry*, *167*, 25–32. doi:10.1016/j.marchem.2014.06.001

Hussain, N., Jaitley, V., & Florence, A. T. (2001). Recent advances in the understanding of uptake of microparticulates across the gastrointestinal lymphatics. *Advanced Drug Delivery Reviews*, *50*(1), 107–142. doi:10.1016/S0169-409X(01)00152-1 PMID:11489336

Ivar Do Sul, J. A., & Costa, M. F. (2014). The present and future of microplastic pollution in the marine environment. *Environmental Pollution*, *185*, 352–364. doi:10.1016/j.envpol.2013.10.036 PMID:24275078

Jambeck, J. R., Geyer, R., Wilcox, C., Siegler, T. R., Perryman, M., Andrady, A., ... Law, K. L. (2015). Plastic waste inputs from land into the ocean. *Science*, *347*(6223), 768–771. doi:10.1126cience.1260352 PMID:25678662

Jang, S. W., Kim, D. H., Seong, K. T., Chung, Y. H., & Yoon, H. J. (2014). Analysis of floating debris behaviour in the Nakdong River basin of the southern Korean peninsula using satellite location tracking buoys. *Marine Pollution Bulletin*, *88*(1–2), 275–283. doi:10.1016/j.marpolbul.2014.08.031 PMID:25261180

Jayasiri, H. B., Purushothaman, C. S., & Vennila, A. (2013). Quantitative analysis of plastic debris on recreational beaches. *Marine Pollution Bulletin*, *77*(1), 107–112. doi:10.1016/j.marpolbul.2013.10.024 PMID:24210947

Jovanović, B. (2017). Ingestion of microplastics by fish and its potential consequences from a physical perspective. *Integrated Environmental Assessment and Management*, *13*(3), 510–515. doi:10.1002/ieam.1913 PMID:28440941

Kashiwada, S. (2006). Distribution of nanoparticles in the see-through medaka (Oryzias latipes). *Environmental Health Perspectives, 114*(11), 1697–1702. doi:10.1289/ehp.9209 PMID:17107855

Kershaw, D. P. J. (2015). *Biodegradable Plastics & Marine Litter. Misconceptions, concerns and impacts on marine environments.* United Nations Environment Programme (UNEP). Retrieved from http://wedocs.unep.org/handle/20.500.11822/7468

Kühn, S., Bravo Rebolledo, E. L., & Van Franeker, J. A. (2015). Deleterious effects of litter on marine life. In Marine Anthropogenic Litter (pp. 75–116). doi:10.1007/978-3-319-16510-3_4

Kumar, A. A., Sivakumar, R., Reddy, Y. S. R., Bhagya Raja, M. V., Nishanth, T., & Revanth, V. (2016). Preliminary study on marine debris pollution along Marina beach, Chennai, India. *Regional Studies in Marine Science, 5*, 35–40. doi:10.1016/j.rsma.2016.01.002

Laist, D. W. (1997). Impacts of Marine Debris: Entanglement of Marine Life in Marine Debris Including a Comprehensive List of Species with Entanglement and Ingestion Records. In J. M. Coe & D. B. Rogers (Eds.), *Marine Debris* (pp. 99–139). Springer Series on Environmental Management. doi:10.1007/978-1-4613-8486-1_10

Lambert, S., Sinclair, C. J., Bradley, E. L., & Boxall, A. B. A. (2013). Effects of environmental conditions on latex degradation in aquatic systems. *The Science of the Total Environment, 447*, 225–234. doi:10.1016/j.scitotenv.2012.12.067 PMID:23384646

Lambert, S., & Wagner, M. (2016). Characterisation of nanoplastics during the degradation of polystyrene. *Chemosphere, 145*, 265–268. doi:10.1016/j.chemosphere.2015.11.078 PMID:26688263

Lavers, J. L., Bond, A. L., & Hutton, I. (2014). Plastic ingestion by flesh-footed shearwaters (Puffinus carneipes): Implications for fledgling body condition and the accumulation of plastic-derived chemicals. *Environmental Pollution, 187*, 124–129. doi:10.1016/j.envpol.2013.12.020 PMID:24480381

Law, K. (2017). Plastics in the marine environment. In Environmental Toxicology and Chemistry (Vol. 33). doi:10.1146/annurev-marine-010816-060409

Lebreton, L. C. M., Greer, S. D., & Borrero, J. C. (2012). Numerical modelling of floating debris in the world's oceans. *Marine Pollution Bulletin, 64*(3), 653–661. doi:10.1016/j.marpolbul.2011.10.027 PMID:22264500

Lebreton, L. C. M., Van Der Zwet, J., Damsteeg, J. W., Slat, B., Andrady, A., & Reisser, J. (2017). River plastic emissions to the world's oceans. *Nature Communications, 8*, 15611. doi:10.1038/ncomms15611 PMID:28589961

Lee, D. I., Cho, H. S., & Jeong, S. B. (2006). Distribution characteristics of marine litter on the sea bed of the East China Sea and the South Sea of Korea. *Estuarine, Coastal and Shelf Science, 70*(1–2), 187–194. doi:10.1016/j.ecss.2006.06.003

Li, J., Yang, D., Li, L., Jabeen, K., & Shi, H. (2015). Microplastics in commercial bivalves from China. *Environmental Pollution, 207*, 190–195. doi:10.1016/j.envpol.2015.09.018 PMID:26386204

Lindberg, M., Lindgren, M., & Packendorff, J. (2014). Quadruple Helix as a Way to Bridge the Gender Gap in Entrepreneurship: The Case of an Innovation System Project in the Baltic Sea Region. *Journal of the Knowledge Economy*, *5*(1), 94–113. doi:10.100713132-012-0098-3

Lithner, D., Larsson, A., & Dave, G. (2011). Environmental and health hazard ranking and assessment of plastic polymers based on chemical composition. *The Science of the Total Environment*, *409*(18), 3309–3324. doi:10.1016/j.scitotenv.2011.04.038 PMID:21663944

Lithner, D., Nordensvan, I., & Dave, G. (2012). Comparative acute toxicity of leachates from plastic products made of polypropylene, polyethylene, PVC, acrylonitrile-butadiene-styrene, and epoxy to Daphnia magna. *Environmental Science and Pollution Research International*, *19*(5), 1763–1772. doi:10.100711356-011-0663-5 PMID:22183785

Liu, T. K., Wang, M. W., & Chen, P. (2013). Influence of waste management policy on the characteristics of beach litter in Kaohsiung, Taiwan. *Marine Pollution Bulletin*, *72*(1), 99–106. doi:10.1016/j.marpolbul.2013.04.015 PMID:23673204

Lobelle, D., & Cunliffe, M. (2011). Early microbial biofilm formation on marine plastic debris. *Marine Pollution Bulletin*, *62*(1), 197–200. doi:10.1016/j.marpolbul.2010.10.013 PMID:21093883

Lusher, A. (2015). Microplastics in the marine environment: Distribution, interactions and effects. In M. Bergmann, L. Gutow, & M. Klages (Eds.), *Marine Anthropogenic Litter* (pp. 245–307)., doi:10.1007/978-3-319-16510-3_10

Martinez, E., Maamaatuaiahutapu, K., & Taillandier, V. (2009). Floating marine debris surface drift: Convergence and accumulation toward the South Pacific subtropical gyre. *Marine Pollution Bulletin*, *58*(9), 1347–1355. doi:10.1016/j.marpolbul.2009.04.022 PMID:19464033

Martins, J., & Sobral, P. (2011). Plastic marine debris on the Portuguese coastline: A matter of size? *Marine Pollution Bulletin*. Retrieved from http://www.sciencedirect.com/science/article/pii/S0025326X1100

Mato, Y., Isobe, T., Takada, H., Kanehiro, H., Ohtake, C., & Kaminuma, T. (2001). Plastic resin pellets as a transport medium for toxic chemicals in the marine environment. *Environmental Science & Technology*, *35*(2), 318–324. doi:10.1021/es0010498 PMID:11347604

Mattsson, K., Adolfsson, K., Ekvall, M. T., Borgström, M. T., Linse, S., Hansson, L. A., ... Prinz, C. N. (2016). Translocation of 40 nm diameter nanowires through the intestinal epithelium of Daphnia magna. *Nanotoxicology*, *10*(8), 1160–1167. doi:10.1080/17435390.2016.1189615 PMID:27181920

Mattsson, K., Ekvall, M. T., Hansson, L. A., Linse, S., Malmendal, A., & Cedervall, T. (2015). Altered behavior, physiology, and metabolism in fish exposed to polystyrene nanoparticles. *Environmental Science & Technology*, *49*(1), 553–561. doi:10.1021/es5053655 PMID:25380515

Mattsson, K., Hansson, L. A., Linse, S., Malmendal, A., & Cedervall, T. (2014). Effect of Nanoparticles in Top Consumers. *Biophysical Journal*, *106*(2), 625a. doi:10.1016/j.bpj.2013.11.3454

Mattsson, K., Johnson, E. V., Malmendal, A., Linse, S., Hansson, L. A., & Cedervall, T. (2017). Brain damage and behavioural disorders in fish induced by plastic nanoparticles delivered through the food chain. *Scientific Reports*, *7*(1), 11452. doi:10.103841598-017-10813-0 PMID:28904346

Maximenko, N., Hafner, J., & Niiler, P. (2012). Pathways of marine debris derived from trajectories of Lagrangian drifters. *Marine Pollution Bulletin*, *65*(1–3), 51–62. doi:10.1016/j.marpolbul.2011.04.016 PMID:21696778

Mazur, S., & Hitchcock, T. (2001). Spontaneous pneumomediastinum, pneumothorax and ecstasy abuse. In *Emergency Medicine* (Vol. 13). CBD Techni. doi:10.1046/j.1442-2026.2001.00190.x

McCauley, S. J., & Bjorndal, K. A. (1999). Conservation implications of dietary dilution from debris ingestion: Sublethal effects in post-hatchling loggerhead sea turtles. *Conservation Biology*, *13*(4), 925–929. doi:10.1046/j.1523-1739.1999.98264.x

Meier, E. (2009). *Material Density*. Retrieved December 20, 2018, from A Psimple Psaltery website: http://www.apsimplepsaltery.com/appendices/material_densities/

Miller, K., McAdam, R., & McAdam, M. (2018). A systematic literature review of university technology transfer from a quadruple helix perspective: Toward a research agenda. *R & D Management*, *48*(1), 7–24. doi:10.1111/radm.12228

Mirenda, P., & Beukelman, D. R. (1987). A Comparison of Speech Synthesis Intelligibility with Listeners from Three Age Groups. *Augmentative and Alternative Communication*, *3*(3), 120–128. doi:10.1080/07434618712331274399

Mohamed Nor, N. H., & Obbard, J. P. (2014). Microplastics in Singapore's coastal mangrove ecosystems. *Marine Pollution Bulletin*, *79*(1–2), 278–283. doi:10.1016/j.marpolbul.2013.11.025 PMID:24365455

Moore, C. J., Moore, S. L., Leecaster, M. K., & Weisberg, S. B. (2001). A comparison of plastic and plankton in the North Pacific Central Gyre. *Marine Pollution Bulletin*, *42*(12), 1297–1300. doi:10.1016/S0025-326X(01)00114-X PMID:11827116

Moore, C. J., Moore, S. L., Weisberg, S. B., Lattin, G. L., & Zellers, A. F. (2002). A comparison of neustonic plastic and zooplankton abundance in southern California's coastal waters. *Marine Pollution Bulletin*, *44*(10), 1035–1038. doi:10.1016/S0025-326X(02)00150-9 PMID:12474963

Moore, E., Lyday, S., Roletto, J., Litle, K., Parrish, J. K., Nevins, H., ... Kell, S. (2009). Entanglements of marine mammals and seabirds in central California and the north-west coast of the United States 2001-2005. *Marine Pollution Bulletin*, *58*(7), 1045–1051. doi:10.1016/j.marpolbul.2009.02.006 PMID:19344921

National Oceanic and Atmospheric Administration. (2012). *How Much Would it Cost to Clean up the Pacific Garbage Patches*. Retrieved August 20, 2016, from Office of Response and Restoration website: http://response.restoration.noaa.gov/about/media/how-much-would-it-cost-clean-pacific-garbage-patches.html

Nelms, S. E., Duncan, E. M., Broderick, A. C., Galloway, T. S., Godfrey, M. H., Hamann, M., ... Godley, B. J. (2016). Plastic and marine turtles: A review and call for research. *ICES Journal of Marine Science*, *73*(2), 165–181. doi:10.1093/icesjms/fsv165

Neves, D., Sobral, P., Ferreira, J. L., & Pereira, T. (2015). Ingestion of microplastics by commercial fish off the Portuguese coast. *Marine Pollution Bulletin*, *101*(1), 119–126. doi:10.1016/j.marpolbul.2015.11.008 PMID:26608506

Nistor, I., Goseberg, N., & Stolle, J. (2017). Tsunami-Driven Debris Motion and Loads: A Critical Review. *Frontiers in Built Environment, 3*. doi:10.3389/fbuil.2017.00002

NOWPAP MERRAC. (2017). *Understanding of floating marine litter distribution in the NOWPAP region.* MERRAC Technical Report No. 35.

O'Hanlon, N. J., James, N. A., Masden, E. A., & Bond, A. L. (2017). Seabirds and marine plastic debris in the northeastern Atlantic: A synthesis and recommendations for monitoring and research. *Environmental Pollution, 231*, 1291–1301. doi:10.1016/j.envpol.2017.08.101 PMID:28917819

Orós, J., Torrent, A., Calabuig, P., & Déniz, S. (2005). Diseases and causes of mortality among sea turtles stranded in the Canary Islands, Spain (1998-2001). *Diseases of Aquatic Organisms, 63*(1), 13–24. doi:10.3354/dao063013 PMID:15759796

Ortega, M. A., & Dorrance, A. E. (2011). Microsporogenesis of Rps8/rps8 heterozygous soybean lines. In Euphytica (Vol. 181). doi:10.100710681-011-0422-1

Passow, U., De La Rocha, C. L., Fairfield, C., & Schmidt, K. (2014). Aggregation as a function of PCO2and mineral particles. *Limnology and Oceanography, 59*(2), 532–547. doi:10.4319/lo.2014.59.2.0532

Passow, U., Ziervogel, K., Asper, V., & Diercks, A. (2012). Marine snow formation in the aftermath of the Deepwater Horizon oil spill in the Gulf of Mexico. *Environmental Research Letters, 7*(3), 1–11. doi:10.1088/1748-9326/7/3/035301

Pearce, A., Jackson, G., & Cresswell, G. R. (2018). Marine debris pathways across the southern Indian Ocean. *Deep-sea Research. Part II, Topical Studies in Oceanography*. doi:10.1016/j.dsr2.2018.06.009

PLASTICS. (2012). *History of Plastics.* Retrieved December 1, 2018, from SPI - The Plastics Industry Trade Association website: http://www.plasticsindustry.org/AboutPlastics/content.cfm?ItemNumber=670&navItemNumber=1117

Porte, C., Janer, G., Lorusso, L. C., Ortiz-Zarragoitia, M., Cajaraville, M. P., Fossi, M. C., & Canesi, L. (2006). Endocrine disruptors in marine organisms: Approaches and perspectives. *Comparative Biochemistry and Physiology. Toxicology & Pharmacology: CBP, 143*(3), 303–315. doi:10.1016/j.cbpc.2006.03.004 PMID:16723279

Program, N. O., & A. A. M. D. (2014). *Report on the Entanglement of Marine Species in Marine Debris with an Emphasis on Species in the United States.* Silver Spring, MD: Academic Press.

Raum-Suryan, K. L., Jemison, L. A., & Pitcher, K. W. (2009). Entanglement of Steller sea lions (Eumetopias jubatus) in marine debris: Identifying causes and finding solutions. *Marine Pollution Bulletin, 58*(10), 1487–1495. doi:10.1016/j.marpolbul.2009.06.004 PMID:19631950

RCO-LIPI. (2018). Kajian Sampah Laut (Marine Debris) dan Dampaknya pada Ekosistem Laut. Jakarta, Indonesia: Author.

Rochman, C. M. (2015). The complex mixture, fate and toxicity of chemicals associated with plastic debris in the marine environment. In Marine Anthropogenic Litter (pp. 117–140). doi:10.1007/978-3-319-16510-3_5

Rochman, C. M., Hoh, E., Kurobe, T., & Teh, S. J. (2013). Ingested plastic transfers hazardous chemicals to fish and induces hepatic stress. *Scientific Reports*, *3*(1), 3263. doi:10.1038rep03263 PMID:24263561

Rochman, C. M., Tahir, A., Williams, S. L., Baxa, D. V., Lam, R., Miller, J. T., ... Teh, S. J. (2015). Anthropogenic debris in seafood: Plastic debris and fibers from textiles in fish and bivalves sold for human consumption. *Scientific Reports*, *5*(1), 14340. doi:10.1038rep14340 PMID:26399762

Rodríguez, B., Bécares, J., Rodríguez, A., & Arcos, J. M. (2013). Incidence of entanglements with marine debris by northern gannets (Morus bassanus) in the non-breeding grounds. *Marine Pollution Bulletin*, *75*(1–2), 259–263. doi:10.1016/j.marpolbul.2013.07.003 PMID:23932474

Rosevelt, C., Los Huertos, M., Garza, C., & Nevins, H. M. (2013a). Marine debris in central California: Quantifying type and abundance of beach litter in Monterey Bay, CA. In Marine Pollution Bulletin (Vol. 71). doi:10.1016/j.marpolbul.2013.01.015

Rosevelt, C., Los Huertos, M., Garza, C., & Nevins, H. M. (2013b). Marine debris in central California: Quantifying type and abundance of beach litter in Monterey Bay, CA. *Marine Pollution Bulletin*, *71*(1–2), 299–306. doi:10.1016/j.marpolbul.2013.01.015 PMID:23499538

Rummel, C. D., Jahnke, A., Gorokhova, E., Kühnel, D., & Schmitt-Jansen, M. (2017). Impacts of biofilm formation on the fate and potential effects of microplastic in the aquatic environment. *Environmental Science & Technology Letters*, *4*(7), 258–267. doi:10.1021/acs.estlett.7b00164

Ryan, P. G. (2015). A brief history of marine litter research. In Marine Anthropogenic Litter (pp. 1–25). doi:10.1007/978-3-319-16510-3_1

Ryan, P. G. (2018). Entanglement of birds in plastics and other synthetic materials. *Marine Pollution Bulletin*, *135*, 159–164. doi:10.1016/j.marpolbul.2018.06.057 PMID:30301025

Sadri, S. S., & Thompson, R. C. (2014). On the quantity and composition of floating plastic debris entering and leaving the Tamar Estuary, Southwest England. *Marine Pollution Bulletin*, *81*(1), 55–60. doi:10.1016/j.marpolbul.2014.02.020 PMID:24613232

Shafiei, S. R., Melville, B. W., Beskhyroun, S., & Shamseldin, A. Y. (2014). Preliminary investigation of the tsunami-borne debris impact on structures: a new method for impact force measurement. *Hydraulic Structures and Society - Engineering Challenges and Extremes*, 1–9. doi:10.14264/uql.2014.44

Sheavly, S. B., & Register, K. M. (2007). Marine debris & plastics: Environmental concerns, sources, impacts and solutions. *Journal of Polymers and the Environment*, *15*(4), 301–305. doi:10.100710924-007-0074-3

Smith, S. D. A. (2012). Marine debris: A proximate threat to marine sustainability in Bootless Bay, Papua New Guinea. *Marine Pollution Bulletin*, *64*(9), 1880–1883. doi:10.1016/j.marpolbul.2012.06.013 PMID:22770700

Stelfox, M., Hudgins, J., & Sweet, M. (2016). A review of ghost gear entanglement amongst marine mammals, reptiles and elasmobranchs. *Marine Pollution Bulletin, 111*(1–2), 6–17. doi:10.1016/j.marpolbul.2016.06.034 PMID:27345709

Sussarellu, R., Suquet, M., Thomas, Y., Lambert, C., Fabioux, C., Pernet, M. E. J., … Huvet, A. (2016). Oyster reproduction is affected by exposure to polystyrene microplastics. *Proceedings of the National Academy of Sciences, 113*(9), 2430–2435. 10.1073/pnas.1519019113

Teuten, E. L., Saquing, J. M., Knappe, D. R. U., Barlaz, M. A., Jonsson, S., Björn, A., ... Takada, H. (2009). Transport and release of chemicals from plastics to the environment and to wildlife. *Philosophical Transactions of the Royal Society of London. Series B, Biological Sciences, 364*(1526), 2027–2045. doi:10.1098/rstb.2008.0284 PMID:19528054

Thompson, R. C. (2015). Microplastics in the marine environment: Sources, consequences and solutions. In Marine Anthropogenic Litter (pp. 185–200). doi:10.1007/978-3-319-16510-3_7

Thompson, R. C., Moore, C. J., Saal, F. S. V., & Swan, S. H. (2009). Plastics, the environment and human health: Current consensus and future trends. *Philosophical Transactions of the Royal Society of London. Series B, Biological Sciences, 364*(1526), 2153–2166. doi:10.1098/rstb.2009.0053 PMID:19528062

Thompson, R. C., Olson, Y., Mitchell, R. P., Davis, A., Rowland, S. J., John, A. W. G., ... Russell, A. E. (2004). Lost at Sea: Where Is All the Plastic? *Science, 304*(5672), 838. doi:10.1126cience.1094559 PMID:15131299

Topçu, E. N., Tonay, A. M., Dede, A., Öztürk, A. A., & Öztürk, B. (2013). Origin and abundance of marine litter along sandy beaches of the Turkish Western Black Sea Coast. *Marine Environmental Research, 85*, 21–28. doi:10.1016/j.marenvres.2012.12.006 PMID:23290790

Turner, J. T. (2015). Zooplankton fecal pellets, marine snow, phytodetritus and the ocean's biological pump. *Progress in Oceanography, 130*, 205–248. doi:10.1016/j.pocean.2014.08.005

Uhrin, A. V., Matthews, T. R., & Lewis, C. (2014). Lobster Trap Debris in the Florida Keys National Marine Sanctuary: Distribution, Abundance, Density, and Patterns of Accumulation. *Marine and Coastal Fisheries, 6*(1), 20–32. doi:10.1080/19425120.2013.852638

UNEP. (2011). *NEP Year book 2011: Emerging Issues in Our Global Environment.* Retrieved from http://wedocs.unep.org/bitstream/handle/20.500.11822/17716/UNEP_Year_Book_Emerging_Issues_in_our_Global.pdf?sequence=1&isAllowed=y

Van Cauwenberghe, L., Claessens, M., Vandegehuchte, M., & Janssen, C. R. (2014). XXII International Pigment Cell Conference (IPCC) "Bringing Colors to Life: Advances in Pigment Cell Research and Translation into Clinical Practice" Organised by the Asian Society for Pigment Cell Research (ASPCR), in partnership with the Dermatological. In *Pigment Cell & Melanoma Research* (Vol. 27). 10.1111/pcmr.12292

Van Cauwenberghe, L., Claessens, M., Vandegehuchte, M. B., & Janssen, C. R. (2015). Microplastics are taken up by mussels (Mytilus edulis) and lugworms (Arenicola marina) living in natural habitats. *Environmental Pollution, 199*, 10–17. doi:10.1016/j.envpol.2015.01.008 PMID:25617854

Van Cauwenberghe, L., Claessens, M., Vandegehuchte, M. B., Mees, J., & Janssen, C. R. (2013). Assessment of marine debris on the Belgian Continental Shelf. *Marine Pollution Bulletin*, *73*(1), 161–169. doi:10.1016/j.marpolbul.2013.05.026 PMID:23790460

Van Cauwenberghe, L., & Janssen, C. R. (2014). Microplastics in bivalves cultured for human consumption. *Environmental Pollution*, *193*, 65–70. doi:10.1016/j.envpol.2014.06.010 PMID:25005888

Van Cauwenberghe, L., Vanreusel, A., Mees, J., & Janssen, C. R. (2013). Microplastic pollution in deep-sea sediments. *Environmental Pollution*, *182*, 495–499. doi:10.1016/j.envpol.2013.08.013 PMID:24035457

Varotto, L., Domeneghetti, S., Rosani, U., Manfrin, C., Cajaraville, M. P., Raccanelli, S., ... Venier, P. (2013). DNA Damage and Transcriptional Changes in the Gills of Mytilus galloprovincialis Exposed to Nanomolar Doses of Combined Metal Salts (Cd, Cu, Hg). *PLoS One*, *8*(1), e54602. doi:10.1371/journal.pone.0054602 PMID:23355883

Vigiak, O., Ribolzi, O., Pierret, A., Sengtaheuanghoung, O., & Valentin, C. (2008). Trapping Efficiencies of Cultivated and Natural Riparian Vegetation of Northern Laos. *Journal of Environment Quality*, 889. doi:10.2134/jeq2007.0251

vom Saal, F. S., & Hughes, C. (2005). An extensive new literature concerning low-dose effects of bisphenol A shows the need for a new risk assessment. *Environmental Health Perspectives*, *113*(8), 926–933. doi:10.1289/ehp.7713 PMID:16079060

Von Moos, N., Burkhardt-Holm, P., & Köhler, A. (2012). Uptake and effects of microplastics on cells and tissue of the blue mussel Mytilus edulis L. after an experimental exposure. *Environmental Science & Technology*, *46*(20), 11327–11335. doi:10.1021/es302332w PMID:22963286

Wabnitz, C., & Nichols, W. J. (2010). Editorial: Plastic Pollution: An Ocean Emergency. *Marine Turtle Newsletter*, *20*(129), 1–4. Retrieved from http://search.proquest.com/docview/924334169?accountid=27795

Wagner, M., Scherer, C., Alvarez-Muñoz, D., Brennholt, N., Bourrain, X., Buchinger, S., ... Reifferscheid, G. (2014). Microplastics in freshwater ecosystems: What we know and what we need to know. *Environmental Sciences Europe*, *26*(1), 1–9. doi:10.118612302-014-0012-7 PMID:28936382

Warkentin, I. G., Sodhi, N. S., Espie, R. H. M., & Poole, A. F. (2005). Merlin (Falco columbarius). *The Birds of North America Online*. doi:10.2173/bna.44

Watters, D. L., Yoklavich, M. M., Love, M. S., & Schroeder, D. M. (2010). Assessing marine debris in deep seafloor habitats off California. *Marine Pollution Bulletin*, *60*(1), 131–138. doi:10.1016/j.marpolbul.2009.08.019 PMID:19751942

Webb, H. K., Crawford, R. J., Sawabe, T., & Ivanova, E. P. (2009). Poly(ethylene terephthalate) Polymer Surfaces as a Substrate for Bacterial Attachment and Biofilm Formation. *Microbes and Environments*, *24*(1), 39–42. doi:10.1264/jsme2.ME08538 PMID:21566352

Wegner, A., Besseling, E., Foekema, E. M., Kamermans, P., & Koelmans, A. A. (2012). Effects of nanopolystyrene on the feeding behavior of the blue mussel (Mytilus edulis L.). *Environmental Toxicology and Chemistry*, *31*(11), 2490–2497. doi:10.1002/etc.1984 PMID:22893562

Welden, N. A., Abylkhani, B., & Howarth, L. M. (2018). The effects of trophic transfer and environmental factors on microplastic uptake by plaice, Pleuronectes plastessa, and spider crab, Maja squinado. *Environmental Pollution*, *239*, 351–358. doi:10.1016/j.envpol.2018.03.110 PMID:29674213

Woodall, L. C., Robinson, L. F., Rogers, A. D., Narayanaswamy, B. E., & Paterson, G. L. J. (2015). Deep-sea litter: A comparison of seamounts, banks and a ridge in the Atlantic and Indian Oceans reveals both environmental and anthropogenic factors impact accumulation and composition. *Frontiers of Materials Science*, *2*. doi:10.3389/fmars.2015.00003

Worm, B., Barbier, E. B., Beaumont, N., Duffy, J. E., Folke, C., Halpern, B. S., ... Watson, R. (2006). Impacts of biodiversity loss on ocean ecosystem services. *Science*, *314*(5800), 787–790. doi:10.1126cience.1132294 PMID:17082450

Wright, S. L., Thompson, R. C., & Galloway, T. S. (2013). The physical impacts of microplastics on marine organisms: A review. *Environmental Pollution*, *178*, 483–492. doi:10.1016/j.envpol.2013.02.031 PMID:23545014

Yawson, R. M. (2009). *The Ecological System of Innovation: A New Architectural Framework for a Functional Evidence-Based Platform for Science and Innovation Policy*. doi:10.2139srn.1417676

Yin, X., Zhang, J., & Wang, X. (2004a). *Sequential injection analysis system for the determination of arsenic by hydride generation atomic absorption spectrometry*. doi:10.1017/CBO9781107415324.004

Yin, X., Zhang, J., & Wang, X. (2004b). Sequential injection analysis system for the determination of arsenic by hydride generation atomic absorption spectrometry. In Fenxi Huaxue (Vol. 32). doi:10.1017/CBO9781107415324.004

ADDITIONAL READING

Bergmann, M., Gutow, L., & Klages, M. (Eds.). (2015). *Marine anthropogenic litter*. Cham: Springer; doi:10.1007/978-3-319-16510-3

Bergmann, M., Tekman, M. B., & Gutow, L. (2017). Marine litter: Sea change for plastic pollution. *Nature*, *544*(7650), 297–297. doi:10.1038/544297a PMID:28425989

Coe, J. M., & Rogers, D. B. (Eds.). (1997). *Marine Debris: Sources, Impacts, and Solutions*. New York, NY: Springer-Verlag New York; doi:10.1007/978-1-4613-8486-1

Derraik, J. G. B. (2002). The pollution of the marine environment by plastic debris: A review. *Marine Pollution Bulletin*, *44*(9), 842–852. doi:10.1016/S0025-326X(02)00220-5 PMID:12405208

Galgani, F. (2015). Marine litter, future prospects for research. *Frontiers of Materials Science*, *2*, 87. doi:10.3389/fmars.2015.00087

Jambeck, J. R., Geyer, R., Wilcox, C., Siegler, T. R., Perryman, M., Andrady, A., ... Law, K. L. (2015). Plastic waste inputs from land into the ocean. *Science*, *347*(6223), 768–771. doi:10.1126cience.1260352 PMID:25678662

Thompson, R. C., Olson, Y., Mitchell, R. P., Davis, A., Rowland, S. J., John, A. W. G., ... Russell, A. E. (2004). Lost at Sea: Where Is All the Plastic? *Science*, *304*(5672), 838. doi:10.1126cience.1094559 PMID:15131299

Wright, S. L., Thompson, R. C., & Galloway, T. S. (2013). The physical impacts of microplastics on marine organisms: A review. *Environmental Pollution*, *178*, 483–492. doi:10.1016/j.envpol.2013.02.031 PMID:23545014

KEY TERMS AND DEFINITIONS

Anthropogenic: Changes in nature originating by human activity, in this case, plastic litter made by people.

Bioaccumulation: The accumulation of toxic substances in various tissue or organ of the living organism.

Bioavailability: Absorption that reaches the living organism system.

Biomagnification: The increasing concentration of a pollutant at higher levels in a food chain.

Ingestion: The consumption process of a substance by a living organism, in this case, plastic litter material.

Marine Plastic Litter: Human created wasted made from synthetic material that deliberately or accidentally to the marine ecosystem and will affect the marine organism.

Microplastic: Microscopic size of the plastic litter, have a size less than 5mm and has dangerous potential compared to larger plastic sizes.

Plastic: A synthetic material made by a human that easily shaped or molded.

Thermoplastic: Plastic substance formed by heating and harden by cooling, able to repeat the process.

Thermosetting: Plastic substance formed set permanently after the heating process.

Chapter 7
Detrimental Impact of Plastic Outcome on Agriculture:
Biggest Threat to Environment

Shivom Singh
ITM University Gwalior, India

Prachi Dixit
ITM University Gwalior, India

Kajal S. Rathore
Government KRG Autonomous College, India

Neha Sharma
Amity University Madhya Pradesh, India

ABSTRACT

Generally, plastic is made up of non-biodegradable chemicals i.e. polyolefin, polyester, and polyurethanes. This is hardly surprising since the use of polythene bags has infiltrated all sectors of economy, agriculture, consumer goods, and especially in packaging, where polythene is increasingly replacing jute, paper, wood, and glass. Polythene bags can release harmful chemicals into the surrounding agricultural soil, which can then seep into ground water or other surrounding water sources. This can cause serious harm to the species that drink this water. Unlike natural organic material they do not disintegrate with time but keep accumulating in the environment. So it is very difficult to dispose of the polythene bags. If the polythene bags burned in agriculture land, they release harmful chemicals like Cd, Pb, CO, NO_X and SO_2, which causes many diseases in animals as well as in human beings. The accumulation of polythene bags also makes agricultural soil sterile/barren as it stops the gaseous exchange. In normal agricultural land, the concentration of oxygen is 3 ppm. Where polythene is present, the concentration of oxygen in soil decreases to 0.001 ppm. In addition, the polythene pollution can adversely affect agricultural lands, waterways, and oceans.

DOI: 10.4018/978-1-5225-9452-9.ch007

INTRODUCTION

At present stage, plastics are everywhere, in our home, school, work, playground, parks, and beaches; life without plastic seems to be impossible due to light in weight, low in cost, durability and easy manufacturing in any shape make it popular in a very short time. Accretion of plastic-based products in the environment shows harmful effects on wildlife, marine life and terrestrial life and human is a main concern for this crisis. The other main quality of plastic is that it is not easily decomposed therefore; chemical structure of most plastics renders them resistant to many natural processes of degradation. Plastic also pollutes without being littered purposely, through the discharge of compounds used in its manufacture. Indeed, pollution of the environment by chemicals leached from plastics into air and water is an emerging area of apprehension.

Number of studies show that, more than six million tons of plastic waste goes un-recycled every year in India. Over the past decade we have produced and consumed extra plastic than the entire century. The plastic pollution can harmfully affect lands, water streams and ocean along with animals that are widely injured or killed by plastic pollution. Plastics are a variety of synthetic or semi-synthetic polymerization goods that can be formed into a permanent article having the possessions of plasticity. Community are using plastic bags, which are environmentally hazardous, for they're on a daily basis requirements generally for shopping purposes as an outcome of which, the environment and agricultural manure are thereby being polluted and contaminated too. Plastic Pollution has numerous harmful effects on the atmosphere such as on birds, fish, turtles, coral reefs, human health, and on tourism and the living of inhabitants. Discarded plastic bags which have also found their means into the land are not solitary extremely harmful but also sincerely detrimental for agriculture. Plastic bags are randomly discarded into millions of landfills wide-reaching which engage trillions of hectors of lands and release hazardous methane and carbon dioxide gases throughout their decaying phases in addition to extremely poisonous leachates from these landfills (Simmons, 2005).

Generally plastic is made up of polyolifins, polyster and polyurethanes, those all there chemicals are petroleum based and non-biodegradable. Big cities, town or even the remote hinterland, plastic is ubiquitous and is causing harm to India's ecological balance which finally comes back to haunt us. Though if seen globally, the crisis in India is relatively less grave but citing the population and increase in usage in plastic over some year. It is used in every field of life as it unaffected by moisture, acids and base. The stability of plastics and their possible for various applications, as well as extensive use as disposable substances were expected, but the troubles linked with plastic trash were not. It is supposed that public began to use plastic bags to hold groceries, foodstuffs and articles by hands or else in the 1970s, (Clapp & Swantoon, 2009) and these Polly bags became popularized speedily in the last part of the 20th century (Sugii, 2008).Thus, plastic bags should be prohibited global and their substitutes which are eco-friendly should be launched in order to determine these unbearable and poisonous troubles.

CONSUMPTION OF PLASTIC IN DIFFERENT AREAS

This is hardly surprising since the use of plastics has infiltrated all sectors of the economy. Infrastructure, agriculture building and construction, telecommunications, consumer's goods and packing are all high growth areas which indicate a spiraling demand for plastics. For instance, in packaging plastics are increasingly replacing jute, paper, wood, glass and metal due to low cost and easy availability. Even traditional areas such as agriculture and marine are also using plastics as a part of modern scientific methods of packaging. Plastics are being used in all sectors of the economy. From 1.88 million tons (1995-96), the domestic demand for plastics is expected to cross 4 million tons by year 2001-2002 and is continuously increasing with time (figure1).

Polythene bags or plastic bags are comprehensively used by the citizens and is referred to as one of the biggest progression of the millennium (Table1). The consequence of plastic pollution is associated with plastics being easy on the pocket and long lasting, which provides to elevated stages of plastics used by human beings (Hester& Harrison, 2011).

According to Greenpeace international report (2014) approximate yearly fabrication of plastic in world is approximately 100 million tons. Total 4% plastic extreme all over world and it has been expected that India's current per capita consumption of 1.6 kg of plastics is expected to rise to around 129% and all inclusive polyethylene demand is predictable to accumulate 8.2 million tons by 2023, up from 3.6 million tons in 2013 that would be largest in Asia (Figure2) (www.buisness-standard.com).

CAUSES OF PLASTIC BAGS USE

Plastic is derived from the Greek word "Plastics" which means "Moulded". However a growing lobby of antiplastic activities worldwide but there is much argues in favor of plastics. They can be moulded into any shape and therefore the material of choice for packaging. They occupy less space and are waterproof. Without plastic 400% more material by weight and 200% more material by volume would be needed to make packaging while the volume of packaging would be more than double.

For every seven trucks needed to deliver paper grocery bags to the store. Only one truck is needed to carry the same number of polythene bags. Using paper bags, the only available alternative to plastic

Figure1. Figure showing the plastic consumption in India
Source: Central Pollution Control Board (CPCB)

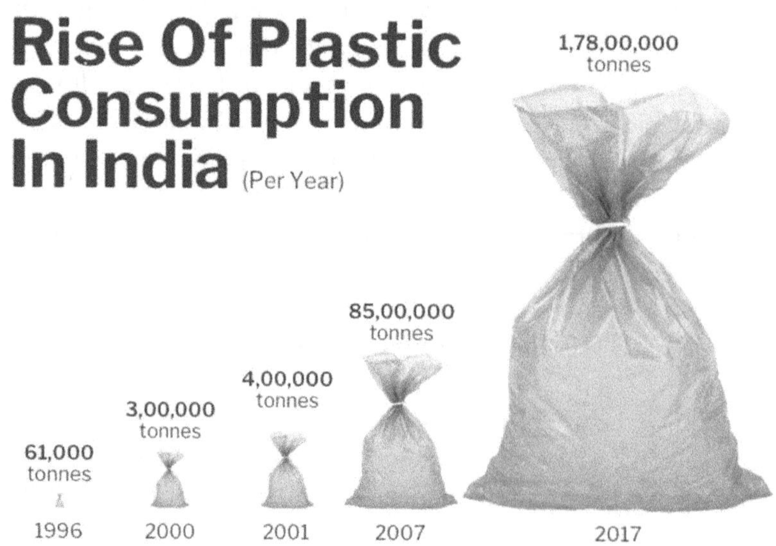

Table1. Different type of plastics and its common uses

S. No.	Polymer type	Short name	Common uses
A.	Polyethylene Terephthalate	PET	Beer and soft drink bottles, water bottles, and carpet, paneling and salad trays.
B.	High Density Polyethylene	HDPE	Milh pouches, agricultural pipes, playground equipments, carry bags, shampoo bottles and recycling bins.
C.	Polyvinyl Chloride	PVC	Non-food bottles, chairs, window and door frames, pipes, fencing and flooring.
D.	Low Density Polyethylene	LDPE	Wash bottles, plastic bags, tubing, packing films, carrier bags and dispensing bottles.
E.	Polypropylene	PP	Fibres and filaments for carpets, margarine tubes, auto parts, food containers and dishware.
F.	Polystyrene	PS	Plastic cutlery, yoghurt pots, egg cartons, protective packaging.
G.	Other References	O	Polycarbonate, laminates and Bakelite.

Figure 2. Different types of plastics
Source: Times of India (TOI), 2018

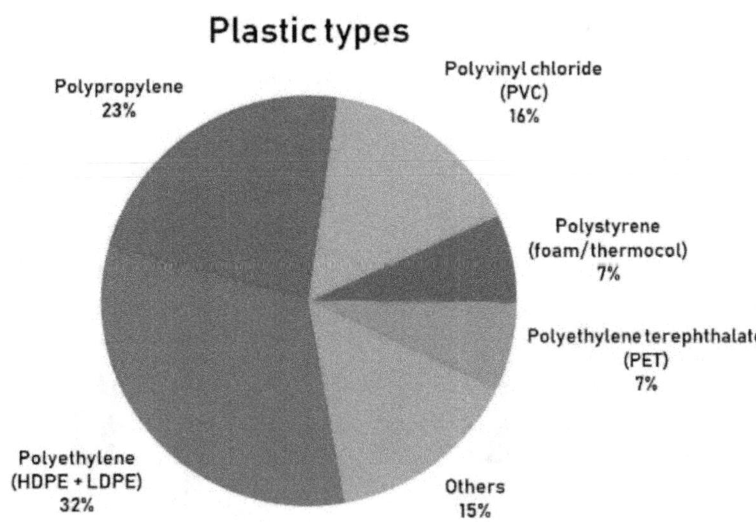

bags, means cutting down more trees. Plastic bags are also much stronger than paper bags. Especially when the kitchen garbage is put into paper bags they tear easily or water which is a major component of kitchen garbage, leaks out.

This is only just surprising since the used of plastic bags has infiltrated all sectors of economy. Infrastructures, agriculture, building and construction, telecommunication, consumer goods and packaging are all high growth areas which indicate a spiraling demand of plastic for instance, in packaging plastics are increasingly replacing jute, paper, wood, glass and metal etc (Figure 3 & 4).

Figure 3.Different uses of plastic in commercial and consumer goods are presented in given below
Source: Anh Nguyen, (2018)

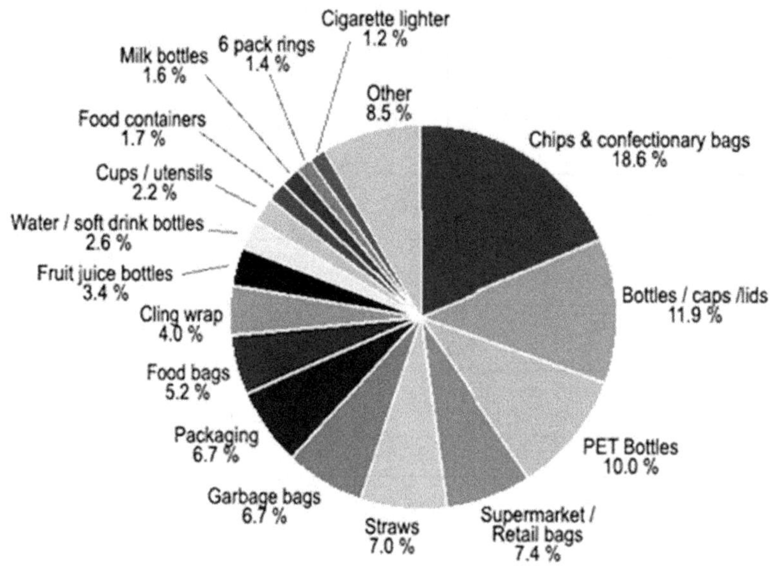

Figure 4. Global plastic packaging market, 2014-2020 in kilo tons
Source: Zion Research Analysis, (2016)

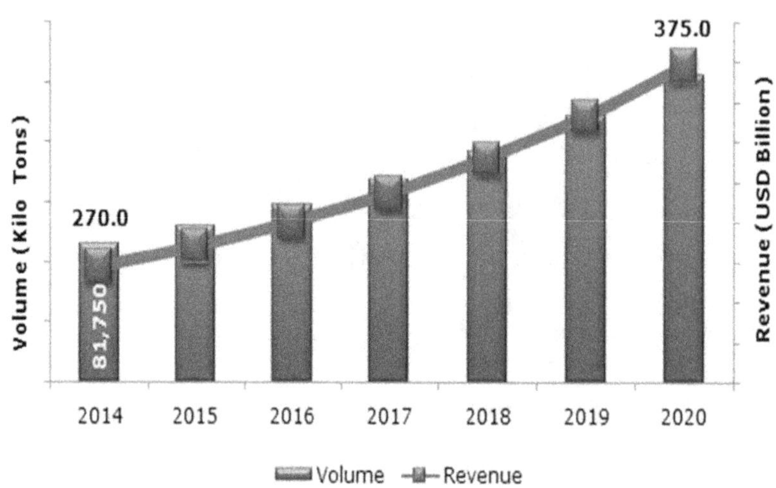

CONSEQUENCE HEALTH HAZARDS OF PLASTIC DEBRIS ON DIFFERENT KIND OF ENVIRONMET AND HUMAN

Plastic is non-biodegradable, lightweight, easy to go and its durability are becoming unavoidable to use in many daily activities of the developing countries such as India. Unlike natural organic material they do not disintegrate with time and keep accumulating in the environment. It is very difficult to dispose off the plastic waste while some is melted and reprocessed, some is burned, some is disposed off in dumps and some is discarded, turning into rivers and field.

The environment has been classified in different classes. It is tremendously terrible information that plastic is presenting poisonous properties on every mankind of environment. Consequences associated with plastic debris on different kind of environment are as follows:

Impact of Plastic Bags on Aquatic Environment

The threat to aquatic environment is caused by aquatic debris of plastic (Webb, Arnott, Crawford & Ivanova, 2013). Due to plastic debris, there has been reduce in aquatic fauna inhabitants, either they tangled through their body or they were ingested by fishes and turtles faulting debris to be kill (Derraik, 2002).According to a report published in Dainik Bhaskar newspaper, 2018,about 32 million tons of plastic is harvested every year in the world. Out of these 1.2 million tons of plastic debris goes into the sea. Besides survey also revealed that, from 1950 to 2018, 8.3 billion tons of plastic was found in aquatic environment. If the current situation of plastic production remains the same, then about 12 billion tons of plastic garbage will be in the atmosphere by 2050. This will be equal to the weight of 10 million blue whales. While there are just 20,000 blue whales in the world right now. Another report of Dainik Bhaskar, 2018 says that annually 10 lakhs of marine animals are being killed by plastic, Whale fish were found dead on the coast of Indonesia. On study it was found that, the cause of death was presence of more than 1000 plastic pieces from its stomach, including 115 cups, 25 plastic bags, 4 plastic bottles and plastic pieces. The list of affected species signifies that oceanic garbage is affecting a considerable figure of species. It affects at least 267 species global, as well as 86% of all sea turtle species, 44% of all seabird species and 43% of all marine mammal species (Laist, 1997). The amassing of such trash can reduce the gas exchange between the overlying waters and the stoma waters of the sediments, and the ensuing hypoxia or anoxia in the benthos can obstruct with the ordinary environment implementation and modify the framework of existence on the aquatic ground (Goldberg, 1994). There is still comparatively diminutive information on the impact of plastic pollution on the aquatic environment. Seeing as the use of plastic continuous to enhances, so the quantity of plastic is polluting the aquatic environment.

Impact of Plastic Bags on Atmosphere

Plastic is composed of main noxious pollutants; it has the latent to origin immense destruction to the atmosphere in the form of air pollution. Smoldering of plastic desecrate in the open air, leads to environmental pollution as a result of the discharge of toxic compounds like, cadmium (Cd), lead (Pb), NO_X, SO_2, CO. The polluted air when inhaled by humans and animal cause respiratory diseases besides other health related problems. Open smoldering of plastics also liberate huge quantity of poisonous components and climate changing pollution due to black carbon, which significantly contribute to climate change. Polycyclic aromatic hydrocarbons (PAHs), polychlorinated biphenyls (PCBs), dioxins and furans are among the most toxic chemicals commonly released into the air when burning plastic waste, chronic exposure cause cancer and interfere with hormone functions (Carisse, 2018). According to the institute of Lifecycle Environmental Assessment (1990), the manufacturing of two plastic bags generates 1.1 kg of atmospheric pollution, which contributes to acid rain and smog. Acid rain is documented as a severe danger to natural and human-made atmospheres, mainly in areas which have traditionally relied greatly on coal. Plastic elements are now being found in the stomach of birds in the Antarctic and sub-Antarctic. Birds with plastic in their stomachs may prevent sensitivity starving, prevent stalking for food, and ultimately starve to fatality, on the other hand, chicks that have ingested plastics can suffer intestinal obstruction and may ulcers. This is a warning sign that plastic pollution is rising since these areas were measured to be unaffected by pollution. An article published in Times of India (TOI) 28 November, waste and garbage pickers live right in front of the gate of Yamuna biodiversity park, Wazirabad and every 2-3 days they burn plastic waste, which cause a lot of pollution and that too in front of the biodiversity park which not only affects humans but also the fauna of the park adversely (Singh, 2018).

Impact of Plastic Bags on Agriculture or Landfill

Plastic is growing day by day is a big threat not only for the environment but also for the human, animals and plants. Once again, the report has been issued for clean cities in the country, but when it comes to garbage management, in the next 30 years, we need 88 sq km of land for waste management only. This information has released from research by ASSOCHAM (Associated Chambers of Commerce and Industry of India). According to a recently released report by the International Organization World Wide Fund, plastic pollution will be doubled by 2030. The number of plastic accumulated during the year 1950 to 2016 is expected to be deposited in the next decade only. With this, plastic waste can reach 300 million tons in the oceans. By the year 2030, carbon dioxide emissions will triple on plastic combustion, which will increase heart disease rapidly. Focusing on Dainik Bhaskar newspaper, India is the third largest plastic consuming country in the world. According to the annual report 2015-16 of the Central Pollution Control Board, more than 1.5 million tons of plastic production in India is produce annually. The total number of plastic-making units in different states is 2243 and there is a plastic composting unit in Uttar Pradesh. In total, 312 non-registered plastic factories are running in Andhra Pradesh, Assam, Jammu and Kashmir, Jharkhand and Uttar Pradesh, there is no restriction on them. In the global scenario, by the year 2020, 12 billion tons of plastic waste will be deposited worldwide, which will be the biggest threat for the environment.

The agricultural impacts of plastic bags are detrimental in numerous characteristics and accordingly these plastic bags grow to be the danger to our food and existence. As a case we may pass on to the Cape Town of South Africa where there were more than 3,000 plastic bags at an assured moment that sheltered each kilometer of path (Ryan & Rice, 1996).

Plastic bags are accidentally discarded into millions of landfill globally which engage trillions of hectors of lands and emanate hazardous methane and carbon dioxide gases for the duration of their decaying stages as well as highly toxic leachates from these landfills (Simmons, 2005). It successfully obstructs sewerage pipes and litters agricultural lands due to agricultural yields cannot cultivate where the plastic bags reside because their roots cannot be in motion around due to the ever there of plastic bags. The most noteworthy harmful impacts of the plastic bags on agriculture such as diminution in agricultural soil productiveness reduce in nitrogen fixation, enormous defeat of nutrients in the soil, diminish in crop yield, disproportion in flora and fauna on soil etc. due to several uncaring factors, approximately 96% of all plastic grocery bags are discarded into agricultural field (Williamson, 2003).

Deposition of plastic bags in the agricultural land can affect the air, water and soil ratio it creates disturbances in aeration process and delaying the growth of plants and crops. "Due to impact on crop growth, yield and efficiency could be affected and, in the long run, pose a hazard to food security" (Times of India; 08 August, 2018).

Impact of Plastic Bags on Health

Discarded plastic bags which have also initiated their mode into the land are not only acutely detrimental but also critically damaging for human and animal or cattle health.

Animal or cattle, especially cow ingest the plastic bags which are dumped by human beings at anywhere and develop health complications. This finally results in their death, "says Gustavo Pinto, a veterinary surgeon, the vets from six animal husbandry hospitals and around twelve dispensaries in rural areas usually carry out postmortems on site only if cattle deaths have medico-legal implications to settle compensation claims. Otherwise, there are no figures of the number of animals dying from plastic in another case Astrid Almeida, veterinary director of the Assagao-based International Animal Rescue (IAR) says that, when they do conduct some surgeries on animals, it is often a shocking revelation for the animal rescuers that, "even an apparently healthy cow could be having a rumen half filled with plastic bags. Actually, the cattle have three non-glandular fore-stomach compartments i.e rumen, reticulum and omasum and the fourth glandular compartment is abomasums also called true stomach because the enzymatic digestion of food is takes place in this compartment. The feed enters from the reticulum to the rumen, omasum and finally the abomasums explains by P K Naik, animal nutritionist at the Indian Council of Agricultural Research (ICAR), (TOI, 3 January 2013) but when the plastic is ingurgitated by cattle it enters from the reticulum to the rumen and cattle may not be capable to absorb the real food due to the blockage of rumen, various pathological conditions that are encountered due to ingestion of plastic bags in animal such as tympani, immunosuppressant and complete or partial anorexia, loss of weight and reduction of milk quantity (Ramaswamy & Sharma, 2011) once plastic bags enters their entrails, it can neither be digested nor vomited as once the plastic is ingested by the cattle and animal there is no technique to remove it, says Amrut Singh, an animal rescuer, suffocation occurs and die a slow death from starvation, infection and sometimes chocking on plastic bags (Alessa, 2016).

Plastic bag usage may build way to cancerous diseases caused by the uncontrolled explosion of carcinogenic materials (Spivey, 2003). Bisphenol A (BPA) and phthalates are common synthetic chemicals which can be released from beverages and food containers and other consumer products that commonly interfere with human endocrine system. These chemicals can leach into food and drinking materials and leaching process is accelerated by again and again process of washing of food and drink containers and leaching increases when plastic material comes in contact with oily foods and when it's heated. As a result, reusable water bottles, baby milk bottles and food cans adversely impact on human health when these items are used to carry food materials. The BPA is considered as a female hormone "estrogen" because it has been associated with many diseases such as rapid puberty, ovarian damage, cardiovascular disorder, endometrial hyperplasia, risk of breast cancer, miscarriages, ovarian syndrome and obesity etc.

BPA and phthalates can easily enter into the body of the newborn baby through breastfeeding and pregnancy so these chemicals will be able to harm them easily. BPA and phthalates can cross the placenta, resulting in growth retardation and neurological harm. There are also evidences to suggest hormonal derangements and cancers in children (Zaman, 2012).

Plastic can be easily entered in the food chain, when fish consume plastics and toxic chemicals leached by plastics, human being eat those contaminated fish. Even if a fish is cleaned before cooking, they may still be contaminated with toxic chemicals in its flesh. Chemicals humans are exposed to due to eating contaminated fish are associated with birth defects, immune system problems, heart, brain and lever diseases and lead, cadmium and mercury poisoning.

POLICY MEASURES AND REGULATIONS FOR REDUCING USAGE OF PLASTIC BAGS

Worldwide it is not easy to inflict absolute ban on plastic bags use but various policy measures are being taken to decrease the consumption of plastic bags in India. Recycled plastics create and convention rules were informed by Government of India in the 1999 and further revised in 2003 to have managed over the manufacture, sale and use of recycled plastic bags and recycled plastic containers. Under these rules, units manufacturing plastic bags were necessary to register with their own State Pollution Control Boards (SPCBs) or Pollution Control Committees (PCCs) prior to the beginning of creation (report published in Toxics Link, 2014).

The Ministry of Environment, Forests and Climate Change (MoEF&CC) has banned the manufacture and use of plastic bags less than 8X12 inches in size and micron in thickness. The central government has recently approved a ruling under the supplies of the Environment Protection Act 1986, confining the sale of some products in plastic bags. Some states like Punjab, Kerala, Madhya Pradesh, etc. are still maintain width of carry bags less than 40 micron, however as per Polythene Waste Management (PWM), 2011, the width of carry bags shall not less than 40 micron. Also some states like Maharashtra and Tamil Nadu has improved width 50 and 60 micron respectively (CPCB, 2013).

Himachal Pradesh Non-biodegradable Garbage (Control) Act, 1995 has been initiated by the Government of Himachal Pradesh. The act suitably predicts prevention of throwing or putting plastic objects in municipal places and to ease the collection through trash in particular and marked trash containers for non-biodegradables, located at convenient places.

Maharashtra, Delhi, Punjab, Rajasthan, Himachal Pradesh, Goa and West Bengal, among others have banned the use of plastic bags. The union territory Chandigarh implemented a complete ban on the manufacture, use, storage and sale of plastic bags in the entire region since 2008. Recently Rajasthan in 2010 and Haryana in 2011 imposed a complete ban on plastic bags. In January 2009, the Delhi government also ordered a whole ban on the use of all plastic bags in market areas (Table 2& Figure 5).

PLASTIC BAGS AND ITS MANAGEMENT

Recycling

Due to throwing polythene or plastic bags on the road, not only sewer lines, drains chalks but due to cattle eating it dies. Recycling of plastic bags by manufacturers has been very successful and has proven economical, but recovering of discarded plastic bags from consumers is more difficult (Ansari, 2017). Plastic materials can be recycled in a variety of ways and the ease of recycling varies among polymer type, package design and product type. For example, rigid containers consisting of a single polymer are simpler and more economic to recycle than multilayer packages. Recycling of plastic bags comprises of some key steps: collection, sorting, size reduction and cleaning, further separation and compatibilization to reduce contamination. In this method collection of plastic wastes can be done by bring schemes then sorting of plastic bags material by manual and automatic method. These methods have the capability to separate polymer by type or grade. In size reduction and cleaning step includes dry cleaning, which cleans surfaces of polymer materials through friction without using water. After size reduction, a range

Table 2.Table showing the different states of India in which plastic has been banned

S. No.	State	Plastic bag ban
1.	Arunachal Pradesh	The use of carry bags have been banned in six districts.
2.	Gujarat	Banned in two districts, Kutch and Junagarh.
3.	Haryana	Yes
4.	Himachal Pradesh	Yes
5.	Jharkhand	Yes
6.	Kerala	Ban on sale and use of carry bags in Sannidhan, Nitakkal and Erumeli.
7.	Madhya Pradesh	The use of plastic carry bags is banned in Gwalior.
8.	Meghalaya	Yes
9.	Nagaland	Yes
10.	Odisha	In pilgrimage centres, use of carry bags has been banned.
11.	Rajasthan	Yes
12.	Sikkim	Yes
13.	Tripura	Yes
14.	Uttar Pradesh	The government has issued a notification on the complete ban on use of plastic carry bags within 2 km from the mid-stream of Ganga river.
15.	West Bengal	Blanket in ecologically sensitive areas and in heritage sites.
16.	Delhi	Yes
17.	Chandigarh	Yes

Source: Toxics Link, (2014)

Figure 5. Figure demonstrating the different states of India in which complete, partial and not banned on usage of plastic carry bags
Source: Central Pollution Control Board (CPCB)

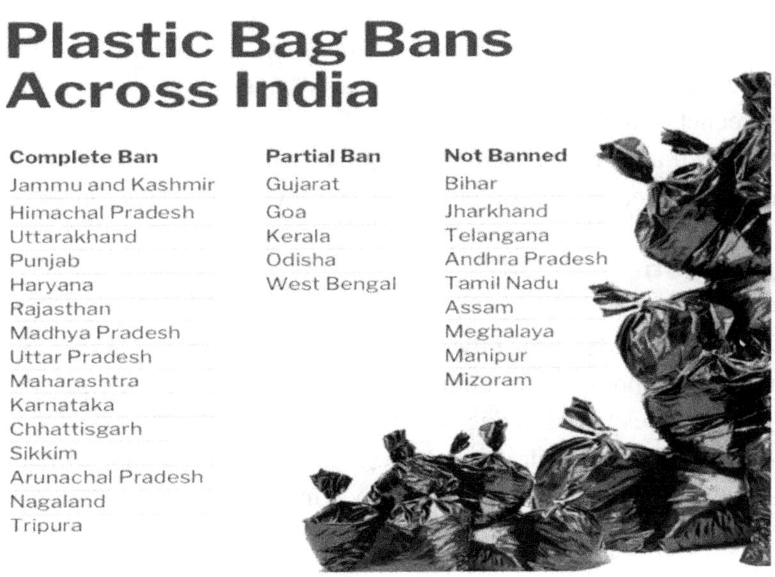
Plastic Bag Bans
Across India
Complete Ban
Jammu and Kashmir
Himachal Pradesh
Uttarakhand
Punjab
Haryana
Rajasthan
Madhya Pradesh
Uttar Pradesh
Maharashtra
Karnataka
Chhattisgarh
Sikkim
Arunachal Pradesh
Nagaland
Tripura
Partial Ban
Gujarat
Goa
Kerala
Odisha
West Bengal
Not Banned
Bihar
Jharkhand
Telangana
Andhra Pradesh
Tamil Nadu
Assam
Meghalaya
Manipur
Mizoram

of separation techniques can be applied for further separation of plastic bags (Hopewell, Dvorak & Kosior, 2009).

About 60% of plastic garbage were used for recycling in every part of the world were accepted. The main institutes of different countries to use these processes are:

- In Japan: Plastic waste management institute and European centre for plastic in Environment.
- In America: Plastic recycling foundation. America plastic council.
- In Canada: National packaging protocol and environmental and plastic institute, Recycling Council of British Plastic Federation.
- In Malaysia: Plastic Waste management, Task Force are main.
- In India at present about 2000 plastic recycling industries were mentions.

A news published in Dainik Bhaskar (01 December, 2018) news paper, Chris and Laura Moriarty, who lives in Washington, US, they make artificial hands by using 3D printing technology from marine plastics and are provided them to the needful persons. They used 15 bottles and spent about 3200 rupees in making of artificial hands. For this work, he has also created an organization named Million Waves Project. According to this, about 2,800 million pounds a year or so, about 1,270 million kg of plastic is available in the sea.

Reduce Use of Plastic Bags

Sometimes it has been observed that not all types of plastic can be recycled. Only 1% of plastic waste generated is recycled as it is a costly process and rest is dumped in dumping grounds, at dumping grounds it takes approximately 300 years for a plastic to naturally degrade in environment (CPCB, 2013). In this step plastic pollution can be reduced by using less plastic bags and switching to alternatives. Reduction of plastic pollution can occur by altering the design, manufacture or use of plastic products and materials (Dara, Terfa & Deng, 2018). These are some of the tips we can follow as individuals to minimize the use of plastic bags:

- Reuse plastic bags for many times to reduce consumption.
- Don't buy convenience food packages in plastic carry bags.
- Avoid buying products using plastic packaging.
- Choose the products that can be reused and recycled.
- Use glass containers instead of plastic bags for storing vegetables and other food items.

Enzymatic Degradation

Some strains that are capable of degrading the plastic bags and materials are*Brevibacillus spp., Bacillus spp.,* where protease is responsible for degradation of polythene (Sivan, 2011). Papain and urease are the two proteolytic enzymes found to degrade medical polyester. Polymer degraded by papain was due to the hydrolysis of urethane and urea linkages producing free amine and hydroxyl group (Phua, Castillo, Anderson & Hiltner,1987). Microbial enzymes induce the rate of biodegradation of plastics very effectively without causing any harm to the environment.

Table 3.Enzymes those are responsible for plastic degradation

S. No.	Enzymes	Microorganisms	References
1.	Manganese peroxidase	*Phanerochaete chrysosporium*	Shimao, (2001).
2.	Cutinase	*Fusarium, Aspergillus oryzae*	Shimao, (2001), Maeda & Yamagata, (2005).
3.	Catalase, protease	*Aspergillus niger*	Tokiwa & Calabia, (2009).
4.	Lipase	*Rhizopus delemar*	Tokiwa & Calabia, (2009).
5.	Glucosidases	*Aspergillus flavus*	Tokiwa & Calabia, (2009).
6.	Lipase	*Penicillium, Rhizopus arrizus*	Tokiwa & Calabia, (2009).
7.	Serine hydrolase	*Pseudomonas stutzeri*	Shimao, (2001).
8.	Extracellular enzyme (not characterized)	*Streptomyces spp.*	Pometto, Lee, &Johnson, (1992).

A report published by US Department of Energy, researchers is trying to improve the enzyme further to allow it to be used industrially to degrade plastic. Researchers made the breakthrough while examining the structure of a natural enzyme, which evolved in a waste recycling centre in Japan. Allowing a bacterium to degrades plastic as a food source. The goal was to determine its structure and how it works. But they ended up engineering an enzyme better than the natural one. It could result in a recycling solution for millions of tons of plastic bags and bottles. This usually takes hundreds of years to biodegrade.

Microbial Degradation

Microorganisms are involved in the degradation of plastics. The microorganisms that are responsible for biodegradation differ from each other and have their own optimal growth conditions (Wackett & Harshberger, 2001.). In this process polythene can be degraded by microbes through two mechanisms, aerobic and anaerobic. In aerobic degradation oxygen gets acts as an electron acceptor and final products are carbon dioxide and water and anaerobic degradation occur in absence of oxygen and therefore microbe use nitrate, sulphate and iron as electron acceptor (Grover, Gupta, Chandra & Kumari et al., 2015).

RECOMMENDATIONS AND ALTERNATIVE SUGGESTIONS OF PLASTIC BAGS

Taking food substitutes in polythene colored bags is like inviting illnesses. According to experts, the chemicals added for polythene color are harmful for health. There are many environment friendly alternatives to plastic bags, such as biodegradable bags, reusable bags, paper bags and jute bags, polymer blended bitumen road construction and bioplastics.

Use of Biodegradable Plastic Bags

The term biodegradable means capable of being decomposed by bacteria or other biological means (Collins, 2000). Biodegradable plastic is made from starch had been marketed as the ultimate be good feel good material. The claims have already been contested as test have shown that even under ideal conditions the plastic mainly disintegrated into very small pieces on land and did not dissolve in sea water on the land plastic carry bag chock the sail. The world of oceans and sea are being affected by plastic bags

Table 4.Microorganisms those are responsible for plastic degradation

S. No.	Microorganism	References
1.	*Bacillus cereus*	Abrusci, Pablos, Corrales, Lopez-Marín, & Marín(2011), Suresh, Maruthamuthu, Palanisamy, Ragunathan, &Pandiyaraj (2011), Aswale (2010).
2.	*Bacillus subtilis*	Priyanka &Archana (2011), Abrusci et al. (2011), Nwachukwu, Obidi, & Odocha(2010).
3.	*Bacillus spp.*	Usha, Sangeetha, &Palaniswamy(2011).
4.	*Bacillus megaterium*	Abrusci et al. (2011).
5.	*Pseudomonas spp.*	Priyanka &Archana (2011), Kathiresan (2003), Nanda, Sahu, & Abraham(2010), Usha et al. (2011).
6.	*Pseudomonas aeruginosa*	Nwachukwu et al. (2010), Kyaw, Champakalakshmi, Sakharkar, Lim, & Sakharkar(2012), Aswale (2010).
7.	*Pseudomonas putida*	Kyaw et al. (2012), Nwachukwu et al. (2010).
8.	*Pseudomonas syringae*	Kyaw et al. (2012).
9.	*Staphylococcus spp.*	Reddy (2008), Kathiresan (2003), Usha et al (2011).
10.	*Staphylococcus aureus*	Priyanka & Archana (2011).
11.	*Staphylococcus epidermis*	Chatterjee, Roy, Roy, & Banerjee (2010).
12.	*Streptococcus spp.*	Reddy (2008), Kathiresan (2003).
13.	*Streptococcus lactis*	Priyanka & Archana (2011).
14.	*Streptococcus aureus*	Aswale (2010).
15.	*Micrococcus spp.*	Reddy (2008), Kathiresan (2003).
16.	*Micrococcus luteus*	Priyanka & Archana (2011).
17.	*Micrococcus lylae*	Aswale (2010).
18.	*Streptomyces spp.*	El-Shafei, Abd El-Nasser, Kansoh, &Ali, (1998), Usha et al (2011).
19.	*Streptomyces vinidosporus T7A*	Lee, Pometto, Fratzke, & Bailey(1991), Pometto et al., (1992).
20.	*Streptomyces badius 252*	Lee, et al., (1991).
21.	*Streptomyces setonii 75 Vi 2*	Lee, et al., (1991).
22.	*Rhodococcus ruber*	Sivan, (2011), Chandra & Rustgi (1997).
23.	*Rhodococcus rhodochrous*	Bonhomme,Cuer,Delort, Lemaire, Sancelme, et al., (2003).
24.	*Proteus vulgaris*	Priyanka & Archana (2011).
25.	*Bravibacillus borstelensis*	Abrusci, et al., (2011).
26.	*Serratia marscence*	Aswale (2010).
27.	*Nocardia steroids*	Bonhomme, et al., (2003).
28.	*Arthrobacter spp.*	Balasubramanian,Natarajan, Hemambika, Ramesh Sumathi, et al., (2010).
29.	*Diplococcus spp.*	Reddy (2008).
30.	*Moraxella spp.*	Reddy (2008), Kathiresan (2003).
31.	*Penicillium spp.*	Priyanka & Archana (2011).
32.	*Aspergillus niger*	Aswale (2010), Priyanka & Archana (2011), Kathiresan (2003), Reddy (2008), Nwachukwu et al., (2010), Aswale (2011).
33.	*Aspergillus ridiculans*	Priyanka & Archana (2011), Reddy (2008), Usha, et al., (2011).
34.	*Aspergillus flavus*	Priyanka & Archana (2011), Reddy (2008), El-Shafei (1998), Usha (2011).
35.	*Aspergillus glaucus*	Priyanka & Archana (2011), Reddy (2008), Kathiresan (2003), Aswale (2010).
36.	*Aspergillus ornatus*	Reddy (2008).
37.	*Aspergillus cremus*	Reddy (2008).
38.	*Aspergillus candidus*	Reddy (2008).
39.	*Aspergillus nidulance*	Kathiresan (2003).
40.	*Phanerochaete chrysosporium*	Lee, et al.,(1991).
41.	*Cladosporium cladosporides*	Bonhomme et al., (2003).

and similar trash to the extent that they kill sea birds. It has been estimated that world merchant ship dump 6,39,000 plastic containers including bags into sea each day.

Sephony Environmental Limited, England were among the first to make biodegradable plastic. According to this institute that new degradable plastic were degraded by many factors like; UV rays, heat, oxygen etc. Water and carbon dioxide cannot degrade these types of plastics and these factors would remain in the environment.

Biodegradable plastic are being heralded as safer than the usage of non biodegradable plastics, nonetheless there are many types of degradable and biodegradable plastics and to make the problem more challenging, not all of the biodegradable and compostable alternative plastics are environment friendly. So it needs to remember that degradable plastics or traditional polythene products are still harmful for agricultural crops and other plants when they decompose into the soil whereas the biodegradable plastics are not (Jalil, 2013).

Use of Biopolymer

Due to increase in plastic garbage disposal problem, the scientists are searching alternatives to remove this problem. Use of biopolymer is one of them. These polymers are extracted from plants and microorganisms. The main qualities of these biopolymers are that they are natural and easily degradable by microorganisms like bacteria in plant cells.

Biopolymers are made by carbohydrates and proteins, lactic acid found in some plants. Bacteria are making lactic acid polymer which is used in the formation of biodegradable polymer. The main row matter used in making of biodegradable plastic is polyhydrate butyrate which is extracted from Allelginise, Eutrots bacteria. These eutrots bacteria produce polyhydroxy butyrate (PHB). This PHB are flexible in nature about 80ºC after some months this is completely degradable and water and carbon dioxide are left.

Polymer Blended Bitumen Road Construction

It is one of the innovative idea of using plastic waste material. The non wetting property of plastic is also being implemented successfully in road construction business. When plastic waste is coated over aggregate, the coating reduces its affinity for water due to non wetting nature of polymer (Dara, 2018). The segregated plastic waste is stored and should be transported to the working site for drying. The dried plastic waste is shredded to 2-4 mm size and added to heated stone aggregate followed by mixing. Further the coated aggregate is mixed with hot bitumen, which is used for lying and compaction. Presently several roads have been constructed by using plastic waste with bitumen in many of the states such as; Himachal Pradesh, Tamil Nadu, West Bengal, Nagaland and Pondicherry (CPCB, 2017). Indonesia is producing 18.27 million tons of plastic waste annually, as well as making roads with recycled plastic.

Jute Bags

Jute bags are biodegradable containers made from plant fiber called jute. Jute bags are manufactured from jute yarn and are used for packing a wide range of industrial and agricultural goods such as; grains, oil seeds, salt and sugar and other food materials. Jute bags are also suitable for shopping and grocery purposes. Jute shopping bags and carriers are increasingly replacing the plastic non woven ones as ecology friendly alternatives. Due to their biodegradable nature jute bags are becoming an ecology friendly alternative (Rahman, 2009).

Paper Bags

It has been scientifically proven that paper bags are not harmful to the environment as plastic bags (ACG, 2006; Though, 2007). The natural fibers of paper and the renewable resource used have a positive image as the increase in volume of the paper bags. Scottish research has demonstrated that a levy on plastic bags can result in an increase of paper bag consumption (Though, 2007).

These are some of the suggestions we can follow as individuals to reduce the use of plastic carry bags in our daily life:

- Reduce the use of polythene wrapped goods.
- Discourages plastic bags production by imposing heavy taxes.
- Segregate waste at home and compost the trash.
- Avoid use plastic bottles.
- Strictly avoid the disposal single use plastic plates, bottles and cups etc.

CONCLUSION

The overall conclusion of this review is that plastic carry bags have been a part of daily life. Of principal concern from a human health perspective are endocrine disrupting properties of plastic components such as; BPA and phthalates. According to scientist Cd, Cr, Pb etc are used to make polythene colorful. Yellow color gets from Cd and Cr. In the colorful polythene, when the liquid food material is kept, these lethal chemicals dissolve in them and reach the human body. The effect of these chemicals is the risk of respiratory diseases. Some people resort to polythene bags because of lack of information and all the people resort to polythene bags to avoid the hassle of getting out of the house, without thinking that they are going to invite the diseases to their family.

Many governments have chosen the route of recycling. The trend of free ticket and shopping is increasing in exchange for plastic waste worldwide. So that people can be made aware of the use of plastic bags. Indonesia and Turkey are one of them, in these countries bus tickets are being given instead of plastic waste. By which people are travelling. Perhaps in a culture where convenience often comes before environmental concern, speaking to consumers pocketbooks may be the only way to effectively deal with this ever-increasing problem. Physical environments and the transportation of plastic bags from their origin to their place of use also contribute significantly to the environmental footprint of this product (Ansari, 2017).

There is a single use plastic ban in 32 countries around the world. It has more than half the African country, where plastic bags have chock the drain system, with these increase cases of malaria. The use of plastic bags in Kenya is a fine of up to Rs 13 lakhs and a prison term of 4 years. The solution to India's problems with plastic waste can be addressed through targeted investments in recycling and ensuring sustained effort to cut down consumption. Scientists believe that present time in the age of challenges is in biology. A plastic trash is a vast challenge of environment. On the roads, on the drain, in the river and tourist places we can face these problems. And the quantity of the plastic garbage increased by consumerism. Today everything is found in plastic polythene. In the present time to control the plastic garbage rules are apply but there are no actual directions to apply these rules.

The biodegradable plastic is better option for reduce use of ordinary plastic but the biodegradable plastic is being costly than ordinary plastic but there is hope due to rapid growth of scientific researches that in the earlier time lower cost biodegradable plastics will be available in India and other developing countries.

REFERENCES

Abrusci, C., Pablos, J. L., Corrales, T., Lopez-Marín, J., Marín, L., & Catalina, F. (2011). Biodegradation of photo-degraded mulching films based on polyethylene and stearates of calcium and iron as pro-oxidant additives. *International Biodeterioration & Biodegradation*, *65*(3), 451–459. doi:10.1016/j.ibiod.2010.10.012

ACG. (2006). *Allen Consulting Group*. ACG.

Alessa, K. (2016). *Environmental impacts of plastic bags: it can be a danger to animal's life*. Academic Press.

Ansari, Y., Chavan, F. I., & Husain, M. (2017). Effect of plastic grocery bags on environment and its reuse. *International Journal of Advance Research, Ideas and Innovations in Technology*, *3*, 3.

Aswale, P. (2010). *Studies on bio-degradation of polythene* (PhD thesis). Dr. Babasaheb Ambedkar Marathwada University, Aurangabad, India.

Balasubramanian, V., Natarajan, K., Hemambika, B., Ramesh, N., Sumathi, C. S., Kottaimuthu, R., & Kannan, V. R. (2010). High-density polyethylene (HDPE)-degrading potential bacteria from marine ecosystem of Gulf of Mannar, India. *Letters in Applied Microbiology*, *51*, 205–211. PMID:20586938

Bhaskar, D. (2019). *88 square kilometer land will be needed only for garbage management*. Academic Press.

Bonhomme, S., Cuer, A., Delort, A. M., Lemaire, J., Sancelme, M., & Scott, G. (2003). Environmental biodegradation of polythene. *Polymer Degradation & Stability*, *81*(3), 441–452. doi:10.1016/S0141-3910(03)00129-0

Carisse, H., Thomas, M., & Sumi, M. (2018). *Combating plastic and air pollution on earth day*. Vital Strategies Environmental Health Division.

Central Pollution Control Board (CPCB). (2013). *Overview of Plastic Waste Management*. Author.

Central Pollution Control Board (CPCB). (2017). *Consolidated guidelines for segregation, collection and disposal of plastic waste*. Author.

Chandra, R., & Rustgi, H. (1998). Biodegradable polymers. *Progress in Polymer Science*, *23*(7), 1273–1335. doi:10.1016/S0079-6700(97)00039-7

Chatterjee, S., Roy, B., Roy, D., & Banerjee, R. (2010). Enzyme-mediated biodegradation of heat treated commercial polyethylene by Staphylococcal species. *Polymer Degradation Stability, 95,* 195-200.

Clapp, J., & Swantoon, L. (2009). Environmental Policies. Centre for International Governance Innovation.

Dara, P. K., Terfa, A. M., & Deng, B. P. (2018). Beating the plastic pollution: A review. *International Journal of Innovative Research in Science, Engineering and Technology, 7,* 6.

Derraik, J. G. B. (2002). The pollution of the marine environment by plastic debris: A review. *Marine Pollution Bulletin, 44*(9), 842–852. doi:10.1016/S0025-326X(02)00220-5 PMID:12405208

El-Shafei, H. A., Abd El-Nasser, N. H., Kansoh, A. L., & Ali, A. M. (1998). Biodegradation of disposable polyethylene by fungi Streptomyces species. *Polymer Degradation & Stability, 62*(2), 361–365. doi:10.1016/S0141-3910(98)00019-6

Fernandes, P. (2018). *Beware, plastic could be in everything you eat.* Academic Press.

Goldberg. (1994). The pollution of the marine environment by plastic debris: a review, *Marine Pollution Bulletin, 44,* 842-852.

Grover, A., Gupta, A., Chandra, S., & Kumari, A., & Khurana, P. S. M. (2015). Polythene and environment. *International Journal of Environmental Sciences, 5,* 6.

Hester, R. E., & Harrison, R. M. (2011). Marine Pollution and Human Health. Royal Society of Chemistry, 84-85.

Hopewell, J., Dvorak, R., & Kosior, E. (2009). Plastics recycling: Challenges and opportunities. *Philosophical Transactions of the Royal Society of London. Series B, Biological Sciences, 364*(1526), 2115–2126. doi:10.1098/rstb.2008.0311 PMID:19528059

Jalil, A., Mian, N., & Rahman, K. M. (2013). Using plastic bags and its damaging impact on Environment and Agriculture: An alternative proposal. *International Journal of Learning & Development, 17,* 3-4.

Kathiresan, K. (2003). Polythene and plastic degrading microbes from mangrove soil. *Revista de Biología Tropical, 51,* 629–633. PMID:15162769

Kyaw, B. M., Champakalakshmi, R., Sakharkar, M. K., Lim, C. S., & Sakharkar, K. R. (2012). Biodegradation of Low Density Polythene (LDPE) by Pseudomonas species. *Indian Journal of Medical Microbiology, 52*(3), 411–419. doi:10.100712088-012-0250-6 PMID:23997333

Laist, D. W. (1997). Impacts of marine debris: Entanglement of marine life in marine debris including a comprehensive list of species with entanglement and ingestion records. In Marine Debris (pp. 99-139). New York, NY: Springer.

Lee, B., Pometto, A. L., Fratzke, A., & Bailey, T. B. (1991). Biodegradation of degradable plastic polyethylene by phanerochaete and streptomyces species. *Applied and Environmental Microbiology, 57,* 678–685. PMID:16348434

Maeda, H., Yamagata, Y., Abe, K., Hasegawa, F., Machida, M., Ishioka, R., ... Nakajima, T. (2005). Purification and characterization of a biodegradable plastic-degrading enzyme from Aspergillus oryzae. *Applied Microbiology and Biotechnology, 67*(6), 778–788. doi:10.100700253-004-1853-6 PMID:15968570

Nanda, S., Sahu, S., & Abraham, J. (2010). Studies on the biodegradation of natural and synthetic polyethylene by Pseudomonas spp. *Journal of Applied Science & Environmental Management*, *14*(2), 57–60. doi:10.4314/jasem.v14i2.57839

Nguyen, A. (2018). *Under the plastic sea, the earth is screaming for help*. Academic Press.

Nwachukwu, S., Obidi, O., & Odocha, C. (2010). Occurrence and recalcitrance of polyethylene bag waste in Nigerian soils. *African Journal of Biotechnology*, *9*, 6096–6104.

Phua, S. K., Castillo, E., Anderson, J. M., & Hiltner, A. (1987). Biodegradation of polyurethane in vitro. *Journal of Biomedical Materials Research*, *21*(2), 231–246. doi:10.1002/jbm.820210207 PMID:3818683

Pometto, A. L., Lee, B., & Johnson, K. E. (1992). Production of an extracellular polyethylene-degrading enzyme(s) by Streptomyces species. *Applied and Environmental Microbiology*, *58*, 731–733. PMID:1610196

Priyanka, N., & Archana, T. (2011). Biodegradability of Polythene and Plastic by the Help of Microorganism: A Way for Brighter Future. *Journal of Environmental & Analytical Toxicology*, *1*(02), 111. doi:10.4172/2161-0525.1000111

Rahman, A. K. M. R. (2009). Jute in South Asia. In *Proceedings of the Symposium on National Fibers* (pp. 19-20). Academic Press.

Ramaswamy, V. & Sharma, H. R. (2011). Plastic bags-Threat to environment and cattle health: A retrospective study from Gondar city of Ethiopia. *Environmental Management for Sustainable Development, 2*, 1.

Reddy, R. M. (2008). Impact of soil composting using municipal solid waste on biodegradation of plastics. *Indian Journal of Biotechnology*, *7*, 235–239.

Ryan, P. G., & Rice, N. (1996). The Free Shopping Bag Debate: Costs and Attitudes. *South African Journal of Science*, *92*(4), 163–164.

Shimao. (2001). Biodegradation of plastics. *Current Opinion in Biotechnology, 12,* 242–247.

Simmons, C. (2005). *It's in the Bag: An Estimate of the Effect of CO2 Emissions of the Irish Plastic Bag Tax*. Academic Press.

Singh, A. (2018). *Plastic waste burning at Yamuna Biodiversity Park*. Academic Press.

Sivan, A. (2011). New perspectives in plastic biodegradation. *Current Opinion in Biotechnology*, *22*(3), 422–426. doi:10.1016/j.copbio.2011.01.013 PMID:21356588

Spivey, A. (2003). Plastic Bags – Prolific Problems. *Environmental Health Perspectives, 111*(4), A208.

Sugii, T. (2008). *Plastic Bag Reduction*. Policies to Reduce Environmental Impact.

Suresh, B., Maruthamuthu, S., Palanisamy, N., Ragunathan, R., Pandiyaraj, K. N., & Muralidharan, V. S. (2011). Investigation on biodegradability of polyethylene by Bacillus cereus strain Ma-Su isolated from compost soil. *International Research Journal of Microbiology*, *2*, 292–302.

Though, R. (2007). Plastic Shopping Bags: Environmental Impacts and Policy Options. New Zealand: Victoria University of Wellington.

Tokiwa, Y., Calabia, B., Ugwu, C., & Aiba, S. (2009). Review: Biodegradability of Plastics. *International Journal of Molecular Sciences*, *10*(9), 3722–3742. doi:10.3390/ijms10093722 PMID:19865515

Toxics Link. (2014). *Report: Plastics and The Environment*. Assessing The Impact of The Complete Ban on Plastic Carry Bag.

Usha, R., Sangeetha, T., & Palaniswamy, M. (2011). Screening of Polyethylene Degrading Microorganisms from Garbage Soil. *Libyan Agriculture Research Center Journal International*, *2*, 200–204.

Wackett, L. P., & Hershberger, C. D. (2001). *Biocatalysis and Biodegradation; Microbial Transformation of Organic Compounds*. Washington, DC: ASM Press.

Webb, H. K., Arnott, J., Crawford, R. J., & Ivanova, E. P. (2013). Plastic Degradation and Its Environmental Implications with Special Reference to Poly (ethylene terephthalate). *Polymers*, *5*(1), 1–18. doi:10.3390/polym5010001

Williamson, L. J. (2003). It's Not My Bag, Baby! *Onearth*, *25*(2), 32–34.

Zaman, T. (2010). *The Prevalence and Environmental Impact of Single Use Plastic Products*. Academic Press.

Zion Research Analysis. (2016). *Plastics: Complex systems problem*. Academic Press.

KEY TERMS AND DEFINITIONS

Agricultural Countries: Of the major cereal and vegetable crops, the United States, China, India, and Russia frequently appear as top producers. It probably won't surprise readers that China is the leading worldwide producer of rice, but it's also the leading producer of wheat and the number two producer of corn, as well as the largest producer of many vegetables including onions and cabbage. In terms of total production, the United States is third in wheat and first in corn and soybeans.

Agricultural Land: Agricultural land is typically land devoted to agriculture, the systematic and controlled use of other forms of life particularly the rearing of livestock and production of crops to produce food for humans. It is thus generally synonymous with farmland or cropland, as well as pasture or rangeland.

Non-Biodegradable: Those materials which cannot be broken down or decomposed into the soil by natural agents are labeled as non-biodegradable. These substances consist of plastic materials, metal scraps, aluminum cans and bottles, hazardous chemicals etc.

Plastic Factories: The plastics industry manufactures polymer materials commonly called plasticsand offers services in plastics important to a range of industries, including packaging, building and construction, electronics, aerospace, and transportation. It is part of the chemical industry.

Plastic Pollution: Plastic pollution is the accumulation of plastic objects (e.g.: plastic bottles and much more) in the Earth's environment that adversely affects wildlife, wildlife habitat, and humans. Plastics that act as pollutants are categorized into micro, meso, or macro debris, based on size. Plastics are inexpensive and durable, and as a result levels of plastic production by humans are high. However, the chemical structure of most plastics renders them resistant to many natural processes of degradation and as a result they are slow to degrade. Together, these two factors have led to a high prominence of plastic pollution in the environment.

Polythene Bag: A plastic bag, polybag, or pouch is a type of container made of thin, flexible, plastic film, nonwoven fabric, or plastic textile. Plastic bags are used for containing and transporting goods such as foods, produce, powders, ice, magazines, chemicals, and waste. It is a common form of packaging. Polythene pollution is mostly created by polythene bags, plastic syringe, pesticide containers, and medicinal bottles.

Polythene Pollution: Polythene pollution is an example of non-biodegradable pollution and they persist on our earth years after years affecting even future generation.

Chapter 8
Plastic Pollution and Its Remedies:
An Indian Scenario

Aparna Satsangi
Dayalbagh Educational Institute, India

ABSTRACT

Anthropogenic activities are causing slow extinction of fauna, flora, and fungi in natural environment through toxic pollution. It is probably due to industrial and technological advancement in recent decades. This pollution may be of air, water, soil, radioactivity, or plastics. Of these, the most widely spread form is pollution by plastics. It is drastically dangerous and harmful for marine life, but it also affects human health. Since plastic is non-biodegradable, one can hardly get rid of it. The harmful chemicals get absorbed in the plastic debris, have a varied and harmful range of chronic effects like endocrine disorders. Therefore, it is high time for the government to take stringent steps to overcome the problems associated with plastic pollution. Policy makers and advisers should sternly follow the steps: never throw plastic bags on roads; always carry bags from home; and, use paper decorative items rather than of plastics as paper can be reused.

DOI: 10.4018/978-1-5225-9452-9.ch008

INTRODUCTION

"India is the fastest-growing economy in the world today. We are committed to realizing the standards of our people in a way that is sustainable and green," Mr. Narendra Modi, Prime Minister, India on World Environment Day

Plastics are materials that are light in weight, strong, durable, and resistant to corrosion and are inexpensive. They also possess thermal and electrical insulation properties. Their diverse and versatile properties have made its use possible in a large variety of products for packing and storage. Plastics are materials which are not used directly but are generally mixed with resins and additives to enhance its applicability (Thompson et al., 2009).

Plastic pollution is emerging as a top threat to ocean ecosystems. By 2025, there could be 1 ton of plastics for every 3 tons of fish in the ocean. -An Earth Law Solution to Ocean Plastic Pollution by Michelle Bender

The Beginning

Age of Plastics came into existence after World War II due to reduction and shortfall in rubber and other natural materials. There was a surplus of synthetic and fossil fuels which caused companies to create market for plastic products. This led to increase in production of synthetic plastics at reduced costs, making them more competitive than natural materials. It successively entered every walk of life becoming a part and parcel of life. Figure 1 shows the rise in plastic consumption in India. Excessive use of plastics became a chaos leading to dumping of piles in grounds due to its non-biodegradable nature.

Approximately 140 million tons of plastics are produced throughout the world each year. In India also around 4-5% of municipal solid waste (MSW) material are post-consumer plastics in comparison to 6-10% in the US, Europe and other developed countries. India recycled 47% of its total plastic waste in contrast to China (11%), the US (3.5%), South Africa (15%), and UK (7%). There are around 20,000

Figure 1: Rise in Plastic Consumption (Source: CPCB, India)

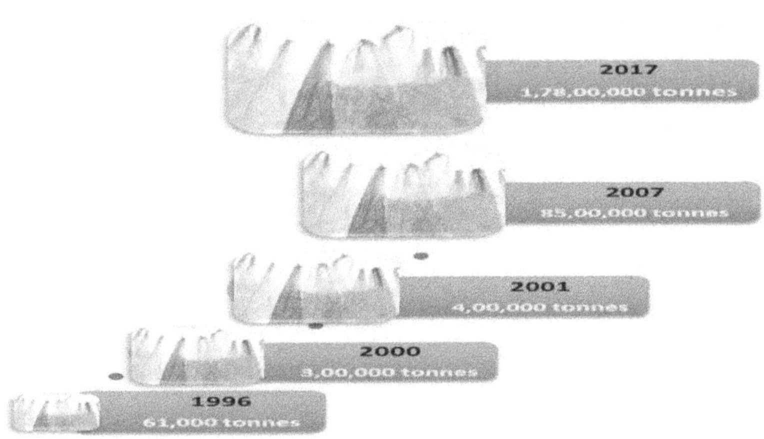

Rise in Plastic Consumption
(Source: Central Pollution Control Board)

Figure 2a: Plastic pollution from different countries

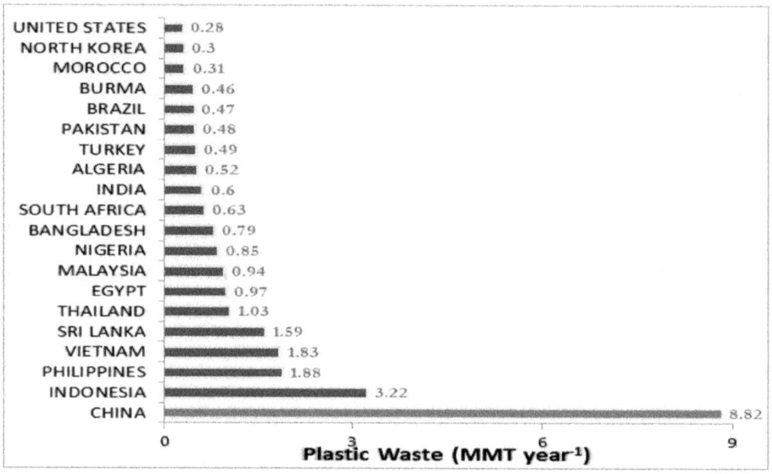

Figure 2b: Reusable percent of plastic products

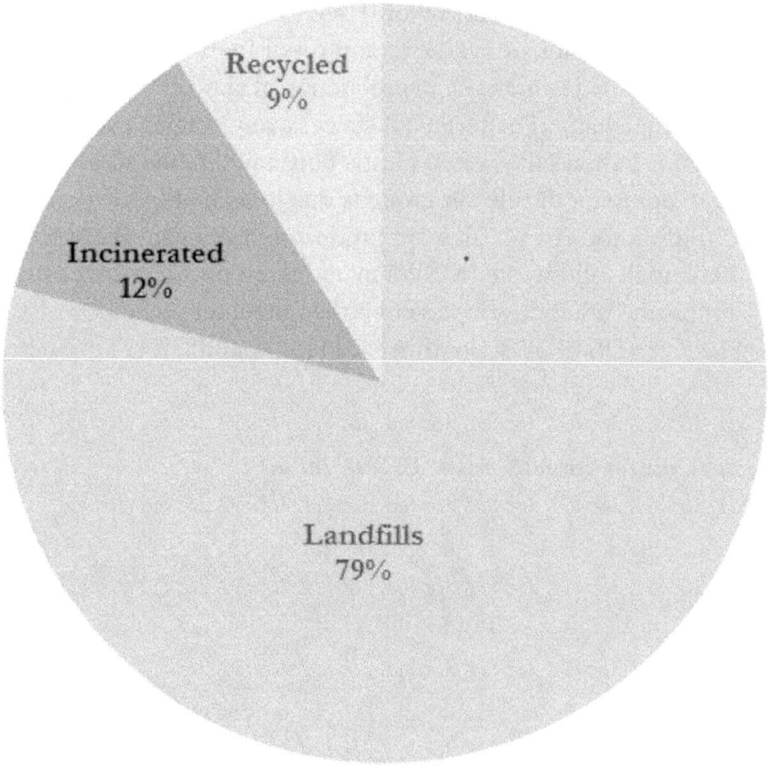

plastics recycling industries in India with a daily capacity of 1,500 tons (Daspatnaik, 2016). Another article states that 8.3 billion metric tons (9.1 billion US tons) of virgin (non-recycled) plastic has been produced to date which has contributed 6.3 billion metric tons (6.9 billion US tons) of plastic waste. Out of this, 9% of the waste has been recycled while 12% of it incinerated. The remaining 79% (5.5 billion US tons) of plastics have accumulated in landfills and the natural environment. This has been represented in Figure 2b. It is estimated that 12 billion metric tons (13.2 billion US tons) will enter the landfills or the environment by 2050 if current production and waste management trends continue at the present rate. Hence, policies and management strategies need to be modified if plastic waste has to be reduced. This seems mandatory as collection of plastic waste would lead to hazardous after effects on mankind.

More plastic waste per person is generated in high-income countries, according to a report on plastic pollution by Hannah Ritchie and Max Roser of Our World in Data. Although these countries are able to manage the waste well but still, plastic waste still enters rivers and oceans, especially from coastal areas. U.S.A. itself produces an alarming plastic litter of 275,000 tons every year with a high risk of polluting surrounding rivers and the ocean.

Plastic waste disposal *has* changed underwent change globally: earlier there was no recycling of plastics prior to 1980, while in 2015, approximately 20% of plastic was recycled and it is expected that recycling may increase to only 44% by 2050 (Dorger, 2019).

INDIAN SCENARIO

Central Pollution Control Board (CPCB) gave a surprising new report which stated that its plastic waste estimate of 660,785.85 tonnes is only from 14 regional pollution boards as compared to 35 in total. This reveals that more than sixty percent of plastic waste produced from other Indian states and union territories has not accounted for in official figures for the period of 2017-18.

It has been reported that Delhi alone produces 10,000 metric tonnes of garbage every day. Dumping of this waste is a severe problem. One of the garbage dump in East Delhi's Ghazipur rises to as high as 65 metres which is very close to the height of Qutub Minar (73 metres). In another metropolitan city of Mumbai, fire broke out in one of the largest landfill site at Deonar on March 26, 2018. Another pollution causing burning activity has been reported from Kolkata where Dhapa dumping ground is burning since November 2018 making the city's polluted air even more toxic. Toxic smoke from a blaze at the Okhla landfill in the national capital has also led to health problems amongst local residents.

Such incidents bring out the major gaps in our knowledge on how to reduce plastic waste which is being produced extensively and causing damage to not only the environment but human health.

CAUSES OF PLASTIC POLLUTION:

As the world's population continues to grow, so does the amount of garbage that people produce. On-the-go lifestyles require easily disposable products, such as soda cans or bottles of water, but the accumulation of these products has led to increasing amounts of plastic pollution around the world. Figure 3 shows various fields were plastics are used. As plastic is composed of major toxic pollutants, it has the potential to cause great harm to the environment in the form of air, water and land pollution. Plastic pollution occurs when plastic has gathered in an area and has begun to negatively impact the natural environment

Figure 3. Uses of Plastic Pollution

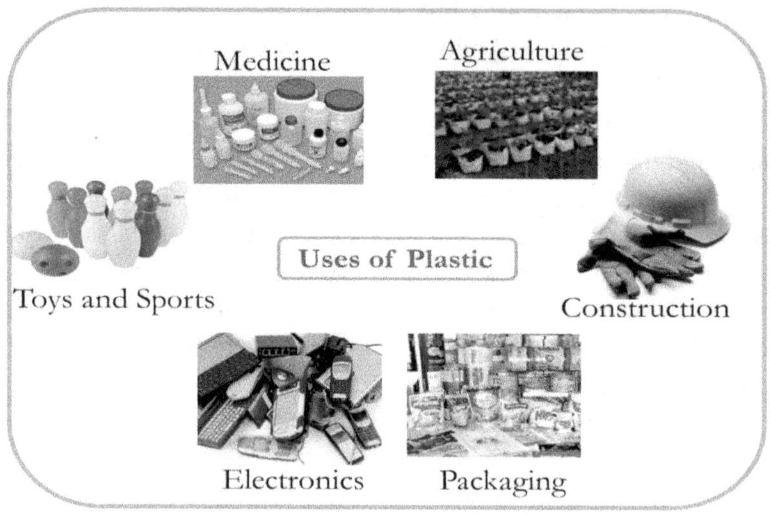

and create problems for plants, wildlife and even human population. Often this includes killing plant life and posing dangers to local animals. Plastic is an incredibly useful material, but its manufacture from toxic compounds and it's non-biodegradable nature are its deleterious effects.

Plastics are chiefly used to bring any item (fruits, vegetables, grocery, clothes or shoes). It is also used to sell packaged products like milk, yogurt, oil, ghee and fruit juice in the market. Fast food products are also sold in packed form. After use, these bags are discarded but they are not processed or recycled in proper manner but dumped in the fields or along with waste and garbage creating a nuisance and threat to environment. These carry bags hinder the photosynthesis process ultimately causing reduction in crop yield in agricultural fields. Medicines and drugs are also wrapped in plastic packets. The consumption of these food items threatens human life and causes harmful diseases.

While plastics have many valuable uses, we have become addicted to single-use or disposable plastic — with severe environmental consequences. Around the world, one million plastic drinking bottles are purchased every minute, while up to 5 trillion single-use plastic bags are used worldwide every year. In total, half of all plastic produced is designed to be used only once — and then thrown away. Plastic waste is now so ubiquitous in the natural environment that scientists have even suggested it could serve as a geological indicator of the Anthropocene era.

TYPES OF PLASTICS (SEVEN TYPES OF PLASTICS):

Table 1 represents the types of plastics and their uses in different fields.

1. **Polyethylene Terephthalate (PETE or PET):** Good gas and moisture barrier properties Mineral Water, fizzy drink and beer bottles High heat resistance Pre-prepared food trays and roasting bags Clear Boil in the bag food pouches Hard Soft drink and water bottles Tough Fibre for clothing and carpets Microwave transparency Strapping Solvent resistant, Water bottles, dispensing containers, biscuit trays.

Table 1. Types of Plastics and their Uses

S. No.	PLASTICS	Abbreviation	Structural unit	Plastic Recycling Symbol	Uses
				Plastic recycling	
1	Polyethylene Terephthalate	PETE or PET	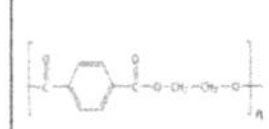	1 PETE Polyethylene terephthalate	to make many common household items like beverage bottles, medicine jars, rope, clothing and carpet fibre
2	High-Density Polyethylene	HDPE	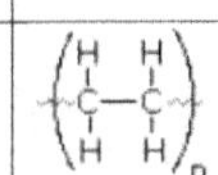	2 HDPE High-density polyethylene	containers for milk, motor oil, shampoos and conditioners, soap bottles, detergents, and bleaches. It is NEVER safe to reuse an HDPE bottle as a food or drink container if it didn't originally contain food or drink
3	Polyvinyl Chloride	PVC	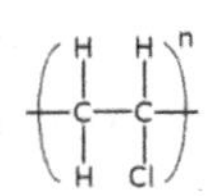	3 PVC/V Polyvinyl chloride	for all kinds of pipes and tiles, but is most commonly found in plumbing pipes. This kind of plastic should not come in contact with food items as it can be harmful if ingested
4	Low-Density Polyethylene	LDPE	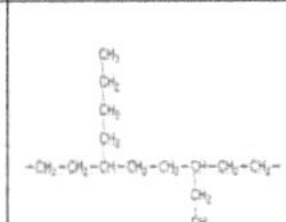	4 LDPE Low-density polyethylene	cling-film, sandwich bags, squeezable bottles, and plastic grocery bags are made from LDPE
5	Polypropylene	PP	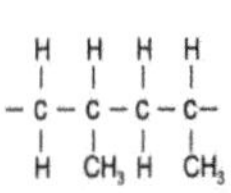	5 PP Polypropylene	used to make lunch boxes, margarine containers, yogurt pots, syrup bottles, prescription bottles. Plastic bottle caps are often made from PP
6	Polystyrene or Styrofoam	PS	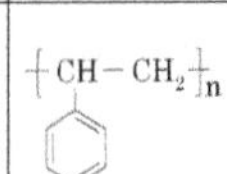	6 PS Polystyrene	disposable coffee cups, plastic food boxes, plastic cutlery and packing foam
7	Polylactic Acid or Polycarbonate	**PLA** **PC**	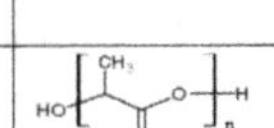	7 O OTHER	baby bottles, compact discs, and medical storage container

2. **High-Density Polyethylene (HDPE):** Excellent moisture barrier properties; used to make detergent, bleach and fabric conditioner bottles. Excellent chemical resistance: Snack food boxes and cereal box liners Hard to semi-flexible and strong Milk and non-carbonated drinks bottles Soft

waxy surface Toys, buckets, rigid pipes, crates, plant pots Permeable to gas Plastic wood, garden furniture HDPE films crinkle to the touch Wheeled refuse bins, compost containers Pigmented bottles stress resistant, Shampoo bottles, milk bottles, freezer bags, ice cream containers.

3. **Polyvinyl Chloride (PVC):** Excellent transparency Credit cards Hard, rigid (flexible when plasticised) Carpet backing and other floor covering Good chemical resistance Window and door frames, guttering Long term stability Pipes and fittings, wire and cable sheathing Good weathering ability Synthetic leather products Stable electrical properties Low gas permeability.
4. **Low-Density Polyethylene (LDPE):** Tough and flexible Films, fertiliser bags, refuse sacks Waxy surface Packaging films, bubble wrap Soft – scratches easily Flexible bottles Good transparency Irrigation pipes Low melting point Thick shopping bags (clothes and produce) Stable electrical properties Wire and cable applications Good moisture barrier properties, Bags, trays, containers, food packaging film.
5. **Polypropylene (PP):** Excellent chemical resistance Most bottle tops High melting point Ketchup and syrup bottles Hard, but flexible Yoghurt and some margarine containers Waxy surface Potato crisp bags, biscuit wrappers Translucent Crates, plant pots, drinking straws Strong Hinged lunch boxes, refrigerated containers. Potato chip bags, microwave dishes, ice cream tubs, bottle caps.
6. **Polystyrene or Styrofoam (PS):** Clear to opaque Yoghurt containers, egg boxes Glassy surface Fast food trays Rigid or foamed Video cases Hard Vending cups and disposable cutlery Brittle Seed trays High clarity Coat hangers Affected by fats and solvents Low cost brittle toys.

7. **Polylactic Acid (PLA):** Polylactic Acid is unique in relation to others. Other (PLA/PC): There are other polymers that have a wide range of uses, particularly in engineering sectors. They are identified with the number 7 and OTHER (or a triangle with numbers from 7 to 19).

IMPORTANCE OF PLASTICS

The versatility of plastic materials comes from the ability to mould, laminate or shape them, and to tailor them physically and chemically. There is a plastic suitable for almost any application. Plastics do not corrode, though they can degrade in UV (a component of sunlight) and can be affected by solvents — for example, PVC plastic is soluble in acetone.

However, because many plastics are so durable and do not corrode, they create considerable disposal problems. They are not good for the landfill as many will persist for hundreds of years and when incinerated, dangerous gases can be produced. Many supermarkets now give us one-time grocery bags — leave them in a cupboard for a year and all you will have left is dust — they are engineered to degrade. Perversely, some plastics can be cured (hardened) by UV — that just goes to show how varied their formulas are. We are getting wiser, though, and now many plastics can be chemically, mechanically, or thermally recycled.

EFFECTS OF PLASTIC POLLUTION

Plastics, being non-biodegradable affect human life and other life forms. It disturbs the food chain, causes land pollution, reaches underground causing groundwater pollution and its accumulation kills animals.

1. **Impact of additive compounds:** The additive materials include a wide variety of compounds which improve the property of plastics. Some of the additives used are inorganic fillers like carbon and silica that reinforce the material, plasticizers are added to render the material elastic, thermal and ultraviolet stabilizers, flame retardants and colourings may also be added. Few such additive chemicals are potentially toxic like lead and tributyl tin added in the manufacture of polyvinyl chloride, PVC. Certain additives like phthalates and bisphenol A, BPA are released from plastic items and cause adverse effects on animal or human populations. The major problem is uptake and accumulation of these additives in plastics by the living organisms (Koch and Calafat 2009; Meeker et al. 2009; Talsness et al. 2009). Most common additives are phthalate plasticizers, BPA, brominated flame retardants and anti-microbial agents. BPA and phthalates are present in good quantity in products like medical devices, food packaging items, perfumes, cosmetics, toys, flooring materials, computers and CDs. Phthalates can easily leach out of products because they are not chemically bound to the matrix of plastics and, thus, are the central attractions because of their high production in volumes for their wide use (Thompson et al. 2009).
2. **Accumulation of Plastic Waste in Natural Environment:** Most polymers are buoyant in water, and since items of plastic debris such as cartons and bottles often trap air, substantial quantities of plastic debris accumulate on the sea surface and may also be washed ashore. As a consequence, plastics represent a considerable proportion (50–80%) of shoreline debris. Discarded plastic also contaminates a wide range of natural terrestrial, freshwater and marine habitats, with newspaper accounts of plastic debris on even some of the highest mountains. There are also some data on littering in the urban environment. There are accounts of inadvertent contamination of soils with small plastic fragments as a consequence of spreading sewage sludge (Zubris& Richards 2005), of fragments of plastic and glass contaminating compost prepared from municipal solid waste (Brinton 2005) and of plastic being carried into streams, rivers and ultimately the sea with rain water and flood events. Kostigen and Magazine (2008) reported that the pill bottles dumped in India along with oil and detergent containers from Russia, Korea, and China have been found on the southern parts of Hawaii.
3. **Effects of Plastic Debris in the Environment and on Wildlife:** Floating plastic debris can rapidly become colonized by marine organisms and since it can persist at the sea surface for substantial periods, it may subsequently facilitate the transport of non-native or 'alien' species (Barnes, 2002; Barnes et al., 2009; Gregory, 2009). However, the problems attracting most public and media attention are those resulting in ingestion and entanglement by wildlife. Over 260 species, including invertebrates, turtles, fish, seabirds and mammals, have been reported to ingest or become entangled in plastic debris, resulting in impaired movement and feeding, reduced reproductive output, lacerations, ulcers and death (Laist 1997; Derraik 2002; Gregory, 2009). The limited monitoring data we have suggest rates of entanglement have increased over time (Ryan et al., 2009). A wide range of species with different modes of feeding including filter feeders, deposit feeders and detritivores are known to ingest plastics. An area of particular concern is the abundance of small plastic fragments or microplastics. Fragments as small as 1.6 mm have been identified in some marine habitats,

and it seems likely there will be even smaller pieces below current levels of detection. However, the extent and consequences of ingestion of microplastics by natural populations are not known. In addition to the physical problems associated with plastic debris, there has been much speculation that, if ingested, plastic has the potential to transfer toxic substances to the food chain. In the marine environment, plastic debris such as pellets, fragments and microplastics have been shown to contain organic contaminants including polychlorinated biphenyls (PCBs), polycyclic aromatic hydrocarbons, petroleum hydrocarbons, organochlorine pesticides (2,20-bis(p-chlorophenyl)-1,1,1 trichloroethane (DDT) and its metabolites; together with hexachlorinated hexane (HCH)), polybrominated diphenylethers (PBDEs), alkylphenols and BPA at concentrations ranging from ng g^{-1} to mgg^{-1}. Some of these compounds are added to plastics during manufacture while others adsorb to plastic debris from the environment.

Molluscs and amphibians appear to be particularly sensitive to these compounds and biological effects have been observed in the low ng l^{-1} to mgl^{-1} range. In contrast, most effects in fish tend to occur at higher concentrations. Most plasticizers appear to act by interfering with hormone function, although they can do this by several mechanisms (Hu et al. 2009). The itinerant plastics end up in animals' stomachs or around their necks, but there is also growing concern that plastics are acting as a medium for invasive species. The hard surfaces of plastics are now an alternate material for invasive species such as barnacles, molluscs, and algae to attach, compared to the natural material which previously carried invasive species for centuries (Gregory, 2009).

4. **Effect on Humans Biomonitoring** (measuring concentration of environmental contaminants in human tissue) provides an integrated measure of an organism's exposure to contaminants from multiple sources. This approach has shown that chemicals used in the manufacture of plastics are present in the human population, and studies using laboratory animals as model organisms indicate potential adverse health effects of these chemicals (Talsness et al., 2009). Body burdens of chemicals that are used in plastic manufacture have also been correlated with adverse effects in the human population, including reproductive abnormalities (Swan et al. 2005; Lang et al. 2008). Interpreting biomonitoring data is complex, and a key task is to set information into perspective with dose levels that are considered toxic on the basis of experimental studies in laboratory animals. Research on experimental animals informs epidemiologists about the potential for adverse effects in humans and thus plays a critical role in chemical risk assessments. The biomonitoring approach has demonstrated phthalates and BPA, as well as other additives in plastics and their metabolites, are present in the human population. It has also demonstrated that the most common human exposure scenario is to a large number of these chemicals simultaneously. Exposure data for BPA are similar but less extensive. While average concentrations of phthalates in selected populations worldwide appear quite similar, there is evidence of considerable variability in daily intake rates among individuals, and even within individuals (Peck et al. 2009). Exposures through ingestion, inhalation and dermal contact are all considered important routes of exposure for the general population (Adibi et al. 2003; Rudel et al. 2003). Koch and Calafat (2009) show that while mean/median exposures for the general population were below levels determined to be safe for daily exposure (USA, EPA reference dose, RfD; and European Union tolerable daily intake, TDI), the upper percentiles of di-butyl phthalate and DEHP urinary metabolite concentrations show that for some people daily intake might be substantially higher than previously assumed and could exceed estimated safe daily

exposure levels. Current 'safe' exposure levels are typically based on the application of traditional toxicological assumptions regarding acute toxicants to calculate daily exposures for chemicals in a range of widely used plastic items. The toxicological consequences of such exposures, especially for susceptible subpopulations such as children and pregnant women, remain unclear and warrant further investigation. However, there is evidence of associations between urinary concentrations of some phthalate metabolites and biological outcomes (Swan et al. 2005; Swan 2008; Thompson et al., 2009).

PLASTIC POLLUTION IN INDIA

Statistics shows that in India, 70 percent of total plastic consumption is discarded as waste. Total amount of plastic generated is about 5.6 million tonnes per annum (TPA) which suggests 15,342 tonnes of plastics is used per day (TPD). Further, 17 states and union territories have completely banned the manufacturing, sale and use of plastic carry bags. Maharashtra produces plastic products worth Rs. 500 billion. The state government announced a ban on most single-use plastics in April 2018. Indian capital, Delhi announced ban on disposable plastics in the year 2017. The use of plastic carry bags has been partially banned at many pilgrimage centres, tourist and historical places located in Andhra Pradesh, Arunachal Pradesh, Assam, Goa, Gujarat, Karnataka, Odisha, Tamil Nadu, West Bengal, Uttar Pradesh and Uttarakhand.

India's first attempt at tackling the menace of plastic waste came in 2011 when the government notified the Plastic Waste (Management and Handling) Rules, 2011. The policy sought to dis-incentivise the use of poly bags by setting up a pricing mechanism for them and also to establish rules for recycling by local authorities. The Rules were replaced with a stronger Plastic Waste Management Rules, 2016 (Venkatesh and Kukreti, 2018). The government formulated Plastic Waste Management Rules, 2016, which regulate manufacture, sale, distribution and use of plastic carry bags including those of compostable plastic, and plastic sheets for packaging or wrapping applications (Ghosh, 2018).

As the implementation of the rules were poor and still being figured out, the government came up with an amendment to the rules earlier in 2018 which has gone quite a way in diluting the effect of the 2016 rules. For one, the rule on explicit pricing of carry bags which required vendors to register and pay an annual fee to urban local bodies was removed. The complete ban on "non-recyclable multilayered plastic" which was implied in the 2016 rules was removed through some clever word play. The term "non-recyclable multilayered plastic if any" has been substituted by "multi-layered plastic which is non-recyclable or non-energy recoverable or with no alternate use" giving producers an escape route by claiming that products can be put to some other use, if not recycled. This type of plastic was supposed to be banned by March 2018, but it is nowhere near a phase-out. While the government has claimed several times that it wants to shut down all small and illegal plastic producing plants, the amendment to the rules seems to dilute this as well (Venkatesh and Kukreti, 2018).

In 2017, Central Pollution Control Board (CPCB), extrapolated data from about 60 major Indian cities, and reported that India generates around 25,940 tonnes of plastic waste per day. About 94 per cent of which is composed of thermoplastics: PET (polyethylene terephthalate) and PVC (polyvinyl chloride) which is recyclable. The remaining plastics belong to thermosetting and other categories of plastics, like sheet molding compounds (SMC), fibre reinforced plastics (FRP) and multi-layer thermocol, which are non-recyclable. According to the latest report on the Implementation of Plastic Waste Management Rules published in 2016, the plastic waste generated across the country (barring six states where data was not available) is close to 1.6 million tonnes a year, with almost half of it coming from Maharashtra and Gujarat. However, the volume of plastic waste generated seems suspiciously low when compared with the data of Plastindia Foundation—a body of major associations, organisations and institutions connected with plastics. The Foundation estimated that in 2017-18 alone, India consumed 16.5 million tonnes of plastic. Worse, according to industry body FICCI, 43 per cent of India's plastics are used in packaging and are single-use plastic. Consumption has clearly outstripped India's capacity to recycle.

RULES FRAMED BY INDIAN GOVERNMENT

Indian Government framed rules to eradicate plastic waste. In this respect, it has been formulated that since there is no eco-friendly product which is a complete substitute of the plastic in all the uses, it is impractical and undesirable to impose a complete ban on the use of plastics all over the country. The real challenge in such a case is to improve plastic waste management systems. Hence, increasing thickness of plastic carry bags from 40 to 50 micron and stipulation 50 micron thickness for plastic sheets would probably increase about 20% cost, thus, the tendency to provide free carry bags will come down and the collection by the waste pickers may also increase to some extent.

Firstly, **Plastic Waste (Management and Handling) Rules, 2011** were framed. According to it, local body was made responsible for plastic waste management system and for performing the associated functions. It could seek financial assistance from producers to set up the Waste Management System and encourage use of plastic waste (PW) for road construction, energy recovery, and other activities. Further, no carry bags shall be made available free of cost by retailers to consumers. The Municipal authority may by notification determine minimum price of carry bags.

These rules were later modified as **Plastic Waste Management (PWM) Rules, 2016.** Figure 4 represents Indian Government Regulations for Plastic Waste Management. PWM Rules 2016 rules apply to every waste generator, local body, Gram Panchayat, manufacturer, importers and producers. According to PWM Rules, 2016, waste generators including institutional generators, event organisers shall not litter plastic waste segregate waste and handover to authorized agency; and pay user fee as prescribed by Urban Local Bodies (ULBs) and spot fine in case of violation. Producers and brand owners require work out modalities for waste collection system for the collection of plastic waste within a period of six months in consultation with local authority / State Urban Development Department and implement with two years thereafter. This plan shall be submitted to the SPCB while applying for Consent to Establish or Operate or Renewal. The responsibility of local body and Gram Panchayat is to promote use of plastic waste for road construction as per Indian Road Congress guidelines or energy recovery or waste to oil. By notification or an order, introduction of collection of plastic waste management fees through pre-registration may be implemented for the producers, importers of plastic carry bags / multilayered packaging and vendors who are selling the same. Plastic waste management fees shall be of minimum rupees forty eight thousand at Rs. 4000 per month. The body may even prescribe higher plastic waste management fees, depending upon the production or sale capacity.

Figure 4: Indian Government Regulations for Plastic Waste Management

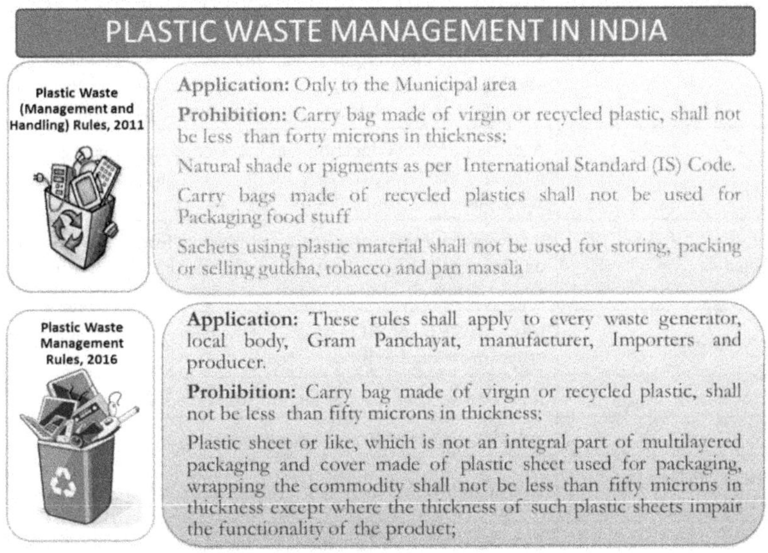
PLASTIC WASTE MANAGEMENT IN INDIA
Plastic Waste (Management and Handling) Rules, 2011
Application: Only to the Municipal area
Prohibition: Carry bag made of virgin or recycled plastic, shall not be less than forty microns in thickness;
Natural shade or pigments as per International Standard (IS) Code.
Carry bags made of recycled plastics shall not be used for Packaging food stuff
Sachets using plastic material shall not be used for storing, packing or selling gutkha, tobacco and pan masala
Plastic Waste Management Rules, 2016
Application: These rules shall apply to every waste generator, local body, Gram Panchayat, manufacturer, Importers and producer.
Prohibition: Carry bag made of virgin or recycled plastic, shall not be less than fifty microns in thickness;
Plastic sheet or like, which is not an integral part of multilayered packaging and cover made of plastic sheet used for packaging, wrapping the commodity shall not be less than fifty microns in thickness except where the thickness of such plastic sheets impair the functionality of the product;

FUTURE ACTIONS THAT MAY BE TAKEN UP FOR PLASTIC WASTE REDUCTION

- Persons generating waste may be charged fees so that the task may not be repeated again
- Segregation of waste into biodegradable and recyclable material at the source may be effective for proper waste management.
- Setting up decentralized composting plants to reduce the load on garbage collectors. For larger cities, units may be setup zone-wise.
- Encouragement for educational institutions to include waste management in their curriculum
- Promoting students to take up projects for waste recycling.
- Non-recyclable single-use polyethylene bags must be banned and development of biodegradable bags must be initiated.
- Recycling of plastic waste or other innovative techniques like conversion of plastics to fuel and plastic waste to energy must be implemented.
- Recirculation of biodegradable waste in landfills must be practiced and encouraged to enhance the stabilization of waste.

Many more (over 100) organizations exist and are coming up for the reduction of plastic and protection of this Earth's environment from 42 different countries.

SOLUTIONS TO PLASTIC POLLUTION

Accumulation of plastic debris in the environment and the associated consequences are largely avoidable. Considerable immediate reductions in the quantity of waste entering natural environments, as opposed

Table 1: Certain major NGOs of the World

S. No.	NGOs	Purpose
1	**5 GYRES**	5 GYRES works to fight against plastic use based on science, education and art; it also has programs through which it lends trawls (scientific equipment) to citizen scientists for the collection of data on plastic pollution.
2	**Algalita**	Algalita provides education and knowledge for reducing plastic pollution; some of its programs are Trash Trackers for the community, ocean waste monitoring and STEM Workshops and Presentations
3	**Clear Blue Sea**	It is working for the eradication of plastics from oceans. Their programs are based on Floating Robot for Eliminating Debris (FRED). It also rescues animals trapped in plastic debris.
4	**Earth Day Network**	It is actively involved in providing awareness for plastic reduction and runs various programs related to it.
5	**Friends of the Earth**	It aims to achieve a better and healthier environment by 2030.
6	**Greenpeace**	It deals with a number of environmental issues.
7	**Natural Resources Defence Council (NRDC)**	It strongly focuses on plastic conservation and preservation.
8	**One Green Planet**	They keenly favour Crush Plastic Movement. Its main focus is to encourage single use of plastics.
9	**Oceans**	It is mainly concerned with cleaning and protection of oceans.
10	**Plastic Change**	It is working by developing awareness and implementing programs for plastic reduction.
11	**Plastic-Pollution.org**	Its mission is to raise awareness, educate and advocate plastic reduction. It also aims to include such programs in school curriculum.
12	**Plastic Pollution Coalition**	It is a network of partners which aim to understand and solve problems related to plastic pollution. Its pledge includes 4Rs (refuse, Reduce, Reuse and Recycle).
13	**Plastic Soup Foundation**	It also works to develop awareness, educate and find solutions for plastic pollution.
14	**Plastic Oceans**	Mission of this NGO: "To change the world's attitude towards plastic within a generation". In this respect, it develops school curriculum and educational films for the budding students.
15	**The Story of Stuff Project**	It works to reduce plastic pollution along with other environmental issues.
16	**Surfrider Foundation**	It protects oceans. It also works for single-use plastic items and recycling it.
17	**World Wild Fund (WWF)**	The WWF is one of the largest global foundations fighting to protect living species and their environments around the world. Its programs focus for healthier oceans with reduced plastics in the environment.

to landfill, could be achieved by better waste disposal and material handling. Littering is a behavioural issue and some have suggested that it has increased in parallel with our use of disposable products and packaging. Perhaps increasing the capacity to recycle will help to reverse this trend such that we start to regard end-of-life materials as valuable feed stocks for new production rather than waste. To achieve this will require better education, engagement, enforcement and recycling capacity. Unfortunately, we were unable to source a contribution on education and public engagement, but it is evident that social research on littering behaviour could be very informative.

One of the most common and simple way of plastic reduction is by burning it in heaps; commonly called 'incineration'. It requires less land but generates toxic gas emissions that contain heavy metals, dioxins, and other volatile organic compounds (VOCs). Hence, this method should not be implemented (Daspatnaik, 2016).

Where plastic debris enters watercourses as a consequence of dumping or littering a range of strategies including catch basin inserts, booms and separators can be used to facilitate removal. Substantial quantities of end-of-life plastics are disposed of to landfill. Waste generation statistics vary among countries and according to the rationale for data collection. For instance, plastics are a small component of waste by weight but a large component by volume. Temporal and spatial comparisons can thus be confounded, and data on quantities of waste recycled can be skewed according to categorization of various wastes.

Efficient treatment approaches are available and are in use in some countries (Teuten et al. 2009). From a waste management perspective, the three R's—reduce, reuse and recycle are widely advocated to reduce the quantities of plastic and especially plastics packaging the waste we generate. Hopewell et al. (2009) outline the benefits and limitations of these strategies. They show that to be effective we need to consider the three R's in combination with each other and together with a fourth 'R', energy recovery. Indeed we also need to consider a 5th 'R', molecular redesign, as an emerging and potentially very important strategy. Hence, the three R's become five: 'reduce, reuse, recycle, recover and redesign'. There are opportunities to 'reduce' usage of raw material by down gauging and there are also some opportunities to 'reuse' plastics, for example, in the transport of goods on an industrial (pallets, crates) and a domestic (carrier bags) scale.

BIOPOLYMERS, DEGRADABLE & BIODEGRADABLE POLYMER SOLUTIONS

Degradable polymers have been advocated as an alternative to conventional oil-based plastics and their production has increased considerably in recent decades. Materials with functionality comparable to conventional plastics can now be produced on an industrial scale; they are more expensive than conventional polymers and account for less than 1 per cent of plastics production (Song et al., 2009). Biopolymers differ from conventional polymers in that their feedstock is from renewable biomass rather than being oil-based. They may be natural polymers (e.g. cellulose), or synthetic polymers made from biomass monomers (e.g. PLA) or synthetic polymers made from synthetic monomers derived from biomass (e.g. polythene derived from bioethanol) (WRAP 2009). They are often described as renewable polymers since the original biomass, for example corn grown in agriculture, can be reproduced.

ACKNOWLEDGMENT

This work is financially supported by Women Scientist Scheme (SR/WOS-A/AS-04/2013, WOS A Project, Department of Science and Technology), India. The authors gratefully acknowledge Director, Dayalbagh Educational Institute and Head, Department of Chemistry for providing necessary facilities.

REFERENCES

Adibi, J. J., Perera, F. P., Jedrychowski, W., Camann, D. E., Barr, D., Jacek, R., & Whyatt, R. M. (2003). Prenatal exposures to phthalates among women in New York City and Krakow, Poland. *Environmental Health Perspectives, 111*(14), 1719–1722. doi:10.1289/ehp.6235 PMID:14594621

Barnes, D. K. A. (2002). Biodiversity—invasions by marine life on plastic debris. *Nature, 416*, 808–809. doi:10.1038/ 416808a

Barnes, D. K. A. (2005). Remote islands reveal rapid rise of southern hemisphere sea debris. *Scientific World Journal, 5*, 915–921.

Brinton, W. F. Jr. (2005). Characterization of man-made foreign matter and its presence in multiple size fractions from mixed waste composting. *Compost Science & Utilization, 13*(4), 274–280. doi:10.1080 /1065657X.2005.10702251

Central Pollution Control Board. (2013). *Overview of Plastic Waste Management, India*. Author.

Central Pollution Control Board. (2015). Assessment & Characterisation of Plastic Waste Generation in 60 Major Cities, India. Author.

Central Pollution Control Board. (2017). India, Life cycle assessment study of plastics packaging products. Author.

Daspatnaik. (2016). Retrieved from http://www.ecoideaz.com/expert-corner/finding-solutions-to-plastic-waste-management-in-india

Derraik, J. G. B. (2002). The pollution of the marine environment by plastic debris: A review. *Marine Pollution Bulletin, 44*(9), 842–852. doi:10.1016/S0025-326X(02)00220-5 PMID:12405208

Dorger. (2019). Retrieved from https://www.thestreet.com/world/countries-most-plastic-waste-14878534

Gregory, M. R. (2009). Environmental implications of plastic debris in marine settings—Entanglement, ingestion, smothering, hangers-on, hitch-hiking and alien invasions. *Philosophical Transactions of the Royal Society of London. Series B, Biological Sciences, 364*(1526), 2013–2025. doi:10.1098/ rstb.2008.0265 PMID:19528053

Hopewell, J., Dvorak, R., & Kosior, E. (2009). Plastics recycling: Challenges and opportunities. *Philosophical Transactions of the Royal Society of London. Series B, Biological Sciences, 364*(1526), 2115–2126. doi:10.1098/rstb.2008.0311 PMID:19528059

Hu, G. X., Lian, Q. Q., Ge, R. S., Hardy, D. O., & Li, X. K. (2009). Phthalate-induced testicular dysgenesis syndrome: Leydig cell influence. *Trends in Endocrinology and Metabolism, 20*(3), 139–145. doi:10.1016/j.tem.2008.12.001 PMID:19278865

Koch, H. M., & Calafat, A. M. (2009). Human body burdens of chemicals used in plastic manufacture. *Philosophical Transactions of the Royal Society of London. Series B, Biological Sciences, 364*(1526), 2063–2078. doi:10.1098/rstb.2008.0208 PMID:19528056

Kostigen, T. M., & Magazine, F. D. (2008). The world's largest dump: the great pacific garbage patch. *Discover Magazine*. Retrieved from http://discovermagazine. com/2008/jul/10theworldslargestdump.

Laist, D. W. (1997). Impacts of marine debris: entanglement of marine life in marine debris including a comprehensive list of species with entanglement and ingestion records. In J. M. Coe, & B. D. Rogers (Eds.), *Marine debris: sources, impacts and solutions* (pp. 99–141). Berlin, Germany: Springer. doi:10.1007/978-1-4613-8486-1_10

Lang, I. A., Galloway, T. S., Scarlett, A., Henley, W. E., Depledge, M., Wallace, R. B., & Melzer, D. (2008). Association of urinary bisphenol A concentration with medical disorders and laboratory abnormalities in adults. *Journal of American Medical Association, 300*, 1303–1310. doi:.11.1303 doi:10.1001/jama.300

Meeker, J. D., Sathyanarayana, S., & Swan, S. H. (2009). Phthalates and other additives in plastics: Human exposure and associated health outcomes. *Philosophical Transactions of the Royal Society of London. Series B, Biological Sciences, 364*(1526), 2097–2113. doi:10.1098/rstb.2008.0268 PMID:19528058

Ministry of Environment. (2016). *Forest and Climate Change*. Plastic Waste Management Rules.

Peck, J. D., Sweeney, A. M., Symanski, E., Gardiner, J., Silva, M. J., Calafat, A. M., & Schantz, S. L. (2009). Intra- and inter-individual variability of urinary phthalate metabolite concentrations in Hmong women of reproductive age. *Journal of Exposure Science & Environmental Epidemiology*. doi:10.1038/jes.2009.4 PMID:19223940

Rudel, R. A., Camann, D. E., Spengler, J. D., Korn, L. R., & Brody, J. G. (2003). Phthalates, alkylphenols, pesticides, polybrominated diphenyl ethers, and other endocrinedisrupting compounds in indoor air and dust. *Environmental Science & Technology, 37*(20), 4543–4553. doi:10.1021/es0264596 PMID:14594359

Ryan, P. G., Moore, C. J., van Franeker, J. A., & Moloney, C. L. (2009). Monitoring the abundance of plastic debris in the marine environment. *Philosophical Transactions of the Royal Society of London. Series B, Biological Sciences, 364*(1526), 1999–2012. doi:10.1098/rstb.2008.0207 PMID:19528052

Song, J. H., Murphy, R. J., Narayan, R., & Davies, G. B. H. (2009). Biodegradable and compostable alternatives to conventional plastics. *Philosophical Transactions of the Royal Society of London. Series B, Biological Sciences, 364*(1526), 2127–2139. doi:10.1098/rstb.2008.0289 PMID:19528060

Swan, S. H. (2008). Environmental phthalate exposure in relation to reproductive outcomes and other health endpoints in humans. *Environmental Research, 108*, 177–184. doi:10.1016/j.envres.2008.08.007

Swan, S. H., Main, K. M., Liu, F., Stewart, S. L., Kruse, R. L., Calafat, A. M., ... Teague, J. L. (2005). Decrease in anogenital distance among male infants with prenatal phthalate exposure. *Environmental Health Perspectives, 113*(8), 1056–1061. doi:10.1289/ehp.8100 PMID:16079079

Talsness, C. E., Andrade, A. J., Kuriyama, S. N., Taylor, J. A., & Vom Saal, F. S. (2009). Components of plastic: Experimental studies in animals and relevance for human health. *Philosophical Transactions of the Royal Society of London. Series B, Biological Sciences, 364*(1526), 2079–2096. doi:10.1098/rstb.2008.0281 PMID:19528057

Teuten, E. L., Saquing, J. M., Knappe, D. R., Barlaz, M. A., Jonsson, S., Bjorn, A., ... Ochi, D. (2009). Transport and release of chemicals from plastics to the environment and to wildlife. *Philosophical Transactions of the Royal Society B: Biological Sciences, 364*(1526), 2027–2045. doi:10.1098/rstb.2008.0284

The Ministry of Environment and Forests. (2011). *Plastic Waste (Management and Handling).* Author.

Thompson, R. C., Moore, C. J., Vom Saal, F. S., & Swan, S. H. (2009). Plastics, the environment and human health: Current consensus and future trends. *Philosophical Transactions of the Royal Society of London. Series B, Biological Sciences, 364*(1526), 2153–2166. doi:10.1098/rstb.2009.0053 PMID:19528062

Venkatesh, S., & Kukreti, I. (2018). *India's plastic consumption increases at over 10 percent year-on-year.* Down to Earth.

WRAP. (2009). *Biopolymer packaging in UK grocery market.* Banbury, UK: WRAP.

Zubris, K. A. V., & Richards, B. K. (2005). Synthetic fibers as an indicator of land application of sludge. *Environmental Pollution, 138*(2), 201–211. doi:10.1016/j.envpol.2005.04.013 PMID:15967553

ADDITIONAL READING

Barnes, S. J. (2019). Understanding Plastics Pollution: The Role of Economic Development and Technological Research. *Environmental Pollution, 249*, 812–821. doi:10.1016/j.envpol.2019.03.108 PMID:30953943

Bonefeld-Jorgensen, E. C., Long, M., Hofmeister, M. V., & Vinggaard, A. M. (2007). Endocrine-disrupting potential of bisphenol A, bisphenol A dimethacrylate, 4-n-nonylphenol, and 4-n-octylphenol in vitro: New data and a brief review. *Environmental Health Perspectives, 115*(Suppl. 1), 69–76. doi:10.1289/ehp.9368 PMID:18174953

Chae, Y., & Youn-Joo, A. (2018). Current Research Trends on Plastic Pollution and Ecological Impacts on the Soil Ecosystem: A Review. *Environmental Pollution, 240*, 387–395. doi:10.1016/j.envpol.2018.05.008 PMID:29753246

Duty, S. M., Singh, N. P., Silva, M. J., Barr, D. B., Brock, J. W., Ryan, L., ... Hauser, R. (2003). The relationship between environmental exposures to phthalates and DNA damage in human sperm using the neutral comet assay. *Environmental Health Perspectives, 111*(9), 1164–1169. doi:10.1289/ehp.5756 PMID:12842768

Halden, R. U. (2010). Plastics and health risks. *Annual Review of Public Health, 31*(1), 179–194. doi:10.1146/annurev.publhealth.012809.103714 PMID:20070188

Hassan, S. (2019). Plastics: A brief review of its disasters and degradation techniques. *Science Proceedings Series, 1*(2), 100–102. doi:10.31580ps.v1i2.698

Liboiron, M. (2016). Redefining pollution and action: The matter of plastics. *Journal of Material Culture, 21*(1), 87–110. doi:10.1177/1359183515622966

North, E. J., & Halden, R. U. (2013). Plastics and environmental health: The road ahead. *Reviews on Environmental Health*, *28*(1), 1–8. doi:10.1515/reveh-2012-0030 PMID:23337043

Tibbetts, J. H. (2015). Managing Marine Plastic Pollution: Policy Initiatives to Address Wayward Waste. *Environmental Health Perspectives*, *123*(4). doi:10.1289/ehp.123-A90 PMID:25830293

KEY TERMS AND DEFINITIONS

Biodegradable: An item which may be degraded into natural materials in the environment without causing harm.

Plastic Waste: Accumulation of plastic materials in the Earth's environment that adversely affects wildlife, wildlife habitat, and humans.

Policy: Plan or principle of action adopted or proposed by an individual, organization, or government.

Reusable: That can be used again or more than once.

Waste Management (or Waste Disposal): Activities or actions taken up to manage waste from its generation to final disposal; it includes collection, transport, treatment, and disposal of waste, together with its monitoring and regulatory action.

Chapter 9
Plastic Pollution and Its Impact on Aquatic Fauna

Yahya Bakhtiyar
University of Kashmir, India

Saima Andrabi
University of Kashmir, India

Mohammad Yasir Arafat
University of Kashmir, India

Hamid Iqbal Tak
Sur College of Applied Sciences, Oman

ABSTRACT

Plastic pollution is the buildup of unwanted plastic products in the environment by its abundant and limitless use by a greedy human population in various ways. Plastics are usually made of chains of monomer units of ethylene and propylene linked together. Plastics are durable and resistant to degradation and tend to accumulate where they are disposed. One more disaster this material causes is the release of toxic chemicals with time which badly affects the ecosystem where it is dumped. Same is the case with aquatic ecosystem, because tons of plastic wastes are dumped into it in one way or the other. The major threats of this menace on aquatic ecosystem include ocean acidification, degradation of water quality, increase in number of invasive species, overfishing, pollution and choking of water bodies, habitat degradation, loss of aesthetic value, blocking of sea routes, and above all, it badly affects plant and animal life there.

INTRODUCTION

Pollution can simply be defined as the introduction of contaminants into the natural environment that causes adverse changes. It is the addition of any unwanted substances to the environment at a faster rate than it can be dispersed, diluted, decomposed or recycled. Pollution is known to be there with the humankind ever since groups of people first congregated and remained for a long time in any one place, but present situation is worse as it has grown to unprecedented levels due to rapid industrialization and

DOI: 10.4018/978-1-5225-9452-9.ch009

advance of science and technology and hence now has become a universal problem. Pollution is often categorized as point source or non-point source. Any substance, as certain chemicals or waste products, that renders the air, soil, water, or other natural resource harmful or unsuitable for a specific purpose is known as pollutant. Pollutants, the components of pollution, can be either foreign substances, energies (such as noise, heat or light) or naturally occurring contaminants (like volcanic eruptions, dust etc).

One of the greatest inventions ever introduced to mankind is the invention of plastic, which has revolutionized every aspect of our world. Its inception dates back to the mid-1800 when chemists all over the world began experimenting with a substance known as rubber. Plastic being low cost, and a synthetic polymer of resin, is highly versatile, durable and resistant to external shocks. Its use over past 50-60 years has escalated too fast and mainly engaged in packaging, building and construction, electrical equipments, automotive components, agriculture and medical equipments, etc. Plastic is being used in almost every item used in our day to day life (Sebille *et al.*, 2016). Its production is continuously increasing, with annual production estimated at 300 million tons and it is expected to increase up to 33 billion tons till 2050 (Sussarellu *et al.*, 2016). The usage of plastic in such enormous quantities is a leading cause of this pollution in almost all types of ecosystems. Pollution of the environment with plastic is a global problem, with plastic debris contaminating habitats from the poles to the equator and from the shoreline and sea surface to the deep sea. Plastic pollution results from a highly heterogeneous mixture of litter types differing in origin, size, shape and polymer type. Some of the items that are thrown away after single-use, discarded ropes and nylon nets etc. form main polluting agents. The majority of this litter originates from the land with rivers providing an important pathway to the sea (Thompson, 2017).

Plastics are usually made of chains of monomer units of ethylene and propylene linked together. These are synthetic polymers, the most common being: polyethylene (PE), polypropylene (PP), polyvinyl chloride (PVC) polyethylene terephthalate (PET) and polystyrene (PS). They can be made into a vast range of inexpensive, light-weight and durable products that bring numerous societal benefits. This has resulted in an exponential increase in global demand, from around 5 million tonnes in the 1950s to over 300 million tones today (Thompson, 2017). These are non-biodegradable and tend to accumulate in the natural environment rather than decomposition (Geyer *et al.*, 2017). Due to this property plastics become long lasting and remain as a sort of "plastic dust", which with the advent of time-release toxic chemicals like cadmium, lead, benzene, dioxins etc and contaminate the environment where it exists. These toxic chemicals are ingested by the fauna present there and result in endocrine disruption and cancer causing mutations and other dreadful disorders. Being used in huge quantities in man's everyday life in different forms, the biggest problem with plastics is its disposal. Though the plastic is dumped off in landfills or in the nearby water bodies, they constitute important source of pollution for the aquatic ecosystem (Pavani and Rajeshwari, 2014). It has been found that marine ecosystems are especially exposed to plastic pollution as tons of plastic wastes are disposed off in rivers and oceans. When plastic reaches the oceans a fraction of its debris is submerged into deep sea floor, while other lighter fractions remain floating and suspended in the water column and accumulate along the coastal belts.

In addition, when these plastic materials on the surface of water are exposed to atmospheric variables like ultra violet rays, sea water and other physical forces such as wave actions, these debris gradually breaks down into micro-sized plastic particles called microplastics, which is even more dangerous for aquatic fauna. Microplastics are classified as plastics that are smaller than 5 mm wide and any plastic debris found over 5 mm wide are classified as macroplastics to help classify samples in studies. Microplastics are also known as primary plastics, which are plastics that are directly disposed into the environment (Mendoza, 2018). Microplastics are almost of the same size as that of food particles and

Figure 1. Microplastic beads polluting sea (Pirolini, 2014) (www.azom.com)
Sources of Plastic Pollution in Aquatic Ecosystems

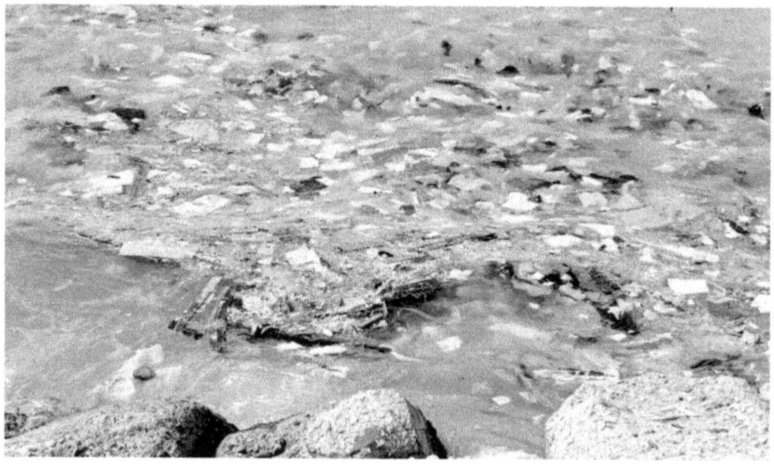

other suspended type materials, and are ingested by fauna mistaken as feed resulting in various physiological abnormalities and even a leading cause of death (Thushari *et al.*, 2017). Microplastics include a combination of chemicals added during manufacture, the so-called additives, that are efficiently sorb (adsorb or absorb) persistent, bioaccumulative and toxic contaminants for the environment. The ingestion of microplastics by aquatic organisms and the accumulation of these toxic compounds have been central to the perceived hazard and risk of microplastics in the marine environment. and aquaculture Microplastics are widespread in the marine environment and have been observed in seawater, lakes, rivers, estuaries, sediments and many species of biota. Small numbers of microplastics have been reported in commercial species of finfish and shellfish from field observations, and in fishery products. Serious issues have been raised about the presence and harmful effects of microplastics, and their associated chemicals, which pose a serious risk on fish productivity, fisheries resources and potentially adverse effects on food safety and may result in contamination of foodstuffs. The presence of microplastics in the environment and in foodstuffs, including fishery and aquaculture products, creates a need for assessing environmental, ecological and human health risks (Lusher *et al.*, 2017). The ingestion of microplastics may cause both direct physical and physiological effects on marine organisms. Physical effects include internal abrasions and gut blockages, which may lead to starvation. Physiological effects are due to toxicity derived from plastic monomers and additives, which may cause carcinogenesis and endocrine disruption. Besides that, microplastics also act as vectors of hazardous chemicals into marine organisms, as POPs (persistent organic pollutants) are absorbed from the surrounding environment and concentrated on the microplastics surfaces (Vendel *et al.*, 2017).With increase in abundance of microplastics in the aquatic ecosystem, the bioavailability will enhance organism's encounter with plastic particles and thus the progressive fragmentation of macroplastic items is likely to increase the amount of particles available for ingestion to a wider range of organisms.

Different sources that cause the accumulation of plastic and thus leading to plastic pollution in aquatic ecosystems are:

- **Poor Waste Management and Unlawful Dumping:** Due to in absence of effective landfills, fragments of plastic from open dumping grounds may be washed away into streams, rivers or directly into the ocean. Also due ineffective waste transportation from collecting ground to landing ground considerable amount is escaped which finally leads to water bodies. In some nations, rivers are sometimes used to dispose off wastes as they do not have any format waste disposal services (Verma *et al.*, 2016).
- **Industries:** Most of the industries lack proper waste disposal mechanisms, so these prefer to release the wastes generated into streams, rivers or the ocean.
- **Inadequate Wastewater Filtration:** Most of the wastewater treatment plants lack the facility of filtering small pollutants like microplastics, such as cosmetic micro beads or fibers from clothing, making wastewater treatment plants a significant source of microplastic pollution.
- **Coastal Littering:** Tourism industry is also one of the main sources of plastic pollution. Beaches form the main tourist destination and also main cause for generation of plastic wastes in the form of plastic wrappings, food and beverage packaging, and plastic beach toys (Steer *et al.*, 2017).
- **Discharge of Flood / Storm Water:** During storms, runoff water can pick up municipal waste, waste from dumpsites, street litter or even landfill waste. This litter is then discharged into streams, rivers or directly into the ocean through the drainage network.
- **Combined Sewage Overflows:** In the event of heavy rainfall, when combined sewage systems (carrying wastewater and storm water) are overflowed, mixed sewage and storm water may be released untreated into nearby rivers or the ocean leading to heavy metal pollution of water bodies (Sebille *et al.*, 2016).
- **Natural Disasters:** Extreme events can result in almost any kind of wastes being released into the ocean. Though they are not so common, such events can cause substantial environmental impacts. Natural disasters include tsunamis, torrential rains etc. Boats, ships and offshore industrial platforms are also potential sources of marine debris (Leberton and Borrero, 2013).

Figure 2. Sources of plastics in marine environment (Safety4sea.com)

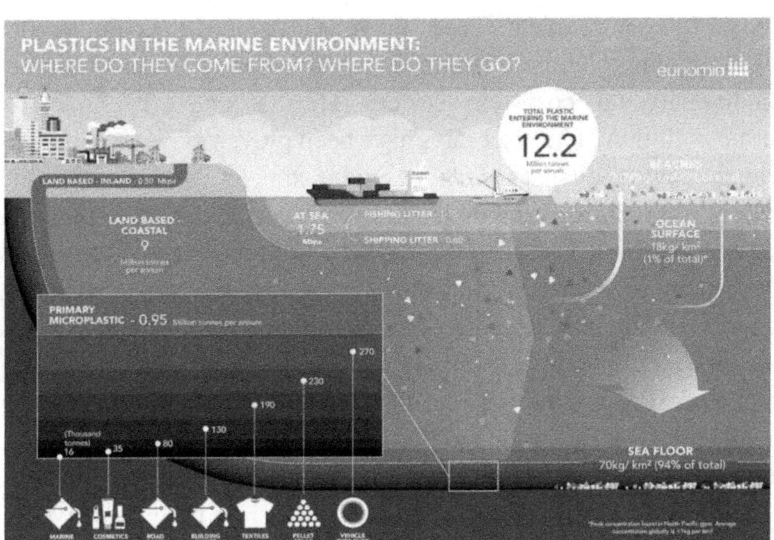

- **Ghost Fishing:** Boats may inadvertently lose or intentionally dump non-functional fishing equipment (nets, lines and rope, etc) into the ocean which remains stranded over there for years resulting in ghost fishing.
- **Shipping:** Cargo ships may discharge litter into the ocean by accident (Steer *et al.*, 2017).
- **Offshore Oil and Gas Platforms, Undersea Exploration:** Like with shipping, litter can accidentally be released into the ocean during any type of operation at sea (Sebille *et al.*, 2016).

Thus, plastic pollution of aquatic ecosystems is becoming an increasingly urgent problem, with the weight of plastic pollution in the oceans predicted soon to outweigh that of the fauna present in this ecosystem.

RATIONALE

Pollution by plastics is a worldwide recognized threat to environment particularly the aquatic one. Fish, amphibians, reptiles, birds and mammals, also other aquatic fauna are worst affected by this nuisance as they are being injured and killed by plastics in their habitats. This is becoming a leading cause of extinction of aquatic organisms. The aim of presenting this book chapter is to highlight the basic issues and effects of plastic pollution in easy possible way so that awareness can be created in common masses about the harmful effects of plastic pollution.

IMPACT ON INVERTEBRATE FAUNA

Effects of plastic ingestion in the form of microplastics have been reported in wide range of invertebrate organisms including crustaceans, insects, lobsters, mollusks etc. many filter feeders such as mussels, oysters and barnacles are investigated for microplastic uptake and most of them were having plastic fibers in their stomach (Devriese *et al.,* 2015). Being persistent in the environment for a long time period without decomposing leads to accumulation of organic pollutants released from it like Poly-chlorinated biphenyl, in the surrounding environment. These toxic pollutants get accumulated in the body tissues of invertebrates as well leading to chronic health risks. Also due to bioaccumulation it has a negative impact on coastal biodiversity and ecosystem services (Thushari *et al.,* 2017).

The impact of plastic pollution of invertebrates have been proven experimentally by different workers as in one such experiment it was seen that *Gammarus pulex* showed a significant reduction in growth due to size selective uptake of microplastics and their slow excretion, leading to depletion of energy reserves. Similarly, in another experiment it was seen that in marine lugworm, *Arenicola marina*, ingestion of microplastic caused weight loss and reduced feeding (Hasselerharm *et al.,* 2018).

Microplastics occur predominantly in sedimentary habitats and thus deposit and detritus feeders are more susceptible to exposure. Amphipods directly mistake microplastics as natural food source causing loss of proper nutrition. The marine polychaete worm, *Arenicola marina,* is capable of size based selectivity, where small plastic particles stick to the mucus lined proboscis papilla and are ingested. The same is seen in benthic holothurians (sea cucumbers), *Thyonella gemmata*, *Holothuria floridana*, *H. grisea* and *Cucumaria frondosa*. Due to retention of plastic debris in their digestive tract these organisms are not able to get proper nourishment and thus vulnerable to b lost forever. Some non-selective benthic

Figure 3. A jellyfish ingesting plastics (Macali et al., 2018) www.nature.com)

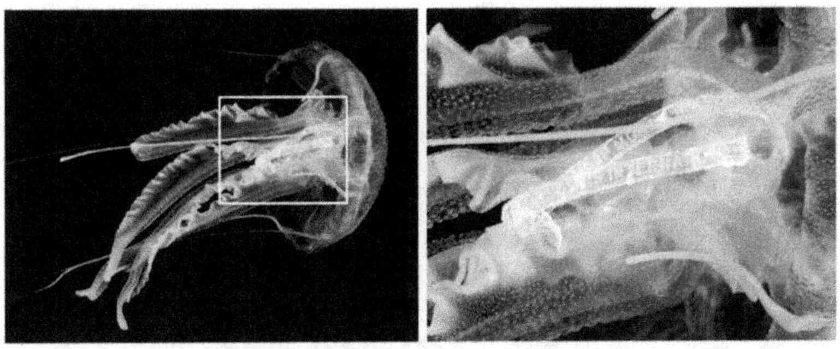

scavengers and predatory crustaceans like *Nephrops norvegicus* have also been shown to ingest small plastic fragments (Wright *et al.,* 2013).

Experimental reports have shown that foregut content analysis of about 83% animals collected from Clyde Sea contained plastic materials especially the tangled nylon strand balls. Also marine ciliates are shown to be capable of engulfing plastics while plastic fragments and monofilaments have been found in tissues of some filter feeding salps like *Thetys vagina*. In China it has been reported that high concentration of spherical microplastics occurs in oysters. It was also seen that microplastic pollution is wide spread in bivalves and that they can be used as indicators of microplastic pollution in coastal waters. The presence of microplastics in commercial bivalves can pose a threat to food safety as they are consumed as human food by a large population throughout the world as sea food (Li *et al.,* 2015).

Thus it can be concluded that the global impact of plastic ingestion on invertebrates include: internal or external abrasions and ulcers, blockage of digestive tract resulting in false satiation, starvation and physical deterioration which in turn leads to reduced reproductive fitness, drowning, diminished predator avoidance, impairment in feeding ability, potential transfer of damaging toxicants from sea water and ultimately death. The most detrimental effect in case of invertebrates is the potential of microplastics to clog and block the feeding appendages and also becoming embedded in tissues (Wright *et al.,* 2013).

IMPACT ON FISH FAUNA

The problems arising from indiscriminate disposal of plastics into global water bodies are chronic rather than acute and long recognized. Most important problems arising from this nuisance include entanglement and ingestion of these particles which are hazardous for the fish population. The ingestion of plastics has been reported in various groups of organisms including fish, leading to internal blockages and injury to the digestive tract. The plastic ingestion has been reported approximately in 150 fish species, including carnivore fishes (*Sillago sihama, Pampus cinereus, Harpodon nehereus* etc), omnivore fishes (*Cyprinus carpio, Carassius auratus, Mugil cephalus*), planktivore ones (*Hyporhamphus intermedius, Hypophthalamichthys molitrix* etc), inhabiting almost all the possible niches in aquatic habitat as pelagic, benthopelagic, demersal and benthic. The severity of plastic pollution has been reported from many parts of world, e.g. North Central Pacific Gyres, North Pacific Subtropical Gyres and the Mediterranean Sea. The highest percentage of plastic pollution has been reported in the sea fish Boops boops and the fresh water fishes *Lepomis macrochirus* and *L. megalotis*. Plastic items have been extracted from the whole

Figure 4. Crab entangled in plastic ropes (www.aquarium.co.za)

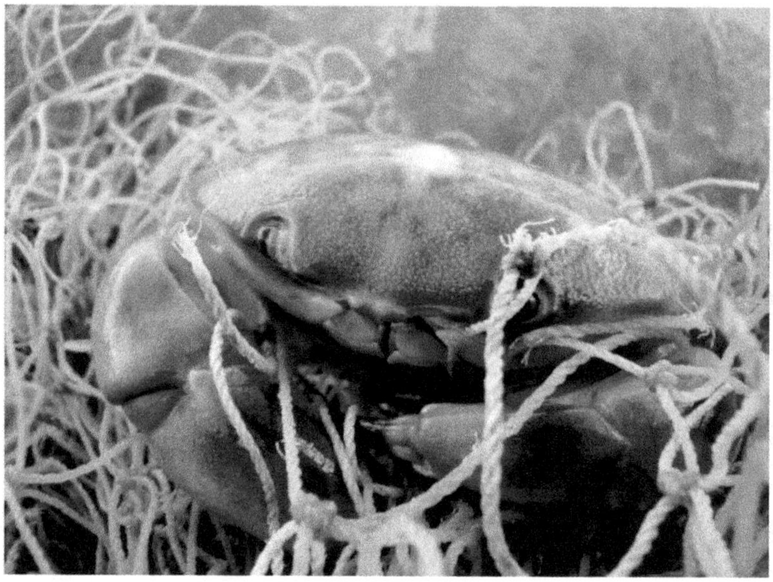

GIT tracts of fishes (Jabeen *et al.,* 2017). Ingested microplastics which are retained in the GIT can lead to formation of clumps or knots, because these are usually in the form of small fibers, resulting in the blockage of feeding appendages and hindrance in passage of food. Some experimental studies suggest that is plastic particles accumulate in higher numbers in the intestines of small animals, they may have similar effect to larger items of debris and clog the digestive system. This also causes decrease in food consumption as the presence of debris gives a false sense of satiation (Lusher *et al.*, 2013).

Plastic pollution has many other negative impacts on fishes, e.g., it significantly affects the survival of fishes during early developmental stages as in *Perca fluviatilis. In Pomatochistus microps* juveniles show a decrease in predatory performance and efficiency after exposure to microplastics (Jabeen *et al.,* 2017).

In addition, the accumulation of plastics inside the body of fishes may lead to adverse health effects because of the fact that with the advent of time the plastics release harmful chemicals like cadmium, lead etc which can be transported through the whole body and cause degradation of fish health e.g., the release of a component from plastics Bisphenol-A can affect the hormonal system and reproductive output of all the aquatic organisms. Other harmful chemicals like persistent organic pollutants (POPs) cause a toxic risk to animals that consume plastics. An endocrine disruptive substance, Nonylphenol, an additive in plastic, has been found in mackerel inhabiting the Pacific Ocean with largest concentration of plastic debris. Also by the ingestion of microplastics by individual organisms at lower trophic levels it gets accumulated and transferred to higher levels by biomagnifications with increased effects at higher levels (Lusher *et al.*, 2013). Above all plastic pollution is a leading cause of fish deaths across the globe. Some species of fish off the British coast were found to contain plastic cups within their guts causing their deaths.

Another tragedy of plastic pollution is in the form of "Ghost nets"- which are lost or abandoned fishing nets that remain suspended in the water column or sink to the bottom. It forms a leading cause of fish death which gets stranded into it and remains entangled until death due to injury and starvation. Sharks are seen to be caught in such nets leading to their death. Tangled masses of relatively intact, but

Figure 5. A plastic band restricts the growth of a blue-striped grunt fish in the Caribbean Sea) (Reddy, 2018) (www.Pewteusts.org)

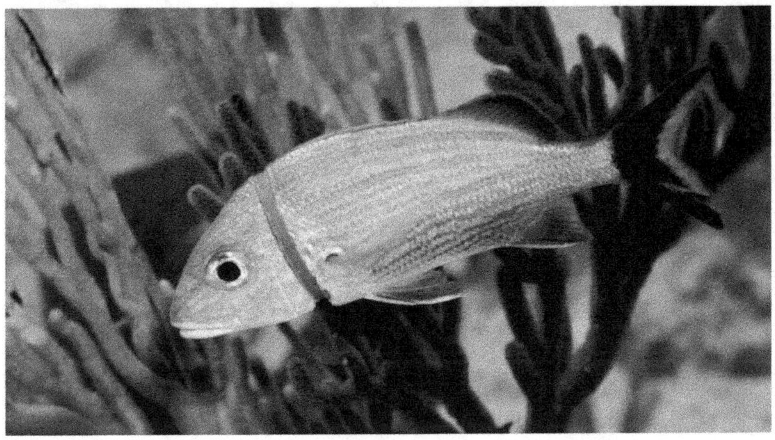

lost and abandoned or derelict, trawl nets, gill nets, webbing and monofilament etc, retain the ability to capture target fish for longer periods resulting in conspicuous mortality and also catch loses (Gregory, 2009; Derraik, 2002).

'Fish predators' interacting with plastic debris is known around the world, carcharhinid sharks seem to be most at risk of entanglement, probably due the high abundance and species diversity in this group. Cliff *et al.* (2002) put forward the observation that with the advent of time plastic entanglement of a carcharhinid species from South Africa has increased considerably, which is leading to a highest risk of negative interactions between floating litter and the animal. Shark species are also likely to be impacted by plastic debris, but the limited number of studies on these underscores that more research is required to determine the full extent of this problem (Thiel *et al.*, 2018).

IMPACT ON AQUATIC REPTILES

Recent concern about apparent declines in amphibian populations in many parts of the world suggests that there is an urgent need for information about how amphibians are impacted by pollutants. Among amphibians the most affected specie is that of sea turtle. Like other aquatic organisms these are also facing difficulties caused by ingestion and entanglement of plastics. These are exposed to a number of anthropogenic stressors among which plastic pollution is holding one of the top positions, as sea turtles live in diverse habitat conditions, have definite migratory behavior, and complex life histories. Litter ingestion and entanglement of plastic fragments have been accepted as serious threats to these species worldwide. It has been reported that five sea turtle species dwelling in the S.E. Pacific (*Caretta caretta, Chelonia mydas, Dermochelys coriacea, Eretmochelys imbricata, and Lepidochelys olivacea*) all are listed from vulnerable to critically endangered on the IUCN Red List and have documented interactions with marine litter (Thiel *et al.*, 2018).

After post mortem examination of various dead sea turtles it has been reported that ingested plastic and tar are the primary culprits of stress and non-natural death for sea turtles. Plastic material obtained from dead turtle digestive tracts included fishing line, ropes, nets, six pack rings, styrofoam, and plastic

Figure 6. A Lemon shark tangled in a plastic band (Grossman et al., 2017) (www.huffingtonpost.in)

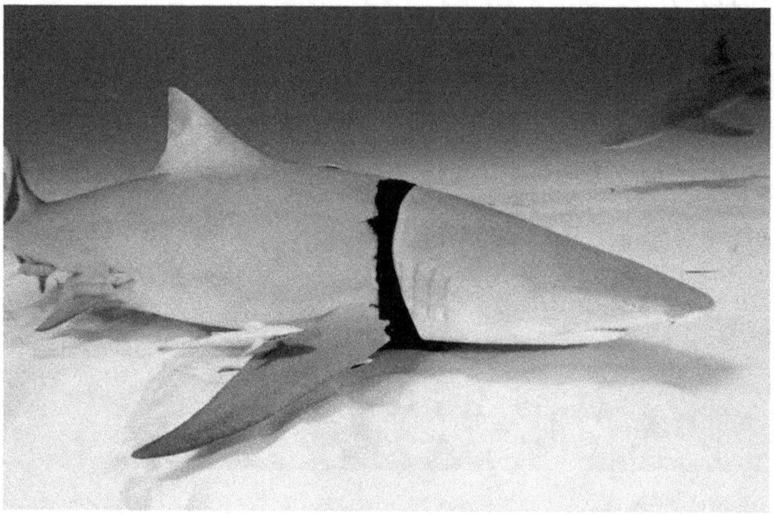

bags. This plastic debris, especially the plastic bags floating in the water strongly resemble the shape of jellyfish, a primary food source for sea turtles, thus resulting in the ingestion of the bags. In another case, 371leatherback turtles were put to autopsy which showed that 37% had plastic in their gastrointestinal tracts. Although it is not known if the plastic ingested was the cause of death, 8.7% of the turtles had a plastic bag presumably blocking the passage of food (Sigler, 2014).Many workers have reported that plastic ingestion has been the cause of death of stranded turtles in Ecuador and Chile.

Entanglement also affects the continued existence of the endangered sea turtles and entanglement has been recognized as a cause of mortality globally, there are quantitative knowledge gaps on rates and population implications. According to recent studies it has been reported that entanglement of plastic occurs across all species, life stages, and ocean basins, with higher vulnerability in pelagic juveniles.

Figure 7. Sea horse entangled in plastics (Ahmad, 2018) (www.waterlogic.com)

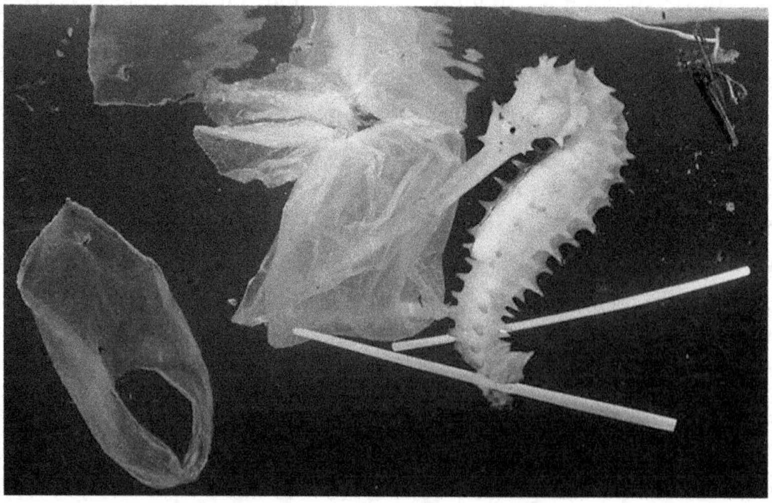

Figure 8. Plastic pollution in the world's oceans is threatening marine life). (Rashid, 2018) (news.un.org)

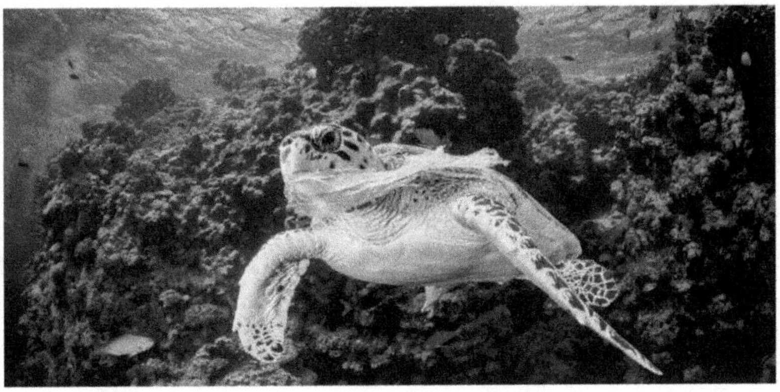

It has been reported that derelict fishing gear contributed globally to the majority of entanglements, while debris from land-based sources contributed to a lesser extent. Entanglements are a greater threat to sea turtles than climate change and direct exploitation, but less of a threat than plastic ingestion and by catches (active gear) (Derraik, 2002).

IMPACT OF PLASTIC POLLUTION ON AQUATIC BIRDS

The fundamental properties and extensive presence of plastic particles in marine environment have intense effect on birds inhabiting the world's oceans and water bodies. The most prevalent form of plastic in marine environment occurs as polystyrene, polypropylene, polyethylene, Styrofoam and polyvinyl chloride. These are having profound and prominent effects on aquatic birds by disturbing their physiological and trophic balance. As sea birds are highly diverse in behavior and adapt variedly to the marine environment, so they come in contact with this deadly material in many ways. Mainly two orders of sea birds have been extensively studied for the effect of this menace on aquatic birds which include: Procellariformes (Petrels, Prions, Shearwaters, Fulmars etc.) and Charadriiformes (Red phalaropes, Gulls, Terns and Waders).

From the study it was seen that birds of the order Procellariiformes are most affected ones due to plastic pollution as they tend to accumulate more plastic than do other species. Birds of order Charadriiformes are usually seen to regurgitate indigestible parts in their food but those of Procellariiformes find it difficult to expel out the indigested food due to a constriction between the gizzard and proventriculus. Less potential of regurgitation of plastic particles along with the smaller gizzard size to accumulate them make Procellariiformes especially susceptible to adverse effects of plastic pollution (Azzarello and Vleet, 1987).

Pattern of feeding also plays a role in the accumulation of plastics in the body of many birds as the ones feeding by pursuit- diving tend to eat more plastic because they are usually present on the surface or in the epiplagic zones, thus mistaken as prey and ingested along with them. Different colored plastic debris found in epiplagic zones resembles the planktonic larvae of some crustaceans and adults of other species and thus are ingested as food by birds. One of the serious issues created by plastic ingestion is injury to internal parts. Consuming plastics may result in complete blockage or internal injury. It has

Figure 9. A dead albatross found on Midway Atoll in the Pacific Ocean with plastic debris in its stomach (greentravelife.com)

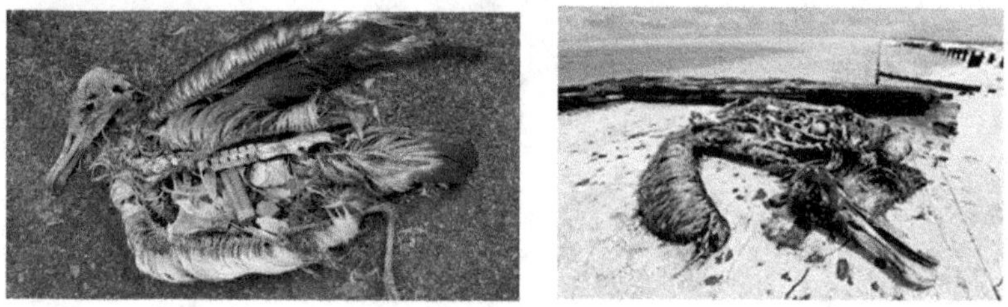

been seen in some young birds (Albatross) that large quantities of indigestible matter contributed to the intestinal obstruction and also bulky particles in the proventriculus had led to ulceration in the mucosa. Also birds which do not vomit out unnecessary or indigested food particles tend to accumulate them in their gizzards, leading to gastrointestinal blockage which in turn affects the feeding stimulus and activity, as hunger and satiety are regulated by hypothalamus on the basis of signals transduced from empty or full stomach respectively (Sigler, 2014). In addition the presence of large quantity of plastic particles in the stomach may alter the secretion of gastric enzymes or the movement of food in the small intestines.

Another huge effect of plastic pollution in birds is reduction of reproduction process because of harmful chemicals and toxins released from plastics with time. These include Dichloro diphenyl trichloro ethane, Polychlorinated biphenyls and other chlorinated hydrocarbons. These affect by lowering the steroid hormone levels causing delayed ovulation. Plastic contamination also may produce physiological effects which threaten the survival as well as reproductive success of birds (Azzarello and Vleet, 1987).

Summing up the major effects of plastic pollution on aquatic birds include, obstruction of the gastro intestine and subsequent passage of food into the intestines, blockage of gastric enzyme secretion, reduced feeding incentive, lowered steroid hormone levels, delayed ovulation and reproductive failure. Thus it can be concluded that plastic pollution has detrimental effects on aquatic birds.

Figure 10. Bird entangled in plastic bag (www.aquarium.co.za)

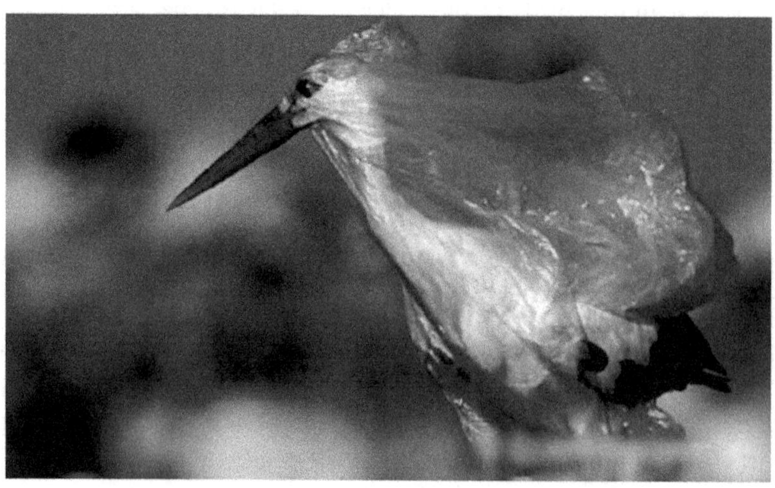

IMPACT ON AQUATIC MAMMALS

In the oceans the threat to marine life comes in various forms, such as over exploitation and harvesting, dumping of waste pollution, alien species, land reclamation, dredging and global climate change. Among marine mammals cetaceans are the ones most affected by plastic pollution including whales, manatees, dolphins. Cetaceans usually live in deeper waters and thus direct intake of plastic is limited, but ingestion is most likely by mixture of debris with desired food. The ingested plastic material gets accumulated in their stomachs resulting in blockage of nutrition process and it is seen that most of the whales die because of blockage of gastrointestinal tracts. It has been reported that entanglement is the main cause of deaths in aquatic mammals followed by ingestion of plastic materials.

Atleast 26 species of cetaceans have been recognized to ingest plastic debris. A young male pygmy sperm whale (*Kogia breviceps*) stranded alive in Texas, USA, died after few days and the necropsy showed that the first two stomach compartments were completely occluded by plastic debris. In Calfornia two sperm whales (*Physeter macrocephalus*) were found off the coast with a large amount of fishing gears in their gastrointestinal tracts, one was having rupture in third compartment of the stomach due to nylon netting while the other had fishing lines and plastic bags completely blocking the stomach from intestines. In Brazil, stomach analysis of a Blainvelle's beaked whale (*Mesoplodon densirostris*) showed the presence of a large bundle of blue plastic thread occupying the main part of the stomach. It is important to know that within the last decade atleast seven endangered migratory humpback whales (*Megaptera novaeangliae*) have been spotted to be tangling with masses of nylon ropes and other debris (Sigler, 2014).

It was reported that the death of an endangered West Indian manatee (*Trichechus manatus*) in 1985 in Florida was caused by a large piece of plastic that blocked its digestive tract. Deaths of the endangered Florida manatee (*Trichechus manatus latirostris*) have too been due to plastic debris in their guts.

A considerable number of pinnipeds, large baleen whales, and Odontocetes (dolphins, porpoises, and toothed whales) have been found to be entangled in fishing gear throughout neritic and oceanic waters off Peru and Chile. Plastic entanglement occurs when large gillnets are deployed at the bottom or drifting near the sea surface, depending on the fishery. Marine mammals swim or dive through the mesh and become entangled. Animals which are usually small in size, such as sea otters and sea lions, may die soon after entanglement, as these species may not have the necessary strength to escape from nets and being air-breathers will consequently drown. The same is probably also the case for dolphins such as the dusky dolphin (*Lagenorhynchus obscurus*), bottlenose dolphin (*Tursiops truncatus*), long-beaked common dolphin (*Delphinus capensis*), and the Burmeister porpoise (*Phocoena spinipinnis*) in Peru. Above the aforesaid species, in Chile the southern right whale dolphin (*Lissodelphis peronii*), Commerson's dolphin (*Cephalorhynchus commersonii*), Chilean dolphin (*Cephalorhynchus eutropia*), and Peale's dolphin (*Lagenorhynchus australis*) also suffer mortality from entanglements (Thiel *et al.*, 2018).

Plastic entanglement can greatly reduce fitness, as it leads to a significant increase in energetic costs of travel. Like incase of northern fur seals (*Callorhinus ursinus*) net fragments over 200 g could result in 4-fold increase in the demand of food utilization to maintain body condition. The decline in the populations of the northern sea lion (*Eumetopias jubatus*), endangered Hawaiian monk seal (*Monachus schauinslandi*) and northern fur seal seems at least aggravated by entanglement of immature or young animals in lost or redundant nets and packing bands. The population in 1976 was declining at a rate of 4–6% a year, and scientists estimated that up to 40,000 fur seals a year were being killed by plastic entanglement. A

Figure 11. (Seals are killed by abandoned fishing nets.) (Owens, 2016) (www.hakaimagazine.com)

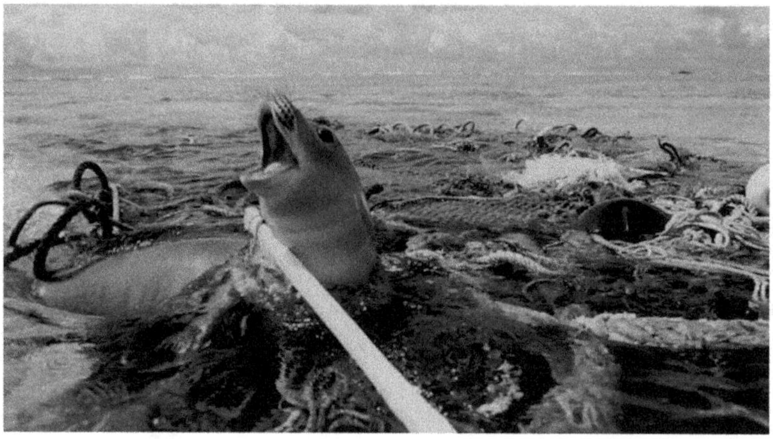

decline due to entanglement also seems to be occurring with Antarctic fur seals (*Arctocephalus gazella*) as well as with Australian fur seals (*Arctocephalus pusillus doriferus*). In one observation at South-east Farallon Island, Northern California, a survey from 1976–1988 showed 914 pinnipeds entangled in or with body constrictions from synthetic materials (Derraik, 2002).

CONCLUSION

Plastic is the wonder product of this century due to their low production costs and specific characteristics like durability and flexibility but it is equally a menace due to its haphazard management by common man. The ultimate drainage of the plastic wastes into the water bodies has extremely bad effect on the fauna in particular and environment as a whole. Due to ingestion or entanglement in plastic debris, over 270 species, including turtles, fish, seabirds, and mammals have experienced impaired movement, starvation or death leading to serious concerns about saving biodiversity. Proper steps should be taken at the earliest at local, national and global level to prevent further damage by this menace, before it takes a serious turn by wiping out the whole aquatic and terrestrial biodiversity.

REFERENCES

Ahmad, S. (2018). *World Environmental Day 2018: Let's beat plastic pollution.* Retrieved from www.waterlogic.com

Alshawafi, A., Analla, M., Alwashali, E., Aheichti, M., & Aksissou, M. (2018). Impacts of Marine Waste, Ingestion of Microplastic in the Fish, Impact on Fishing Yield, M'diq, Morocco. *International Journal of Marine Biology and Research,* 2475-4706.

Antonelis, K., Huppert, D., Velasquez, D., & June, J. (2011). Dungeness crab mortality due to lost traps and a cost–benefit analysis of trap removal in Washington State waters of the Salish Sea. *North American Journal of Fisheries Management*, *31*(5), 880–893. doi:10.1080/02755947.2011.590113

Table 1: Compilation of various studies on the effect of plastic pollution on some aquatic fauna

Invertebrates			
Organism	**Encounter Pathways**	**Effect**	**Reference**
Bivalve mollusks (Lab study)	Ingestion and accumulation of miroplastics in digestive cavity and tubules	Reduced feeding	Browne *et al.*, 2008
Arenicola marina (Lab study)	Exposure and ingestion of polystyrene microplastic	Weight loss, loss of feeding activity	Besseling *et al.*, 2012
Crab and octopus	Caught in derelict traps	Death due to stress, injuries or starvation	Antonelis *et al.*, 2011
Daphnia (Lab study)	Direct exposure and ingestion of nanopolystyrene	Changing in feeding and reproduction	Nasser & Lynch, 2016
Copepods (Lab study)	ingestion of nano and microplastic particles	Death	Lee *et al.*, 2013
Sessile invertebrates (coral reefs)	Direct contact with plastic hooks	Tissue abrasions	Chiappone *et al.*, 2005
Marine insects	Direct interaction with microplastic substrates	Increased population size	Goldstein *et al.*, 2012
Crustaceans	Caught in lost gill nets and traps	Death due to suffocation, predation, starvation and cannibalism	Kruse and Kimker, 1993
Vertebrates			
Fish			
Harpodon nehereus and *Pampus cinereus*	Ingestion of micro and mesoplastic particles	Blockage of gastrointestinal tract	Jabeen *et al.*, 2017
Decapterus muroadsi and *Cheilopogon rapanouienesis*	Microplastics ingestion mistaken as food particles	Blocked intestines, reduced feeding	Thiel *et al.*, 2016
Kyphosus sandwicensis and *Acanthurus leucopareius*	Entangled in derelict fishing net	Death	Thiel *et al.*, 2016
Micromesistius poutassou, Trachurus trachurus, Trisopterus minutes and *Zeus faber*	Ingestion of plastic debris especially the synthetic nylon fibers	Blocked of GIT	Lusher *et al.*, 2013
Juviniles of blue shark, *Prionace glauca*	Plastic straps entangled around gill region	Injuries to dorsal musculature, pectoral fins and obstructing gill slits	Colmenero, 2017
Diplodus cervinus and Auxis thazard.	Ingestion of micro plastics	Death	Alshawafi *et al.*, 2018
Carassius carassius (lab study)	Ingestion of *Daphnia magna* (previously fed on nanoparticles of polysterene)	Reduced feeding activity, behavioural changes, liver and brain damage	Mattsson *et al.*, 2015
Reptiles			
Caretta caretta, Chelonia mydas, Dermochelys coriacea, Eretmochelys imbricata, and *Lepidochelys olivacea*	Ingestion of plastic in the form of plastic bags, monofilament nylon, rope, and fishing nets	Stomach and intestinal blockage, Death	Thiel *et al.*, 2016
C. caretta	Entanglement	Death	Thiel *et al.*, 2016
Sea turtles	Entanglement in fishing gear	Death	Vélez-Rubio *et al.*, 2013
Sea snake, *Hydrophis elegans*	Entanglement	Starvation by restricting the food passage	Udyawer *et al.*, 2013
Birds			
Petrels, Prions, Shearwaters, Fulmars	Accumulation of plastic in gizzard and proventriculus	Reduced feeding potential and blocked internal organs, reduced satiety	Azzarello and Vleet, 1987
Albatross	Ingestion of plastic debris	Intestinal obstruction, death	Sigler, 2014
Prions, gulls, albatross	Ingestion of plastic particles, pellets	Perforated gut	Carey, 2011
Penguins	Ingestion of plastic particles	Perforated gut, death	Brandão *et al.*, 2011
Mammals			
Sperm whales	Ingestion of plastic debris	Gastric rupture, gut impaction, death	Jacobsen *et al.*, 2010
Pinnipeds	Ingestion of plastic fishing hooks	Internal wound	Dau *et al.*, 2009
Manatees	Ingestion and entanglement in MF line, fish hooks, other debris	Intestinal blockage, death	Beck & Barros, 1991
Whales	Entanglement	Dermal wound	Woodward *et al.*, 2006
Fur seals	Entanglement in Trawl nets	Death due to dermal wound	Fowler, 1987

Azzarello, M. Y., & Van Vleet, E. S. (1987). Marine birds and plastic pollution. *Marine Ecology Progress Series*, *37*, 295–303. doi:10.3354/meps037295

Beck, C. A., & Barros, N. B. (1991). The impact of debris on the Florida manatee. *Marine Pollution Bulletin*, *22*(10), 508–510. doi:10.1016/0025-326X(91)90406-I

Besseling, E., Wegner, A., Foekema, E. M., Van Den Heuvel-Greve, M. J., & Koelmans, A. A. (2012). Effects of microplastic on fitness and PCB bioaccumulation by the lugworm Arenicola marina (L.). *Environmental Science & Technology*, *47*(1), 593–600. doi:10.1021/es302763x PMID:23181424

Brandão, M. L., Braga, K. M., & Luque, J. L. (2011). Marine debris ingestion by Magellanic penguins, *Spheniscus magellanicus* (Aves: Sphenisciformes), from the Brazilian coastal zone. *Marine Pollution Bulletin*, *62*(10), 2246–2249. doi:10.1016/j.marpolbul.2011.07.016 PMID:21864861

Browne, M. A., Dissanayake, A., Galloway, T. S., Lowe, D. M., & Thompson, R. C. (2008). Ingested microscopic plastic translocates to the circulatory system of the mussel, *Mytilus edulis* (L.). *Environmental Science & Technology*, *42*(13), 5026–5031. doi:10.1021/es800249a PMID:18678044

Carey, M. J. (2011). Intergenerational transfer of plastic debris by Short-tailed Shearwaters (Ardenna tenuirostris). *Emu-Austral Ornithology*, *111*(3), 229–234. doi:10.1071/MU10085

Chiappone, M., Dienes, H., Swanson, D. W., & Miller, S. L. (2005). Impacts of lost fishing gear on coral reef sessile invertebrates in the Florida Keys National Marine Sanctuary. *Biological Conservation*, *121*(2), 221–230. doi:10.1016/j.biocon.2004.04.023

Cliff, G., Dudley, S. F., Ryan, P. G., & Singleton, N. (2002). Large sharks and plastic debris in KwaZulu-Natal, South Africa. *Marine & Freshwater Research*, *53*(2), 575–581. doi:10.1071/MF01146

Colmenero, A. I., Barría, C., Broglio, E., & García-Barcelona, S. (2017). Plastic debris straps on threatened blue shark Prionace glauca. *Marine Pollution Bulletin*, *115*(1-2), 436–438. doi:10.1016/j.marpolbul.2017.01.011 PMID:28089553

Dau, B. K., Gilardi, K. V., Gulland, F. M., Higgins, A., Holcomb, J. B., Leger, J. S., & Ziccardi, M. H. (2009). Fishing gear–related injury in California marine wildlife. *Journal of Wildlife Diseases*, *45*(2), 355–362. doi:10.7589/0090-3558-45.2.355 PMID:19395745

Derraik, J. G. (2002). The pollution of the marine environment by plastic debris: A review. *Marine Pollution Bulletin*, *44*(9), 842–852. doi:10.1016/S0025-326X(02)00220-5 PMID:12405208

Devriese, L. I., van der Meulen, M. D., Maes, T., Bekaert, K., Paul-Pont, I., Frère, L., & Vethaak, A. D. (2015). Microplastic contamination in brown shrimp (*Crangon crangon*, Linnaeus 1758) from coastal waters of the Southern North Sea and Channel area. *Marine Pollution Bulletin*, *98*(1-2), 179–187. doi:10.1016/j.marpolbul.2015.06.051 PMID:26456303

Fowler, C. W. (1987). Marine debris and northern fur seals: A case study. *Marine Pollution Bulletin*, *18*(6), 326–335. doi:10.1016/S0025-326X(87)80020-6

Geyer, R., Jambeck, J. R., & Law, K. L. (2017). Production, use, and fate of all plastics ever made. *Science Advances*, *3*(7), e1700782. doi:10.1126ciadv.1700782 PMID:28776036

Goldstein, M. C., Rosenberg, M., & Cheng, L. (2012). Increased oceanic microplastic debris enhances oviposition in an endemic pelagic insect. *Biology Letters*, *8*(5), 817–820. doi:10.1098/rsbl.2012.0298 PMID:22573831

Greentravelife. (2016). *Midway Island: An Environmental Tragedy.* Retrieved from Greentravelife.com.

Gregory, M. R. (2009). Environmental implications of plastic debris in marine settings entanglement, ingestion, smothering, hangers-on, hitch-hiking and alien invasions. *Philosophical Transactions of the Royal Society of London. Series B, Biological Sciences*, *364*(1526), 2013–2025. doi:10.1098/rstb.2008.0265 PMID:19528053

Grossman, S. R., Dahlem, D., & Huffington Post. (2017). *Heartbreaking photos show what your trash does to animals.* Retrieved from www.huffingtonpost.in

Hasselerharm, R. P. E., Falahudin, D., Peeters, E. T., & Koelmans, A. A. (2018). Microplastic effect thresholds for freshwater benthic macroinvertebrates. *Environmental Science & Technology*, *52*(4), 2278–2286. doi:10.1021/acs.est.7b05367 PMID:29337537

Jabeen, K., Su, L., Li, J., Yang, D., Tong, C., Mu, J., & Shi, H. (2017). Microplastics and mesoplastics in fish from coastal and fresh waters of China. *Environmental Pollution*, *221*, 141–149. doi:10.1016/j.envpol.2016.11.055 PMID:27939629

Jacobsen, J. K., Massey, L., & Gulland, F. (2010). Fatal ingestion of floating net debris by two sperm whales (*Physeter macrocephalus*). *Marine Pollution Bulletin*, *60*(5), 765–767. doi:10.1016/j.marpolbul.2010.03.008 PMID:20381092

Kruse, G. H., & Kimker, A. (1993). *Degradable escape mechanisms for pot gear: a summary report to the Alaska Board of Fisheries.* Alaska Department of Fish & Game, Division of Commercial Fisheries.

Law, K. L. (2017). Plastics in the Marine Environment. *Annual Review of Marine Science*, *9*(1), 205–229. doi:10.1146/annurev-marine-010816-060409 PMID:27620829

Lebreton, L. C. M., & Borrero, J. C. (2013). Modeling the transport and accumulation floating debris generated by the 11 March 2011 Tohoku tsunami. *Marine Pollution Bulletin*, *66*(1-2), 53–58. doi:10.1016/j.marpolbul.2012.11.013 PMID:23219397

Lee, K. W., Shim, W. J., Kwon, O. Y., & Kang, J. H. (2013). Size-dependent effects of micro polystyrene particles in the marine copepod *Tigriopus japonicus*. *Environmental Science & Technology*, *47*(19), 11278–11283. doi:10.1021/es401932b PMID:23988225

Li, J., Yang, D., Li, L., Jabeen, K., & Shi, H. (2015). Microplastics in commercial bivalves from China. *Environmental Pollution*, *207*, 190–195. doi:10.1016/j.envpol.2015.09.018 PMID:26386204

Lusher, A., Hollman, P., & Mendoza-Hill, J. (2017). Microplastics in fisheries and aquaculture. *FAO Fisheries and Aquaculture Technical Paper (FAO) eng no. 615.*

Lusher, A. L., Mchugh, M., & Thompson, R. C. (2013). Occurrence of microplastics in the gastrointestinal tract of pelagic and demersal fish from the English Channel. *Marine Pollution Bulletin*, *67*(1-2), 94–99. doi:10.1016/j.marpolbul.2012.11.028 PMID:23273934

Macali, A., Semenov, A., Venuti, V., Crupi, V., D'Amico, F., Rossi, B., & Bergami, E. (2018). Episodic records of jellyfish ingestion of plastic items reveal a novel pathway for trophic transference of marine litter. *Scientific Reports*, *8*(1), 6105. doi:10.103841598-018-24427-7 PMID:29666447

Mattsson, K., Ekvall, M. T., Hansson, L. A., Linse, S., Malmendal, A., & Cedervall, T. (2015). Altered behavior, physiology, and metabolism in fish exposed to polystyrene nanoparticles. *Environmental Science & Technology*, *49*(1), 553–561. doi:10.1021/es5053655 PMID:25380515

Mendoza, A. (2018). The Impacts of Plastic Pollution in the Great Lakes. California State University, Sacramento ENVS 190.

Nasser, F., & Lynch, I. (2016). Secreted protein eco-corona mediates uptake and impacts of polystyrene nanoparticles on Daphnia magna. *Journal of Proteomics*, *137*, 45–51. doi:10.1016/j.jprot.2015.09.005 PMID:26376098

Owens, B. (2016). *The ghosts of fishers past*. Coastal Science & Societies. Retrieved from www.hakaimagazine.com

Pavani, P., & Raja Rajeswari, T. (2014). Impact of plastics on environmental pollution. *Journal of Chemical and Pharmaceutical Sciences,* 2087-2093.

Pirolini, A. (2014). *Impact of microplastics/microbeads accumulation on the marine environment.* Retrieved from www.azom.com

Rashid, S. (2018). *Plastic pollution in the world's oceans is threatening marine life.* Retrieved from News.un.org.

Reddy, S. (2018). *Plastic pollution affects sea life throughout the ocean.* Retrieved from www.pewtrust.org

Safety4sea. (2018). *How plastic affects marine life.* Retrieved from Safety4sea.com

Sigler, M. (2014). The effects of plastic pollution on aquatic wildlife: Current situations and future solutions. *Water, Air, and Soil Pollution*, *225*(11), 2184. doi:10.100711270-014-2184-6

Steer, M., Cole, M., Thompson, R. C., & Lindeque, P. K. (2017). Microplastic ingestion in fish larvae in the western English Channel. *Environmental Pollution*, *226*, 250–259. doi:10.1016/j.envpol.2017.03.062 PMID:28408185

Sussarellu, R., Suquet, M., Thomas, Y., Lambert, C., Fabioux, C., Pernet, M. E. J., ... Corporeau, C. (2016). Oyster reproduction is affected by exposure to polystyrene microplastics. *Proceedings of the National Academy of Sciences of the United States of America*, *113*(9), 2430–2435. doi:10.1073/pnas.1519019113 PMID:26831072

Thiel, M., Luna-Jorquera, G., Álvarez-Varas, R., Gallardo, C., Hinojosa, I. A., Luna, N., ... Portflitt-Toro, M. (2018). Impacts of Marine Plastic Pollution From Continental Coasts to Subtropical Gyres—Fish, Seabirds, and Other Vertebrates in the SE Pacific. *Frontiers in Marine Science, 5*(238).

Thompson, R. C. (2017). *Future of the Sea: Plastic Pollution.* Foresight, Government Office for Science.

Thushari, G. G. N., Senevirathna, J. D. M., Yakupitiyage, A., & Chavanich, S. (2017). Effects of microplastics on sessile invertebrates in the eastern coast of Thailand: An approach to coastal zone conservation. *Marine Pollution Bulletin*, *124*(1), 349–355. doi:10.1016/j.marpolbul.2017.06.010 PMID:28760587

Two Oceans Aquarium. (2018). *The plastic problem: How does plastic pollution affect wildlife*. Retrieved from www.aquarium.co.za

Udyawer, V., Read, M. A., Hamann, M., Simpfendorfer, C. A., & Heupel, M. R. (2013). First record of sea snake (*Hydrophis elegans*, Hydrophiinae) entrapped in marine debris. *Marine Pollution Bulletin*, *73*(1), 336–338. doi:10.1016/j.marpolbul.2013.06.023 PMID:23809333

Van Sebille, E., Spathi, C., & Gilbert, A. (2016). The ocean plastic pollution challenge: Towards solutions in the UK. *Grant. Brief. Pap*, *19*, 1–16.

Vélez-Rubio, G. M., Estrades, A., Fallabrino, A., & Tomás, J. (2013). Marine turtle threats in Uruguayan waters: Insights from 12 years of stranding data. *Marine Biology*, *160*(11), 2797–2811. doi:10.100700227-013-2272-y

Vendel, A. L., Bessa, F., Alves, V. E. N., Amorim, A. L. A., Patrício, J., & Palma, A. R. T. (2017). Widespread microplastic ingestion by fish assemblages in tropical estuaries subjected to anthropogenic pressures. *Marine Pollution Bulletin*, *117*(1-2), 448–455. doi:10.1016/j.marpolbul.2017.01.081 PMID:28214011

Verma, R., Vinoda, K. S., Papireddy, M., & Gowda, A. N. S. (2016). Toxic Pollutants from Plastic Waste-A Review. *Procedia Environmental Sciences*, *35*, 701–708. doi:10.1016/j.proenv.2016.07.069

Woodward, B. L., Winn, J. P., Moore, M. J., & Peterson, M. L. (2006). Experimental modeling of large whale entanglement injuries. *Marine Mammal Science*, *22*(2), 299–310. doi:10.1111/j.1748-7692.2006.00020.x

Wright, S. L., Thompson, R. C., & Galloway, T. S. (2013). The physical impacts of microplastics on marine organisms: A review. *Environmental Pollution*, *178*, 483–492. doi:10.1016/j.envpol.2013.02.031 PMID:23545014

Chapter 10
Analyses of the Recycling Potential of Medical Plastic Wastes

Nasreena Sajjad
University of Kashmir, India

Sumaya Hassan
https://orcid.org/0000-0002-9658-6936
University of Kashmir, India

Jasfeeda Qadir
University of Kashmir, India

Rohaya Ali
University of Kashmir, India

Durdana Shah
University of Kashmir, India

ABSTRACT

Medical wastes have been historically disposed of either in landfills or treated in poorly-designed or inadequately-controlled incinerators that leads to the release of a significant quantity of hazardous pollutants, such as dioxins and heavy metals including Cd, Hg and Pb in the environment. This has led to increased public concerns over the disposal of medical wastes. Plastic is one of the most important components of the medical waste. The plastic content (20–25% by weight) of medical waste is significantly higher than that of municipality solid waste. Therefore, recycling of plastics should be increased to save landfill space and also to reduce expensive disposal cost of medical wastes. The recycling issues like risk of transmitting infections, improper collection and separation, can be resolved by proper management, education and innovative waste collection and disposal policies. Analysis and use of alternative products should always be considered as an important part of any recycling program.

DOI: 10.4018/978-1-5225-9452-9.ch010

INTRODUCTION

Medical waste management is one of the challenging problems worldwide. Medical waste is classified by the World Health Organization (WHO) as "waste that is generated in the diagnosis, treatment or immunization of human beings or animals." If the medical waste is not properly disposed off it causes various hazardous outputs (Pandey et al., 2016). It affects both biotic and abiotic components of environment (Nie and Wu, 2016). Therefore it is a worldwide concern of disposal of medical waste. The United States tops the list of higher production of medical waste and it alone creates over 3.5 million tonnes of medical waste per year with an average disposal cost of $790 per tonne (Lee et al., 2004). In the developing nations, the medical waste is increasing owing to better medical services. Medical wastes have been historically disposed off either in landfills or treated in poorly designed or inadequately controlled incinerators that leads to release of significant quantity of hazardous pollutants, such as dioxins, furans and heavy metals including Cd, Hg and Pb in the environment. It has led to greater public concerns over the disposal of medical wastes. Plastic is one of the most important components of the waste that occupies landfill space, therefore, recycling of plastics should be increased to save landfill space, to preserve natural resources and to reduce expensive disposal cost of medical wastes (Thompson et al., 2009). The plastic content (20–25% by weight) of medical waste is significantly higher than that of municipality solid waste. The main obstacle in the development of recycling programs for medical wastes is the potential risk of transmitting infections and improper classification of medical wastes (Aljabre, 2002). However, increased cost of medical disposal and limited availability of landfill has lead to efforts that encourage waste recycling.

MEDICAL WASTE

Medical waste is a wider term. It comprises of many different types of wastes including medical waste, regulated medical waste, infectious medical waste and hospital waste. In other words medical waste refers to all waste that is generated at any healthcare or healthcare-related facility (Khajuria et al., 2007). Contaminated syringes and needles represent a particular threat, as the failure to dispose them safely may lead to dangerous recycling and repackaging which lead to unsafe reuse. Contaminated injection equipment may be scavenged from waste areas and dumpsites and either reused or sold to be used again (Gyawali et al., 2013). Biomedical waste may be defined as any waste in the form of solid or liquid, which is generated during the treatment, diagnosis and immunization of human beings and animals in research (Baghotia, 2009). Many synonyms to medical waste exist and they are currently used interchangeably (Mehala et al., 2018). According to Moritz (1995) some of the easily used synonyms are clinical waste, hospital waste and biomedical waste. The WHO uses the term "healthcare waste" in reports and other official publications. The United States Medical Waste Tracking act of 1988 defines medical waste as "any solid waste that is generated in the diagnosis, treatment, or immunization of human beings or animals, in research pertaining thereto, or in the production or testing of biologicals". It is estimated by the World Health Organization (WHO) that 20 percent of these medical wastes can be classified as hazardous materials that may be infectious, toxic, or radioactive (Brichard, 2002).

Figure 1. Classification of hospital waste

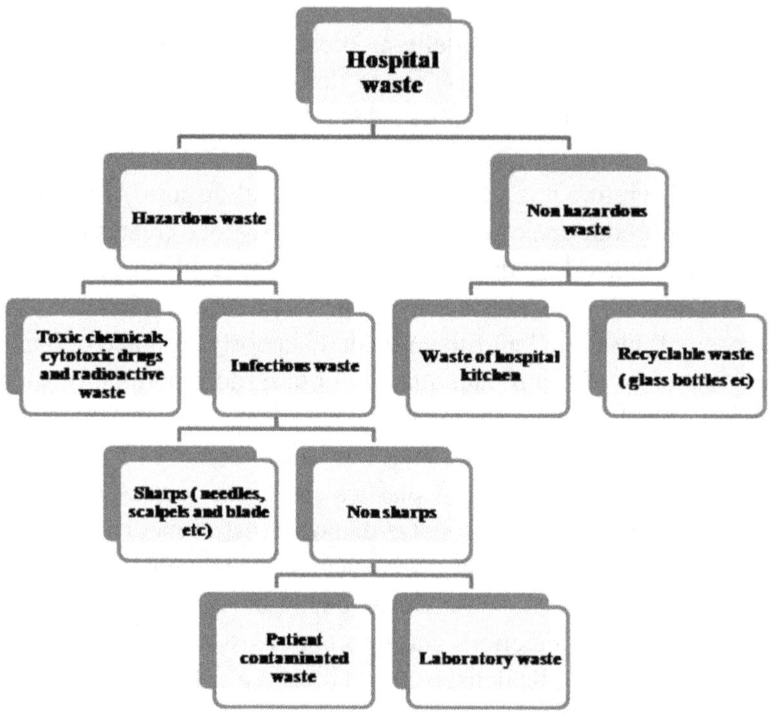

Production of Medical Waste

Medical waste is on increase in its type and amount by different Health Care centers. The hospital waste imposes risk for workers and personnel who handle them and also poses a threat to public health and their environment. According to the quantities of waste production, Prüss et al., 1999, classified the sources of health care waste into two groups as major and minor. These are listed below:

Major Sources

Major sources for biomedical waste production:

- Waste produced from medical colleges, paramedical services and from research centers.
- Waste produced from govt. hospitals, nursing homes, dispensaries and private hospitals.
- Waste generated from mortuaries, blood banks and autopsy centers.
- Waste also generated from production units.
- Waste produced from biotechnology institutions.
- Waste produced from primary health centers.
- Waste from veterinary colleges and animal research centers.

Minor Sources

Following are the minor sources for biomedical waste production:

- Waste from physicians and dentists clinics.
- Waste produced from blood donation camps.
- Waste from psychiatric clinics, acupuncturists and cosmetic piercing centers.
- Waste from animal houses and slaughter houses.
- Waste from vaccination centers.
- Waste from institutions for physically challenge.

Categories of Medical Waste

Medical wastes constitute a larger part of hazardous wastes (Jang et al., 2006). The generation of these wastes is a continuous phenomenon. Hospital waste is sub-divided into health care general waste (HCGW) and health care risk waste (HCRW). The health care system is under enormous pressure to dispose of health care waste, as there are unnecessarily high levels of environmental degradation. The aim of health care facilities worldwide is a beginning to subscribe to the social goals of a cleaner and safer environment (Datta et al., 2018). Determining which portion or component of clinical waste is infectious is challenged by its inherent heterogeneous nature and definitional problems. The U.S.EPA, 1986 and Centers for Disease Control, despite their discrepancies in clarifying the term infectious waste, have designated pathological waste, blood and blood products, contaminated sharps (scalpels, needles and blades) and microbiological waste (cultures and stocks) as infectious (OTA, 1998). In general, for waste to be infectious, it has to contain enough virulence capable of causing an infectious disease including a portal of entry in a susceptible host. The amount of medical waste produced at various healthcare centers is of apparent interest, with many studies done on the subject. The quantity and composition of medical waste generated is reliant on many factors, with a medical waste study focusing on Italian hospitals finding that the type of sanitary service offered greatly impacts the amount of infectious waste produced (Windfeld et al., 2015).

The study has found that 52% of overall infectious medical waste production comes from short-term patients in rehabilitation service, followed by analytical laboratories (23%), surgeries (14%), dialyses (7%) and first aid (4%) (Windfeld et al., 2015). A similar study done in Taiwan found that the dialysis unit generate the greatest amount of infectious medical waste i.e., (23%), followed by the intensive care unit (17%), the emergency care unit and the outpatient clinic (12% each) (Cheng et al., 2009). In evaluating medical waste generation, it is helpful to use a common basis for quantification, so that data from different regions can be compared.

According to Eigenheer & Zanon (1991) and Biomedical Waste (Handling & Management Rules, 1998) amended in 2000, biomedical waste has been categorized under 10 categories with respect to its collection. According to Prüss et al., 1999, The Department of Health, Government of India, 2011 and The Royal College of nursing, 2007, hospital wastes may be categorized into the following groups:-

Figure 2. Categories of biomedical waste

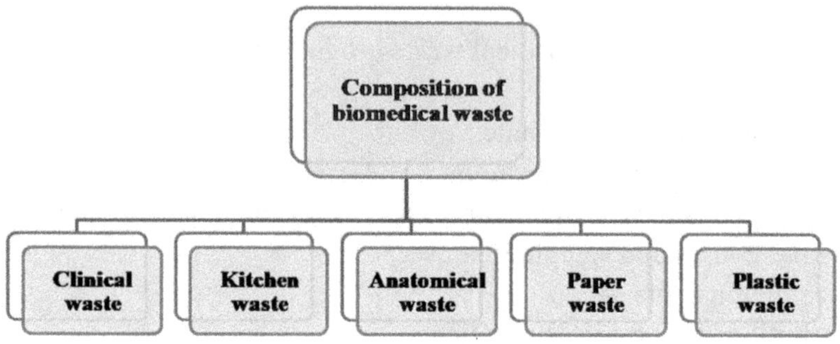

Infectious Waste

The waste which consists of pathogens in major concentrations and cause diseases to humans. Some examples of the infectious wastes are;

- Discarded syringes and needles used to draw blood or give vaccination to the patients.
- Production of culture dishes, petriplates, glassware, test tubes and other glass instruments used in laboratory work.
- Discarded surgical gloves and surgical instruments.
- Contaminated blood-soaked bandages and cotton plugs.
- Swabs used to inoculate cultures and stocks.
- Blood contaminated materials, sharps and other instruments etc
- Removed body organs like placenta, limbs, appendices, uterus and other body parts etc.
- Specimens and laboratory cultures etc.

Chemical Wastes

This type of waste category includes discarded liquid, solid and gaseous chemicals which are used in disinfecting the products, cleaning and in housekeeping.

Pathological Wastes

It includes body organs, human foetus, placenta, blood and body fluids etc.

Sharps

It includes those waste materials which could be infectious to people taking care of it. Sharps can also cut or puncture the skin. They can include blades, needles, nails, saws, scalpels and broken glasses etc.

Radioactive Waste

It consists of radionuclide in the form of solid, liquid and gaseous form used in *in-vitro* analysis of body tissues and body fluid and *in vivo* body organ imaging, tumor location and therapeutic procedures.

Pharmaceutical Wastes

It comprises of outdated drugs and chemicals which have been discarded from different wards.

General Waste

This type of waste is mainly consists of household wastes such as Packaging material, wrappers, kitchen waste, plastics and paper etc. It is to human beings.

Hospital Plastic Waste

Plastics being increasingly utilized for the storage and delivery of life saving fluids. Although, virgin polymer is generally considered safe due to its inertness, however, the plastic products could be harmful due to migration of certain chemical additives like plasticizers, stabilizers, pigments and unreacted monomers into the stored commodity (Koushal et al., 2014). Therefore, plastic products intended for storage and delivery of life saving fluids must be evaluated for their safety. (Andrady et al., 2009). The authority principally responsible for regulating medical devices in India, however, is the Central Drugs Standards Control Organization (CDSCO) under MoHFW. Companies must register all products with the CDSCO before introducing its product into the Indian market. Different countries have laid down different safety assessment tests and guidelines for the suitability and quality of the plastics. Indian climatic conditions are quite different than that of western countries. The guidelines provided by the Bureau of Indian Standards, New Delhi has recommended the test for Global migration residue for safety assessment of plastics. Several International regulatory agencies have also recommended tests for the presence of heavy metals, UV absorbing materials and oxidizable materials in the plastics used in biomedical devices as well as food packaging. Plastic and polymeric products are now being a part of our life and living without them is almost beyond thoughts (Halden, 2010).

Plastic products are generally widely accepted because of various reasons mainly due to their light weight, moldability, non-corrosive in nature, variety of colors, save the use of plant woods for house hold furniture and above all reusability etc (Zaman, 2010). The applications of plastic are rapidly increasing all over the world (Lee et al., 2002). Plastics are being used in a variety of other consumer and industrial products viz. textile, fibers, packaging, automobiles, paints, alternate building materials etc. Plastics are being widely used in electronic devices such as television, air conditioners, refrigerators, agricultures etc. due to their versatile properties (Li et al., 2009).

In the present scenario, we find the plastic usage pattern in various sectors like 33% of plastic is being used for the packaging purpose, 20% in building construction, 10% in electrical and electronic items, 7% in automobiles, 5% in agriculture and 25% in the other sectors such as medical and leisure (Banerjee et al., 2012). In hospital, plastic medical devices are being used for storage and transfusion of life saving fluids, syringes, blood bags, biomedical implants, tubing and heart valves for the cardiac patients (Al-Khatib et al, 2009). Plastic use is dominated by single use or short term use, and at the same time most plastics are extremely persistent in the environment. Plastics are important in our society and extend many benefits for human health and the environment, for instance:

1. Plastic packaging protects food from contamination and hence saves it from wastage.
2. The light weight packaging material saves fuel and decreases emissions during transportation.
3. Plastic water supply systems and storage containers/tanks provide clean water. Light plastic materials in cars and aircraft save fuel and decreases emissions.
4. Plastic protective clothing and safety equipment (e.g. fire proof materials, helmets, air bags) protects from injury.
5. Plastic products for medical applications contribute to improved heath (e.g. blood pouches, tubings, disposable syringes, prosthesis).
6. The plastic industries in India started with the introduction of products like-cellulose acetate, acrylics and vinyl. The newer plastics, such as polyethylene, polypropylene, polystyrene, polycarbonate, polymethyl methacrylate, polyurethane, polyester and silicones joined polystyrene and PVC in wide applications.

More recently, because of better understanding of the importance of surface, avoidance of contamination, and control of molecular weight and molecular weight distribution, the use of synthetic polymers in the biomedical sciences is increasing (Ren, 2003). Polymers are viewed as important biomedical materials for a number of reasons, some of which appear contradictory but only because of different uses require different properties (Pandey et al., 2016). Various important properties are the ability surface control, strength, flexibility, rigidity, inertness/reactivity, ease of fabrication, lightweight, ability to achieve a high degree of purity, compatibility and the ability of some of them to withstand long term exposure to the human body-a truly hostile environment (Shah et al., 2008). A number of new materials have been developed because of the health fears associated with the monomer Bisphenol A, which is the commoner for most polycarbonates, butanediol (Vandenburg et al., 2007). The global medical device industry shows a tremendous growth (Gregory, 2009). Germany is the largest market in Europe followed by France, Italy, and the United Kingdom. Japan is the second largest country by market share next to the U. S. The rest of the world comprises regions like China, India, and Latin America. These regions are seeing 10-15% annual growth rates in the medical device market.

Medical devices are of many types ranging from simple devices such as depressors, syringes, and bandages to highly complex imaging machines and long term surgical implants. It include MRI machines, surgical instruments, catheters, coronary stents, pacemakers, X-ray machines, artificial hips, prosthetic limbs, surgical gloves, knees, and bandages. Devices are classified into three classes: Class I, Class II, and Class III depending upon their risk and criticality.

Examples of **Class I devices** include tongue depressors, bandages, gloves, and simple surgical devices. **Class II devices** are wheel-chairs, X-ray machines, MRI machines, surgical needles, catheters, and diagnostic equipment. **Class III devices** are used inside the body. Most implants are Class III devices. Examples include stents, heart valves, silicone implants, implanted pacemakers and hip and bone implants (Laurence, 2014).

Medical devices can be grouped into two major categories i.e., disposables and non disposables. Disposable devices include gloves, bandages, blood bags, colostomy bags, syringes, catheters, IV kits, and tubing. There is a wide spectrum of requirements that apply to materials used in medical device applications. It is important to understand these requirements and design the right part with the right material that fits the intended use and the processing and assembly of the finished device. Materials that are used in design, production, and assembly of medical devices include ceramics, glass, metals, and plastics. Among these, plastics have superior design flexibility compared to metals, ceramics, and glass. Their properties can be tailored to meet a wide spectrum of physical, mechanical, chemical, and biocompatibility requirements (Shemwell et al., 2011). Elastomers are loosely cross linked polymers and have the characteristics of rubber in terms of elasticity and flexibility e.g. styrene butadiene block copolymers, natural rubber, polyisoprene, polybutadiene, ethylene propylene rubber, fluoroelastomers, polyurethane elastomers, silicone elastomers and nitrile rubbers (Vert, 2011).

Poly (Ethylene Terephthalate) – PET or PETE

It is clear, tough and has good gas and moisture barrier properties making it ideal for carbonated beverages, food containers and life saving fluid bottles etc.

Poly (Vinyl Chloride) – PVC or V

It has chemical resistant, excellent transparency, stable electrical properties and long term stability. Vinyl products can be broadly divided into rigid and flexible materials. The application varies from water pipes and fittings to windows, laminates, blood bags, medical tubing etc.

Polypropylene – PP

It is commonly used in packaging due to its excellent chemical resistance and high melting point making it ideal for hot fill liquids. Like other plastics PP has excellent resistance to water, salts and acids that are destructive to metals. Typical applications include ketchups bottles, medicine bottles and automobile battery casings.

Polystyrene – PS

PS is used in the making of variety of containers, including those known as Styrofoam plates, dishes, cups, biomedical devices etc.

Other Plastics

Beside these, various specialized plastic products can also be seen in the market such as Nylon, polyester, polycarbonate, polymethyl methacrylate, Glass fiber reinforced plastics, Teflon, ABS copolymers, blends and multilayered combinations (Elias,2005). Products are frequently composed of components; however simple examples are a disposable syringe (needle, barrel, plunger, lubricant, and stopper etc.). Changing a component can significantly alter the biocompatibility of a product, and certain components, by the nature of both their composition and exposure to patients, are more likely to present biocompatibility problems (Li et al., 2015). An example is the common disposable plastic syringe, of which 14 billion are used each year. For the syringe, the most likely problem component is the stopper—the flexible piece at the end of the plunger. The stopper is most commonly made of natural rubber, and has direct contact with fluids entering the body (and frequently a fluid path).

Plastics used in medical device applications must meet stringent performance requirements through production, packaging, shipping, end use, and disposal. Many devices and device kits are sterilized before they are shipped for use (Gundarov et al., 2001). The devices also come in contact with various chemicals solvents, bodily fluids, skin, organs, and tissues during manufacturing (Rai et al., 2011). The materials used in medical devices must be resistant to the sterilization methods, chemicals, and fluids that they encounter, be compatible with bodily fluids, skin and tissues and still maintain their safety, effectiveness, and functionality. Requirements for plastics use in medical device include the following:

- Chemical and lipid resistance
- Material Characterization
- Sterilization Resistance
- Shelf life and Stability
- Biocompatibility and Haemocompatibility
- Extractables and Leachables Characterization

Various devices need to be sterilized and packaged either before distribution or before use. Examples of such devices are surgical gloves, specimen cups, clean room, garments, wound care products, needles, syringes, sutures, catheters, drain bags, IV bags, fluid delivery systems, dialysis equipments, implants, dental instruments, surgical instruments, surgery supplies, and combination products.

All materials used in such medical devices including the plastics must be capable of being sterilized without losing performance.

The main sterilization methods used in medical devices are:

- Autoclaving (Steam, Dry Heat)
- Ethylene oxide (EtO)
- Radiation like Gamma Radiation, Electron Beam Radiation etc.

Gamma radiation can negatively affect plastics in the following ways:

- Formation of radicals leading to chain scission and degradation
- Formation of radicals leading to cross linking
- Color change

Transparent polymers like polyvinyl chloride, acrylics, polycarbonates, and polyurethanes have a tinting agent and some polymers also require free radical scavengers or quenchers to prevent degradation. Plastics used in medical devices can come into contact with various solvents and chemicals either during the manufacturing process or during end use (Chanprateep, 2010). The medical devices must maintain their integrity, performance, and aesthetics when exposed to such solvents and chemicals. Chemical can react with the additives causing them to leach out of the part or form unwanted byproducts.

The following are some of the sources of possible toxic substances in medical device materials.

Residual Monomers

Polymerization results in a distribution of molecular weights. Although monomers are usually toxic, the toxicity of the polymeric unit generally decreases with increase in molecular weight (Vroman and Tighzert, 2009). Residual monomers result from incomplete polymerization; their concentration can be controlled by carefully regulating polymerization conditions.

Residual Solvents

Solvents are an integral part of manufacturing and may remain behind in fluid materials such as adhesives, barrier pastes, adhesive removers, lubricants or gels. Some acrylate adhesive systems are now water-based, which eliminates the concern for residual solvents (Middleton and Tipton 1998). When the solvent is an integral component of the final product, as with adhesive removers and certain barrier pastes, its presence and potential transdermal absorption must be addressed in labeling.

Degradation Products

Materials may undergo degradation during manufacture, sterilization, or storage, or after application to or implantation in the body. During manufacture, heat may thermally degrade a material; especially polyvinyl chloride which is susceptible to heat and may release hydrochloric acid, resulting in an autocatalytic unzipping process. During sterilization, polytetrafluorethylene is susceptible to irradiation breakdown, resulting in the release of hydrofluoric acid. Stored materials exposed to light and oxygen may suffer ultraviolet degradation or oxidation.

PLASTICS AND THEIR ADDITIVES

The finished plastic material is made by the chemical chain called as monomer and several other chemicals are added to it to give its desired shape, color and several other properties which are known as additives (Muller et al., 2017). There are about 2000 additives utilized in various types of plastic and can be divided in following common major classes: Antioxidants, plasticizers, light Stabilizers, heat stabilizers, antimicrobial agents, anti blocking agents, Coloring agents, antistatic agents, impact modifiers, fillers, mold release agents, Slip agents, preservatives etc.

Antioxidants

Antioxidants are additives that inhibit or retard the oxidative degradation of the plastic material within the intended processing and usage limits of the materials. Degradation is initiated by the action of highly reactive free radicals caused by heat, radiation, metallic impurities or mechanical shear. The initiation of free radicals may occur during processing, polymerization, or fabrication. Once the first step of initiation occurs, propagation follows. The function of an antioxidant is to prevent the propagation steps of oxidation. It must be effective at low concentration, non toxic, conveniently and safely handled, and low in cost. In addition to this, it must not impart undesirable characteristics to the system in which it is used (Hahladakis et al., 2018). Depending upon the method by which they prevent oxidation, antioxidants are classified as primary and secondary antioxidants. The most widely used antioxidants in plastics are phenolics. Phenolics are mainly used in polyolefins, styrenics, and engineering resins and are generally stain resistant and include simple phenolics (BHT), various bisphenolics and polyphenolics (Al-Salem et al., 2009). A phenolic antioxidant may then be used for long term protection. Primary antioxidants are generally radical scavengers or H-donors i.e. hindered phenols such as BHT, Irganox1010, or Irganox 1076, cyanox 2246 and 425 and bisphenol A. Long term protection for the polymer, secondary antioxidants is typically hydroperoxide decomposers i.e. trivalent phosphorus compounds such as tris-nonylphenyl phosphate (TNPP) is the most commonly used organophosphite followed by tris (2, 4-di-tert-butylphenyl) phosphate (Irgafos 168). Organophosphite are used in polyolefins, styrenics, and engineering resins (Achilias et al., 2007). Phosphite can improve colour and engineering resins stability, but can be corrosive if hydrolysed. Thioesters act as secondary antioxidants and also provide high heat stability to a variety of polymers (polyolefins and styrenics). Secondary antioxidants are typically used in synergistic combination with primary antioxidants. Lactone stabilizers are a new class of materials that are reputed to stop the autoxidation process before it starts.

Plasticizers

According to the ASTM D-883 definition, a plasticizer is a material incorporated into a plastic to increase its flexibility, workability, or dispensability. The addition of a plasticizer may lower the melt viscosity, elastic modulus. It should be relatively non volatile, non-mobile, inert, nontoxic, inexpensive and compatible with the system to be plasticized. The plasticizers are stable organic solvents or low melting solids which are stable both chemically and thermally and which when mixed with a polymer modifies its flow as well as the mechanical and electrical properties (Lim and Hoag, 2013). According to the chemical constitution of plasticizers, they are broadly classified into four types:

- Phthalates
- Aliphatic esters
- Phosphates
- Miscellaneous.

The development of plasticizers has been plagued with toxicity problems. Thus, the use of highly toxic polychlorinated biphenyls (PCBs) has been discontinued. Phthalic acid esters, such as DEHP, may be extracted from blood stored in plasticized PVC blood bags and tubing (Rowdhwal and Chen, 2018). These problems have been solved by using non migrating plasticizers or oligomeric polyester instead of DEHP, in appropriate situation. Recently, some limited tests have indicated a relationship of prenatal exposure to phthalates and reproductive abnormalities of male babies.

Stabilizers

Stabilizers are used to prevent the degradation of a material due to high processing temperatures and extent of their life stability under degrading environmental conditions. The effectiveness of a stabilizer also depends on the presence of oxygen i.e. some are effective in its presence while other are less effective (Marinova et al., 2017). The effectiveness of a stabilizer is very much dependent upon the grade of resin (degree of polymerization) in which they are compounded. Some stabilizers are highly effective in one grade of PVC but only moderate in another. A judicious choice of stabilizers is therefore very important in the formulation of plastic (Saliba et al.,2016) The presence of other additives such as plasticizers and fillers also sometimes strongly influence the efficiency of a stabilizer for example Phosphates and chlorinated extenders often reduce the efficiency of a stabilizer. The major classes of stabilizers are mixed metal salt blends, epoxy compounds, polyfunctional alcohols, alkyl/aryl organophosphate etc.

Light Stabilizers

Light stabilizers are used to protect plastics, especially polyolefin's, polystyrenes, from discoloration, embrittlement, and degradation by UV light. The major classes of light stabilizers are:

UV absorbers, excited state quenchers, and free radical terminators.

UV absorbing materials

UV absorbing materials are the substances which give characteristic absorption peak in UV region. The commonly used UV absorbing materials are derivatives of benzotriazoles, benzophenones, diphenylacrylates, phenyl esters (Shang et al., 2003).

Benzophenones

It is a type of UV absorbers which have been used for many years in polyolefin's, PVC, and other resins. Some important benzophenones are, 2-hydroxy4methoxybenzophenone, 2-hydroxy4-noctoxybenzophenone, 2, 4-dihydroxy-4-n-dodecycloxybenzophenone (Huang et al., 2016).

Benzotriazoles

It is a type of UV absorbing material which is highly effective in high temperature resins such as acrylics and polycarbonate. Some important benzotriazole are: 2-(2-hydroxy-5-methylphenyl) benzotriazole, 2, 2-(2-hydroxy-5-tert-octylphenyl) benzotriazole, 2-(32-tert-butyl-2-hydroxy-5 methylphenyl) etc (Nakagawa & Suzuki, 2002). Nickel compounds are used as excited state quenchers and hindered amine light stabilizers (HALS) are used as free radical terminator.

Health Sustainability

Another aspect of addressing medical waste is through sustainability efforts, specifically recycling of items that can be diverted from the waste stream. While there often is much recycling going on in healthcare facilities, often there is little to no data. It's important to track, even if roughly, the amount of recyclables removed from the facility. So whether it's paper or corrugated cardboard bales, pallets, electronics or mixed plastics, organizations should track the materials as it leaves the facility (North and Halden, 2013).

Plastics have become a vital asset for humanity. Though extensive research and new technologies have led to the invention of newer and safer plastics, but drawbacks and challenges of plastics have never been resolved and impact is on the rise (Hopewell et al., 2009). Some of the major compounds like dioxins vinyl chloride, and plasticizers are causative factors of reproductive dysfunction, hormone-disruption, testicular cancers and breast growth. The harmful effects are also pronounced in newborns via mothers during pregnancy or young children exposed directly (Street et al., 2018).

Recycling Potential of Plastic Medical Waste

Plastic waste is a major environmental and public health problem in India particularly in the urban areas. Plastic shopping or carrier bags are one of the main sources of plastic waste in our country. Due to the problems of misuse and overuse, Plastic bags of all sizes and colors cover the city's landscape. Besides this visual pollution, plastic bag wastes contribute to blockage of drains and gutters. Moreover they are threat to aquatic life when they find their way to water bodies, and can cause livestock deaths when the livestock consume them. Furthermore, when filled with rainwater, plastic bags become breeding grounds for mosquitoes, which cause malaria (Sigler, 2014). Plastic has become prevalent because of its inexpensive quality and can be engineered with a wide range of properties (Thompson et al., 2009). Plastics have become a critical material in the modern economy. The annual volume of plastics produced exceeds that volume of steel.

The kind of recycling practiced in India is quite different from what is practiced in the rest of the world, in that state of the art technologies are not employed here. The starting point is the sorting of plastic waste (based on colour, transparency, hardness, density and opacity of the scrap. (Ruj et al., 2015). The sorted waste is then sent to the granulators to obtain granules with the traditional mechanical and grinding techniques. The converters use these granules to make finished plastic products. The majority of such units like granulators and convertors are often located in slums, and function single machine extruding units. Scrap storage is done in the backyards, and washing is done in open drums. These activities are often termed as backyard recycling (Singh et al., 2017). The technologies used in these industries are also old and local. Of the types of plastics recycled in India, PVC (polyvinyl chloride) accounts for 45%, LDPE (low density polyethylene) for 25%, HDPE (high density polyethylene) for 20%, PP (polypropylene) for 7.6% and other polymers such as PS (polystyrene) for 2.4% (Banerjee et al., 2014).

The final stage in the life cycle of plastics is disposal. In India, there are three common ways of getting rid of plastics they are as under:

1. By dumping them in landfills,
2. By burning them in incinerators
3. By littering them.

In case of littering, plastic wastes fail to reach landfills or incinerators. It is the improper way of disposing plastics and is identified as the cause of manifold ecological problems. Incineration of plastic wastes also significantly reduces the volume of waste requiring disposal. It is believed that the volume reduction brought about by incineration ranges from 80 to 95%. But the burning of these chlorine-containing substances releases toxic heavy metals and emits noxious gasses like dioxins and furans (Shiri et al., 2015).

Recycling is one of the most convenient and easiest ways. Smarter sorting, energy efficient ways, developing smarter plastics and research to develop certain fungi and bacteria that hasten degradation of conventional plastics are some of the present era needs. Source reduction (Reduce and Reuse) can occur by altering the design, manufacture or reduced use of plastic products (Koushal et al., 2014). Biodegradable plastics are similar to conventional plastics, with the additional quality of being able to naturally decompose and break into natural and safe byproducts. Bioplastics, nature derived plastics, are derived from biological sources such as sugar cane, cellulose etc. and these either degrade in open air or are made to compost using fungi, bacteria or enzymes (Song et al., 2009).

As we have discussed above, plastics play vital role in hospitals and medical field as they are used on large scale in hospitals and medical field. The daily plastic waste generation includes disposable syringes, I.V sets, disposable plastic aprons; glucose bottles, cannulas, catheters etc. are disposed of on daily basis (Gokhale, 2017). The increased use and production of plastic in developing and emerging countries is a particular concern, as the sophistication of their waste management infrastructure may not be developing at an appropriate rate to deal with their increasing levels of plastic waste (Thompson et al., 2009). Generally, there are two kinds of commercial plastics i.e., thermoplastic (reheated, melted, and molded into different shapes) and thermosetting plastics which degrade and turn into other substances if reheated after molding. Today, there are many different types of plastics manufactured in the plastic industry (Anastas et al., 2000).

The plastics are usually non-biodegradable and remain in the environment as a waste for pretty long time. But if they are broken into small pieces the microorganisms will be able to degrade them. However, the breakdown process is too long for most of the traditional plastics, if there is no any artificial processing before being thrown in a landfill is involved. Therefore, before the plastics degrade themselves naturally, more plastics will be manufactured, causing increasing plastic pollution around the world (Song et al., 2009). Plastic waste also has the ability to attract contaminants, such as persistent organic pollutants (POPs). Plastic could potentially transport these chemicals to otherwise clean environments and, when ingested by wildlife, plastic could cause the transfer of chemicals into the organism's system. However, in some conditions plastic could potentially act as a sink for contaminants, making them less available to wildlife, particularly if they are buried on the seafloor (Hartmann and Rolim, 2002).

Recycling techniques deals with the tones of plastic waste that is choking earth. So, in addition to developing smarter plastics that takes the place of conventional plastics, there is emergent need to deal with the immense quantities of toxic wastes already out there and hurting humans and the environment as well (Balakrishnan et al., 2017). Smarter sorting of plastic Wastes, energy efficient ways of getting rid of the plasticizers and increasing the scale of this entire process is very vital to overcome this challenge. Recent reports of discovery of certain fungi and bacteria that hasten degradation of conventional plastics have received a lot of scientific attention. In this process, the byproducts of this natural way of decomposition are safe for the environment and there are no hidden adverse consequences of this approach (Musdalslien and Sandberg, 2002). Each year, an estimated 500 billion to 1 trillion plastic bags are consumed worldwide. That comes out to over one million per minute. Billions end up as litter each year or in landfills. Now focus on another important part of eco-friendly living: reduce your use of plastic. Source reduction (Reduce and Reuse) can occur by altering the design, manufacture, or use of plastic products and materials.

Through a study of the analysis of recycling potential of medical plastic wastes, the major components of total plastic wastes were medical packaging, cafeteria plastics, sharps, blood bags, IV bags and tubing. The major sources of plastic wastes generated by the hospitals were facilities, operating rooms, cafeterias and laboratories. Hospital cafeterias were the easiest recycling source and had the highest plastics recycling potential. This is mainly due to a very slight infection probability and efforts to purchase a single plastic, PS (Lee et al., 2002). The plastic content of wastes in the hospital cafeterias varied from hospital to hospital. Although plastic generated by operating rooms and laboratories generally are not considered for plastic recycling and are handled as RMW, some of the plastics generated by emergency rooms and ambulance services can be considered for plastics recycling (Aljabre, 2002). The total plastic content of these wastes was above 30% due to the high plastic content included in biomedical wastes. In particular, the total plastic content of medical wastes generated from the ambulance service was about 49%. This high plastic content was due to the increased use of plastic products for emergency patient care outside the hospital. To increase recycling of medical plastics, modification of the regulations and guidelines of RMW concept or definition, proper source separation of infected or non infected wastes, development of a recycling infrastructure, education of workers and managers, and efforts of the entire hospital staff to increase recycling of wastes should be pursued (Koushal et al., 2014).

A recent study on the state of healthcare in Asia found that very few developing nations in Asia have specific, integrated legislation governing the collection, treatment and disposal of infectious medical waste (Ananth et al., 2010). Where medical waste legislation does exist, it is frequently relegated to a sub-section of other waste legislation, rather than specifically addressed in a dedicated piece of legislation (Ananth et al., 2010).Even when a developing nation has enacted medical waste legislation, there is often a marked disconnect between the thoroughness of the legislation and the reality of medical waste management in that country

Biodegradable Plastics (BDP): This is one of the options to the conventional plastics. One of the common constituents of BDP is polyhydroxyalkanoate (PHA). The BDP are similar to conventional plastics in all aspects with the additional quality of being able to naturally decompose and break into natural and safe byproducts. Hence if all plastics in the city waste were biodegradable, it could simply be allowed to decompose along with the food and other non-recyclable but biodegradable articles like wet paper and cotton fibers (Miller, 2005).

Since the technologies to manufacture BDPs are relatively new and not widely prevalent, the production cost is higher. Therefore, further research in areas of more cost effective and energy efficient manufacturing methods for biodegradable plastics is the call of an hour. The incorporation of BDP is a progressive approach to a greener, healthier, and a better environment (Mohee, 2008). The progressive development of several biopolymers over the years has stirred the plastic industry. The induction of biodegradable plastics is a promising and progressive prospect and will greatly reduce the dependence on fossil fuels (Murphy & Bartle, 2004).

The fact that sets biodegradable plastics one step ahead of conventional plastics is that they can be manufactured by using renewable biomass instead of biofuels. This will be of huge advantage because as "renewable biomass", will include "agro-industrial" wastes that are not only cheap, but their conversion solves another problem by turning waste materials into useful products. This makes production of biodegradable plastics possible even in the countries that lack the scope for crop expansion (Narayan, 2006). In return, they are being benefitted economically and ecologically. At present biodegradable polymer technology can only offer a limited range of materials. It is due to this limitation that biodegradable plastics have not been able to go mainstream yet.

A bioplastic is a plastic that is made partly or wholly from polymers derived from biological sources such as potato starch, sugar cane or the cellulose from trees, cotton and straw. Some bioplastics degrade in an open air while others are made so that they compost in an industrial composting plant, aided by bacteria, fungi and enzymes. Others mimic the robustness and durability of conventional plastics such as polyethylene or PET. However, that does not imply that bioplastics can naturally decompose like biodegradable plastics (Shamsuddin et al., 2017). Hence, further research should focus on developing bioplastics that are both biodegradable and also energy efficient to produce. Recycling is more energy efficient and releases less carbon dioxide than making a new product. One major problem with efforts to recycle bioplastics is that if they become mixed with petroplastics they can contaminate the whole batch (Gill, 2014).

CONCLUSION

Medical waste disposal is a field that requires further study to meet the growing global demand for medical waste disposal. Rising healthcare usage, driven by a variety of factors, is increasing medical waste production which in turn is putting stress on current disposal systems. Current disposal strategies involve sorting waste at disposal end within healthcare facilities, and then transporting the infectious medical waste to a safe disposal site, where it is treated by incineration or autoclaving and the residual product is used for landfilling. Both incineration and autoclave treatment methods have drawbacks, with incineration undesirable atmospheric emissions are created which cause adverse health and environmental impacts. Autoclave treatment is not able to handle all types of wastes nor it produces a treated product that is universally accepted at landfills. The best way to control the impact of medical waste is to produce less, and one of the most effective ways to do this is to ensure that only infectious medical waste is sent for treatment and other hospital waste should be treated in the same manner as municipal household waste. This could be accomplished through better training of healthcare workers along with the implementation of standardized medical waste streams and disposal bin colors. Further, there are a number of approaches that governments could make to reduce the problems of excess infectious medical waste generation and to improve treatment and disposal of all types of medical waste. Firstly, governments should provide highly explicit, standardized definitions of infectious and non-infectious medical waste and should tightly regulate the disposal of infectious waste to prevent illegal dumping of waste. Secondly, governments should provide healthcare facilities with incentives, monetary or otherwise, to reduce medical waste production. These incentives will help convince local healthcare facility management to make waste reduction, particularly infectious medical waste production, a priority. Finally, governments should seek to increase research in the area of medical waste reduction and treatment though research grants and industry research partnerships. In particular, priority should be given to research with medical equipment suppliers to develop and produce products that release negligible amounts of dioxins or mercury when incinerated. These products will be particularly valuable to developing nations where many waste disposal facilities lack the advanced pollution control technologies used in the developed world to prevent the release of toxic substances produced by waste incineration. As such, these incineration-safe medical products reduce the risk of exposing populations in developing nations to the harmful emissions produced by the incineration of infectious medical waste.

REFERENCES

Achilias, D. S., Roupakias, C., Megalokonomos, P., Lappas, A. A., & Antonakou, E. V. (2007). Chemical recycling of plastic wastes made from polyethylene (LDPE and HDPE) and polypropylene (PP). *Journal of Hazardous Materials*, *149*(3), 536–542. doi:10.1016/j.jhazmat.2007.06.076 PMID:17681427

Al-Khatib, I. A., Al-Qaroot, Y. S., & Ali-Shtayeh, M. S. (2009). Management of healthcare waste in circumstances of limited resources: A case study in the hospitals of Nablus city, Palestine. *Waste Management & Research, 27*(4), 305–312. doi:10.1177/0734242X08094124 PMID:19423582

Al-Salem, S. M., Lettieri, P., & Baeyens, J. (2009). Recycling and recovery routes of plastic solid waste (PSW): A review. *Waste Management (New York, N.Y.), 29*(10), 2625–2643. doi:10.1016/j.wasman.2009.06.004 PMID:19577459

Aljabre, S. H. (2002). Hospital generated waste: A plan for its proper management. *Journal of Family & Community Medicine, 9*(2), 61–65. PMID:23008674

Alzahrani, M. A., Alshanshouri, M. A., & Fakhri, Z. I. (1998). *Guide of healthcare waste management.* Riyadh, Saudi Arabia: Ministry of Health.

Ananth, A. P., Prashanthini, V., & Visvanathan, C. (2010). Healthcare waste management in Asia. *Waste Management (New York, N.Y.), 30*(1), 154–161. doi:10.1016/j.wasman.2009.07.018 PMID:19726174

Anastas, P. T., Bickart, P. H., & Kirchhoff, M. M. (2000). Designing safer polymers New York. New York, NY: John Wiley and Sons, Wiley-Interscience.

Andrady, A. L., & Neal, M. A. (2009). Applications and societal benefits of plastics. *Philosophical Transactions of the Royal Society of London. Series B, Biological Sciences, 364*(1526), 1977–1984. doi:10.1098/rstb.2008.0304 PMID:19528050

Baghotia, K. S. (2009). Biomedical waste management-Delhi experience. *Indian Soc Hosp Waste Management, 7-8*(1), 29–34.

Balakrishnan, A., & Flora, R. M. N. (2017). The Environmental Impact of Plastics and Recycling of Plastic Waste. *International Journal of Engineering Research and Reviews* (Online) *5*(3), (14-20).

Banerjee, T., Srivastava, R. K., & Hung, Y. T. (2012). Plastics waste management in India: an integrated solidwaste management approach. Handbook of Environmental and Waste Management, 2.

Birchard, K. (2002). Out of sight, out of mind...the medical waste problem. *Lancet, 359*(9300), 56. doi:10.1016/S0140-6736(02)07256-2 PMID:11809202

Chanprateep, S. (2010). Current trends in biodegradable polyhydroxylakanoates. *Journal of Bioscience and Bioengineering, 110*(6), 621–632. doi:10.1016/j.jbiosc.2010.07.014 PMID:20719562

Cheng, Y. W., Sung, F. C., Yang, Y., Lo, Y. H., Chung, Y. T., & Li, K.-C. (2009). Medical waste production at hospitals and associated factors. *Waste Management (New York, N.Y.), 29*(1), 440–444. doi:10.1016/j.wasman.2008.01.014 PMID:18359619

Datta, P., Mohi, G. K., & Chander, J. (2018). Biomedical waste management in India: Critical appraisal. *Journal of Laboratory Physicians, 10*(1), 6–14. doi:10.4103/JLP.JLP_89_17 PMID:29403196

Eigenheer, E., & Zanon, U. (1991). O quefazer com osresiduoshospitaleres. Propostaparaclassificacao, embalagem, coleta e destinacao final. *Arquivos Brasileiros de Medicina, 65*(3), 233–237.

Elias, H. G. (2005). *Plastics, General Survey.* Ullmann's Encyclopedia of Industrial Chemistry.

Gill, M. (2014). Bioplastic: A better alternative to plastics. *International Journal of Research in Applied Natural Sciences*, *2*(8), 115–120.

Gokhale, S. (2017). How safe is your hospital - doctor? *Medical Journal, Armed Forces India*, *52*(2), 120–123. doi:10.1016/S0377-1237(17)30858-4 PMID:28769360

Gregory, M. R. (2009). Environmental implications of plastic debris in marine settings-entanglement ingestion smothering hangers-on hitch-hiking and alien invasions. *Philosophical Transactions of the Royal Society of London. Series B, Biological Sciences*, *364*(1526), 2013–2025. doi:10.1098/rstb.2008.0265 PMID:19528053

Gundarov, V. P., & Kavalerov, G. I. (2001). Development of standardization and certification of the quality of medical devices. *Meditsinskaia Tekhnika*, (3): 4–8. PMID:11515269

Gyawali, S., Rathore, D. S., Shankar, P. R., & Kumar, K. V. (2013). Strategies and challenges for safe injection practice in developing countries. *Journal of Pharmacology & Pharmacotherapeutics*, *4*(1), 8–12. doi:10.4103/0976-500X.107634 PMID:23662018

Hahladakis, J. N., Velis, C. A., Weber, R., Iacovidou, E., & Purnell, P. (2018). An overview of chemical additives present in plastics: Migration, release, fate and environmental impact during their use, disposal and recycling. *Journal of Hazardous Materials*, *344*, 179–199. doi:10.1016/j.jhazmat.2017.10.014 PMID:29035713

Halden, R. U. (2010). Plastics and health risks. *Annual Review of Public Health*, *31*(1), 179–194. doi:10.1146/annurev.publhealth.012809.103714 PMID:20070188

Hartmann, L., & Rolim, A. (2002). Post-consumer plastic recycling as a sustainable development tool: a case study. *GPEC 2002: plastics impact on the environment, Conf. Proc.*, 431–438.

Hopewell, J., Dvorak, R., & Kosior, E. (2009). Plastics recycling: Challenges and opportunities. *Philosophical Transactions of the Royal Society of London. Series B, Biological Sciences*, *364*(1526), 2115–2126. doi:10.1098/rstb.2008.0311 PMID:19528059

Huang, Z., Ding, A., Guo, H., Lu, G., & Huang, X. (2016). Construction of Nontoxic Polymeric UV-Absorber with Great Resistance to UV-Photoaging. *Scientific Reports*, *6*(1), 25508. doi:10.1038rep25508 PMID:27138547

Jang, Y. C., Lee, C., Yoon, O. S., & Kim, H. (2006). Medical waste management in Korea. *Journal of Environmental Management*, *80*(2), 107–115. doi:10.1016/j.jenvman.2005.08.018 PMID:16338054

Kaiser, B., Eagan, P. D., & Shaner, H. (2001). Solutions to Health Care Waste: Life-Cycle Thinking and "Green" Purchasing. *Environmental Health Perspectives*, *109*(3), 205–207. doi:10.1289/ehp.01109205 PMID:11333178

Khajuria, A., & Kumar, A. (2007). Assessment of healthcare waste generated by government hospitals in Agra. *Our Nature*, *5*(1), 25–30. doi:10.3126/on.v5i1.794

Koushal, V., Sharma, R., Sharma, M., Sharma, R., & Sharma, V. (2014). Plastics: Issues Challenges and Remediation. *Int J Waste Resources*, *4*, 134. doi:10.4172/2252-5211.1000134

Lee, B. K., Ellenbecker, M. J., & Moure-Ersaso, R. (2004). Alternatives for Treatment and Disposal Cost Reduction of Regulated Medical Wastes. *Waste Management (New York, N.Y.)*, *24*(2), 143–151. doi:10.1016/j.wasman.2003.10.008 PMID:14761753

Li, N., Mahat, D., & Park, S. (2009). *Reduce Reuse and Replace: A Study on Solutions to Plastic Wastes.* An Interactive Qualifying Project Submitted to the faculty of Worcester Polytechnic Institute.

Li, W., Zhou, J., & Xu, Y. (2015). Study of the *in vitro* cytotoxicity testing of medical devices. *Biomedical Reports*, *3*(5), 617–620. doi:10.3892/br.2015.481 PMID:26405534

Lim, H., & Hoag, S. W. (2013). Plasticizer effects on physical-mechanical properties of solvent cast Soluplus® films. *AAPS PharmSciTech*, *14*(3), 903–910. doi:10.120812249-013-9971-z PMID:23689959

Marinova, N., Franckevičius, M., Matulaitienė, I., Devižis, A., Niaura, G., Gulbinas, V., & Delgado, J. L. (2017). Hindered Amine Light Stabilizers Increase the Stability of Methylammonium Lead Iodide Perovskite Against Light and Oxygen. *ChemSusChem*, *10*(19), 3760–3764. doi:10.1002/cssc.201700707 PMID:28762644

McKeen, L., W. (2013). 3 Plastics Used in Medical Devices. *Handbook of Polymer Applications in Medicine and Medical Devices, 21.*

Mehala, D., & Venkatesh, S. (2018). A study on bio medical waste disposal in medicare enviro systems in thanjavur. *IJCESR*, *5*(4), 2394–0697.

Middleton, J. C., & Tipton, A. J. (1998). Synthetic biodegradable polymers as medical devices. *Med. Plastics Biomater. Mag*, *3*, 30.

Miller, R. (2005). The landscape for biopolymers in packaging. Miller-Klein Associates report Summary and Full Report.

Mohee, R., Unmar, G. D., Mudhoo, A., & Khadoo, P. (2008). Biodegradability of biodegradable/degradable plastic materials under aerobic and anaerobic conditions. *Waste Management (New York, N.Y.)*, *28*(9), 1624–1629. doi:10.1016/j.wasman.2007.07.003 PMID:17826972

Moritz, J. M. (1995). Current legislation governing clinical waste disposal. *The Journal of Hospital Infection*, *30*(supplement), 521–530. doi:10.1016/0195-6701(95)90058-6 PMID:7560993

Müller, K., Bugnicourt, E., Latorre, M., Jorda, M., Echegoyen Sanz, Y., Lagaron, J. M., ... Schmid, M. (2017). Review on the Processing and Properties of Polymer Nanocomposites and Nanocoatings and Their Applications in the Packaging, Automotive and Solar Energy Fields. *Nanomaterials (Basel, Switzerland)*, *7*(4), 74. doi:10.3390/nano7040074 PMID:28362331

Murphy, R., & Bartle, I. (2004). *Summary report, biodegradable polymers and sustainability: insight from life cycle assessment*. National Non Food Crops Centre.

Musdalslien, M., & Sandberg, P. (2002, April). Energy and HCL recovery from PVC in municipal solid waste incineration. In *PVC 2002: towards a sustainable future Conf. Proc.* London, UK: IOM Communications.

Nakagawa, Y., & Suzuki, T. (2002). Metabolism of 2-hydroxy-4-methoxybenzophenone in isolated rat hepatocytes and xenoestrogenic effects of its metabolites on MCF-7 human breast cancer cells. *Chemico-Biological Interactions*, *139*(2), 115–128. doi:10.1016/S0009-2797(01)00293-9 PMID:11823001

Narayan, P. (2001). *Analyzing Plastic Waste Management in India: Case study of Polybags and PET bottles.* Lund University.

Narayan, R. (1994). In Y. Doi, & K. Fukuda (Eds.), *Biodegradable plastics and polymers* (p. 261). New York, NY: Elsevier. doi:10.1016/B978-0-444-81708-2.50026-9

Narayan, R. (2006a). Biobased and biodegradable polymer materials: rationale, drivers, and technology exemplars. *American Chemical Society Symposium Ser., 939*(18), 282. 10.1021/bk-2006-0939.ch018

Nie, L., & Wu, H. (2016). Investigation and Analysis of Rural Medical Waste Management. *Journal of Environmental Protection*, *07*(01), 93–98. doi:10.4236/jep.2016.71009

North, E. J., & Halden, R. U. (2013). Plastics and environmental health: The road ahead. *Reviews on Environmental Health*, *28*(1), 1–8. doi:10.1515/reveh-2012-0030 PMID:23337043

Northwest Regional Delegation of Public Health. (2005). *Annual Report*. Author.

Office of Technology Assessment (OTA). (1988, October). Issues in medical waste management (Background paper). Washington, DC: U.S. Government Printing Office. (OTA-BP-O-49)

Pandey, A., Ahuja, S., Madan, M., & Asthana, A. K. (2016). Bio-Medical Waste Management in a Tertiary Care Hospital: An Overview. *Journal of Clinical and Diagnostic Research: JCDR*, *10*(11), DC01–DC03. doi:10.7860/JCDR/2016/22595.8822 PMID:28050362

Pandey, E., Srivastava, K., Gupta, S., Srivastava, S., & Mishra, N. (2016). Some biocompatible materials used in medical practices- A review. *International Journal of Pharmaceutical Sciences and Research.* doi:10.13040/IJPSR.0975-8232.7(7).2748-55

Pruss, A., Giroult, E., & Rushbrook, P. (1999). *Safe Management of Wastes from Health-Care Activities*. Geneva, Switzerland: World Health Organization.

Rai, R., Keshavarz, T., Roether, J. A., Boccaccini, A. R., & Roy, I. (2011). Medium chain length polyhydroxyalkanoates, promising new biomedical medical devices for the future. *Medical devices Science and Engineering: R. Reports*, *72*(3), 29–47. doi:10.1016/j.mser.2010.11.002

Ren, X. (2003). Biodegradable plastics: A solution or a challenge? *Journal of Cleaner Production*, *11*(1), 27–40. doi:10.1016/S0959-6526(02)00020-3

Rowdhwal, S. S., & Chen, J. (2018). Toxic Effects of Di-2-ethylhexyl Phthalate: An Overview. *BioMed Research International*. doi:10.1155/2018/1750368

Ruj, B., Pandey, V., Jash, P., & Srivastava, V. K. (2015). Sorting of plastic waste for effective recycling. *Int. Journal of Applied Sciences and Engineering Research*, *4*(4). doi:10.6088/ijaser.04058

Saliba, M., Matsui, T., Seo, J. Y., Domanski, K., Correa-Baena, J. P., Nazeeruddin, M. K., ... Grätzel, M. (2016). Cesium-containing triple cation perovskite solar cells: Improved stability, reproducibility and high efficiency. *Energy & Environmental Science*, *9*(6), 1989–1997. doi:10.1039/C5EE03874J PMID:27478500

Shah, A. A., Hasan, F., Hameed, A., & Ahmed, S. (2008). Biological degradation of plastics: A comprehensive review. *Biotechnology Advances*, *26*(3), 246–265. doi:10.1016/j.biotechadv.2007.12.005 PMID:18337047

Shamsuddin, I. M., Jafar, J. A., Shawai, A. S. A., Yusuf, S., Lateefah, M., & Aminu, I. (2017). Bioplastics as Better Alternative to Petroplastics and Their Role in National Sustainability: A Review. *Advances in Bioscience and Bioengineering*, *5*(4), 63–70. doi:10.11648/j.abb.20170504.13

Shang, J., Chai, M., & Zhu, Y. (2003). Photocatalytic degradation of polystyrene plastic under fluorescent light. *Environmental Science & Technology*, *37*(19), 4494–4499. doi:10.1021/es0209464 PMID:14572106

Shemwell, B. E., & Levendis, Y. A. (2000). Particulates generated from combustion of polymers. *JAPCA J Air Waste Ma*, 27, *50*(1), 94–102.

Shiri, N. D., Kajava, P. V., Ranjan, H. V., Pais, N. L., & Naik, V. M. (2015). Processing of Waste Plastics into Building Materials Using a Plastic Extruder and Compression Testing of Plastic Bricks. *Journal of Mechanical Engineering and Automation.*, *5*(3B), 39–42. doi:10.5923/c.jmea.201502.08

Sigler, M. (2014). The Effects of Plastic Pollution on Aquatic Wildlife: Current Situations and Future Solutions. *Water, Air, and Soil Pollution*, *225*(11), 2184. doi:10.100711270-014-2184-6

Singh, N., Hui, D., Singh, R., Ahuja, I. P. S., Feo, L., & Fraternali, F. (2017). Recycling of plastic solid waste: A state of art review and future applications. *Composites. Part B, Engineering*, *115*, 409–422. doi:10.1016/j.compositesb.2016.09.013

Song, J. H., Murphy, R. J., Narayan, R., & Davies, G. B. (2009). Biodegradable and compostable alternatives to conventional plastics. *Philosophical Transactions of the Royal Society of London. Series B, Biological Sciences*, *364*(1526), 2127–2139. doi:10.1098/rstb.2008.0289 PMID:19528060

Street, M. E., Angelini, S., Bernasconi, S., Burgio, E., Cassio, A., & Catellani, C., … Amarri, S. (2018). Current Knowledge on Endocrine Disrupting Chemicals (EDCs) from Animal Biology to Humans, from Pregnancy to Adulthood: Highlights from a National Italian Meeting. *International Journal of Molecular Sciences*, *19*(6), 1647. doi:10.3390/ijms19061647

Thompson, R. C., Moore, C. J., vom Saal, F. S., & Swan, S. H. (2009). Plastics, the environment and human health: Current consensus and future trends. *Philosophical Transactions of the Royal Society of London. Series B, Biological Sciences*, *364*(1526), 2153–2166. doi:10.1098/rstb.2009.0053 PMID:19528062

Vandenburg, L. N., Hauser, R., Marcus, M., Olea, N., & Welshons, W. V. (2007). Human exposure to bisphenol A (BPA). *Reproductive Toxicology (Elmsford, N.Y.)*, *24*(2), 139–177. doi:10.1016/j.reprotox.2007.07.010 PMID:17825522

Vert, M. (2011). Not any new functional polymer can be for medicine: What about artificial biopolymers? *Macromolecular Bioscience*, *11*(12), 1653–1661. doi:10.1002/mabi.201100224 PMID:22052691

Vroman, I., & Tighzert, L. (2009). Biodegradable Polymers. *Materials (Basel)*, *2*(2), 307–344. doi:10.3390/ma2020307

Wilson, A. S. (1995). *Plasticizers. Principles and practices*. Cambridge, MA: The Institute of Materials.

Windfeld, E. S., & Brooks, M. S. (2015). Medical Waste Management – A Review. *Journal of Environmental Management*, *163*, 98–108. doi:10.1016/j.jenvman.2015.08.013 PMID:26301686

Zaman, T. (2010). *The Prevalence and Environmental Impact of Single Use Plastic Products*. Academic Press.

KEY TERMS AND DEFINITIONS

Biodegradable Plastics (BDP): This is one of the options to the conventional plastics. The BDP are similar to conventional plastics in all aspects with the additional quality of being able to naturally decompose and break into natural and safe byproducts.

Bioplastic: A bioplastic is a plastic that is made partly or wholly from polymers derived from biological sources such as potato starch, sugar cane or the cellulose from trees, cotton and straw. Some bioplastics degrade in an open air while others are made so that they compost in an industrial composting plant, aided by bacteria, fungi and enzymes.

Medical Waste: Medical waste is a wider term. It comprises of many different types of wastes including medical waste, regulated medical waste, infectious medical waste and hospital waste. In other words medical waste refers to all waste that is generated at any healthcare or healthcare-related facility.

Plasticizer: Plasticizer is a material incorporated into a plastic to increase its flexibility, workability, or dispensability.

Chapter 11
Alternatives for Treatment and Disposal Cost Reduction of Regulated Medical Waste

Sobiya Gul
SKUAST-K, India

Tasaduq Hussain Shah
SKUAST-K, India

Hafsa Javeed
SKUAST-K, India

ABSTRACT

The link between human health and environmental quality is made clearer; the commitment to safeguarding the natural environment is growing in major institutions as the health care industry. New and greater opportunities will open up to reinforce our primary institutional mission-that of caring for the health needs of the community we serve, which include caring for the environment. Developing and implementing effective programs to reduce, recycle and minimize the toxicity of hospital generated wastes (even wastes generated in the care and treatment of patients can be reduced) is one of the most significant environmental challenges the health care industry faces. Hospitals generate one of the most diverse and difficult to manage waste. The amount of medical waste produced by hospitals may vary due to a number of factors, including the hospital type and size, occupancy rate, in- and outpatient ratio, geographic location, state and local waste handling regulations, and hospital waste disposal policies.

INTRODUCTION

It is important to point out that the term 'medical waste' has often been used interchangeably with other terms such as 'hospital waste' and 'infectious waste' around the world. Hospital waste is a broader definition and refers to all wastes generated by hospitals including infectious and noninfectious waste materials, hazardous wastes and chemicals, and other non-hazardous wastes. Medical waste is often considered

DOI: 10.4018/978-1-5225-9452-9.ch011

to be a subcategory of hospital waste and indicates 'potentially' infectious waste that is produced from healthcare facilities (Klangsin & Harding, 1998; Levendis, et al., 2001). Medical waste refers to any potentially infectious wastes that are generated in the diagnosis, treatment, examination, or research by general hospitals, clinics, veterinary, and research centres. It is defined in Section 3 of the Medical Waste Tracking Act of 1988 as "any solid waste that is generated in the diagnosis, treatment, or immunization of human beings or animals, in research pertaining thereto, or in the production or testing of biological.

A medical waste generator is typically a person or business involved in the following activities: the diagnosis, treatment, or immunization of human beings or animals, research pertaining to the aforementioned activities, and the production and testing of biological agents. The following are examples of businesses considered to be generators of medical waste: clinics and hospitals, medical and dental buildings/offices, surgery centres, laboratories/research laboratories, unlicensed and licensed health facilities, chronic dialysis clinics, education and research facilities, veterinary offices, and trauma scene waste management practitioners.

Understanding Your Waste

The first step to improving a facility's waste management is to understand its overall waste stream. Non-regulated waste, which makes up around 85 percent of a hospital's total waste stream, is no different from the waste generated by a hotel, where up to 60 percent is either recyclable or compostable. Regulated medical waste (sharps, pathological waste, trace chemo, and so on) makes up about 5–15 percent and hazardous chemical waste makes up a smaller percentage (less than 5 percent) of a health care organization's waste by total volume Figure 1

Regulated Medical Waste (RMW) means that portion of waste generated in health care facilities as defined above requires special handling and treatment prior to disposal these include Pathological and microbiological waste containing blood or OPIM, contaminated items that would release blood or OPIM in a liquid or semi-liquid state if compressed, Sharps, animal infectious waste, liquid or semi-

Figure 1. Main Categories of HealthCare Waste

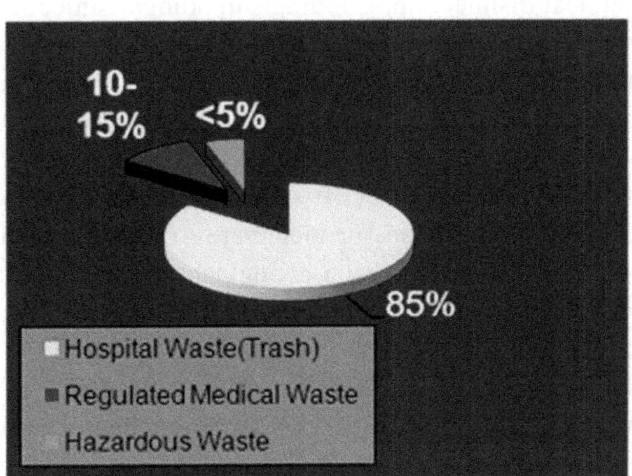

liquid blood or OPIM, Items that are caked with dried blood or OPIM and are capable of releasing these materials during handling.

Examples of regulated medical waste include the following: Bloodborne Pathogens. Pathogenic microorganisms that are present in human blood and can cause disease in humans. These include, but are not limited to, hepatitis B virus and human immunodeficiency virus. Pathological and Anatomical Waste includes Tissues, organs, body parts, and body fluids removed during surgery and autopsy.

Human blood and blood products: Includes waste blood, serum, plasma, bloodproducts, and other potentially infectious materials.

Cultures and stocks of infectious agents also called microbiological waste includes specimens from medical and pathology laboratories; culture dishes and devices used to transfer, inoculate, and mix; and discarded live and attenuated vaccines.

Sharps including but not limited to contaminated hypodermic needles, syringes, scalpel blades, Pasteur pipettes, and broken glass.

Isolation Waste. Generated by hospitalized patients who are isolated to protect othersfrom communicable disease.

Contaminated Animal Carcasses, Body Parts, and Bedding. Also includes related wastes that may have been exposed to infectious agents during research or pharmaceutical testing.

In order to fulfil the medical ethic to "do no harm," it is the responsibility of the health care industry to create and implement waste disposal polices for all of these waste streams that include worker safety, public health and environmental considerations, as well as regulatory compliance. Fulfilling this ethic also calls for a cultural shift to consider disposal technologies and services as part of a total waste management system. This system should include upstream waste management (elimination or minimization of some wastes, reuse and recycling of others) and the proper, accountable operation of all disposal equipment, post-treatment technology management and services (e.g., shredding, landfilled material, incineration ash, air and water emissions). Regulated medical wastes are treated or decontaminated to reduce the microbial load in or on the waste and to render the by-products safe for further handling and disposal. From a microbiologic standpoint, waste need not be rendered "sterile" because the treated waste will not be deposited in a sterile site. In addition, waste need not be subjected to the same reprocessing standards as are surgical instruments. Historically, treatment methods involved steam-sterilization (i.e., autoclaving), incineration, or interment (for anatomy wastes). Alternative treatment methods developed in recent years include chemical disinfection, grinding/shredding/disinfection methods, energy-based technologies (e.g., microwave or radio wave treatments), and disinfection/encapsulation methods.

There are many technologies for the treatment of medical wastes (Park & Jeong, 2001; Yoon, 2001). According to the treatment studies of medical wastes, about 59–60% of RMWs are treated through incineration, 37–20% by steam sterilization, and 4–5% by other treatment methods (Park & Jeong, 2001; Hyland et al., 1994). Currently, the proportion of off-site treatment and disposal has been increasing up to 84% due to severe regulations concerning on-site incineration (Park and Jeong, 2001; Senatore, 1994). New technologies being considered by RMW disposal engineers include microwaving, autoclaving, radiowaving, and electrotechnologies, which incorporate electron-beam irradiation, pyrolysis and oxidation, steam sterilization, and steam detoxification (WastePrevention Association, 2003; Park & Jeong, 2001; Salkin & Krisiunas, 1998; O'Connor, 1994.) Hospitals have faced financial difficulties and some of them have tried to merge with other hospitals in order to overcome their financial problems. Therefore, they are trying to find some cost-effective treatment or disposal means of their wastes. For examples, a few hospitals and companies have investigated alternative disposal methods through recycling of their medical plastic wastes (Lee et al., 2002; Anderson et al., 1999; Marrack and Meyers, 1994; Batholomew et al., 1994). The main reasons that recycling programs of medical plastic waste should be developed are because the plastic content of medical waste is significantly higher than that of municipal solid waste (MSW) and plastic wastes require significant costs for transportation to disposal facilities (US EPA, 2002; Lee et al., 1995). In addition, the total costs for treatment and disposal of RMW were much more expensive than those of NRMW or MSW (Park & Jeong, 2001; Lee et al., 1995).

Regulated medical waste can cost between five to 10 times more than solid waste, over-use of red bag waste receptacles is like throwing away dollars. Depending on current practices, hospitals have saved thousands, tens of thousands and even hundreds of thousands of dollars by addressing container over-use.

Ten Recommendations for Improving Medical Waste Management

1. **Clearly Define the Problem:** If the primary goal of "managing" waste from medical facilities is to prevent the accidental spread of disease, then it must first be acknowledged that there is only a small percentage of the waste stream that is contaminated in a manner that renders it capable of transmitting disease, and that the only documented transmission of disease from medical waste has been from contaminated sharps (syringes, etc.). In the United States we differentiate the waste stream from medical facilities in three major categories: (A) Hospital Waste - all waste generated from a facility (including cafeteria, office, and construction wastes) (B) Medical Waste (A subset of hospital waste) - waste generated as a result of patient diagnosis, treatment, or immunization of human beings or animals (C) Potentially Infectious Waste (A subset of medical waste) - that portion of medical waste that has the potential to transmit an infectious disease.
2. **Focus on Segregation First:** The current waste management practice observed at many hospitals is that all wastes, potentially infectious, office, general, food, construction debris, and hazardous chemical materials are all mixed together as they are generated, collected, transported and finally disposed of. As a result of this failure to establish and follow segregation protocols and infrastructure, the waste leaving hospitals, as a whole is both potentially infectious and potentially hazardous (chemical). At greatest risk are the workers who handle the wastes (hospital workers, municipal workers and rag pickers). The risk to the general public is secondary and occurs in three ways: (1) accidental exposure from contact with wastes at municipal disposal bins; (2) exposure to chemical or biological contaminants in water; (3) exposure to chemical pollutants (e.g., mercury, dioxin) from incineration of the wastes.
3. **Institute a Sharps Management System:** Of the 10 percent or less portion of the waste stream that is potentially infectious or hazardous, the most immediate threat to human health (patients, workers, public) is the indiscriminate disposal of sharps (needles, syringes, lancets, and other invasive tools). Proper segregation of these materials in rigid, puncture proof containers which are then monitored for safe treatment and disposal is the highest priority for any health care institution. If proper sharps management were instituted in all health care facilities most of the risk of disease transmission from medical waste would be solved. This would include proper equipment and containers distributed everywhere that sharps are generated (needle cutters and needle boxes), a secure accounting and collection system for transporting the contaminated sharps for treatment and final disposal, and proper training of all hospital personnel on handling and management of sharps and personal protection.

4. **Keep Focused on Reduction:** Hospitals in the Third World generate significantly less volumes of waste than U.S. hospitals. In part this is a result of a decision to maintain a system that relies on reprocessing and reuse of materials. Establishing clear guidelines for product purchasing that emphasized waste reduction will keep waste management problems in focus. New emphasis needs to be put on waste reduction of hazardous materials. For example, hospital waste management would benefit from a policy of a phase out of mercury-based products and technologies. Digital and electronic technology is available to replace mercury-based diagnostic tools.
5. **Ensure Worker Safety Through Education, Training and Proper Personal Protective Equipment:** Workers who handle hospital wastes are at greatest risk from exposure to the potentially infectious wastes and chemical hazardous wastes. This process starts with the clinical workers who generate the wastes without proper knowledge of the exposure risks or access to necessary protective gear, and includes the workers who collect and transport the wastes through the hospital, the staff who operates a hospital incinerator or who take the waste to municipal bins, the municipal workers who collect wastes at the municipal bins and transport it to city dumping sites, and the rag pickers, who represent the informal waste management sector, but play an important role in reducing the amount of waste destined for ultimate disposal. Proper education and training must be offered to all workers from doctors to ward boys, to labourers and rag pickers to ensure an understanding of the risks that wastes pose, how to protect themselves, and how to manage wastes (especially how to properly segregate). Education and training programs must be developed which speak to each population in a way that will best meet the needs and build understanding and change behaviour in that population. There is no "one" way to educate all workers.
6. **Provide Secure Collection and Transportation:** If the benefits of segregation are to be realized then there must be secure internal and external collection and transportation systems for waste. If waste is segregated at the point of generation only to be mixed together by labourers as they collect it, or if a hospital has segregated its waste and secured it in separate containers for ultimate disposal only to have municipal workers mix it together upon a single collection, then the ultimate value is lost. While worker safety may have been enhanced, the ultimate cost to the environment and the general public is still the same.
7. **Require Plans and Policies:** To ensure continuity and clarity in these management practices, health care institutions should develop clear plans and policies for the proper management and disposal of wastes. They need to be integrated into routine employee training, continuing education, and hospital management evaluation processes for systems and personnel. In the U.S. the Joint Commission for the Accreditation of Health Care Organizations has been developing a set of standards on the "Environment of Care" which includes plans and policies for the proper management of hazardous materials and workers' safety, without which a hospital cannot be accredited.
8. **Invest in Training and Equipment For Reprocessing Of Supplies:** The science of the reprocessing of equipment and materials for reuse in medical facilities is well established in India and should be supported. Professional health care associations should be urged to firmly support judicious reuse of materials, and should begin to set standards for reprocessing. Maintenance of this effort within hospitals will provide quality products and thwart efforts to increase reliance on disposables. Disposables are costly, increase waste generation, and do not necessarily provide for decreases in infection rates in hospitals. A reprocessing industry must however be supported with investment in proper equipment and training so that it is carried on in a safe and efficient manner.

9. **Invest in Environmentally Sound & Cost Effective Medical Waste Treatment and Disposal Technologies:** The rush to incinerate medical waste in countries around the world as an ultimate solution to a problem without definition is doing a great injustice to the community, the public health of its people, and the environment. Of the eleven recommendations that we are making, it is no accident in giving attention to treatment technologies as ninth. Without proper attention being paid to one through eight on this list, whatever decisions being made for treatment and disposal will be insufficient, if not counterproductive. The mass incineration of hospital waste given current practices of waste disposal will not reduce risk to workers (this is where the greatest risk of disease transmission or chemical exposure exists) and will actually create a greater threat to the general public as mercury and other heavy metals are spewed out into the general air, or dioxins and furans are created from the combustion of plastics such as PVC which is growing in use in medical packaging. Additionally, the ash generated from incineration of medical waste is also tainted with heavy metals and other toxic residues. Lesser risks are associated with the treatment of unsegregated wastes through other treatment technologies such as autoclaving, hydroclaving, microwaving and chemical disinfection, which affect workers more than the general public, and contaminate water sources rather than air if improperly operated. Choices of treatment technologies should be made in line with a clear knowledge of the waste stream to be managed and the goal to be achieved through treatment. If the technology is to be environmentally sound, the waste stream should be able to be treated (disinfected) without creating other hazardous by-products.
10. **Develop an infrastructure for the safe disposal and recycling for hazardous materials:** There was little or no observable capacity for the management, treatment, recycling or final disposal of hazardous wastes in most countries (e.g. chemicals, mercury, batteries). Hospitals seeking to segregate hazardous wastes are left with little or no option for safe disposal. The development of an industry which is capable of managing hazardous waste (chemicals) is essential. On-site reprocessing technology is available for hospitals for materials such as xylene or formalin, and recovery technology for silver from developing solution. These technologies may be cost prohibitive at this time. Pollution prevention and the choice of nonhazardous or less hazardous material is the only real option left to hospitals, which should be followed regardless of the existence of a hazardous waste industry.

INCINERATION

This is the process of burning of waste in temperatures ranging from 1,800°F to 2,000°F (982°C to 1093°C). On-site incineration provides the advantage of a quick, easy disposal method, but there are emissions concerns. While some states and localities actively encourage incineration as the preferred method of treatment, others have enacted moratoriums on incinerators to suspend permitting until further information on the safety of the option is available. Historically, incineration has been used as an important treatment method for RMW. That is because incineration has many advantages including putrefaction prevention and sterilization of pathological or anatomic wastes, volume reduction, and waste heat recovery (Hyland, 1993). Many hospitals are employing on-site incineration for treatment of their RMWs (MPCA, 1991). However, RMW includes significant quantities of chlorine containing wastes, such as polyvinylchloride (PVC) or disinfectants, and it might be incinerated with status lacking proper controls and emission reduction devices.

Medical waste incinerators emit dioxins, furans and heavy metals including lead, mercury and cadmium, fine dust particles, hydrogen chloride, sulphur dioxide, carbon monoxide, nitrogen oxides, PICs (Products of Incomplete Combustion) and many other pollutants into the atmosphere. These compounds have serious negative impacts on the health of incineration plant personnel, the public and the environment. Non-incineration treatment technologies can be classified in many ways - such as according to size, purchase price, types of waste handled, or market share The four basic processes are:

1. Low-heat thermal processes
2. Chemical processes
3. Irradiative processes
4. Biological processes

LOW-HEAT THERMAL PROCESSES

In general, low-heat thermal technologies operate between 93°C to about 177°C. Two basic categories of low-heat thermal processes are wet heat (steam) and dry heat (hot air) disinfection. Wet heat treatment involves the use of steam to disinfect and sterilise waste and is commonly done in an autoclave. Microwave treatment is essentially a steam disinfection process since water is added to the waste and destruction of micro-organisms occurs through the action of moist heat and steam generated by microwave energy1. In dry heat processes, no water or steam is added. Instead, the waste is heated by conduction, natural or forced convection, and/or thermal radiation using infrared heaters.

CHEMICAL PROCESSES

Chemical processes employ disinfectants such as dissolved chlorine dioxide, bleach (sodium hypochlorite), peracetic acid, or dry inorganic chemicals. To enhance exposure of the waste to the chemical agent, chemical processes often involve shredding, grinding, or mixing. In liquid systems, the waste may go through a dewatering section to remove and recycle the disinfectant. Besides chemical disinfectants, there are also encapsulating compounds that can solidify sharps, blood, or other body fluids within a solid matrix prior to disposal. One developing technology uses ozone to treat medical waste and others utilise catalytic oxidation. A novel system uses alkali to hydrolyse tissues in heated stainless steel tanks.

IRRADIATIVE PROCESSES

Irradiation-based technologies involve electron beams, Cobalt-60, or UV irradiation. These technologies require shielding to prevent occupational exposures. Electron beam irradiation uses a shower of high-energy electrons to destroy micro-organisms in the waste by causing chemical dissociation and rupture of cell walls. The pathogen destruction efficacy depends on the dose absorbed by the mass of waste, which in turn is related to waste density and electron energy. Germicidal ultraviolet radiation (UV-C) has been used as a supplement to other treatment technologies. Irradiation does not alter the waste physically and would require a grinder or shredder to render the waste unrecognisable.

BIOLOGICAL PROCESSES

Biological processes employ enzymes to destroy organic matter. Only a few non-incineration technologies have been based on biological processes.

MECHANICAL PROCESSES

Mechanical processes - such as shredding, grinding, hammermill processing, mixing, agitation, liquid solid separation, conveying (using augers2, rams, or conveyor belts), and compaction – supplement other treatment processes. Mechanical destruction can render the waste unrecognisable and is used to destroy needles and syringes so as to minimise injuries or to render them unusable. In the case of thermal- or chemical-based processes, mechanical devices such as shredders and mixers can also improve the rate of heat transfer or expose more surfaces to chemical disinfectants. Mechanical processes can add significantly to the level of maintenance required. A mechanical process is supplementary and cannot be considered a treatment process per se. Unless shredders, hammermills, and other mechanical destruction processes are an integral part of a closed treatment system, they should not be used before the waste is decontaminated. Otherwise, workers would be exposed to pathogens released to the environment by mechanical destruction. If mechanical processes are part of a system, the technology should be designed in such a way that the air in and from the mechanical process is disinfected before being released to the surroundings. It is especially important for air to be drawn into the mechanical process (away from the inlet) when waste is being fed. This is often done using a draft fan that maintains a negative pressure in the mechanical processing chamber; air taken from the mechanical process passes through the disinfection chamber or through a high efficiency particulate air (HEPA) filter before being released to the environment. These technologies range from small units for use at or near the point of generation to high-capacity systems for large medical centres or regional facilities.

STEAM DISINFECTION

Steam disinfection, a standard process in hospitals for sterilising reusable instruments, has been adapted for medical waste treatment. There are two traditional types of equipment used for steam treatment: autoclaves and retorts. Other steam-based systems, sometimes referred to as advanced autoclaves, have been developed in recent years. One unique design of a steam-based process is a microwave unit that achieves disinfection or sterilisation by means of moist heat and steam. An autoclave consists of a metal chamber sealed by a charging door and surrounded by a steam jacket. Steam is introduced into both the outside jacket and the inside chamber which is designed to withstand elevated pressures. Heating the outside jacket reduces condensation in the inside chamber wall and allows the use of steam at lower temperatures. Because air is an effective insulator, the removal of air from the chamber is essential to ensure penetration of heat into the waste. This is done in two general ways: gravity displacement or pre-vacuuming. A gravity-displacement (or downward-displacement) autoclave takes advantage of the fact that steam is lighter than air; steam is introduced under pressure into the chamber forcing the air downward into an outlet port or drain line in the lower part of the chamber. A more effective method is the use of a vacuum pump to evacuate air before introducing steam, as is done in pre-vacuum autoclaves. Pre-vacuum (or high-vacuum) autoclaves need less time for disinfection due to their greater efficiency in taking out air. Some autoclaves may use pressure pulsing with or without gravity displacement to evacuate air. A retort is similar to an autoclave except that it has no steam jacket. It is cheaper to construct but requires a higher steam temperature than an autoclave. Retort-type designs are found in largescale applications. Autoclaving, which is also known simply as steam sterilization, is the most commonly utilized alternative to incineration. It is both less costly and carries no documented health impacts. In this method, wastes are sterilized or disinfected prior to disposal in a landfill. Bags of waste are placed in a chamber and steam is introduced for a determined period of time at a specified pressure and temperature. This assures the destruction of microorganisms.

Approximately 90% of regulated medical wastes are suitable for autoclaving, particularly microbiological wastes. Autoclaves are not suitable, however, for pathological, cytotoxic, or other toxic chemical wastes.

GAS STERILIZATION

In this process, medical waste is fed into an evacuated air-tight chamber and treated with a sterilizing agent (such as ethylene oxide or formaldehyde). The gas that comes into contact with the waste will kill harmful, infectious agents.

It's important to note that the EPA does not recommend ethylene oxide for treating infectious wastes because of its toxicity.

CHEMICAL DISINFECTION

This process involves the use of chemical agents for disinfection, such as chlorine. In the past, the most common chemical disinfectants for treating medical waste were chlorine-based because of the ability of chlorine and hypochlorite to inactivate a broad range of micro-organisms. Solutions of sodium hypochlorite(bleach) were regularly used. In recent years however, concerns have been raised about small amounts of toxic by-products associated with the use of large quantities of chlorine and hypochlorite (such as in the pulp and paper industry). Apparently, no studies have been done to establish whether or not this problem exists downstream of chemical treatment facilities for medical waste. It is believed however, that reactions between chlorine/hypochlorite and organic matter produce trihalomethanes, haloacetic acids, and chlorinated aromatic compounds that are toxic. Chemical disinfection processes are most appropriate for liquid wastes, although they can still be used to treat solid wastes. There are a number of factors that should be considered regarding the effective usage, including: the types and biology of microorganisms in the wastes, degree of contamination, type of disinfectant used as well as its concentration and quantity, contact time, and mixing requirements. Another option is the grinding of medical waste before exposing it to a liquid chemical disinfectant. Grinding ensures sufficient exposure of the chemical agent to all parts of the waste and assists in easy disposal of any residues. The resulting liquids are placed into the sewer system, while solid residues are disposed in landfills.

MICROWAVE

The application of microwave technology treatment also can disinfect waste. Waste is first shredded, and then mixed with water and internally heated to neutralize all present biologicals. Computerized controls are employed to ensure the minimum parameters for disinfection and proper equipment function. As with autoclaving, approximately 90% of medical wastes can be treated with this process. The shredding process results in a volume reduction, and energy use is reportedly lower than that of an incinerator. Microwaving might be economically competitive with incineration and applicable to continuous—or batch operation (CEC, 1993). Wastes are microwaved for 30min in a preheated treatment chamber and then held at a minimum temperature of 93–95 _C to ensure proper disinfection. However, microwaving is not sufficient for sterilization temperature above 120 _C. By microwaving spores are activated and some spores may survive (Chaand Carlisle, 2001; CEC, 1993).

IRRADIATION

This method involves sterilizing waste by exposing it to a cobalt source. Cobalt gives out gamma radiations that destroy all microbes in waste. The high cost of cobalt and high operating costs, however, have discouraged commercial ventures from using the technology for the treatment and management of medical waste. Ionising radiation can be obtained using radioactive materials, such as Cobalt-60, that emit highspeed gamma rays. UV-C or ultraviolet radiation in the C range (253.7 nm), also known as germicidal or short wave UV, is another kind of ionising radiation that can destroy cells under the proper conditions. UV-C can be generated using special lamps and has been employed as a supplement to alternative treatment technologies to inactivate aerosolised pathogens from shredders and other mechanical devices. Another technique for producing ionizing radiation is to use an “electron gun” from which a beam of high-energy electrons is propelled at high speed to strike against a target. A product of the nuclear and defence industries, electron beam (or e-beam) technology has been around for a few decades. It is also used in other applications, such as polymer processing, tyre manufacturing, and sterilisation of medical products. Unlikecobalt-60, e-beam technology does not use radioactive sources and has no residual radiation once the e-beam system is turned off. One area of debate, however, is the issue of induced radioactivity. E-beam manufacturers argue that radioactivity cannot be induced unless very high energies are used, e.g., above 10 or 16 MeV (mega-electron volts). Others have stated that low levels of radioactivity may be induced at much lower energies. This argument has arisen in the context of the public controversy over food irradiation using e-beam technology. There also have been some questions raised about the actual process of radiating the material and achieving adequate disinfection. As with autoclaving and microwave methods, it is not recommended for pathological wastes.

THERMAL INACTIVATION

This process involves heating waste to temperatures at which infectious agents are killed. It is used for treating large volumes of liquid clinical wastes. A chamber is preheated to an intense, specified temperature and held for a specified time, then released.

Before adopting a medical waste disposal strategy, make sure your business knows the applicable regulatory requirements. Assess capabilities, costs, and associated health and environmental risks. Bear in mind that some special treatment issues warrant consideration regarding specific pieces of the regulated medical waste stream, such as sharps (check out Special Treatment Considerations: Sharps for more information).

Flexibility for the generators to meet their management needs and comply with requirements will allow for adoption of the most suitable treatment options, as well as ensure safe and compliant management of medical wastes.

CONCLUSION

Within the healthcare community, it is widely acknowledged that biomedical wastes have reached colossal levels across the world. Medical device manufacturers and hospitals' management have been compelled to increase awareness of the issue, step up waste management initiatives, and accelerate technological advancements in this space. With such incredible, massive amounts of dangerous medical wastes produced each year, hospitals need safe, effective ways to dispose of them. Each of these methods ensures that infections aren't spread to staff, patients, or the general public. With the EPA imposing tighter regulations in the US, the number of hospital, medical, and infectious waste incinerators (HMIWI) have reduced drastically since 1997. In accordance to the new guidelines, medical care professionals are no longer allowed to dispose certain pharmaceuticals that are potentially reactive, toxic, corrosive, or ignitable. Besides conventional technologies being deployed across geographies, many companies are also focusing on alternatives such as microwave technologies, autoclaving, electro-pyrolysis, and chemical mechanical systems. These treatments ensure medical wastes are non-infectious, so that they can be disposed in incinerators or landfills as regular solid waste. By careful exclusion of non-RMW from RMW waste streams, hospitals can reduce the RMW volume that requires special treatment and reduce disposal costs.

REFERENCES

Anderson, J., Curmen, R., & Miripori, J. (1999). Alternatives to Current Blood Bag Plastic and Plasticizer Materials. *US Department of Health and Human Services Workshop on Plasticizers.*

Batholomew, P., Cycyota, M., Petrilli, L., Rosauer, D., Scharf, M., & Giovanetto, S. (1994). Recycling post-consumer hospital wastes. In *87th Annual Meeting and Exhibition, Air & Waste Manage. Assoc.* (Paper No. 94-FA-154.02)

Cha, C. Y., & Carlisle, C. T. (2001). Microwave process for volatile organic compound abatement. *Journal of the Air & Waste Management Association*, *51*(12), 1628–1641. doi:10.1080/10473289.2001.10464389 PMID:15666467

Citizens Environmental Coalition (CEC). (1993). Managing Medical Waste, CEC Fact Sheet #6. Albany, NY: CEC.

Hyland, R. G. (1993). Regulatory developments affecting medical waste disposal. In *86th Annual Meeting and Exhibition.* Air & Waste Manage. Assoc. (Paper No. 93-TA-47.03)

Hyland, R. G., Drum, D. A., & Bulley, M. (1994). Disposal medical wastes. In *87th Annual Meeting and Exhibition.* Air & Waste Manage. Assoc. (Paper No. 94-RP-123B.02)

Klangsin, P., & Harding, A. (1998). Medical waste treatment and disposal methods used by hospitals in Oregon, Washington and Idaho. *Journal of the Air & Waste Management Association*, *48*(6), 516–526. doi:10.1080/10473289.1998.10463706 PMID:9949738

Lee, B. K., Ellenbecker, M. J., & Moure-Eraso, R. (2002). Analyses of the recycling potential of medical plastic wastes. *Waste Management, 22*(5), 461–470.

Lee, B. K., Moure-Eraso, R., & Ellenbecker, M. J. (1995). Potential dioxin and furan sources from hospital solid waste streams: a pilot study. *J. Korea Air Pollution Research Assoc.*, *11*(E), 13–21.

Levendis, Y., Atal, A., Carlson, J., & Quintana, M. (2001). PAH and soot emissions from burning components of medical waste: Examination/surgical gloves and cotton pads. *Chemosphere*, *42*(5-7), 775–783. doi:10.1016/S0045-6535(00)00251-4 PMID:11219703

Marrack, D., & Meyers, D. (1994). *PP/PE medical syringe recycling system: sharps away. In 87th Annual Meeting and Exhibition.* Air & Waste Manage. Assoc. (Paper No. 94-RP-123B.01)

O'Connor, L. (1994). Improving medical waste disposal. *Mechanical Engineering (New York, N.Y.)*, *116*(5), 56–59.

Park, H. S., & Jeong, J. W. (2001). Recent trends on disposal technologies of medical waste. *J. Korean Solid Wastes Engineering Soc*, *18*(1), 18–27.

Salkin, I. F., & Krisiunas, E. (1998). Alternatives to medical waste incinerators. *Journal of Solid Waste Technology Management*, *25*(1), 9–13.

Senatore, P. J. (1994). Medical waste disposal alternatives: selection and implementation. In *87th Annual Meeting and Exhibition.* Air & Waste Manage. Assoc. (Paper No. 94-RP123B.03)

US EPA. (2002). *Municipal Solid Waste in the United States: 2000 Facts and Figures (EPA-530-R-02-001).* US Environmental Protection Agency.

Waste Prevention Association. (2003). *Medical Waste Treatment Technologies-Alternatives to Incineration.* Available from http://www.otzo.most.org.pl/en/docs/med_tech.pdf

Yoon, O. S. (2001). Disposal measures and problems of medical waste. *Journal of Korean Solid Wastes Engineering Soc*, *18*(1), 1–12.

KEY TERMS AND DEFINITIONS

Environmental Protection Agency (EPA): The Environmental Protection Agency (EPA) is an independent agency of the United States federal government for environmental protection.

Gas Sterilization: Sterilization by means of a bactericidal gas, frequently used for items that are heat and moisture sensitive.

Incineration: Incineration is a waste treatment process that involves the combustion of organic substances contained in waste materials.

Irradiation: The use of high-energy radiation from x-rays, gamma rays, neutrons, and other sources to kill cancer cells and shrink tumors. Radiation may come from a machine outside the body (external-beam radiation therapy) or from materials called radioisotopes.

Other Potentially Infectious Materials (OPIM): The following human body fluids: semen, vaginal secretions, cerebrospinal fluid, synovial fluid, pleural fluid, pericardial fluid, peritoneal fluid, amniotic fluid, saliva in dental procedures, any body fluid that is visibly contaminated with blood, and all body fluids in situations where it is difficult or impossible to differentiate between body fluids.

Radio Waves: Radio waves are a type of electromagnetic radiation with wavelengths in the electromagnetic spectrum longer than infrared light. Radio waves have frequencies as high as 300 gigahertz (GHz) to as low as 30 hertz (Hz).

Regulated Medical Waste: Regulated medical waste (RMW), also known as 'biohazardous' waste or 'infectious medical' waste, is the portion of the waste stream that may be contaminated by blood, body fluids or other potentially infectious materials, thus posing a significant risk of transmitting infection.

Thermal Radiation: Also known as heat, is the emission of electromagnetic waves from all matter that has a temperature greater than absolute zero. It represents the conversion of thermal energy into electromagnetic energy.

Section 2
Plastics and Human Health

Chapter 12
Association between Urinary Bisphenol A Concentration and Obesity Prevalence in Children and Adolescents:
Bisphenol A and Its Effects on Humans

Sajad Hussain Mir
https://orcid.org/0000-0002-4655-7846
Kashmir University, India

Attiya Baddar
University of Kashmir, India

ABSTRACT

Bisphenol A is an organic compound that serves as a building block of polycarbonate plastics and epoxy resins. Being the world's highest-volume chemicals in use today in the form of medical devices, water and infant bottles, food cans, kitchen utensils, water supply pipes, compact devices, etc., this compound—after gaining an access to the body of an individual by way of leaching into food and water supplies—acts as an obesogen and disrupts the body weight regulation by either promoting adipogenesis or triggering the differentiation of fibroblasts into adipocytes. The other adverse effects of bisphenol A include insulin resistance, adipocyte differentiation or aromatase-mediated transformation of androgen into estrogen, cardiovascular diseases, liver function abnormalities, alterations in the circulating thyroid hormone levels, association with diabetes and carcinogenic effect. Its other aspects on health individually as well as in combination with other chemicals are worth mentioning.

DOI: 10.4018/978-1-5225-9452-9.ch012

INTRODUCTION

The plastic monomer bisphenol A is one of the highest volume chemicals produced worldwide, with over 6 billion pounds produced each year and over 100 tons released into the atmosphere by yearly production. Humans are widely exposed to bisphenol A and animal studies have linked bisphenol A to obesity (Golub, *et al.,* 2010; Newbold, 2010; Rubin, 2011). Emerging evidence linking the worldwide obesity epidemic to increased exposures to environmental endocrine disruptors, collectively called ''environmental obesogens'' (Heindel, 2003; Wang and Lobsttein, 2006; Newbold, 2008; Heindel and Vom, 2009), one such important potential obesogen is bisphenol A. Although it was first recognized in the 1930's as a potential synthetic estrogen (Dodds and Lawson, 1938), bisphenol A is contained in a variety of consumer products from baby bottles, plastic containers, and the resin lining of cans for food and beverages, to dental sealants (National Toxicology Program USDOHAHS, 2008). Bisphenol A was detected in about 93%–100% of children and adolescents in Northern America, some European nations, Egypt, Australia, and Asian countries (Dodds and Lawson, 1938; Newbold, 2007; National Toxicology Program USDOHAHS, 2008; Heindel and Vom, 2009; Golub *et al.,* 2010; Newbold, 2010; Rubin, 2011). In Thailand Bisphenol A was detected in 52.8% of adults in serum samples (Calafat *et al.,* 2008).

In recent decades, both developing countries such as China as well as developed countries have witnessed an alarming increase in the prevalence of obesity (Chen, 2008; *et al.,* 2008; Shan *et al.,* 2010). The most troubling aspect of this increase is the acceleration in the prevalence of obesity and overweight among children. The prevalence of obesity in U.S. children is close to 20% (Barlow, 2007; Kosti and Panagiotakos, 2006; Wang and Lobsttein, 2006). This is especially alarming given the well-known consequences of overweight and obesity which include type 2 diabetes, hyperinsulinemia, insulin resistance, coronary heart disease, hypertension, stroke, and liver and kidney diseases among many other adverse health effects. Bisphenol A could both accelerate girls' pubertal development and weight gain during this period. The acceleration of growth by Bisphenol A may impact both weight and height, leading to a slightly weaker bisphenol A effect on Body Mass Index measurement. It has been hypothesized that human exposure to Bisphenol A in the early stage of development could also lead to the onset of obesity and other metabolic syndrome (Rubin *et al.,* 2001; Somm *et al.,* 2009).

Research studies have reported an association between urine bisphenol A level and obesity in human populations (Carwile and Michels, 2011; Wang *et al.,* 2012). Urine is an appropriate specimen with which to determine BISPHENOL A exposure because BISPHENOL A and its metabolites are present in urine for several weeks or months (Volkel *et al.,* 2002; Stahlhut *et al.,* 2009). Bisphenol A is rapidly eliminated from plasma within 24 hours after ingestion (Stahlhut *et al.,* 2009). Urinary bisphenol A levels are reported to be associated with food in plastic containers (Nahar *et al.,* 2012), bottled milk feeding (Rhie *et al.,* 2014), and eating canned food (Casas *et al.,* 2013). One study reported an association between urine bisphenol A level and metabolic diseases including diabetes (Lang *et al.,* 2008). In a recent study, an association between urine bisphenol A and obesity among children and adolescents has been reported (Trasande *et al.,* 2012) using U.S. National Health and Nutrition Examination Survey (NHANES) data. In a U.S. representative sample, bisphenol A was detected in more than 92% of urine samples including those from children (Heffeman *et al.,* 2013; Calafat *et al.,* 2008) and in populations of many other countries (Kim *et al.,* 2003; Matsumoto *et al.,* 2003; Silva *et al.,* 2004; Miyamoto and Kotake, 2006; Li *et al.,* 2011). One of the troubling aspects of bisphenol A exposure is that younger children generally have higher urine bisphenol A level than adults indicating a heavier biological burden likely due to a higher bisphenol A exposure or slower metabolic process or both among young children (Calafat *et al.,* 2008).

In 2011, a population-based study to examine the relationship between urine bisphenol A and obesity in school-age children was conducted. Bisphenol A was detected in about 93%–100% of children and adolescents in Northern America, some European nations, Egypt, Australia, and Asian countries (Calafat *et al.,* 2008; Becker *et al.,* 2009; Bushnik *et al.,* 2010; Zhang *et al.,* 2011; Pirard *et al.,* 2012; Frederiksen *et al.,* 2013; Frederiksen *et al.,* 2013; Casas *et al.,* 2013; Ha *et al.,* 2014; Nahar *et al.,* 2012; Heffeman *et al.,* 2013). It was observed that high urine bisphenol A level was associated with overweight among female students aged 9–12 years old (likely in pubertal developmental stages) (Sun *et al.,* 2012), but not in male students.

WORLDWIDE PRODUCTION OF BISPHENOL A

The world's consumption in 2009 of bisphenol A as a monomer in the manufacture of polycarbonates was 2768 kiloton and as a precursor or a starting material for monomers of certain epoxy resins it was 1093 kiloton. The bisphenol A production increased with 64% in EU from the years 1996/1999 to 2005/2006. Observation from Sweden, Norway, Denmark and Finland showed an overall quite stable use up to about 1000 tonnes/year/country from year 2000 till 2010. In 2011, the global bisphenol A production recorded 5.25% YoY growth and reached approximately 4.4 million tonnes. In 2012, it grew by just over 372,000 tonnes if compared to the previous year and surpassed the 4.6 million tonnes mark. Meanwhile, the global operating rate of the Bisphenol A production was at the 80% level. Asia is the dominant bisphenol A manufacturer with nearly 53% share of the overall production volume, which is equal to slightly over 2.4 million tonnes. It is followed by Europe and North America, holding 25% and 18% market shares, respectively. The USA, Taiwan, China, South Korea and Japan are the top five bisphenol A producers worldwide. In 2012, their combined contribution to the world bisphenol A production volume was more than 2.7 million tonnes. As of 2013, global annual production capacity of bisphenol A stands at more than 6.2 million tonnes. Asia Pacific captures just over 57.5% share of the global capacity, which is equal to over 3.58 million tonnes. The USA, South Korea, Taiwan, China and Japan are the top five countries in terms of annual production capacity of bisphenol A. Asia-Pacific is the leading bisphenol A consumer, accounting for over half of the global consumption volume. The bisphenol A market is highly dependent on the overall economic environment as the product's derivatives are mainly used in such end-use sectors as construction, electronic and automotive industries. Around 70% of the global bisphenol A supply volume is used in polycarbonates' production. Epoxy resins industry is another important bisphenol A application area. Over 3 thousand million kilograms of bisphenol A are produced each year.

HISTORY

Bisphenol A is not found naturally in the environment and is therefore, a manmade molecule. It was discovered in 1891 by Russian Chemist Alexander Pavlovich Dianin while carrying out studies on phenols. Dianin's method for preparing Bisphenol A involves the catalyzed condensation of a 2:1 mixture

Figure 1.

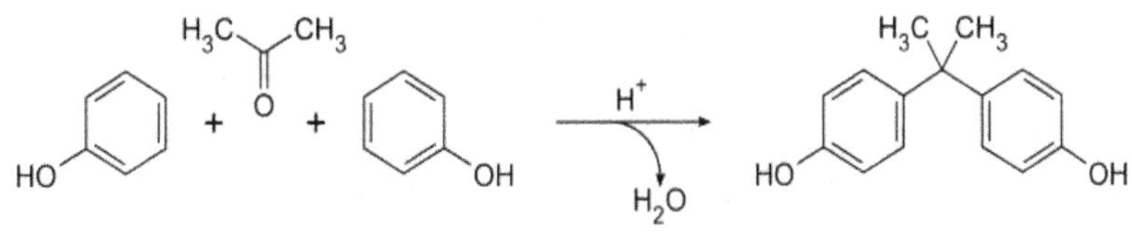

of phenol and acetone in the presence of concentrated hydrochloric acid or sulfuric acid. The reaction proceeds readily at room temperature producing a crude product containing a great variety of side products in a matter of hours, with water as the only by-product.

Mechanistically, the acid catalyst converts the acetone to a carbenium ion that undergoes an electrophilic aromatic substitution reaction with the phenol, producing predominantly para-substituted products. A second carbenium species is produced by protonation and loss of the aliphatic hydroxyl group, leading to bisphenol A (4, 4'-isopropylidenediphenol) after a second aromatic substitution reaction. It was later investigated in the 1930s by Charles Dodds (British Chemist) as a synthetic estrogen but was never developed for pharmaceutical purposes. In the 1950's, bisphenol A began to be used in the production of polycarbonate plastics and epoxy resins, and production has increased steadily since that time.

Bisphenol A is a moderately water-soluble compound (300 mg L-1 at room temperature) and it dissociates in an alkaline environment (Rykowska and Wasiak, 2006). This organic compound has a molecular weight of 228.29 and it melts at 158-159°C (Ozdal and Yesilcubuk, 2014).

USES OF BISPHENOL A

Bisphenol A is an organic chemical compound which functions as the building block for epoxy resins and polycarbonate (PC) plastic. Bisphenol A may be used in the manufacture of modified polyamide, and tetrabromo-bisphenol A. Other products/articles that may contain bisphenol A include protective window glazing, building materials, optical lenses and dyes. Thus, bisphenol A is sometimes also found in PVC products/articles. In a study 5 out of 48 PVC sub samples in toys (approximately 10%) bisphenol A was detected. It was probably used as chain-terminator to end the polymerization of PVC or as an antioxidant for polymers or plasticizers (Voedsel en Waren Autoriteit, 2005). Bisphenol A is also present in recycled paper (WHO, 2010). Other uses that include flame retardants, unsaturated polyester resins, polysulfone (PS) resins and polyetherimides (PEIs). It is primarily used as a monomer in the manufacture of polycarbonates and as a monomer, precursor or a starting material for monomers of certain epoxy resins and as such used in a wide variety of consumer products and articles. Over 95% of the world consumption of Bisphenol A in 2009 was of PC resins (about 75%) and epoxy resins.

Polycarbonate is a highly versatile, durable, heat- and shatter-resistant and clear thermoplastic that is the material of choice for a wide range of end-user applications. Polycarbonate is used in compact disc manufacture, food and beverage contact containers, medical devices, and in glazing applications and film. Polycarbonate blends are used in the electric and electronics industries and in the automotive industry.

Epoxy resins are used primarily as coatings for consumer and industrial applications. They are used in protective coatings, structural composites, electrical laminates, electrical applications and adhesives. Epoxy-phenolic resins are used as liners in metal cans for foods and beverages and as coatings on metal lids for glass jars and bottles. Epoxy resins are used in automotive electro-coating and in automotive and industrial primer and topcoat applications as well as in coatings (e.g. for water pipes) and dental materials/epoxy adhesives.

Bisphenol A is also used in the production of phenolplast, phenolic and unsaturated polyester resins, thermal paper, polyvinylchloride (PVC), alkoxylated Bisphenol A and polyols/polyurethane. Bisphenol A may be used in the manufacture of modified polyamide, and tetrabromobisphenol A. Other articles that may contain Bisphenol A include protective window glazing, building materials, optical lenses and dyes as well as recycled paper (Lise Moller, Frank, Fotel, Poul and Larsen, 2012).

BISPHENOL A MIGRATION TO FOOD

Individuals working in the manufacture of bisphenol A containing products can be exposed to bisphenol A at the workplace. Bisphenol A can leach from polycarbonate plastic food containers and Bisphenol A coated metallic cans. More specifically, exposure to bisphenol A can arise under conditions where residual monomer in the polymer migrates into food and beverages, or where the polymer itself hydrolyses, thereby releasing bisphenol A. Bisphenol A migration from polycarbonates to liquids is resulted by hydrolysis diffusion catalyzed by hydroxides (Hoekstra, and Simoneau, 2013). Recent studies have shown that dietary ingestion is a major route (99%) of human exposure to bisphenol A contamination, especially from canned foods (Braun *et al.,* 2011; Rhie *et al.,* 2014). Other routes are microwave containers, soft drinks, smoking, alcohol consumption, dental sealants (Olea *et al.,* 1996), medical procedures (Duty *et al.,* 2013), and plastic tubing (Silver *et al.,* 2011).

Metallic food and beverage cans are protected from rusting and corrosion by the application of epoxy resins as inner coatings. The synthesis of many of these resins requires the condensation of bisphenol A with epichlorohydrin to create bisphenol A diglycidyl ether. When incomplete polymerization occurs, residual bisphenol A leaches from the epoxy resin. High temperatures and exposure to acidic or basic solutions can also increase leaching of bisphenol A from coatings and plastics, even when complete polymerization has occurred. Temperature has been reported to be more effective for migration of bisphenol A from cans than heating time. According to recent studies, in polycarbonate-based materials; temperature, heat treatment time, destruction, water hardness and pH effect migration. Le et al. found that at room temperature, leaching of bisphenol A occurred into the contained fluid, which increased 55-fold if boiling water was added (Le *et al.,* 2008). Other common sources of ingestion include foods stored in food cans, which are lined with BISPHENOL A epoxy resin films to prevent corrosion (Sajiki *et al.,* 2007; Grumetto *et al.,* 2008; Cao *et al.,* 2010), thermal printing paper commonly used in cash register receipts (Biedermann *et al.,* 2010; Lunder *et al.,* 2010), and bisphenol A containing dental composites and sealants (Olea *et al.,* 1996; Zimmerman-Downs *et al.,* 2010).

In epoxy based resins; lacquering type, amount of lac used, process parameters (temperature and time), contents of the contact food material (amount of salt and oil) factors effect migration (Munguia-Lopez and Soto-Valtez, 2001; Maragoua *et al.,* 2008; Hoekstra and Simoneau, 2013). In polycarbonate bottles, pH is increased while water is boiling according to increased solubility of lime and these results in increased bisphenol A migration. Considering the food groups, it is observed that bisphenol A migration occurs in canned meat/fishery products and instant soups, especially when their salt and oil content is high (Goodson *et al.,* 2002; Thomson, and Grounds, 2005). Besides, alkaline detergent residues after washing in the dishwasher also increase bisphenol A migration. Similarly, food preparation methods that cause increase in pH also gives same effect.

Bisphenol A migration in canned foods is directly affected by storage time and it was observed that bisphenol A firstly migrates to liquid in can and later to solid food materials. Migration occurs during the storage time even if heat treatment is finished (Kang *et al.,* 2006). It was also observed that in plastic containers especially in polycarbonate baby bottles according to excessive usage and scratches and also effect of sterilization resulted in high levels of bisphenol A migration. It was observed that new polycarbonate baby bottles contain below 1.0-3.5 ppb bisphenol A content, whereas it was measured 10-28 ppb levels in used and scratched baby bottles (Kang *et al.,* 2006).

Another study found that exposure levels increased not only with temperature, but also with repeated use of a container (Thomson, and Grounds, 2005). Medical equipment is also raising concerns about bisphenol A levels as a study of newborns found that those who regularly spent time in a neonatal intensive care unit had significantly higher serum bisphenol A levels than the general population—thought to be due to exposure to plastics in medical devices (Calafat *et al.,* 2008). Likewise, dialysis patients appear to have higher rates of exposure, which may be attributable to circulating solvents which expedite the leaching of bisphenol A from polycarbonate hemodialysis equipment (Kanno *et al.,* 2007; Murakami *et al.,* 2007).

Bisphenol A has also been detected in a variety of environmental samples, including water, sewage leachates, indoor and outdoor air samples, and dust (Vandenberg et al. 2007). It is also found in papers and in implanted medical devices and other medical equipment (Welshons and others, 1999). Other, relatively minor sources of consumer exposure to bisphenol A are dental fissure sealants, epoxy-based surface coatings, adhesives, printing inks and thermal paper. Some researches indicate that skin contact may also contribute to human exposure of bisphenol A (Zalko *et al.,* 2011).

Heat treatment, storage conditions, and the presence of damage are the principal factors influencing bisphenol A migration. Goodson and his associates (2004) filled empty epoxy phenolic coated cans with 4 different foods and a simulated food. After filling, the cans were sealed and processed using the usual conditions of heat and duration. To evaluate the effect of damage on bisphenol A migration, half the cans were dented and then all the cans (damaged and undamaged) were stored at different temperature and time intervals. The authors found that 80% to 100% of the bisphenol A present in the coating migrated into the food during the sterilization process. Contrary to it, Errico and his associates (2014) while storing canned tomatoes and different temperatures after denting some cans found that the bisphenol A migration level increased with increasing storage temperature and the presence of damage increased the bisphenol A migration by more than 30% to 40%. The controversial results of these 2 studies can be explained by the different time/temperature conditions employed during the sterilization process. In fact, the drastic heat process used by Goodson and his associates (2004) determined an almost total release of bisphenol A from the internal coating of the cans, therefore the subsequent storage and presence of damage proved inconsequential. However, Errico and his associates (2014) observed increased bisphenol A concentration in the food during storage and in the presence of damage due to low pH of tomato products and the milder heat processing conditions. Similar findings were observed by Munguia-Lopez and his associates in 2005 who also studied the effect of heating on bisphenol A migration in canned jalapen˜o peppers and tuna fish.

EFFECTS ON HUMAN HEALTH

Obesity Prevalence in Children and Adults

Although the tolerable daily intake of bisphenol A has been specified as 0.01mg/kg of body weight/day (Scientific Committee on Food of the European Commission) but the recent findings suggest that the current levels of human exposure to bisphenol A from all sources (food products, synthetic polycarbonates and epoxy resins) exceeds the daily dose and has been estimated to be from 0.48 to 1.6μm kg-1 body mass per day for adults and children respectively. The highest bisphenol A intake in infants and children than adults has been attributed to the fact that they eat, drink, and breathe more per pound of their body weight, and they may ingest more bisphenol A because they explore objects orally (12; Rykowska and Wasiak, 2006). In one study the association between obesity and urinary bisphenol A detection was conducted wherein the bisphenol A detection rate in students with normal weight was significantly higher in the group with bisphenol A <0.05 ng/mL than in the group with bisphenol A >0.05 ng/mL (86.5% vs 77.3%, P = 0.015). The bisphenol A detection rate in obese students was significantly higher in the group with bisphenol A >0.05 ng/mL than in the group with bisphenol A <0.05 ng/mL (13.7% vs 4.5%, P = 0.03). Obesity was significantly associated with bisphenol A detection with an OR of 3.42 (95% CI 1.18–9.95, P = 0.02). Once ingested in the body, bisphenol A is mainly conjugated with glucuronic acid in the liver and is primarily excreted into the bile. However, unconjugated (bioactive) bisphenol A can be found in the blood and, in its glucuronidated form, in urine (Vandenberg *et al.,* 2007). Urinary Bisphenol A concentrations do not decline rapidly with fasting time, suggesting that the compound accumulates in fat and other physiological compartments (Stahihut *et al.,* 2009). Although the relationship between bisphenol A exposure and urinary bisphenol A concentration is complex, Leonardo and others (2012) reported that the higher urinary bisphenol A levels could be due to the release of bisphenol A from stored fat in obese children. An extensive review conducted in 2007 concluded that bisphenol A levels in human blood and/or urine are within the range shown to be dangerous in animals and are therefore likely to be biologically active in humans (Vandenberg *et al.,* 2007). Increasing numbers of studies in humans showed that a higher concentration of urinary bisphenol A is associated with younger age (Calafat *et al.,* 2008; Zhang *et al.,* 2011), female sex, non-Hispanic black, low family income (Calafat *et al.,* 2008), low education, and smoking (Wang *et al.,* 2012; Casas *et al.,* 2013). Unconjugated bisphenol A circulating in blood indicates an internal exposure to the compound, as does its presence in urine, but in this latter case it also suggests a failure of first-pass conjugation and removal or deconjugation. A fraction of the absorbed bisphenol A may also be distributed to body storage site(s) such as adipose tissue, followed by a slow, low-level release of bisphenol A into the bloodstream (Fernandez *et al.,* 2007). In the NHANES 2003–2004 study sample that included 694 men and 761 women, Lang, Li, Chen, and others (2012) found a linear, positive, and statistically significant relationship between urinary BISPHENOL A and body mass index. Pooling NHANES 2003–2004 and 2005–2006 data on 2,747 adult US participants, Carwile and Michels (2012) reported a similar positive association of urinary bisphenol A with general and central obesity in the adult population. Another study by Wang, Li, Chen, and others (2012) among 3,390 Chinese adults also reported a positive and significant association of urinary bisphenol A concentration with generalized and abdominal obesity. Other studies on multiple linear regression analysis showed that high urine bisphenol A and daily intake estimate were significantly associated with an increase in BMI value in all subjects. Specific gravity correction weakened the association, especially after stratified by age or sex. It was reported that overweight and obese subjects might have less urine output (Inoue *et al.,*

2003), which might lead to a higher urine bisphenol A concentration, and similarly a higher urine SG. In this respect, urine SG correction was appropriate. However, there is also a possibility that urine solute excretion increases urine SG in overweight or obese subjects (Yokota *et al.,* 1999), and urine SG correction might result in an underestimation of true urine bisphenol A concentrations in overweight or obese subjects and therefore weaken the association with BMI. Small sample size could be another important reason for non-significant association when stratified by sex and age. One study detected unconjugated bisphenol A accumulation in half the studied women (Fernandez *et al.,* 2007). Furthermore, age, sex, liver function, and physiological status (e.g., pregnancy) could influence bisphenol A metabolism.

There is increasing evidence suggesting that bisphenol A can act as obesogens and interfere with body's natural weight control mechanisms by disrupting adipose tissue biology, endocrine hormone systems, or central hypothalamic-pituitary-adrenal axis (Gruen and Blumberg, 2009; Thayer *et al.,* 2012). Animal and cell studies have demonstrated that bisphenol A can promote adipogenesis (Gruen and Blumberg, 2009; Thayer *et al.,* 2012) by interacting with specialized nuclear receptors (such as steroid hormone receptors or thyroid hormone receptors) for promoting adipogenesis (Casals-Casas and Desvergne, 2011) or by binding to estrogen receptors (ERs) (Rubin, 2011). Soriano et al. found that bisphenol A behaved as a strong estrogen via nuclear ERβ by using pancreatic β-cell from ERβ-/- mice at 1 nM of bisphenol A exposure level (Soriano *et al.,* 2012). Bisphenol A also stimulated calcium influx and prolactin secretion in rat pituitary tumor cells by membrane estrogen receptor α at as low as pM level (Wozniak *et al.,* 2005). Three human cell lines (Ishikawa, HeLa and HepG2) were used to evaluate the estrogenic promoter activity of bisphenol A on estrogen receptors α and β, and bisphenol A were found to act as cell type specific agonists or antagonists at different concentration levels ranging from 1 nM to 1000 nM (Matthews *et al.,* 2001). Sargis and his associates (2010) reported that bisphenol A significantly stimulated glucocorticoid receptor (GR) to promote adipogenesis without significant activation of the peroxisome proliferator-activated receptor-γ in the 3 T3-L1 Cell Line at an incubation concentration of 100 nM. In-vitro studies have indicated that bisphenol A exposure triggers the differentiation of fibroblasts into adipocytes (Masuno *et al.,* 2002). Fibroblasts treated with bisphenol A showed an increase in triglyceride content, lipoprotein lipase activity, and glycerol phosphate dehydrogenase activity (Masuno *et al.,* 2002). Masuno and his associates (2002) has reported that bisphenol A simulates and accelerates the adipocyte conversion process. Secondly, bisphenol A enhances basal and insulin-stimulated glucose uptake (Sakurai *et al.,* 2004). BISPHENOL A exposure of cell suspensions causes lipid accumulation in adipocytes and hepatoma cell lines, associated with obesity and metabolic syndrome (Wada *et al.,* 2007).

Bisphenol A, with its two benzene rings and two (4, 4′)-OH substituents, fits in the ER binding pocket. Biochemical assays have examined the kinetics of bisphenol A binding to ER and have determined that bisphenol A binds both ERα and ERβ, with approximately 10-fold higher affinity to ERβ (Gould *et al.,* 1998; Kuiper *et al.,* 1998). Extensive biochemical studies of ERα have identified two distinct gene trans-activating regions, termed AF1 (found in the amino terminus) and AF2 (located in the carboxyl terminus) (Gould *et al.,* 1998). ER agonists are subdivided based on their ability to activate these regions. Binding of xenoestrogens to the ERs alters their ability to recruit co-activators that may be important for differences in tissue-dependent responses. For instance, biochemical analyses indicate that bisphenol A is able to induce greater changes in downstream gene expression in cells containing ERβ where TIF2 is the main co-activator, but may be equally effective in cells expressing either ERα or ERβ if the steroid receptor coactivator-1a is present (Routledge *et al.,* 2000). Based on these biochemical studies, it has been proposed that differences in the ability of ERα or ERβ to recruit co-activators when bisphenol A is bound may contribute to the complex tissue-specific responses to bisphenol A exposure (Wetherill *et al.,* 2007).

In the recent gender based study on obesity, a statistically significant positive association with obesity among boys but not in girls was found. Similarly, in a stratified analysis by race/ethnicity, it was found that the observed association between urinary bisphenol A and obesity is primarily present in non-Hispanic white boys. Although the exact reasons for these observed gender and racial/ethnic differences in the bisphenol A–obesity association are not clear but animal studies attribute this gender difference in bisphenol A concentrations to a lower rate of BISPHENOL A glucuronidation and subsequent renal clearance in male rats (Takeuchi *et al.,* 2004), potentially resulting in higher free serum bisphenol A concentrations and therefore higher biological action (Matthews *et al.,* 2001; Williams, 2012). Second, estrogens have been reported to have a role in the pathogenesis of obesity (Williams, 2010). It is possible that the relative estrogenic activity of bisphenol A may vary by the levels of endogenous estrogen levels, which are known to vary by gender (lower in males) and race/ethnicity [lower in non-Hispanic whites (Rohrmann *et al.,* 2007)]. It is possible that bisphenol A may act as an estrogenic agonist in the presence of low endogenous estrogen levels (males and non-Hispanic whites), whereas as an antagonist in the presence of higher endogenous estrogen levels (females and other race/ethnicities) (Xu *et al.,* 2011). It is also possible that the effect of bisphenol A on mechanisms related to obesity, such as insulin resistance, adipocyte differentiation, or aromatase-mediated transformation of androgen into estrogen, is different by gender and race/ethnicity (Xu *et al.,* 2011). Further, these observed gender and racial differences in the bisphenol A–obesity association could be due to unmeasured confounding or a chance finding. Moreover, a role for sex steroid hormones in regulating adipocyte hypertrophy and hyperplasia was confirmed by knockout models of sex steroid pathway components (Grun and Blurnberg, 2009).

Thyroid function is critical to the maintenance of basal metabolism, and bisphenol A may influences thyroid hormone. It has been supposed that bisphenol A influences thyroid hormone metabolism, acting either as an agonist or antagonist on the thyroid hormone receptor (Moriyama, Tagami *et al.,* 2002). In the perinatal period, bisphenol A exposed rats had elevated T4 levels during development, and upregulation of a thyroid hormone-responsive gene in the brain, without significant changes in TSH levels (Zoeller *et al.,* 2005). A large cross-sectional study from Denmark found that thyroid function, was associated with BMI (Knudsen *et al.,* 2005). Fox and his associates (2008) found that thyroid function within the reference range, as assessed by serum thyroid stimulating hormone concentration, is associated with body weight in both sexes using data from Framingham Offspring Study. Moreover, Moriyama et al. observed that bisphenol A could inhibit the binding of T3 to the rat hepatic thyroid hormone receptors with an inhibition constant (Ki) of 200 μM and suppress the transcriptional activities mediated by endogenous thyroid hormone receptors at as low as 100 nM (Moriyama *et al.,* 2002).The relationship between urinary bisphenol A concentrations and serum thyroid hormones was evaluated in 1346 adults and 329 adolescents (older than 12-19 years) from the NHANES 2007 to 2008 (Meeker and Ferguson, 2011). In adults, an inverse relationship between urinary bisphenol A and total T4 and TSH was observed, supporting previous reports concerning the association between bisphenol A and altered thyroid hormones (Meeker *et al.,* 2010). In conclusion, human exposure to bisphenol A may be associated with alterations in circulating thyroid hormone levels, as demonstrated in cross-sectional studies.

Moreover, interference with the production and signaling of sex hormones has led to neurological impairment (Leranth *et al.,* 2008; Zhou *et al.,* 2008). Synapse formation during development is regulated by estrogen and androgens; however with exposure to bisphenol A, a recent study found that levels deemed safe by the US Environment Protection Agency, completely abolish the response of synapses to estrogen in the prefrontal cortex and hippocampus (Leranth *et al.,* 2008). Epigenetic effects of BISPHENOL A have been associated with an increased risk of cancer, particularly breast and prostate malignancies (Murray *et al.,* 2007; Jenkins *et al.,* 2009; Weng *et al.,* 2010). The exposure of breast epithelial cells to bisphenol A was found to alter gene expression of 170 genes and increase their vulnerability to other carcinogens (Jenkins *et al.,* 2009; Weng *et al.,* 2010). Additionally, there was silencing of lysosomal-associated membrane protein 3, as occurs in ERα-positive breast cancer (Weng *et al.,* 2010). Similar effects have been seen with respect to prostatic disease, as exposure to bisphenol A has been repeatedly shown to modify methylation of implicated genes (Prins, 2008; Prins *et al.,* 2008). However, most of the studies about the association of bisphenol A, one of focused EDCs, with obesity are lab researches (Tang-Peronard *et al.,* 2011; Vom *et al.,* 2012). For example, Huc et al observed that lipid accumulation in HepG2 cells was induced by bisphenol A at 10-4-10-12 M level (Huc *et al.,* 2012).

In fact, recent evidence suggests that at low concentrations, while most plasma bisphenol A (about 95%) is bound to serum proteins, BISPHENOL A has lipophilic affinity with a fat: blood coefficient of 3.3 (Csan´ady *et al.,* 2002). Furthermore, bisphenol A appears to have a disproportionate affinity to fat in comparison to other tissues such as kidney, muscle, and other sites; "in fat, the accumulation of bisphenol A was about three times higher than in other tissues" (Csan´ady *et al.,* 2002). With evidence of potential bioaccumulation, bisphenol A has the prospect of exerting ongoing metabolic effects.

While studying the bisphenol A exposure in 259 Chinese school children (older than 8-15 years), the authors found that high urine bisphenol A concentration and a daily intake estimate of bisphenol A were significantly associated with an increment in body mass index (BMI) in all the participants (He *et al.,* 2009). These findings reinforce the concept that not only hormones and neurotransmitters, but also endocrine disrupting substances, exert effects at very low exposure levels. Similarly, in 1326 Chinese students (older than 4-12 years), high urine bisphenol A levels were associated with overweight, but only among female students older than 9-12 years (most likely in pubertal developmental stages) (Sun *et al.,* 2012). The association between bisphenol A exposure and obesity was also examined in the United States on 2200 children older than 6-18 years who participated in the National Health and Nutrition Examination Survey (NHANES) in 3 study cycles, 2003–2004, 2005–2006, and 2007–2008, analyzing gender and race/ethnicity separately. The authors found a positive association between increasing levels of urinary bisphenol A and obesity, independent of age, sex, race/ethnicity, and other social and life style variables like education and physical activity level. Children in the highest quartile of BISPHENOL A (>5.4 ng mL_1) had a multivariable odds ratio for obesity of 2.55 (Jiang *et al.,* 2007). These results confirmed the conclusion of the study previously conducted on 6- to 19-year-olds recruited in the same nationally representative survey (Wang *et al.,* 2012).

Bisphenol A has estrogenic activity and binds to the α- and, to a lesser extent, β-estrogen receptors (ER) in vitro and in vivo (Welshons *et al.,*1999). Moreover, bisphenol A can also inhibit the activity of endogenous estrogens and/or disrupt estrogen nuclear hormone receptor action (Laws *et al.,* 2000). There is additional clear evidence of a 17β-estradiol, bisphenol A, and diethylstilbestrol (DES) membrane binding site with a pharmacologic profile that differs from the classical ER. This membrane receptor may be implicated in triggering non-genomic actions of xenoestrogens and it has been demonstrated its existence both in pancreatic β cells and in pancreatic α cells (Papaconstantinou *et al.,* 2000). Bisphenol

A also affects other relevant endocrine activities, including the thyroid hormone pathway and binding to glucocorticoid and androgen receptors as well as more complex interferences with the central nervous system and immune system (Villalobos *et al.,* 1995; Laws *et al.,* 2000).

At present, many lines of evidence revealed that bisphenol A could interact with many nuclear hormone receptors such as estrogen receptor (Okada *et al.,* 2008; Maire *et al.,* 2010; Li *et al.,* 2010), human estrogen-related receptor (Takayanagi *et al.,* 2006; Matsushima *et al.,* 2007), human pregnane X receptor or steroid and xenobiotic receptor (Sui *et al.,* 2012), androgen receptor (Sohoni and Sumpter, 1998; Takayanagi *et al.,* 2006), human peroxisome proliferator activated receptor (Riu *et al.,* 2011) and thyroid hormone receptor (Moriyama *et al.,* 2002; Zoeller *et al.,* 2005). Therefore, bisphenol A could disturb the normal function of nuclear receptors. Nuclear receptors are a class of proteins within cells that are responsible for sensing hormones. Nuclear receptors are ligand-inducible transcription factors specifically regulate the expression of target genes involved in metabolism, development, and reproduction (Mckenna *et al.,* 1999). They are of major importance for intercellular signaling in animals because they transmit different intra and extracellular signals on the regulation of genetic programs. Endogenous hormones such as progestins, estrogens, androgens, glucocorticoids, vitamin D3, thyroid and retinoid hormones can activate the normal function of nuclear receptors. Meanwhile, endocrine disruptors from exogenous environment can also interact with nuclear receptors ligand binding domains (LBDs) and then give rise to disorder of downstream signaling pathways. Because nuclear receptors regulate the expression of a large number of genes, chemicals that could activate these receptors would have profound effects on the organisms. Many of these regulated genes are associated with various diseases such as cancer, osteoporosis, obesity (Junichiro *et al.,* 2008; Judit *et al.,* 2012). Nearly 13% targets of U. S. Food and Drug Administration (FDA) approved drugs are nuclear receptors (Overington *et al.,* 2006). It would lead to serious consequence when the normal function of nuclear receptors was obstructed by exogenous small molecules.

Bisphenol A may play a role in the development of obesity not only when exposure occurs after birth but also when it occurs ''in utero''. Specifically, it has been hypothesized that the obesogenic effect of bisphenol A may be modulated by the availability of methyl donors (e.g, folates) for DNA methylation, this could mean that the programming of adipogenesis, appetite, and energy metabolism may be permanently damaged and, consequently, increase risk in later life obesity (Dolinoy *et al.,* 2007). The epigenetic effects of bisphenol A exposure during development could interfere with complex differentiating endocrine signalling pathways and cause adverse consequences later in life, leading to the concept of ''developmental origins of adult disease'' (Barker *et al.,* 2002). On adipocytes, in vitro studies have shown disruptive effects of bisphenol A on normal adipocyte development as well as 2 Dose-Response: An International Journal on the homeostatic control of adipogenesis and early energy balance (Grun and Blumberg, 2006; Grun *et al.,* 2006). Specifically, it has been observed that low concentrations of bisphenol A induce lipid accumulation mediated by the production of reactive oxygen species in the mitochondria of HepG2 cells (Huc *et al.,* 2012). Moreover, bisphenol A seems to promote adipogenesis, stimulating glucocorticoid receptors in the 3 T3-L1 Cell Line (mouse fibroblasts that can differentiate into adipocytes) and, in combination with insulin, promoting adipocyte formation (Masuno *et al.,* 2002; Sargis *et al.,* 2010). Recently, bisphenol A effects on human adipocytes, taken from breast, subcutaneous, and visceral adipose tissues, were investigated on more than twenty participants. The authors reported that bisphenol A between 1 and 10 nmol/L concentrations interfered with adipocyte metabolism by inhibiting adiponectin release and stimulating the release of two inflammatory cytokines, interleukin (IL-6) and tumor necrosis factor a (TNF-a), showing a 'U' shaped dose–response curve and suggesting that bisphenol A can also act at low dosage (Ben-Jonathan *et al.,* 2009). Adiponectin is one of the most abundant circulating adipokines, exerting an effect on glucose and lipid metabolism and modulating insulin sensitivity by stimulating glucose utilization and fatty acid oxidation (Kadowaki *et al.,* 2006). Moreover, it also has an anti-inflammatory activity, which together with the effect on the pro-inflammatory cytokines TNF-a and IL-6, may be the link between several non-communicable diseases (CVD and type 2 diabetes mellitus) and bisphenol A exposure (Hugo *et al.,* 2008; Ben-Jonathan *et al.,* 2009).

Bisphenol A Exposure and Type 2 Diabetes Mellitus

Initially, the possible association of type 2 diabetes mellitus and bisphenol A was studied cross-sectionally, implying the tested hypothesis that diabetes is concomitant, but not necessarily consequent to bisphenol A exposure. Since 2003, various NHANES cohorts in the United States have been studied repeatedly to confirm this hypothesis, but the results have often been discrepant. Lang et al. were the first to report a positive association with self-reported diabetes, whose odds were 1.4 per 1-standard deviation increment in urinary bisphenol A concentration in the 2003 to 2004 cohort: 1455 adult participants older than 18 to 74 years. They further supported their findings when they repeated the study on 1493 patients in the 2005 to 2006 cohort. Note that in this cohort (2005 to 2006), the association with diabetes did not reach significance, but the pooled estimates of the 2003 to 2008 cohorts remained significant (Melzer *et al.,* 2010). The authors reported that in the second cohort, urinary bisphenol A was 30% lower, with a geometric mean value of 1.79 compared with the earlier mean of 2.49 ng mL_1. The greater range of the patients' bisphenol A exposure in the first NHANES cycle could have influenced the detection of bisphenol A association with diabetes. It was argued that self-reported diabetes could underestimate the true prevalence of diabetes (Molenaar *et al.,* 2007). This modality of diabetes recognition could have subtracted statistical power from the former investigations. Thus, in 2011 a new study included a third cycle (2007-2008) in the analysis and defined diabetes according to glycated hemoglobin (HbA1c) measurements. Overall, urinary bisphenol A and HbA1c were significantly associated in 4389 adult participants, though when the analysis was replicated within each of the 3 cycles, it was recognized that it was the first NHANES cycle that drove the correlation (Silver *et al.,* 2011). In the same year, another analysis (Shankar and Teppala, 2011) was conducted in the same 3 cohorts using recent guidelines of the American Diabetes Association (2011) for diabetes criteria, that is, a serum glucose greater than 126 mg dL_1 after fasting for a minimum of 8 hours, a serum glucose greater than 200 mg dL_1 for those who fasted less than 8 hours before their NHANES visit, an HbA1c value greater than 6.5% or self-reported current use of oral hypoglycemic medication or insulin. Using the full spectrum of the possibilities to diagnose diabetes, this study found that there was a positive association between serum bisphenol A levels and diabetes mellitus in this nationally representative sample of US adults. In subsequent stratified analyses, the observed association was found to be present among both normal weight and overweight/obese adults. The NHANES saga was finally enriched by Sabanayagam and his associates, (2013) whose study examined the association between urinary bisphenol A levels and prediabetes in 3516 participants from the 3 cycles between 2003 and 2008. Again, prediabetes was defined according to ADA criteria (fasting glucose concentration 100-125 mg dL_1 or 2-hour glucose concentration of 140 199 mg dL_1 or an HbA1c value of 5.7%-6.4%). This work associated bisphenol A with prediabetes, more strongly for women and obese patients. In summary, with the exception of one study, all the investigators who evaluated the association of bisphenol A and diabetes or prediabetes in the NHANES cohorts between 2003 and 2008 found at least some evidence of positive association.

The association of bisphenol A and diabetes has drawn attention also in nonwestern countries, where the current diabetes epidemic is of major concern. In a cross-sectional study from China, there was no detection of a clear association between urinary bisphenol A concentrations and objective measures of impaired glucose regulation, including type 2 diabetes mellitus. The study, involving 3423 participants selected from 10 185 candidates, was a representation of normotolerant, impaired glucose regulation, and diabetes subjects. Caution is raised by the authors because the study did not assess diet or treatment of existing diabetes (Ning *et al.*, 2011). A cross-sectional study of 1210 middle aged Koreans failed to detect an association between self-reported diabetes and urinary bisphenol A (Kim and Park, 2013). The bisphenol A urinary concentrations in Korean patients were comparable to these in the US samples; nonetheless, as noted above, the methodology to assess diabetes may have underestimated its prevalence. More recently, higher bisphenol A exposure, reflected in higher urinary concentrations of bisphenol A, was associated with diabetes in the Iran general adult population in a small study of 119 cases of type 2 diabetes mellitus controlled with 120 non-diabetic participants (Ahmadkhaniha *et al.*, 2014). Finally, 2581 patients from the Thai National Health Examination Survey (2009) were investigated for the association between serum bisphenol A concentrations and impaired fasting glucose or diabetes, the latter being defined on the basis of either fasting plasma glucose or a physician's diagnosis. Serum bisphenol A concentrations were associated with diabetes and not with impaired fasting glucose (Aekplakorn *et al.*, 2015). Most studies were cross-sectional in nature, with an inherent limitation in the possibility of detecting a temporal relationship between exposure and subsequent clinical manifestations that support a causal relationship. bisphenol exposure contributes to the development of diabetes, and the first of such studies in this field was published only recently (Sun *et al.*, 2015). The study involves 2 cohorts of the Nurses Health Study (NHS): one composed of postmenopausal women (average age 66 years—NHS1), the other of younger, premenopausal women (average age 46 years—NHS2). From the 2 cohorts, the authors measured bisphenol A and 8 major phthalate metabolites among 971 incident type 2 diabetes mellitus case–control pairs. Interestingly, a clear association was found between bisphenol A and incident diabetes in the premenopausal women but not in the post-menopausal women. The authors speculated that this difference in susceptibility to diabetes from exposure to bisphenol A, according to menopausal status, could be explained according to the hypothesis that the bisphenol A endocrine interference of estrogen receptors of pancreatic b cells would be enhanced in premenopausal women. Thus, the findings of this first longitudinal study strengthen the idea that bisphenol A exposure could increase diabetes risk, despite the often discrepant results from the many cross-sectional studies conducted worldwide.

Association with Insulin Resistance

It could be that bisphenol A contributes to type 2 diabetes mellitus by increasing insulin resistance. This led to a Korean study of 950 individuals living in urban areas, and such an association was supported by the study reporting a significant positive relationship of urinary bisphenol A with plasma glucose concentrations (Hong *et al.*, 2009). In 2012, a large cross sectional study included 3390 adults aged 40 years or older in China (Wang *et al.*, 2012). After adjusting for BMI, waist circumference, smoking, alcohol intake, education levels, systolic blood pressure, high-density lipoprotein, low-density lipoprotein, total cholesterol, triglycerides, highly sensitive C-reactive protein, alanine transaminase, and g-glutamyl transferase, the fourth quartile of urinary bisphenol A concentration significantly increased the prevalence of insulin resistance by 37% compared with the first quartile. Interestingly, this association was driven by the normal-weight individuals rather than by the overweight ones, suggesting that the effect of higher BMI may overwhelm that of bisphenol A on insulin resistance in participants with higher BMI. More recently, in overweight or obese Ohio children aged 3 to 8 years, the bisphenol A levels were associated with insulin resistance, (Khalil, Ebert, Wang and others, 2014) providing further evidence for the potentially diabetogenic effects of bisphenol A starting at a young age.

Bisphenol A and Carcinogenic Effect

Several studies indicated that BISPHENOL A exposure increases the risk for cancer (Cavalieri and Rogan, 2010; Soto, and Sonnenschein, 2010). There are studies in the literature about BISPHENOL A cause cancer types of testis, prostate, uterus, ovary cancers (Vandenberg et al., 2007). Besides, as bisphenol A has estrogenic characteristics it was indicated that bisphenol A may cause breast cancer (Keri et al., 2007). Cancer types such as breast, uterus, testis and prostate increase in all over the world was correlated with endocrine disruptors (Darbre and Charles, 2010; Soto, and Sonnenschein, 2010; Walvoord, 2010).

Secretory Pathway Ca2+ ATPase's (SPCAs) also mediates accumulation of Ca2+ in the Golgi apparatus. In mammals the SPCA1 isoform is mainly located on the trans-Golgi compartment of cells (Missiaen et al., 2007). Calcium is required in the post-translational modification of proteins being trafficked through the Golgi. Bisphenol A has been shown to inhibit SPCA1 in the cisternal membrane of Golgi apparatus (Lai and Michelangeli, 2012). The role of intracellular Ca2+ has been studied which reasons that Ca2+ is a ubiquitous signal and that altered expression of specific Ca2+ channels and pumps is a characteristic feature of many cancers (Monteith et al., 2007). It hypothesize that bisphenol A (an inhibitor of SPCA1) can be a potential inhibitory drug that not only blocks the post-translational modification process but may also have a direct role in breast cancers via this very inhibition. The signaling pathways that are Ca2+ dependent are assumed to also undergo modifications in the downstream targeting of respective signal proteins (Missiaen et al., 2007; Monteith et al., 2007; Lai and Michelangeli, 2012).

Bisphenol A and Metabolic Syndrome

Components, and Coronary Disease Risk Factors Among the many risk factors for coronary disease, there appears to be strong evidence of an association between bisphenol A and hypertension. In their analysis of the first NHANES cycle (2003-2004) Shankar and his associates (2012) found a positive association between the increasing levels of urinary bisphenol A of 1380 participants and hypertension, independent of confounding factors such as age, gender, race/ethnicity, smoking, BMI, type 2 diabetes mellitus, and total cholesterol levels. The odds of blood pressure-reducing medication use and/or blood pressures >140/ 90 mm Hg increased by 1.50 between the extreme tertiles of bisphenol A exposure. The same positive association was found in 560 elderly citizens from Korea even though the odds of being hypertensive significantly increased, more than doubled, only in the individuals without previous history of hypertension (Bae *et al.,* 2012). In 2014, the participants in NHANES 2003 to 2008 showed increasing levels of urinary bisphenol A positively associated with metabolic syndrome (Teppala *et al.,* 2012). In contrast, in the Prospective Investigation of the Vasculature in the Uppsala Seniors study, weaker associations were observed for coronary risk assessed by the Framingham Risk Score together with circulating serum levels of bisphenol A (Olsen *et al.,* 2012). Similar findings were also found in a European investigation of 591 patients participating in The Metabolomics and Genomics in Coronary Artery Disease (MaGiCAD) study (Melzer *et al.,* 2012). The bisphenol A exposure was higher in those with severe coronary artery stenosis compared to those with no vessel disease.

The incidence of coronary disease after bisphenol A exposure was also studied prospectively in NHANES 2003 to 2006 participants during the 10 years of follow-up and showed trends similar to previously reported cross-sectional findings in the more highly exposed participants, providing stronger support for the hypothesis of adverse cardiovascular effects of bisphenol A exposure (Melzer *et al.*, 2012).

Further, exposure to bisphenol A has been linked with a number of developmental and reproductive pathologies in both animal models and human subjects. These include abnormalities in reproductive organ function (irregular cycles, multiple ovarian cysts, reduction in primordial follicles (Darbre and Charles, 2010; Keri *et al.*, 2007; Vandenberg *et al.*, 2007), placental dysfunction, increased incidence of miscarriage and neonatal mortality (ICIS, 2008; National Institute of Health (Washington) US, 2008), precocious puberty (FDA, 2012), and sexual dysfunction such as erectile dysfunction, decreased libido, and ejaculation difficulties (European Union, 2008; Williams *et al.*, 2008; Plastics Europe, 2012). In experimental studies, bisphenol A has been shown to affect many reproductive indices, such as ovary, uterus and vagina weights (indicating estrogenic action); egg shape; fertilization rate; number of live-born neonates per litter; distance between the genital pore and the anus in newborns (indicating the degree of masculinization or feminization of external genitalia); time of vaginal opening (indicating the start of female puberty); and onset of the estrous cycle (indicating sexual maturity) (Richter *et al.*, 2007; Cabaton *et al.*, 2011; Nah *et al.*, 2011).The evidence in the literature suggests that bisphenol A exposure in humans may impair fertility (Ehrlich *et al.*, 2012).

Furthermore, Ronn and his associates (2014) while studying association of Bisphenol A with the circulating levels of adiponectin, leptin and ghrelin reported that bisphenol A concentrations in serum are associated with levels of key hormones involved in hunger and satiety.

CONCLUSION

From the perusal of research conducted on the diverse aspects of bisphenol A that include its migration into food and its subsequent health effects from foetus to adults it has been established that this chemical is responsible for causing different deleterious effects in humans that range from metabolic diseases to behavioural and genetic disorders. In several research studies it has been clearly reported that Bisphenol A is ingested in diet from canned food, soft drinks, fishery products, baby bottles, dental sealants etc. and this migration of Bisphenol A into food is affected by temperature, pH, amount of salt and oil, packaging materials and other such factors. The harsh debate among scientists, industry, and regulatory agencies on whether bisphenol A should be banned from use in food packaging has ultimately led to its ban in certain countries. In March 2010, Canada banned bisphenol A from plastic baby bottles and formulas and in September declared it as a toxic substance harmful to health and environment. In April 2010, Denmark was the first European country to ban bisphenol A from materials in contact with food for children older than 0 to 3 years. In January 2011, the European Commission (EC) prohibited the use of bisphenol A for the manufacture of polycarbonate infant feeding bottles. In India concrete steps need to be taken to either develop alternatives to bisphenol A for its use or must be banned like other countries so as to prevent it harmful effects on humans.

ACKNOWLEDGMENT

The authors are highly thankful to Najam-us-Saqib for providing technical assistance during the compilation of this chapter.

REFERENCES

Aekplakorn, W., Chailurkit, L. O., & Ongphiphadhanakul, B. (2015). Relationship of serum Bisphenol A with diabetes in the Thai population, National Health Examination Survey IV, 2009. *Journal of Diabetes*, *7*(2), 240–249. doi:10.1111/1753-0407.12159 PMID:24720399

Ahmadkhaniha, R., Mansouri, M., Yunesian, M., Omidfar, K., Jeddi, M., Larijani, B., ... Rastkari, N. (2014). Association of urinary Bisphenol A concentration with type-2 diabetes mellitus. *Journal of Environmental Health Science & Engineering*, *12*(1), 64. doi:10.1186/2052-336X-12-64 PMID:24625016

American Diabetes Association (ADA). (2011). Diagnosis and classification of diabetes mellitus. *Diabetes Care*, *34*(1), S62–S69. PMID:21193628

Arenholt-Bindslev, D., Breinholt, V., Preiss, A., & Schmalz, G. (1999). Time-related bisphenol-A content and estrogenic activity in saliva samples collected in relation to placement of fissure sealants. *Clinical Oral Investigations*, *3*(3), 120–125. doi:10.1007007840050089 PMID:10803122

Bae, S., Kim, J. H., Lim, Y. H., Park, H. Y., & Hong, Y. C. (2012). Associations of Bisphenol A exposure with heart rate variability and blood pressure. *Hypertension*, *60*(3), 786–793. doi:10.1161/HYPERTENSIONAHA.112.197715 PMID:22851732

Ballesteros-Gomez, A., Rubio, S., & Perez-Bendito, D. (2009). Analytical methods for the determination of Bisphenol A in food. *Journal of Chromatography. A*, *1216*(3), 449–469. doi:10.1016/j.chroma.2008.06.037 PMID:18635192

Barker, D. J., Eriksson, J. G., Forsen, T., & Osmond, C. (2002). Fetal origins of adult disease: Strength of effects and biological basis. *International Journal of Epidemiology*, *31*(6), 1235–1239. doi:10.1093/ije/31.6.1235 PMID:12540728

Barlow, S. E. (2007). Expert committee recommendations regarding the prevention, assessment, and treatment of child and adolescent overweight and obesity: Summary report. *Pediatrics*, *120*(Supplement 4), S164–S192. doi:10.1542/peds.2007-2329C PMID:18055651

Becker, K., Goen, T., Seiwert, M., Conrad, A., Pick-Fuss, H., Muller, J., & .... (2009). Gere's IV: Phthalate metabolites and Bisphenol A in urine of German children. *International Journal of Hygiene and Environmental Health*, *212*(6), 685–692. doi:10.1016/j.ijheh.2009.08.002 PMID:19729343

Ben-Jonathan, N., Hugo, E. R., & Brandebourg, T. D. (2009). Effects of Bisphenol A on adipokine release from human adipose tissue: Implications for the metabolic syndrome. *Molecular and Cellular Endocrinology*, *304*(1-2), 49–54. doi:10.1016/j.mce.2009.02.022 PMID:19433247

Biedermann, S., Tschudin, P., & Grob, K. (2010). Transfer of Bisphenol A from thermal printer paper to the skin. *Analytical and Bioanalytical Chemistry*, *398*(1), 571–576. doi:10.100700216-010-3936-9 PMID:20623271

Braun, J. M., Kalkbrenner, A. E., Calafat, A. M., Baneft, J. T., Pornkunwilai, S., Ye, X., Silva, M. J., … Lanphear, B. P. (2011). Variability and predictors of urinary Bisphenol A concentrations during pregnancy. *Environmental and Health Perspective, 119*(1), 131-137.

Braunrath, R., Podlipna, D., Padlesak, S., & Cichna-Markl, M. (2005). Determination of Bisphenol A in canned foods by immunoaffinity chromatography, HPLC, and fluorescence detection. *Journal of Agricultural and Food Chemistry*, *53*(23), 8911–8917. doi:10.1021/jf051525j PMID:16277382

Bushnik, T, Haines, D., Levallois, P., Levesque, J., van Oostdam, J., & Viau, C. (2010). Lead and Bisphenol A concentrations in the Canadian population. *Health Reproduction,* 217-218.

Cabaton, N. J., Wadia, P. R., Rubin, B. S., Zalko, D., Schaeberle, C. M., Askenase, M. H., ... Soto, A. M. (2011). Perinatal exposure to environmentally relevant levels of Bisphenol A decreases fertility and fecundity in CD-1 mice. *Environmental Health Perspectives*, *119*(4), 547–552. doi:10.1289/ehp.1002559 PMID:21126938

Calafat, A. M., Weuve, J., Ye, X., Jia, L. T., Hu, H., Ringer, S., ... Hauser, R. (2009). Exposure to Bisphenol A and other phenols in neonatal intensive care unit premature infants. *Environmental Health Perspectives*, *117*(4), 639–644. doi:10.1289/ehp.0800265 PMID:19440505

Calafat, A. M., Ye, X., Wong, L. Y., Reidy, J. A., & Needham, L. L. (2008). Exposure of the U.S. population to Bisphenol A and 4-tertiary-octylphenol: 2003–2004. *Environmental Health Perspectives*, *116*(1), 39–44. doi:10.1289/ehp.10753 PMID:18197297

Cao, X. L., & Corriveau, J. (2008). Migration of Bisphenol A from polycarbonate baby and water bottles into water under severe conditions. *Journal of Agricultural and Food Chemistry*, *56*(15), 6378–6381. doi:10.1021/jf800870b PMID:18636679

Cao, X. L., Corriveau, J., & Popovic, S. (2009). Levels of Bisphenol A in canned soft drink products in Canadian markets. *Journal of Agricultural and Food Chemistry*, *57*(4), 1307–1311. doi:10.1021/jf803213g PMID:19170636

Cao, X. L., Corriveau, J., & Popovic, S. (2010). Bisphenol A in canned food products from canadian markets. *Journal of Food Protection*, *73*(6), 1085–1089. doi:10.4315/0362-028X-73.6.1085 PMID:20537264

Cao, X. L., Corriveau, J., Popovic, S., Clement, G., Beraldin, F., & Dufresne, G. (2009). Bisphenol A in baby food products in glass jars with metal lids from Canadian markets. *Journal of Agricultural and Food Chemistry*, *57*(12), 5345–5351. doi:10.1021/jf9006888 PMID:19459630

Carwile, J. L., & Michels, K. B. (2011). Urinary Bisphenol A and obesity: NHANES 2003–2006. *Environmental Research*, *111*(6), 825–830. doi:10.1016/j.envres.2011.05.014 PMID:21676388

Casals-Casas, C., & Desvergne, B. (2011). Endocrine disruptors: From endocrine to metabolic disruption. *Annual Review of Physiology*, *73*(1), 135–162. doi:10.1146/annurev-physiol-012110-142200 PMID:21054169

Casas, M., Valvi, D., Luque, N., Ballesteros-Gomez, A., Carsin, A. E., Fernandez, M. F., ... Vrijheid, M. (2013). Dietary and sociodemographic determinants of Bisphenol A urine concentrations in pregnant women and children. *Environment International*, *56*, 10–18. doi:10.1016/j.envint.2013.02.014 PMID:23542682

Cavalieri, E. L., & Rogan, E. G. (2010). Is Bisphenol A a weak carcinogen like the natural estrogens and diethylstilbestrol? *IUBMB Life*, *62*(10), 746–751. doi:10.1002/iub.376 PMID:20945454

Chen, C. M. (2008). Overview of obesity in Mainland China. *Obesity Reviews*, *9*(1), 14–21. doi:10.1111/j.1467-789X.2007.00433.x PMID:18307694

Csan'ady, G., Oberste-Frielinghaus, H., Semder, B., Baur, C., Schneider, K., & Filser, J. (2002). Distribution and unspecific protein binding of the xenoestrogens Bisphenol A and daidzein. *Archives of Toxicology*, *76*(5-6), 299–305. doi:10.100700204-002-0339-5 PMID:12107647

Darbre, P. D., & Charles, A. K. (2010). Environmental oestrogens and breast cancer: Evidence for combined involvement of dietary, household and cosmetic xenoestrogens. *Anticancer Research*, *30*, 815–827. PMID:20393002

Delfosse, V., Grimaldi, M., Pons, J. L., Boulahtouf, A., le Maire, A., Cavailles, V., ... Balaguer, P. (2012). Structural and mechanistic insights into bisphenols action provide guidelines for risk assessment and discovery of Bisphenol A substitutes. *Proceedings of the National Academy of Sciences of the United States of America*, *109*(37), 14930–14935. doi:10.1073/pnas.1203574109 PMID:22927406

Dianin, A. P. (1891). "О продуктах конденсации кетонов с фенолами" [Condensation of ketones with phenols]. Журнал Русского Физико-Химического Общества. *Journal of the Russian Physical and Chemical Society*, *23*, 488–517.

Dodds, E. C., & Lawson, W. (1938). Molecular structure in relation to oestrogenic activity. Compounds without a phenanthrene nucleus. *Proceedings of the Royal Society*, *125*, 222–232.

Dolinoy, D. C., Huang, D., & Jirtle, R. L. (2007). Maternal nutrient supplementation counteracts Bisphenol A-induced DNA hypomethylation in early development. *Proceedings of the National Academy of Sciences of the United States of America*, *104*(32), 13056–13061. doi:10.1073/pnas.0703739104 PMID:17670942

Duty, S. M., Mendonca, K., Hauser, R., Calafat, A. M., Ye, X., Meeker, J. D., ... Ringer, S. (2013). Potential sources of Bisphenol A in the neonatal intensive care unit. *Pediatrics*, *131*(3), 483–489. doi:10.1542/peds.2012-1380 PMID:23420909

Ehrlich, S., Williams, P. L., Missmer, S. A., Flaws, J. A., Ye, X., Calafat, A. M., ... Hauser, R. (2012). Urinary Bisphenol A concentrations and early reproductive health outcomes among women undergoing IVF. *Human Reproduction (Oxford, England)*, *27*(12), 3583–3592. doi:10.1093/humrep/des328 PMID:23014629

Errico, S., Bianco, M., Mita, L., Migliaccio, M., Rossi, S., Nicolucci, C., ... Diano, N. (2014). Migration of Bisphenol A into canned tomatoes produced in Italy: Dependence on temperature and storage conditions. *Food Chemistry*, *160*, 157–164. doi:10.1016/j.foodchem.2014.03.085 PMID:24799222

EuropeP. (2012). *The Plastics Portal.* Retrieved from http://www. plasticseurope.org/

European Union. (2008). *European Union Risk Assessment Report e Bisphenol A. EINECS No: 201-245-8.* Retrieved from http://esis.jrc.ec.europa.eu/doc/existingchemicals/risk_assessment/REPORT/bisphenolareport325

FDA. (2012). *Bisphenol A (BPA): Use in Food Contact Application.* Retrieved from http://www.fda.gov/newsevents/ publichealthfocus/ucm064437

Fernandez, M. F., Arrebola, J. P., Taoufiki, J., Navalón, A., Ballesteros, O., Pulgar, R., ... Olea, N. (2007). Bisphenol-A and chlorinated derivatives in adipose tissue of women. *Reproductive Toxicology (Elmsford, N.Y.), 24*(2), 259–264. doi:10.1016/j.reprotox.2007.06.007 PMID:17689919

Fernandez, M. F., Arrebola, J. P., Taoufiki, J., Navalon, A., Ballesteros, O., Pulgar, R., ... Olea, N. (2007). Bisphenol-A and chlorinated derivatives in adipose tissue of women. *Reproductive Toxicology (Elmsford, N.Y.), 24*(2), 259–264. doi:10.1016/j.reprotox.2007.06.007 PMID:17689919

Fox, C. S., Pencina, M. J., D'Agostino, R. B., Murabito, J. M., Seely, E. W., Pearce, E. N., & Vasan, R. S. (2008). Relations of thyroid function to body weight: Cross-sectional and longitudinal observations in a community-based sample. *Archives of Internal Medicine, 168*, 587–592. doi:10.1001/archinte.168.6.587 PMID:18362250

Frederiksen, H., Aksglaede, L., Sorensen, K., Nielsen, O., Main, K. M., Skakkebaek, N. E., ... Andersson, A.-M. (2013). Bisphenol A and other phenols in urine from Danish children and adolescents analyzed by isotope diluted TurboFlow- LC-MSMS. *International Journal of Hygiene and Environmental Health, 216*(6), 710–720. doi:10.1016/j.ijheh.2013.01.007 PMID:23491025

Frederiksen, H., Nielsen, J. K., Morck, T. A., Hansen, P. W., Jensen, J. F., Nielsen, O., ... Knudsen, L. E. (2013). Urinary excretion of phthalate metabolites, phenols and parabens in rural and urban Danish mother-child pairs. *International Journal of Hygiene and Environmental Health, 216*(6), 772–783. doi:10.1016/j.ijheh.2013.02.006 PMID:23528233

Golub, M. S., Wu, K. L., Kaufman, F. L., Li, L. H., Moran-Messen, F., Zeise, L., ... Donald, J. M. (2010). Bisphenol A: Developmental toxicity from early prenatal exposure. *Birth Defects Research. Part B, Developmental and Reproductive Toxicology, 89*(6), 441–466. doi:10.1002/bdrb.20275 PMID:21136531

Goodson, A., Robin, H., Summerfield, W., & Cooper, I. (2004). Migration of Bisphenol A from can coatings – effects of damage, storage conditions and heating. *Food Additives and Contaminants, 21*(10), 1015–1026. doi:10.1080/02652030400011387 PMID:15712526

Goodson, A., Summerfield, W., & Cooper, I. (2002). Survey of Bisphenol A and Bisphenol F in canned foods. *Food Additives and Contaminants, 19*(8), 796–802. doi:10.1080/02652030210146837 PMID:12227943

Gould, J. C., Leonard, L. S., Maness, S. C., Wagner, B. L., Conner, K., Zacharewski, T., ... Gaido, K. W. (1998). Bisphenol A interacts with the estrogen receptor _ in a distinct manner from estradiol. *Molecular and Cellular Endocrinology, 142*(1-2), 203–214. doi:10.1016/S0303-7207(98)00084-7 PMID:9783916

Grumetto, L., Montesano, D., Seccia, S., Albrizio, S., & Barbato, F. (2008). Determination of Bisphenol A and bisphenol B residues in canned peeled tomatoes by reversed-phase liquid chromatography. *Journal of Agricultural and Food Chemistry*, *56*(22), 10633–10637. doi:10.1021/jf802297z PMID:18959420

Grun, F., & Blumberg, B. (2006). Environmental obesogens: Organotins and endocrine disruption via nuclear receptor signaling. *Endocrinology*, *147*(6), S50–S55. doi:10.1210/en.2005-1129 PMID:16690801

Grun, F., & Blurnberg, B. (2009). Endocrine disrupters as obesogens. *Molecular and Cellular Endocrinology*, *304*(1-2), 19–29. doi:10.1016/j.mce.2009.02.018 PMID:19433244

Grun, F., Watanabe, H., Zamanian, Z., Maeda, L., Arima, K., Cubacha, R., ... Blumberg, B. (2006). Endocrine-disrupting organotin compounds are potent inducers of adipogenesis in vertebrates. *Molecular Endocrinology (Baltimore, Md.)*, *20*(9), 2141–2155. doi:10.1210/me.2005-0367 PMID:16613991

Ha, M., Kwon, H. J., Leem, J. H., Kim, H. C., Lee, K. J., Park, I., ... Lee, B.-E. (2014). Korean Environmental Health Survey in Children and Adolescents (KorEHS-C): Survey design and pilot study results on selected exposure biomarkers. *International Journal of Hygiene and Environmental Health*, *217*(2-3), 260–270. doi:10.1016/j.ijheh.2013.06.001 PMID:23831304

He, Y., Miao, M., Herrinton, L. J., Wu, C., Yuan, W., Zhou, Z., & Li, D. K. (2009). Bisphenol A levels in blood and urine in a Chinese population and the personal factors affecting the levels. *Environmental Research*, *109*(5), 629–633.

Heffeman, A. L., Aylward, L. L., Toms, L. M., Eaglesham, G., Hobson, P., Sly, P. D., & ... (2013). Age related trends in urinary excretion of Bisphenol A in Australian children and adults: Evidence from a pooled sample study using samples of convenience. *Journal of Toxicology and Environmental Health*, *76*(18), 1039–1055. doi:10.1080/15287394.2013.834856 PMID:24188190

Heindel, J. J. (2003). Endocrine disruptors and the obesity epidemic. *Toxicological Sciences*, *76*(2), 247–249. doi:10.1093/toxsci/kfg255 PMID:14677558

Heindel, J. J., & vom Saal, F. S. (2009). Role of nutrition and environmental endocrine disrupting chemicals during the perinatal period on the etiology of obesity. *Molecular and Cellular Endocrinology*, *304*(1-2), 90–96. doi:10.1016/j.mce.2009.02.025 PMID:19433253

Hoekstra, E. J., & Simoneau, C. (2013). Release of Bisphenol A from polycarbonate-a review. *Critical Reviews in Food Science and Nutrition*, *53*(4), 386–402. doi:10.1080/10408398.2010.536919 PMID:23320909

Hong, Y. C., Park, E. Y., Park, M. S., Ko, J. A., Oh, S.-Y., Kim, H., ... Ha, E.-H. (2009). Community level exposure to chemicals and oxidative stress in adult population. *Toxicology Letters*, *184*(2), 139–144. doi:10.1016/j.toxlet.2008.11.001 PMID:19049859

Huc, L., Lemarie, A., Gueraud, F., & H'elie's-Toussaint, C. (2012). Low concentrations of Bisphenol A induce lipid accumulation mediated by the production of reactive oxygen, species in the mitochondria of HepG2 cells. *Toxicology In Vitro*, *26*(5), 709–717. doi:10.1016/j.tiv.2012.03.017 PMID:22515966

Hugo, E. R., Brandebourg, T. D., Woo, J. G., Loftus, J., Alexander, J. W., & Ben-Jonathan, N. (2008). Bisphenol A at environmentally relevant doses inhibits adiponectin release from human adipose tissue explants and adipocytes. *Environmental Health Perspectives*, *116*(12), 1642–1647. doi:10.1289/ehp.11537 PMID:19079714

Inoue, H., Yuki, G., Yokota, H., & Kato, S. (2003). Bisphenol A glucuronidation and absorption in rat intestine. *Drug Metabolism and Disposition: the Biological Fate of Chemicals*, *31*(1), 140–144. doi:10.1124/dmd.31.1.140 PMID:12485963

Jenkins, S., Raghuraman, N., Eltoum, I., Carpenter, M., Russo, J., & Lamartiniere, C. A. (2009). Oral exposure to Bisphenol A increases dimethyl benzanthraceneo-induced mammary cancer in rats. *Environmental Health Perspectives*, *117*(6), 910–915. doi:10.1289/ehp.11751 PMID:19590682

Jiang, Y., Cole, T., Pan, H., Lin, Z., Ju, M., & … . (2007). Construction of height and weight percentile references for Shanghai children and adolescents. *Shanghai Journal of Preventive Medicine*, *19*, 544–547.

Kadowaki, T., Yamauchi, T., Kubota, N., Hara, K., Ueki, K., & Tobe, K. (2006). Adiponectin and adiponectin receptors in insulin resistance, diabetes, and the metabolic syndrome. *The Journal of Clinical Investigation*, *116*(7), 1784–1792. doi:10.1172/JCI29126 PMID:16823476

Kang, J. H., Kito, F., & Katayama, Y. (2006). Human exposure to Bisphenol A. *Toxicology*, *226*(2-3), 79–89. doi:10.1016/j.tox.2006.06.009 PMID:16860916

Kanno, Y., Okada, H., Kobayashi, T., Takenaka, T., & Suzuki, H. (2007). Effects of endocrine disrupting substance on estrogen receptor gene transcription in dialysis patients. *Therapeutic Apheresis and Dialysis*, *11*(4), 262–265. doi:10.1111/j.1744-9987.2007.00472.x PMID:17661831

Keri, R. A., Ho, S.-M., Hunt, P., Knudsen, K., Soto, A. M., & Prins, G. S. (2007). An evaluation of evidence for the carcinogenic acivity of Bisphenol A. *Reproductive Toxicology (Elmsford, N.Y.)*, *24*(2), 240–252. doi:10.1016/j.reprotox.2007.06.008 PMID:17706921

Khalil, N., Ebert, J. R., Wang, L., Belcher, S., Lee, M., Czerwinski, S. A., & Kannan, K. (2014). Bisphenol A and cardio-metabolic risk factors in obese children. *Science of the Total Environment*, 470-471, 726-732.

Kim, K., & Park, H. (2013). Association between urinary concentrations of Bisphenol A and type 2 diabetes in Korean adults: A population based cross-sectional study. *International Journal of Hygiene and Environmental Health*, *216*(4), 467–471. doi:10.1016/j.ijheh.2012.07.007 PMID:22921714

Kim, Y. H., Kim, C. S., Park, S., Han, S. Y., Pyo, M. Y., & Yang, M. (2003). Gender differences in the levels of Bisphenol A metabolites in urine. *Biochemical and Biophysical Research Communications*, *312*(2), 441–448. doi:10.1016/j.bbrc.2003.10.135 PMID:14637157

Knudsen, N., Laurberg, P., Rasmussen, L. B., Bulow, I., Perrild, H., Ovesen, L., & Jorgensen, T. (2005). Small differences in thyroid function may be important for body mass index and the occurrence of obesity in the population. *The Journal of Clinical Endocrinology and Metabolism*, *90*(7), 4019–4024. doi:10.1210/jc.2004-2225 PMID:15870128

Knudsen, N., Laurberg, P., Rasmussen, L. B., Bulow, I., Perrild, H., Ovesen, L., & Jorgensen, T. (2005). Small differences in thyroid function may be important for body mass index and the occurrence of obesity in the population. *The Journal of Clinical Endocrinology and Metabolism*, *90*(7), 4019–4024. doi:10.1210/jc.2004-2225 PMID:15870128

Kosti, R. I., & Panagiotakos, D. B. (2006). The epidemic of obesity in children and adolescents in the world. *Central European Journal of Public Health*, *14*(4), 151–159. doi:10.21101/cejph.a3398 PMID:17243492

Kuiper, G. G., Lemmen, J. G., Carlsson, B., Corton, J. C., Safe, S. H., Van Der Saag, P. T., ... Gustafsson, J. A. (1998). Interaction of estrogenic chemicals and phytoestrogens with estrogen receptor β. *Endocrinology*, *139*(10), 4252–4263. doi:10.1210/endo.139.10.6216 PMID:9751507

Lai, P., & Michelangeli, F. (2012). Bis(2-hydroxy-3-tert-butyl-5-methyl-phenyl)-methane (bisphenol) is a potent and selective inhibitor of the secretory pathway Ca2+ ATPase (SPCA1). *Biochemical and Biophysical Research Communications*, *424*(3), 616–619. doi:10.1016/j.bbrc.2012.07.004 PMID:22796571

Lang, I. A., Galloway, T. S., Scarlett, A., & ... . (2008). Association of urinary Bisphenol A concentration with medical disorders and laboratory abnormalities in adults. *Journal of the American Medical Association*, *300*(11), 1303–1310. doi:10.1001/jama.300.11.1303 PMID:18799442

Laws, S. C., Carey, S. A., Ferrell, J. M., Bodman, G. J., & Cooper, R. L. (2000). Estrogenic activity of octylphenol, nonylphenol, Bisphenol A and methoxychlor in rats. *Toxicological Sciences*, *54*(1), 154–167. doi:10.1093/toxsci/54.1.154 PMID:10746942

Le, H. H., Carlson, E. M., Chua, J. P., & Belcher, S. M. (2008). Bisphenol A is released from polycarbonate drinking bottles and mimics the neurotoxic actions of estrogen in developing cerebellar neurons. *Toxicology Letters*, *176*(2), 149–156. doi:10.1016/j.toxlet.2007.11.001 PMID:18155859

le Maire, A., Bourguet, W., & Balaguer, P. (2010). A structural view of nuclear hormone receptor: Endocrine disruptor interactions. *Cellular and Molecular Life Sciences*, *67*(8), 1219–1237. doi:10.100700018-009-0249-2 PMID:20063036

Leranth, C., Hajszan, T., Szigeti-Buck, K., Bober, J., & MacLusky, N. J. (2008). Bisphenol A prevents the synaptogenic response to estradiol in hippocampus and prefrontal cortex of ovariectomized nonhuman primates. *Proceedings of the National Academy of Sciences of the United States of America*, *105*(37), 14187–14191. doi:10.1073/pnas.0806139105 PMID:18768812

Leranth, C., Szigeti-Buck, K., MacLusky, N. J., & Hajszan, T. (2008). Bisphenol A prevents the synaptogenic response to testosterone in the brain of adult male rats. *Endocrinology*, *149*(3), 988–994. doi:10.1210/en.2007-1053 PMID:18048497

Li, D. K., Zhou, Z., Miao, M., He Y., Wang, J., Ferber, J., ... Yuan, W. (2011). Urine bisphenol-A (BISPHENOL A) level in relation to semen quality. *Fertility and Sterility, 95,* 625–630. doi:10.1016/j.fertnstert.2010.09.026

Li, Q.A., Li, H., Du, G.F., Xu, Z. H. (2010). Electrochemical detection of Bisphenol A mediated by [Ru(bpy)(3)](2+) on an ITO electrode. *Journal of Hazardous Materials, 180,* 703–709. doi:10.. doi:10.1016/j.jhazmat

Lunder, S., Andrews, D., & Houlihan, J. (2010). *Synthetic estrogen Bisphenol A coats cash register receipts*. Retrieved from http://www.ewg.org/BisphenolA-in-store-receipts

Maragoua, N. C., Makria, A., Lampib, E. N., Thomaidisa, N. S., & Koupparisa, M. A. (2011). Migration of Bisphenol A from polycarbonate baby bottles under real use conditions. *Food Additives and Contaminants*, *25*(3), 373–383. doi:10.1080/02652030701509998 PMID:18311628

Masuno, H., Kidani, T., Sekiya, K., & … . (2002). Bisphenol A in combination with insulin can accelerate the conversion of 3T3-L1 fibroblasts to adipocytes. *Journal of Lipid Research*, *43*(5), 676–684. PMID:11971937

Matsumoto, A., Kunugita, N., Kitagawa, K., Isse, T., Oyama, T., Foureman, G. L., … Kawamoto, T. (2003). Bisphenol A levels in human urine. *Environmental Health Perspectives*, *111*(1), 101–104. doi:10.1289/ehp.5512 PMID:12515686

Matsushima, A., Kakuta, Y., Teramoto, T., Koshiba, T., Liu, X., Okada, H., … Shimohigashi, Y. (2007). Structural evidence for endocrine disruptor Bisphenol A binding to human nuclear receptor ERR gamma. *Journal of Biochemistry*, *142*(4), 517–524. doi:10.1093/jb/mvm158 PMID:17761695

Matthews, J. B., Twomey, K., & Zacharewski, T. R. (2001). In vitro and in vivo interactions of Bisphenol A and its metabolite, Bisphenol A glucuronide, with estrogen receptors α and β. *Chemical Research in Toxicology*, *14*(2), 149–157. doi:10.1021/tx0001833 PMID:11258963

Mckenna, N. J., Lanz, R. B., & O'malley, B. W. (1999). Nuclear Receptor Coregulators: Cellular and Molecular Biology. *Endocrinology Review*, *20*, 321–344. PMID:10368774

Meeker, J. D. (2010). Exposure to environmental endocrine disrupting compounds and men's health. *Maturitas*, *66*(3), 236–241. doi:10.1016/j.maturitas.2010.03.001 PMID:20347536

Meeker, J. D., Calafat, A. M., & Hauser, R. (2010). Urinary Bisphenol A concentrations in relation to serum thyroid and reproductive hormone levels in men from an infertility clinic. *Environmental Science & Technology*, *44*(4), 1458–1463. doi:10.1021/es9028292 PMID:20030380

Meeker, J. D., & Ferguson, K. K. (2011). Relationship between urinary phthalate and Bisphenol A concentrations and serum thyroid measures in U. S. adults and adolescents from the National Health and Nutrition Examination Survey (NHANES) 2007-2008. *Environmental Health Perspectives*, *119*(10), 1396–1402. doi:10.1289/ehp.1103582 PMID:21749963

Melzer, D., Gates, P., Osborne, N. J., & … ., & Grainger, D. (2012). Urinary Bisphenol A concentration and angiography-defined coronary artery stenosis. *PLoS One*, *7*(8), 43378. doi:10.1371/journal.pone.0043378 PMID:22916252

Melzer, D., Osborne, N. J., Henley, W. E., Cipelli, R., Young, A., Money, C., … Galloway, T. S. (2012). Urinary Bisphenol A concentration and risk of future coronary artery disease in apparently healthy men and women. *Circulation*, *125*(12), 1482–1490. doi:10.1161/CIRCULATIONAHA.111.069153 PMID:22354940

Melzer, D., Rice, N. E., Lewis, C., Henley, W. E., & Galloway, T. S. (2010). Association of urinary Bisphenol A concentration with heart disease: Evidence from NHANES 2003/06. *PLoS One*, *5*(1), 8673. doi:10.1371/journal.pone.0008673 PMID:20084273

Mendum, T., Stoler, E. V., & Warner, J. (2010). *Concentration of Bisphenol A in thermal paper*. Retrieved from http://advancinggreenchemistry.org /?p=1176

Missiaen, L., Dode, L., Vanoevelen, D., Raeymaekers, L., & Wuytack, F. (2007). Calcium in the Golgi apparatus. *Cell Calcium*, *41*(5), 405–416. doi:10.1016/j.ceca.2006.11.001 PMID:17140658

Miyamoto, K., & Kotake, M. (2006). Estimation of daily Bisphenol A intake of Japanese individuals with emphasis on uncertainty and variability. *Environmental Sciences*, *13*, 15–29. PMID:16685249

Molenaar, E. A., Van Ameijden, E. J., Grobbee, D. E., & Numans, M. E. (2007). Comparison of routine care self-reported and biometrical data on hypertension and diabetes: Results of the Utrecht Health Project. *European Journal of Public Health*, *17*(2), 199–205. doi:10.1093/eurpub/ckl113 PMID:16887835

Moller, L., Leck, F., Og, F., Bo, P., & Larsen, D. H. I. (2012). *Survey of Bisphenol A and Bisphenol A diglycidylether polymer.* The Danish Environmental Protection Agency Strandgade Copenhagen K, Denmark. Retrieved from www.mst.dk/english

Monteith, G. R., McAndrew, D., Faddy, H. M., & Roberts-Thomson, S. J. (2007). Calcium and cancer: Targeting Ca2+ transport. *Nature Reviews. Cancer*, *7*(7), 519–530. doi:10.1038/nrc2171 PMID:17585332

Moriyama, K., Tagami, T., Akamizu, T., Usui, T., Saijo, M., Kanamoto, N., ... Nakao, K. (2002). Thyroid hormone action is disrupted by Bisphenol A as an antagonist. *The Journal of Clinical Endocrinology and Metabolism*, *87*(11), 5185–5190. doi:10.1210/jc.2002-020209 PMID:12414890

Munguia-Lopez, E. M., Gerardo-Lugo, S., Peralta, E., Bolumen, S., & Soto-Valdez, H. (2005). Migration of Bisphenol A (BISPHENOL A) from can coatings into a fatty-food simulant and tuna fish. *Food Additives and Contaminants*, *22*(9), 892–898. doi:10.1080/02652030500163674 PMID:16192075

Munguia-Lopez, E. M., & Soto-Valtez, H. (2001). Effect of heat processing and storage time on migration of Bisphenol A (BISPHENOL A) and Bisphenol A diglycidyl ether (BADGE) to aqueous food stimulant from Mexican can coatings. *Journal of Agricultural and Food Chemistry*, *49*(8), 3666–3671. doi:10.1021/jf0009044 PMID:11513645

Murakami, K., Ohashi, A., Hori, H., Hibiya, M., Shoji, Y., Kunisaki, M., ... Sugiyama, S. (2007). Accumulation of Bisphenol A in hemodialysis patients. *Blood Purification*, *25*(3), 290–294. doi:10.1159/000104869 PMID:17622711

Murray, T. J., Maffini, M. V., Ucci, A. A., Sonnenschein, C., & Soto, A. M. (2007). Induction of mammary gland ductal hyperplasias and carcinoma in situ following fetal Bisphenol A exposure. *Reproductive Toxicology (Elmsford, N.Y.)*, *23*(3), 383–390. doi:10.1016/j.reprotox.2006.10.002 PMID:17123778

Nah, W. H., Park, M. J., & Gye, M. C. (2011). Effects of early prepubertal exposure to Bisphenol A on the onset of puberty, ovarian weights, and estrous cycle in female mice. *Clinical and Experimental Reproductive Medicine*, *38*(2), 75–81. doi:10.5653/cerm.2011.38.2.75 PMID:22384422

Nahar, M. S., Soliman, A. S., Colacino, J. A., Calafat, A. M., Battige, K., Hablas, A., ... Rozek, L. S. (2012). Urinary Bisphenol A concentrations in girls from rural and urban Egypt: A pilot study. *Environmental Health, 11*(1), 20. doi:10.1186/1476-069X-11-20 PMID:22472083

National Toxicology Program USDOHAHS (2008). *NTP-CERHR Monograph on the Potential Human Reproductive and Developmental Effects of Bisphenol A. 08–5994*. Author.

Newbold, R. R. (2010). Impact of environmental endocrine disrupting chemicals on the development of obesity. *Hormones (Athens, Greece), 9*(3), 206–217. doi:10.14310/horm.2002.1271 PMID:20688618

Newbold, R. R., Padilla-Banks, E., Jefferson, W. N., & Heindel, J. J. (2008). Effects of endocrine disruptors on obesity. *International Journal of Andrology, 31*(2), 201–208. doi:10.1111/j.1365-2605.2007.00858.x PMID:18315718

Newbold, R. R., Padilla-Banks, E., Snyder, R. J., Phillips, T. M., Jefferson, W. N. (2007). Developmental exposure to endocrine disruptors and the obesity epidemic. *Reprod Toxicol., 23*. 290–296. doi:10.1016/j.reprotox

Ning, G., Bi, Y., Wang, T., Xu, M., Xu, Y., Huang, Y., … Wu, Y. (2011). Relationship of urinary Bisphenol A concentration to risk for prevalent type 2 diabetes in Chinese adults: a cross-sectional analysis. *Ann Intern Med., 155*(6), 368-374.

Okada, H., Tokunaga, T., Liu, X. H., Takayanagi, S., Matsushima, A., & Shimohigashi, Y. (2008). Direct evidence revealing structural elements essential for the high binding ability of Bisphenol A to human estrogen-related receptor-gamma. *Environmental Health Perspectives, 116*(1), 32–38. doi:10.1289/ehp.10587 PMID:18197296

Olea, N., Pulgar, R., P'erez, P., Olea-Serrano, F., Rivas, A., Novillo-Fertrell, A., ... Sonnenschein, C. (1996). Estrogenicity of resinbased composites and sealants used in dentistry. *Environmental Health Perspectives, 104*(3), 298–305. doi:10.1289/ehp.96104298 PMID:8919768

Olea, N., Pulgar, R., Perez, P., Olea-Serrano, F., Rivas, A., Novillo-Fertrell, A., … Sonnenschein, C. (1996). Estrogenicity of resin-based composites and sealants used in dentistry. *Environ Health Perspect., 104*(3), 298-305.

Olsen, L., Lind, L., & Lind, P. M. (2012). Associations between circulating levels of Bisphenol A and phthalate metabolites and coronary risk in the elderly. *Ecotoxicol Environ Saf., 80*, 179-183.

Osz, J., Brelivet, Y., Peluso-Iltis, C., Cura, V., Eiler, S., Ruff, M.,, & … . Moras, D. (2012). Structural basis for a molecular allosteric control mechanism of cofactor binding to nuclear receptors. *Proceedings of the National Academy of Sciences of the United States of America, 109*(10), 588–594. doi:10.1073/pnas.1118192109 PMID:22203987

Overington, J. P., Al-Lazikani, B., & Hopkins, A. L. (2006). How many drug targets are there? *Nature Reviews. Drug Discovery, 5*(12), 993–996. doi:10.1038/nrd2199 PMID:17139284

Ozdal, T., & Yesilcubuk, N. S. (2014). Toxicity of Bisphenol A: Effects on health and regulations. *International Scholarly and Scientific Research and Innovation, 8*(6), 553–557.

Papaconstantinou, A. D., Umbreit, T. H., Fisher, B. R., Goering, P. L., Lappas, N. T., & Brown, K. M. (2000). Bisphenol A-induced increase in uterine weight and alterations in uterine morphology in ovariectomized B6C3F1 mice: role of the estrogen receptor. *Toxicol Sci, 56*, 332–339.

Pirard, C., Sagot, C., Deville, M., Dubois, N., &Charlier, C. (2012). Urinary levels of Bisphenol A, triclosan and 4- nonylphenol in a general Belgian population. *Environ Int., 48,* 78-83.

Prins, G. S. (2008). Endocrine disruptors and prostate cancer risk. *Endocrine-Related Cancer, 15*(3), 649–656. doi:10.1677/ERC-08-0043 PMID:18524946

Prins, G. S., Tang, W. Y., Belmonte, J., & Ho, S. M. (2008). Developmental exposure to Bisphenol A increases prostate cancer susceptibility in adult rats: Epigenetic mode of action is implicated. *Fertility and Sterility, 89*(2), 41. doi:10.1016/j.fertnstert.2007.12.023 PMID:18308059

Rhie, Y. J., Nam, H. K., Oh, Y. J., Kim, H. S., & Lee, K. H. (2014). Influence of bottle-feeding on serum Bisphenol A levels in infants. *Journal of Korean Medical Science, 29*(2), 261–264. doi:10.3346/jkms.2014.29.2.261 PMID:24550655

Richter, C. A., Birnbaum, L. S., Farabollini, F., Newbold, R. R., Rubin, B. S., Talsness, C. E., ... Vom Saal, F. S. (2007). In vivo effects of Bisphenol A in laboratory rodent studies. *Reproductive Toxicology (Elmsford, N.Y.), 24*(2), 199–224. doi:10.1016/j.reprotox.2007.06.004 PMID:17683900

Riu, A., Grimaldi, M., le Maire, A., Bey, G., Phillips, K., Boulahtouf, A., ... Balaguer, P. (2011). Peroxisome proliferator-activated receptor gamma is a target for halogenated analogs of Bisphenol A. *Environmental Health Perspectives, 119*(9), 1227–1232. doi:10.1289/ehp.1003328 PMID:21561829

Rohrmann, S., Nelson, W. G., Rifai, N., Brown, T. R., Dobs, A., Kanarek, N., ... Platz, E. A. (2007). Serum estrogen, but not testosterone, levels differ between black and white men in a nationally representative sample of Americans. *The Journal of Clinical Endocrinology and Metabolism, 92*(7), 2519–2525. doi:10.1210/jc.2007-0028 PMID:17456570

Ronn, M., Lind, L., Örberg, J., Kullberg, J., Söderberg, S., Larsson, A., ... Lind, P. M. (2014). Bishenol A is related to circulating levels of adiponectin, leptin and ghrelin, but not to fat mass or fat distribution in humans. *Chemosphere, 112*, 42–48. doi:10.1016/j.chemosphere.2014.03.042 PMID:25048886

Routledge, E. J., White, R., Parker, M. G., & Sumpter, J. P. (2000). Differential effects of xenoestrogens on coactivator recruitment by estrogen receptor (ER) α and ER β. *The Journal of Biological Chemistry, 275*(46), 35986–35993. doi:10.1074/jbc.M006777200 PMID:10964929

Rubin, B. S. (2011). Bisphenol A: an endocrine disruptor with widespread exposure and multiple effects. *Journal of Steroid Biochemistry and Molecular Biology, 127,* 27–34. doi:10.1016/j.jsbmb.2011.05.002

Rubin, B. S., Murray, M. K., Damassa, D. A., King, J. C., & Soto, A. M. (2001). Perinatal exposure to low doses of Bisphenol A affects body weight, patterns of estrous cyclicity, and plasma LH levels. *Environmental Health Perspectives, 109*(7), 675–680. doi:10.1289/ehp.01109675 PMID:11485865

Rubin, B. S., & Soto, A. M. (2009). Bisphenol A: Perinatal exposure and body weight. *Mol Cell Endocrinol, 304*(1-2), 55–62. doi:10.1016/j.mce.2009.02.023

Rykowska, I., & Wasiak, W. (2006). Properties, threats and methods of analysis of Bisphenol A and its derivatives. *Acta Chromatographica*, *16*, 7–27.

Sabanayagam, C., Teppala, S., & Shankar, A. (2013). Relationship between urinary Bisphenol A levels and prediabetes among subjects free of diabetes. *Acta Diabetologica*, *50*(4), 625–631. doi:10.100700592-013-0472-z PMID:23636267

Sajiki, J., Miyamoto, F., Fukata, H., Mori, C., Yonekubo, J., & Hayakawa, K. (2007). Bisphenol A (BISPHENOL A) and its source in foods in Japanese markets. *Food Additives and Contaminants*, *24*(1), 103–112. doi:10.1080/02652030600936383 PMID:17164221

Sakurai, K., Kawazuma, M., Adachi, T., Harigaya, T., Saito, Y., Hashimoto, N., & Mori, C. (2004). Bisphenol A affects glucose transport in mouse 3T3-F442A adipocytes. *British Journal of Pharmacology*, *141*(2), 209–214. doi:10.1038j.bjp.0705520 PMID:14707028

Salehi, A., Gustafsson, J., Quesada, I., & Nadal, A. (2012). Rapid insulinotropic action of low doses of Bisphenol-A on mouse and human islets of langerhans: Role of estrogen receptor β. *PLoS One*, *7*(2), 31109. doi:10.1371/journal.pone.0031109 PMID:22347437

Sargis, R. M., Johnson, D. N., Choudhury, R. A., & Brady, M. J. (2010). Environmental endocrine disruptors promote adipogenesis in the 3T3- L1 cell line through glucocorticoid receptor activation. *Obesity (Silver Spring, Md.)*, *18*(7), 1283–1288. doi:10.1038/oby.2009.419 PMID:19927138

Sargis, R. M., Johnson, D. N., Choudhury, R. A., & Brady, M. J. (2010). Environmental endocrine disruptors promote adipogenesis in the 3 t3-l1 cell line through glucocorticoid receptor activation. *Obesity (Silver Spring, Md.)*, *18*(7), 1283–1288. doi:10.1038/oby.2009.419 PMID:19927138

Shan, X. Y., Xi, B., Cheng, H., Hou, D. Q., Wang, Y., & Mi, J. (2010). Prevalence and behavioral risk factors of overweight and obesity among children aged 2–18 in Beijing, China. *International Journal of Pediatric Obesity; IJPO*, *5*(5), 383–389. doi:10.3109/17477160903572001 PMID:20233154

Shankar, A., & Teppala, S. (2011). Relationship between urinary Bisphenol A levels and diabetes mellitus. *The Journal of Clinical Endocrinology and Metabolism*, *96*(12), 3822–3826. doi:10.1210/jc.2011-1682 PMID:21956417

Shankar, A., & Teppala, S. (2012). Urinary Bisphenol A and hypertension in a multiethnic sample of US adults. *Journal of Environmental and Public Health*, *2012*, 481–641. doi:10.1155/2012/481641 PMID:22363351

Shankar, A., Teppala, S., & Sabanayagam, C. (2012). Bisphenol A and peripheral arterial disease: Results from the NHANES. *Environmental Health Perspectives*, *120*(9), 1297–1300. doi:10.1289/ehp.1104114 PMID:22645278

Shelby, M. D. (2008). *NTP-CERHR Monograph on the Potential Human Reproductive and Developmental Effects of Bisphenol-A. National Toxicology Program, US Department of Health and Human Services. Center for the Evaluation of Risks to Human Reproduction*. Washington, DC: CERHR-NTP.

Silva, M. J., Barr, D. B., Reidy, J. A., Malek, N. A., Hodge, C. C., Caudill, S. P., ... Calafat, A. M. (2004). Urinary levels of seven phthalate metabolites in the U.S. population from the National Health and Nutrition Examination Survey (NHANES) 1999–2000. *Environmental Health Perspectives*, *112*(3), 331–338. doi:10.1289/ehp.6723 PMID:14998749

Silver, M. K., O'Neill, M. S., Sowers, M. R., & Park, S. K. (2011). Urinary Bisphenol A and type-2 diabetes in U.S. adults: data from NHANES 2003–2008. *PlOS 1, 6*, 26868.

Sohoni, P., & Sumpter, J. P. (1998). Several environmental estrogens are also anti-androgens. *The Journal of Endocrinology*, *158*(3), 327–339. doi:10.1677/joe.0.1580327 PMID:9846162

Somm, E., Schwitzgebel, V. M., Toulotte, A., Cederroth, C. R., Combescure, C., Nef, S., ... Hüppi, P. S. (2009). Perinatal exposure to Bisphenol A alters early adipogenesis in the rat. *Environmental Health Perspectives*, *117*(10), 1549–1555. doi:10.1289/ehp.11342 PMID:20019905

Soriano, S., Alonso-Magdalena, P., García-Arévalo, M., Novials, A., Muhammed, S. J., Stahlhut, R. W., ... Swan, S. H. (2009). Bisphenol A data in NHANES suggest longer than expected half-life, substantial nonfood exposure, or both. *Environmental Health Perspectives*, *117*(5), 784–789. doi:10.1289/ehp.0800376 PMID:19479022

Soto, A. M., & Sonnenschein, C. (2010). Environmental causes of cancer: Endocrine disruptors as carcinogens. *Nature Reviews. Endocrinology*, (6): 364–371. PMID:20498677

Sui, Y., Ai, N., Park, S. H., Rios-Pilier, J., Perkins, J. T., Welsh, W. J., & Zhou, C. (2012). Bisphenol A and its analogues activate human pregnane X receptor. *Environmental Health Perspective, 120,* 399–405. doi:.1104426 doi:10.1289/ehp

Sun, Q., Cornelis, M. C., Townsend, M. K., Tobias, D. K., Eliassen, A. H., Franke, A. A., ... Hu, F. B. (2014). Association of urinary concentrations of Bisphenol A and phthalate metabolites with risk of type 2 diabetes: A prospective investigation in the Nurses' Health Study (NHS) and NHSII cohorts. *Environmental Health Perspectives*, *122*(6), 616–623. doi:10.1289/ehp.1307201 PMID:24633239

Sun, Y., Tao, F. B., Su, P. Y., Mai, J. C., Shi, H. J., Han, Y.-T., ... Liu, J. (2012). National estimates of the pubertal milestones among urban and rural Chinese girls. *The Journal of Adolescent Health*, *51*(3), 279–284. doi:10.1016/j.jadohealth.2011.12.019 PMID:22921139

Takayanagi, S., Tokunaga, T., Liu, X., Okada, H., Matsushima, A., & Shimohigashi, Y. (2006). Endocrine disruptor Bisphenol A strongly binds to human estrogen-related receptor gamma (ERRgamma) with high constitutive activity. *Toxicology Letters*, *167*(2), 95–105. doi:10.1016/j.toxlet.2006.08.012 PMID:17049190

Takeuchi, T., Tsutsumi, O., Nakamura, N., Ikezuki, Y., Takai, Y., Yano, T., & Taketani, Y. (2004). Gender difference in serum Bisphenol A levels may be caused by liver UDP glucuronosyl transferase activity in rats. *Biochemical and Biophysical Research Communications*, *325*(2), 549–554. doi:10.1016/j.bbrc.2004.10.073 PMID:15530427

Tang-Peronard, J. L., Andersen, H. R., Jensen, T. K., & Heitmann, B. L. (2011). Endocrine disrupting chemicals and obesity development in humans: A review. *Obesity Reviews*, *12*(8), 622–636. doi:10.1111/j.1467-789X.2011.00871.x PMID:21457182

Teppala, S., Madhavan, S., & Shankar, A. (2012). Bisphenol A and metabolic syndrome: Results from NHANES. *International Journal of Endocrinology*, (5): 98–180. PMID:23251154

Thayer, K. A., Heindel, J. J., Bucher, J. R., & Gallo, M. A. (2012). Role of environmental chemicals in diabetes and obesity: A national toxicology program workshop review. *Environmental Health Perspectives*, *120*(6), 779–789. doi:10.1289/ehp.1104597 PMID:22296744

Thomson, B. M., & Grounds, P. R. (2005). Grounds, Bisphenol A in canned foods in New Zealand: An exposure assessment. *Food Additives and Contaminants*, *22*(1), 65–72. doi:10.1080/02652030400027920 PMID:15895613

Trasande, L., Attina, T. M., & Blustein, J. (2012). Association between urinary Bisphenol A concentration and obesity prevalence in children and adolescents. *JAMA*, *308*, 1113–1121. doi:10.1001/2012.jama.11461

Vandenberg, L. N., Hauser, R., Marcus, M., Olea, N., & Welshons, W. V. (2007). Human exposure to Bisphenol A (BISPHENOL A). *Reproductive Toxicology (Elmsford, N.Y.)*, *24*(2), 139–177. doi:10.1016/j.reprotox.2007.07.010 PMID:17825522

Vandenberg, L. N., Hauser, R., Marcus, M., Olea, N., & Welshons, W. V. (2007). Human exposure to Bisphenol A (BISPHENOL A). *Reproductive Toxicology (Elmsford, N.Y.)*, *24*(2), 139–177. doi:10.1016/j.reprotox.2007.07.010 PMID:17825522

Villalobos, M., Olea, N., Brontons, J. A., Olea-Serrano, M. F., & Pedraza, V. (1995). The E-screen assay: A comparison of different MCF7 cell stocks. *Environmental Health Perspectives*, *103*(9), 844–850. doi:10.1289/ehp.95103844 PMID:7498097

Volkel, W., Colnot, T., Csanady, G. A., Filser, J. G., & Dekant, W. (2002). Metabolism and kinetics of Bisphenol A in humans at low doses following oral administration. *Chemical Research in Toxicology*, *15*(10), 1281–1287. doi:10.1021/tx025548t PMID:12387626

Vom Saal, F. S., Nagel, S. C., Coe, B. L., Angle, B. M., & Taylor, J. A. (2012). The estrogenic endocrine disrupting chemical Bisphenol A (BISPHENOL A) and obesity. *Molecular and Cellular Endocrinology*, *354*(1-2), 74–84. doi:10.1016/j.mce.2012.01.001 PMID:22249005

Wada, K., Sakamoto, H., Nishikawa, K., Sakuma, S., Nakajima, A., Fujimoto, Y., & Kamisaki, Y. (2007). Lifestyle-related diseases of the digestive system: Endocrine disruptors stimulate lipid accumulation in target cells related to metabolic syndrome. *Journal of Pharmacological Sciences*, *105*(2), 133–137. doi:10.1254/jphs.FM0070034 PMID:17928741

Walvoord, E. C. (2010). The Timing of Puberty: Is it changing? Does it matter? *The Journal of Adolescent Health*, *47*(5), 433–439. doi:10.1016/j.jadohealth.2010.05.018 PMID:20970077

Walvoord, E. C. (2011). The Timing of Puberty: Is it changing? Does it matter? *The Journal of Adolescent Health*, *47*(5), 433–439. doi:10.1016/j.jadohealth.2010.05.018 PMID:20970077

Wang, H. X., Zhou, Y., Tang, C. X., Wu, J. G., Chen, Y., & Jiang, Q. W. (2012). Association between Bisphenol A exposure and body mass index in Chinese school children: A cross sectional study. *Environmental Health*, *11*(1), 79. doi:10.1186/1476-069X-11-79 PMID:23083070

Wang, T., Li, M., Chen, B., Xu, M., Xu, Y., Huang, Y., ... Ning, G. (2012). Urinary Bisphenol A (BISPHENOL A) Concentration Associates with Obesity and Insulin Resistance. *The Journal of Clinical Endocrinology and Metabolism*, *97*(2), E223–E227. doi:10.1210/jc.2011-1989 PMID:22090277

Wang, Y., & Lobstein, T. (2006). Worldwide trends in childhood overweight and obesity. *International Journal of Pediatric Obesity; IJPO*, *1*(1), 11–25. doi:10.1080/17477160600586747 PMID:17902211

Welshons, W. V., Nagel, S. C., Thayer, K. A., Judy, B. M., & Vom Saal, F. S. (1999). Low-dose bioactivity of xenoestrogens in animals: Fetal exposure to low doses of methoxychlor and other xenoestrogens increases adult prostate size in mice. *Toxicology and Industrial Health*, *15*(1), 12–25. doi:10.1191/074823399678846745 PMID:10188188

Weng, Y. I., Hsu, P. Y., Liyanarachchi, S., Liu, J., Deatherage, D. E., Huang, Y.-W., ... Cheng, A.-L. (2010). Epigenetic influences of low-dose Bisphenol A in primary human breast epithelial cells. *Toxicology and Applied Pharmacology*, *248*(2), 111–121. doi:10.1016/j.taap.2010.07.014 PMID:20678512

Wetherill, Y. B., Akingbemi, B. T., Kanno, J., McLachlan, J. A., Nadal, A., Sonnenschein, C., ... Belcher, S. M. (2007). In vitro molecular mechanisms of Bisphenol A action. *Reproductive Toxicology (Elmsford, N.Y.)*, *24*(2), 178–198. doi:10.1016/j.reprotox.2007.05.010 PMID:17628395

Williams, E. S., Panko, J., & Paustenbach, D. J. (2008). The European Union's REACH regulation: A review of its history and requirements. *Critical Reviews in Toxicology*, *39*(7), 553–575. doi:10.1080/10408440903036056 PMID:19650717

Williams, G. (2012). Aromatase up-regulation, insulin and raised intracellular oestrogens in men, induce adiposity, metabolic syndrome and prostate disease, via aberrant ER-α and GPER signalling. *Molecular and Cellular Endocrinology*, *351*(2), 269–278. doi:10.1016/j.mce.2011.12.017 PMID:22233684

Williams, G. P. (2010). The role of oestrogen in the pathogenesis of obesity, type 2 diabetes, breast cancer and prostate disease. *European Journal of Cancer Prevention*, *19*(4), 256–271. doi:10.1097/CEJ.0b013e328338f7d2 PMID:20535861

Wozniak, A. L., Bulayeva, N. N., & Watson, C. S. (2005). Xenoestrogens at picomolar to nanomolar concentrations trigger membrane estrogen receptor-alphamediated Ca2+ fluxes and prolactin release in GH3/B6 pituitary tumor cells. *Environmental Health Perspectives*, *113*(4), 431–439. doi:10.1289/ehp.7505 PMID:15811834

Xu, X., Tan, L., Himi, T., Sadamatsu, M., Tsutsumi, S., Akaike, M., & Kato, N. (2011). Changed preference for sweet taste in adulthood induced by perinatal exposure to Bisphenol A—A probable link to overweight and obesity. *Neurotoxicology and Teratology*, *33*(4), 458–463. doi:10.1016/j.ntt.2011.06.002 PMID:21704699

Yokota, H., Iwano, H., Endo, M., Kobayashi, T., Inoue, H., Ikushiro, S., & Yuasa, A. (1999). Glucuronidation of the environmental oestrogen Bisphenol A by an isoform of UDP-glucuronosyl transferase, UGT2B1, in the rat liver. *The Biochemical Journal*, *340*(2), 405–409. doi:10.1042/bj3400405 PMID:10333482

Zalko D, Jacques C, Duplan H, Bruel S, Perdu E. (2011). Viable skin efficiently absorbs and metabolizes Bisphenol A. *Chemosphere, 82,* 424–430. doi.: PMID. 21030062 doi:10.1016/j.chemosphere.2010.09.058

Zhang, Z., Alomirah, H., Cho, H. S., Li, Y. F., Liao, C., Minh, T. B., ... Kannan, K. (2011). Urinary Bisphenol A concentrations and their implications for human exposure in several Asian countries. *Environmental Science & Technology*, *1*(45), 7044–7050. doi:10.1021/es200976k PMID:21732633

Zhang, Z., Alomirah, H., Cho, H. S., Li, Y. F., Liao, C., Minh, T. B., ... Kannan, K. (2011). Urinary Bisphenol A concentrations and their implications for human exposure in several Asian countries. *Environmental Science & Technology*, *1*(45), 7044–7050. doi:10.1021/es200976k PMID:21732633

Zhou, R., Zhang, Z., Zhu, Y., Chen, L., Sokabe, M., & Chen, L. (2009). Deficits in development of synaptic plasticity in rat dorsal striatum following prenatal and neonatal exposure to lowdose Bisphenol A. *Neuroscience*, *159*(1), 161–171. doi:10.1016/j.neuroscience.2008.12.028 PMID:19162132

Zimmerman-Downs, J. M., Shuman, D., Stull, S. C., & Ratzlaff, R. E. (2010). Bisphenol A blood and saliva levels prior to and after dental sealant placement in adults. *Journal of Dental Hygiene*, *84*(3), 145–150. PMID:20579427

Zoeller, R. T., Bansal, R., & Parris, C. (2005). Bisphenol A- an environmental contaminant that acts as a thyroid hormone receptor antagonist in vitro, increases serum thyroxine, and alters RC3/neurogranin expression in the developing rat brain. *The Journal of Endocrinology*, *146*(2), 607–612. doi:10.1210/en.2004-1018 PMID:15498886

KEY TERMS AND DEFINITIONS

Bioaccumulation: The accumulation of toxic substances in various tissue or organ of the living organism.

Bisphenol A: An organic synthetic compound having chemical formula of 2,2-bis(4- hydroxyphenyl) propane. It is a colourless solid that is soluble in organic solvents but poorly soluble in water. It is widely known for its tendency to leach from those products which has made it a subject of public health and environmental concern.

Diabetes Mellitus: It is a disorder of carbohydrate metabolism in which there is impaired insulin secretion and/or insulin resistance leading to high blood sugar level (Hyperglycaemia).

Epoxy Resins: Also known as polyepoxides, are a class of reactive prepolymers and polymers which contain epoxide groups. These low molecular substance normally contain at least two epoxide groups-sometimes referred to as a glycidyl or oxirane group.

Insulin: It is a hormone secreted by the beta cells of pancreatic islets whose role in the body is to trigger cells to take up glucose so that the cells can use this energy yielding sugar.

Obesity: Abnormal or excessive accumulation of fat in the body that presents a risk to health.

Obesogen: A foreign chemical compound that inappropriately disrupts normal development and balance of lipid metabolism. Obesogens cause weight gain by altering lipid homeostasis to promote adipogenesis and lipid accumulation.

Plastic: A synthetic material made by a human that easily shaped or molded.

Polycarbonate: A group of thermoplastic polymers containing carbonate groups in their chemical structures. Compound discs, riot shields, vandal proof glazing, baby feeding bottles, electric components, safety helmets and headlamp lenses etc. are all typical applications for polycarbonates.

Thermoplastic: Plastic substance formed by heating and harden by cooling, able to repeat the process.

Chapter 13
Historical Perspective of Bisphenol A and Phthalates in the Environment and Their Health Effects

Rayees Ahmad Bhat
Jiwaji University, India

D. Kumar
Jiwaji University, India

Sajood Maqbool Bhat
Sanjay Gandhi Smriti Government P. G. College Sidhi, India

Irfan R Sofi
Jiwaji University, India

ABSTRACT

Plastics are widely used in modern life, and their unbound chemicals Bisphenol A and Phthalates, which are important chemical-building blocks, can leach out into the surrounding environment. They are also ubiquitous contaminants in the human body, wildlife, and the environment. BPA and PAEs have recently attracted the special attention of the scientific community, regulatory agencies, and the general public because of their high-production volume, widespread use of plastics, and endocrine-disrupting effects.

DOI: 10.4018/978-1-5225-9452-9.ch013

INTRODUCTION

In recent years, the impact of environmental exposure to chemicals and their immunological effects, including the development of allergy has been a topic of great interest. Epidemiologic studies indicate that exposure to endocrine disrupting chemicals produced in high volumes, including bisphenol A (BPA) and phthalates are omnipresent. The links between their exposure and the development of allergy, asthma and immune dysfunction have been studied *in vitro*, *in vivo* and through human cohort studies.

BISPHENOL A

BPA is (4,4-isopropylidenediphenol 2,2-bis(4- hydroxyphenyl)-propane). an organic synthetic compound with the chemical formula $(CH_3)_2C(C_6H_4OH)_2$ belonging to the group of diphenylmethane derivatives and bisphenols, with two hydroxyphenyl groups. It contains two functional phenol groups that allow the chemical to interact with estrogen and androgen receptors as both an agonist and antagonist. (Michalowicz J. 2014) BPA is classified as a xenoestrogen (environmental estrogen). Its ability to stimulate the estrogen receptor further classifies it as an endocrine disrupting chemical (EDC). (Vandenberg LN, et al.2007. Vandenberg LN, et al. 2009) (The estrogenic activity of BPA has been estimated to be 1/1,000 to 1/10,000 of that of 17β- estradiol. (Guo H, et al.2010)

BPA is contained in polycarbonate plastics and epoxy resins and is used in the production of polyvinyl chloride. (Rosenfeld CS. 2015) Items containing BPA include children's toys, dental sealants, lining of water pipes, food and beverage containers such as plastic water bottles, food packaging and the inner coating of cans and bottles. (Konieczna A, Rutkowska A, Rachon D. 2015) It estimated that each year greater than 15 billion pounds of BPA are produced and over 100 tons are released into the atmosphere. The primary route of exposure of BPA is oral, mainly from eating or drinking from products containing BPA. Other potential exposures include inhalation from dust particles and atmospheric exposure. Once the compound is introduced via the oral route it is absorbed in the gastrointestinal tract and undergoes hepatic metabolism including oxidation and hydrolysis, which leads to the production of several metabolites including BPA monosulfate, BPA glucuronide, and BPA disulfate. (Matthews JB, Twomey K, Zacharewski TR, 2001) These metabolites then undergo conjugation and can be excreted in the urine and feces. The presence of BPA and its metabolites can be measured in bodily fluids, including urine and serum, by using the combined techniques of solid-phase extraction coupled with isotope dilution high-performance liquid chromatography and mass spectrometry.(Vandenberg LN, et al. 2010) Small studies have estimated the half-life of excretion of urinary BPA to approximate 4-5 hours.(Stahlhut RW,

Figure 1.

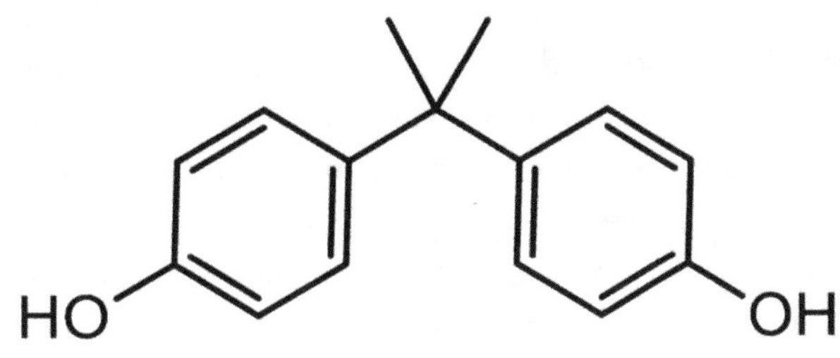

Welshons WV, Swan SH. 2009)Subsequent pharmacokinetic analyses suggest that the rate of excretion of BPA is not greatly affected by fasting, implying that either BPA is excreted slowly from the body or there exists other significant areas of exposure beyond dietary routes.

PHTHALATES

Phthalates are synthetic diesters of phthalic acid- dialkyl- or alkyl/aryl esters of 1,2-benzenedicarboxylic acid. (North ML, et al. 2014). The chemical structures of each individual phthalate vary, mostly according to their side chains and molecular weight. They can be grouped into two broad categories: low molecular weight and high molecular weight. Low molecular weight phthalates include dimethyl phthalate (DMP), diethyl phthalate (DEP), and dibutyl phthalate (DBP). High molecular weight phthalates include diethyl hexyl phthalate (DEHP), diisononyl phthalate (DINP), diisodecyl phthalate (DIDP) and benzyl butyl phthalate (BBzP).

Phthalates are similarly produced in high volumes and are used as plasticizing agents. Low molecular weight phthalates are commonly found in cosmetics and personal care products, whereas high molecular weight phthalates are mostly associated with plastics, particularly polyvinyl chloride (PVC) containing building materials. (Buckley JP, et al, 2012, Carlstedt F, Jönsson B, Bornehag C. 2013, Duty SM, et al. 2005) They serve to increase the stability and flexibility of compounds. Dietary exposures are likely the most common source of exposure, especially to the high molecular phthalates, and frequently occur due to exposure to food and beverage packaging containing PVC. (Koch HM, et al.,2013, Whyatt RM, et al.,2014, Rudel RA, et al,2011) Inhalation exposure occurs through dust from vinyl flooring, carpet backing and consumer products such as fragrances, dryer sheets, air fresheners and sunscreens. (Just AC, et al.2015, Dodson RE, et al. 2012) The phthalate most often linked to indoor air and dust is DEHP, followed by BBzP.(Kolarik B, et al,2008) Exposure through dermal contact also occurs with the use of phthalate-containing personal care products such as sunscreens, lotions and cosmetics.(Li J, et al.,2014) Environmental exposures to phthalates are increased further due to the lack of covalent binding of phthalates in compounds; this property allows phthalates to leach out of the products and into the air, food, beverage or personal care product. (Wormuth M, et al. m,2006) Once phthalates enter the body, they are metabolized to their monoester forms through a variety of enzymatic conversions. These monoesters and other metabolites are then excreted in the urine. Phthalates and their metabolites can be measured in the urine through a combination of solid phase extraction coupled with high performance liquid chromatography–isotope dilution and tandem spectrometry.

TOXICOLOGICAL HISTOGRAPHY

Standard toxicology testing in the 20th century for high production volume industrial chemicals such as BPA and phthalates involved high-dose adult animal studies to evaluate general toxicity (Krewski *et al.*, 2010). Once the no observable adverse effect level (NOAEL) was determined, a safety threshold of 100–1000× was added at which the chemical was presumed safe for humans. Carcinogenicity and occupational exposure risk were also assessed using high doses. The estrogen mimicking properties of BPA were established in the 1930s, but were not considered problematic and were not further investigated until the 1990s after the discovery of nuclear hormone receptors (Dodds and Lawson, 1936). High-dose testing in the 1950s identified only mild dermatitis from occupational exposure to BPA as a toxic effect (Hine *et al.*, 1958). Due to rising production, carcinogenicity assays on BPA using rats were undertaken in the 1970s to investigate occupational exposure (NTP, 1982). The initial study was problematic due to maintenance issues, poor pathology practices, and chemical and animal handling practices that could lead to contamination (United States Government Accountability Office, 1979). In an effort to avoid adulteration of future studies on BPA, pesticides, and other chemicals, the government adopted "Good Laboratory Practice" (GLP) protocols in 1978. GLP includes guidelines for animal care, data collection, and many other organizational aspects of research studies to prevent misconduct and expedite regulation (Services, 2000).

The tendency of phthalates to migrate out of plastics into the environment was first observed in 1970, whereas for BPA, this discovery did not occur until the 1990s (Jaeger and Rubin, 1970; Krishnan and Stathis, 1993). After the realization that phthalates readily leach, studies were conducted to assess if leaching could result in human exposure; phthalates were detected in blood transfusion patients, healthy human volunteers, environmental waters, fish, and even in unmanned NASA spacecraft (Gross and Colony, 1972; Marcel and Noel, 1970; Marx, 1972). Publications on phthalate toxicity surged following these observations. Previous high-dose toxicity analyses had indicated low chronic toxicity for phthalates, but new research indicated "subtle" developmental toxicity in animal models (Autian, 1973). However, these effects were considered to be innocuous because the mode of action was unknown and indicators that subtle early effects could lead to permanent biological changes were undiscovered (Tepper, 1973).

The discovery in 1993 of estrogenic BPA leachate and emerging concern over environmental estrogens brought BPA and phthalates to the attention of the new field of endocrine disruption (Colborn *et al.*, 1993). Endocrine disruptors mimic or disrupt the action of endogenous hormones, which are active at low doses in the body and frequently have multiphasic dose response curves (Gore *et al.*, 2015). Suddenly, the estrogenicity of BPA, which in the 1930s was considered favorable with potential for pharmaceutical application, became an important property to study. Thus, began investigation into the low-dose effects of BPA and phthalates in a significant break from traditional toxicology, which focused on high doses and linear dose response curves.

Low-dose effects, defined as effects present at or below the levels of average human exposure, are often accompanied by NMDRCs, in which the slope of the dose-response curve changes sign (Vandenberg *et al.*, 2012). Although these characteristics are common for natural hormones and pharmaceuticals, they are a newer concept in toxicology (Vandenberg *et al.*, 2009, 2013). NMDRCs disobey the principle of the dose makes the poison; the fact that low-level exposure may be more hazardous than high exposure means that high doses can no longer be considered predictive, especially for any suspected reproductive toxicants. These counterintuitive dose response curves can occur when, for example, different mechanisms of action are at play at different doses. Hormone disrupting toxicity is typically observed within the physiologic concentration of hormones in the body (picomolar to nanomolar), which is also similar to environmental exposure levels (Vandenberg *et al.*, 2012).

More hormones in the body exist than just estrogen and these hormones can be disrupted by mimics. For example, BPA can bind to estrogen, androgen, thyroid, estrogen-related, and peroxisome proliferator-activated receptors (Vandenberg *et al.*, 2012). Phthalates, of which there are more than 10 congeners in commerce and countless metabolites, can also interact with multiple hormone systems. Endocrine disrupting action may or may not be receptor driven and may be agonistic, antagonistic, or a mixture of both.

In addition to the plethora of mechanisms, endocrine disrupting effects also vary widely depending on age of exposure and species. Arguably, timing of exposure is even more critical than dose. Pre- and perinatal exposure can contribute to lifelong disease outcomes that adult toxicity testing cannot predict (Bern, 1992). Critical windows of development, including sex determination and organ formation, are especially vulnerable to insult by low doses of xenobiotics (Heindel and Vandenberg, 2015). Historically, high-dose toxicity tests were performed on adult male animals only, but sex specific effects are also so important that the National Institutes of Health now requires reporting of both sexes in all proposals (Clayton and Collins, 2014). Effects also vary widely by species, as some model animals are well known to be less sensitive to estrogens than other models (Vandenberg *et al.*, 2013). All of these factors are important to consider when designing toxicity studies to understand chemicals like BPA and phthalates.

A unique characteristic of BPA and phthalates compared with persistent organic pollutants (POPs) is their quick metabolism and lack of persistence and bioaccumulation. The estimated half-life of both BPA and phthalate metabolites in the human body is on the order of days (Hauser and Calafat, 2005; Stahlhut *et al.*, 2009). The rapid metabolism of these chemicals in the human body made us quick to discount their potential toxicity (Shaffer *et al.*, 1945). However, we now know that exposure is constant and that the metabolites are the true toxic agents (Heudorf *et al.*, 2007; Stahlhut *et al.*, 2009; Vandenberg *et al.*, 2010). Additionally, rapid metabolism complicates biomonitoring because the timing of sample collection can result in huge variations in metabolite detection (Hormann *et al.*, 2014; Koch *et al.*, 2004). Phthalate esters with long side chains also have more metabolites, which can lead to underestimation of exposure if only a few are measured as biomarkers (Koch *et al.*, 2005).

Another factor that has further complicated the understanding BPA and phthalate toxicity is GLP (Good Laboratory Practise) (Myers *et al.*, 2009). GLP includes strict standards for data collection and provides uniformity to studies to facilitate regulatory interpretation, but is independent of study design. For example, perfect execution of GLP guarantees that comprehensive records were kept, but not that proper controls were included (Myers *et al.*, 2009). Policymakers generally place high weight on GLP studies. However, academic labs often do not follow GLP because of the high cost and excessive paperwork and instead rely on peer review to evaluate research quality. As a result, a divide in the endocrine disruption literature exists between academic and regulatory studies. The Consortium Linking Academic and Regulatory Insights on BPA Toxicity (CLARITY-BPA) project, a consortium between government and academic researchers, was designed to surmount this problem by combining the rigor of GLP with the specialization of academic methods (Schug *et al.*, 2013). In one branch of the project, animals were dosed in a government facility following GLP and the tissues were sent to academic labs for analysis. Academic CLARITY-BPA results from this study published or under review report low-dose effects on gene expression and hormone signaling in the developing brain, ovarian follicle counts, and prostate stem cell differentiation, with many more endpoints yet to be published (Arambula *et al.*, 2016, 2018; Heindel *et al.*, 2015; Patel *et al.*, 2017). Data from another branch of the study performed solely at the FDA under GLP have not been peer reviewed yet, but preliminary data show some low-dose effects that the FDA has dismissed as "minimal" (National Toxicology Program, 2018; vom Saal *et al.*, 2018).

Regulatory and academic scientists must reconverge for the field to move forward and to protect human health and the environment. In the case of BPA and phthalates, the public has not been protected as we have grappled with this over the past 50 years, as exemplified by the accompanying review (Strakovsky and Schantz). It is vital that we do not repeat history as we continue to develop replacements, as current replacements such as bisphenols S and F and the long chain phthalate diisononyl phthalate (DiNP) have proven to have many of the same toxicities (Gray *et al.*, 2000; Rochester and Bolden, 2015). Effective collaboration between risk assessors, government researchers, and academic researchers will be key to properly assessing the low-dose toxicity of future chemical products.

EXPERIMENTAL INCENTIVES

Epidemiologic studies performed in multiple countries found widespread exposure to BPA. For example, a study from Korea published in 2011 showed that 99.8% of the adult population has detectable urinary BPA. A higher concentration of urinary BPA was found in those who resided in rural areas than urban areas. They did not find evidence of significantly different levels of BPA in the urine based on sex, educational level, income or body mass index.(Kim K, et al. 2011) A study of 1016 residents of Sweden, all 70 years or older, examined the serum for levels of BPA and several phthalates metabolites and again confirmed widespread exposure.(Olsén L, et al.,2012) In the United States the National Health and Nutrition Examination Survey (NHANES) study conducted from 2003-2004, levels tended to be higher among children and adolescents than adults.(LaKind JS, Naiman DQ.,2011) A large cross-sectional study analyzed urine samples among 1890 Canadian women in the Maternal-Infant Research on Environmental Chemicals (MIREC) study cohort in their first trimester of pregnancy for the presence of BPA or its metabolite glucuronide of BPA. BPA or its metabolites were detected in up to 95% of urine samples. The highest concentrations of these compounds were measured in the urine of women who were less than 25 years of age, classified as low socioeconomic status or current smokers. (Arbuckle TE, et al., 2015). A review of greater than 80 exposure and toxicology studies again confirmed the ubiquitous exposure to BPA as measured by the presence of conjugated BPA in the vast majority of urine samples. In addition, levels of free unconjugated and therefore active form of BPA were often detected at levels of nanograms per millimeter in serum samples.

As with BPA, the personal exposure to phthalates appears ubiquitous. According to the CDC's Fourth National Report on Human Exposure to Environmental Chemicals of urine samples from 2,636 participants in the NHANES study there was evidence of phthalate metabolites in the urine of almost all participants. A study of 200 women and their newborn infants found evidence of phthalate exposure in cord blood and meconium.(Li LX, et al.,2013) A study of exposures in Europe found high levels of phthalate metabolites common to products such as makeup, shampoo and lotion (including dimethyl phthalate (DMP), DEP, BBzP, DINP, and DIDP) in the urine of women. Our research group at the Columbia Center for Children's Environmental Health (CCCEH) detected levels of phthalates among almost all children. Interestingly, CCCEH found higher levels of urinary phthalate metabolites of BBzP, DnBP, DEHP and DEP among boys when compared to girls; but levels did not differ by age.

The mechanisms by which BPA predisposes to immune deregulation including allergy have not yet been elucidated; only scant direct mechanistic links have been detected. For example, two studies examined the ability of BPA to activate proallergic T helper (TH) cytokines. One *in vitro* study showed that BPA upregulated the TH2 pathway and production of interleukin (IL)-4. (Tian X, Takamoto M, Sugane K.,2003) In another in vitro study examining the effect on dendritic cells after exposure to BPA versus

17- β estradiol, both with administration of tumor necrosis factor (TNF)-alpha, BPA induced greater production of pro-allergic TH2 chemokines and cytokines, including CC chemokine ligand (CCL) -1, IL-10, IL-5 and IL-13. The expression of Th2 transcription factor GATA binding protein 3 (GATA3) also was increased.

There has been growing interest in the effects of exposure to both BPA and phthalates on the alteration of immune function and the development of allergic diseases and asthma. *In vitro* studies indicate that BPA acts on the estrogen and androgen receptors. (Kuiper GG, et al.,2003, Hiroi H, et al.,1999) Its activation of estrogen receptors has been well-documented in studies that showed effects on gene expression, activation of the nuclear estrogen receptor-dependent signaling pathways, and selective estrogen receptor modulation.(Richter CA, et al., 2007, Welshons WV, Nagel SC, Saal FSv.,2006) As an environmental estrogen, BPA may enhance antigen presentation and induce the degranulation of mast cells,(Bonds RS, Midoro-Horiuti T., 2013) or promote dendritic cell maturation.(Uemura Y, et al.,2008) BPA also has aromatase-like activity with the ability to convert testosterone to estrogen, and to activate the aryl hydrocarbon receptor involved in synthesis and degradation of steroid hormones.(Bonefeld-Jorgensen EC, et al.,2007) These BPA-estrogen receptor interactions have been proposed as possible explanations underlying some of the epidemiological associations between estrogen activity and asthma. These include studies that have shown a rise in rates and severity in asthma as women enter puberty and into adulthood. The severity of asthma has been linked to changes in estrogen levels during the menstrual cycle with one study indicating that up to 40% of asthmatic women experiencing exacerbations during the peri-menstrual period.(Thornton J, et al.,2012) Furthermore a Danish study showed that ever using exogenous estrogen in the form of hormone replacement therapy was associated with an increased risk of asthma related hospitalizations (hazard ratio 1.46; 95% CI 1.21-1.76).(Bønnelykke K, et al.,2015) However, due to the paucity of research in this area no clear mechanism of action has been defined for BPA that fully explains its ability to alter allergic or other immune functions.

While not fully characterized, there has been more investigation into the cellular mechanisms of phthalate effects on allergy. Diethyl phthalate (DEP) also can induce the production of pro-allergic TH-2 cytokines including IL-4 and TNF-alpha in human macrophages. When human macrophages are exposed to the diethyl hexyl phthalate (DEHP), the production of non-allergic pro-inflammatory chemokines and cytokines in human macrophages was increased.(Ochiai S, et al.,2012)DEHP can cause mast cell to degranulate and release histamine and beta-hexoaminidase.

In murine studies of the effect of BPA on the development of allergic airway inflammation, prenatal exposure to BPA (0, 0.5, 5, 50 or 500 μg BPA/kg/day) induced variable effects on allergic lung inflammation for the offspring, depending on route of exposure and sex of the offspring. Evidence of increased allergic airway inflammation in those mice exposed prenatally and throughout life to BPA was not evident(Kuo CH, et al.,2012)In mice exposed during weaning to BPA (50 ng, 50 μg or 50 mg of BPA/kg) through the dam's diet there was evidence of increased systemic inflammatory cytokines in the spleen and serum IgE without increased airway inflammation on bronchoalveolar lavage or histologic sections of lung parenchyma.(O'Brien E, et al,2014)

Effects of BPA on ovalbumin-induced allergic airway inflammation reportedly varied based on timing and duration of exposure. Specifically, mice exposed to either water containing 5 μg/ml of BPA or regular water during two distinct time periods-prenatally and perinatally through age 21 days or from birth through age 9 weeks. No significant difference in the development of allergic asthma phenotype was seen in mouse pups exposed to BPA via drinking water in the prenatal and perinatal period. However, mice exposed to BPA from birth through age 9 weeks developed higher levels of airway eosinophils, increased airway hyperreactivity and increased levels of serum IgE.(Petzold S, et al.,2014) Paradoxical effects were observed if BPA intake occurred only during the sensitization period.Some of these results are corroborated in another experimental study that found that the mouse pups who displayed the asthma phenotype, defined as presence of airway eosinophilia and airway hyperreactivity, were those that were exposed both during the prenatal and postnatal periods to 10 µg/ml of BPA in the maternal drinking water. Those only exposed in the postnatal period did not exhibit the asthma phenotype.(Nakajima Y, Goldblum RM, Midoro-Horiuti T.,2012)Hence, ultimately, environmental exposure to BPA may be linked to the development of airway inflammation and possibly even allergic sensitization; however the effects of BPA exposure are likely modified by time period and by duration of exposure.

The majority of animal model studies on phthalates have focused on one major phthalate, DEHP, and its metabolites. Multiple studies have suggested DEHP's role as an adjuvant leading to an enhanced allergic response *in vivo*. In one, DEHP's effect on follicular T cells and the allergic response in mice following exposure to DEHP gavage at doses of 0, 30, 300, 3000 µg/kg with ovalbumin (OVA) vs sham sensitization was studied. Those mice exposed to DEHP and OVA sensitized had increased levels of IgE, IgG1, IL-21 and IL-4, supporting the role of DEHP as an adjuvant.(Han Y, et al.,2014) In another, mice sensitized to OVA in the presence or absence of DEHP (30 µg/kg/day, 300 µg/kg/day, 3000 µg/kg/day) via oral gavage were compared. Those exposed to DEHP + OVA exhibited higher levels of proallergic IgE, IL-4, IFN-γ and eosinophilia when compared to those mice exposed to OVA alone ($p<0.05$).(Guo J, et al.,2012) In experimental studies of the links between perinatal effects of exposure to DEHP and the development of airway inflammation, mice were exposed during gestation and for 21 days in the postnatal period to 2500 ppm DEHP via the diet. Airway inflammation was assessed by measurements of mucus and inducible nitric oxide synthase (iNOS), a marker of airway inflammation. Paradoxically, exposure to DEHP was associated with protection from airway inflammation.(Shin IS, et al.,2014) Dermal exposure to another phthalate, dibutyl phthalate (DBP), also upregulated TH-2 cytokines via increases in thymic stromal lymphopoietin (TSLP) in lymph node cells.(Shigeno T, et al.,2009)In a model of allergic rhinitis, mice sensitized mice to OVA with and without DEHP did not differ in levels of neutrophils or eosinophils in the nasal mucosa, but the additional exposure to DEHP did increase the production of IL-13.(He M, et al.,2013)

CONCLUSION

In the past decade, researchers begun to examine the relationships between common chemical exposures, including BPA and phthalates, and their links to the development of allergy, asthma and immune dysfunction. It is clear from multiple epidemiologic studies that human exposure to these chemicals is ubiquitous due to their use in a wide range of consumer products, food production and building materials. The attempts at elucidating the mechanisms by which these chemicals are potentially immune modifying have been sparse and their results are fairly inconclusive. While the biochemical effects of phthalates have been studied more extensively when compared to BPA, no clear consensus has been made about the underlying mechanisms of allergy and asthma. Although DEHP has been studied more extensively in mouse models and most studies do seem to support some role as an adjuvant.

The studies performed in human subjects draw no clear conclusion about the roles that BPA and phthalates play in the rising incidence of allergy and asthma, but they appear to substantiate a link between these chemical exposures and asthma outcomes. Several studies found increased exposure to BPA was associated with the development of wheeze or atopy. They also suggest that the timing and duration of exposure to BPA alter the clinical phenotype. Many of the studies are limited by the analysis of spot urine samples and use of self-reported questionnaires to determine the development of allergy, asthma, wheeze or eczema. Many of the population-based human studies confirm the relationship with phthalates, specifically DEHP, with the increased risk of developing wheeze, asthma and allergy. The associations between other phthalates and allergy are less clear. The most vulnerable time for exposure to these chemicals also has not yet been determined, although the prenatal period seems to be especially important.

Future research should focus on defining the mechanism of action of these chemicals and the dose at which these effects occur. It will be imperative to discern the key time period for exposure to these chemicals, as well as characterize the most susceptible populations in which immune changes take place. Ultimately, if the research continues to support the existence of a relationship between these chemicals and immune deregulation, it will be necessary to determine methods to limit further exposure to these chemicals.

REFERENCES

Arambula, S. E., Belcher, S. M., Planchart, A., Turner, S. D., & Patisaul, H. B. (2016). Impact of low dose oral exposure to bisphenol A (BPA) on the neonatal rat hypothalamic and hippocampal transcriptome: A CLAIRTY-BPA Consortium study. Endocrinology, 157(10), 3856–3872. doi:10.1210/en.2016-1339 PubMed doi:10.1210/en.2016-1339 PMID:27571134

Arambula, S. E., Jima, D., & Patisaul, H. B. (2018). Prenatal bisphenol A (BPA) exposure alters the transcriptome of the neonate rat amygdala in a sex-specific manner: A CLARITYBPA consortium study. Neurotoxicology, 65, 207–220. doi:10.1016/j.neuro.2017.10.005 PubMed doi:10.1016/j.neuro.2017.10.005 PMID:29097150

Arbuckle, T. E., Marro, L., Davis, K., Fisher, M., Ayotte, P., Bélanger, P., . . . Fraser, W. D. (2015). Exposure to free and conjugated forms of bisphenol A and triclosan among pregnant women in the MIREC Cohort. Environmental Health Perspectives, 123(4), 277–284. doi:10.1289/ehp.1408187 PubMed doi:10.1289/ehp.1408187 PMID:25494523

Autian, J. (1973). Toxicity and health threats of phthalate esters: Review of the literature. Environmental Health Perspectives, 4, 3–26. doi:10.1289/ehp.73043 PubMed doi:10.1289/ehp.73043 PMID:4578674

Bauer, S. M., Roy, A., Emo, J., Chapman, T. J., Georas, S. N., & Lawrence, B. P. (2012). The effects of maternal exposure to bisphenol A on allergic lung inflammation into adulthood. Toxicological Sciences, 130(1), 82–93. doi:10.1093/toxsci/kfs227 PubMed doi:10.1093/toxsci/kfs227 PMID:22821851

Bern, H. (1992). The fragile fetus. In T. Colborn, & C. Clement (Eds.), Chemically-Induced Alterations in Sexual and Functioal Development: The Wildlife/Human Connection. Princeton, NJ: Princeton Scientific Publishing Co.

Bonds, R. S., & Midoro-Horiuti, T. (2013). Estrogen effects in allergy and asthma. Current Opinion in Allergy and Clinical Immunology, 13(1), 92–99. doi:10.1097/ACI.0b013e32835a6dd6 PubMed doi:10.1097/ACI.0b013e32835a6dd6 PMID:23090385

Bonefeld-Jorgensen, E. C., Long, M., Hofmeister, M. V., & Vinggaard, A. M. (2007). Endocrine-disrupting potential of bisphenol A, bisphenol A dimethacrylate, 4-n-nonylphenol, and 4-n-octylphenol in vitro: New data and a brief review. Environmental Health Perspectives, 115(Suppl 1), 69–76. doi:10.1289/ehp.9368 PubMed doi:10.1289/ehp.9368 PMID:18174953

Bønnelykke, K., Raaschou-Nielsen, O., Tjønneland, A., Ulrik, C. S., Bisgaard, H., & Andersen, Z. J. (2015). Postmenopausal hormone therapy and asthma-related hospital admission. The Journal of Allergy and Clinical Immunology, 135(3), 813–816.e5. doi:10.1016/j.jaci.2014.11.019 PubMed doi:10.1016/j.jaci.2014.11.019 PMID:25579482

Buckley, J. P., Palmieri, R. T., Matuszewski, J. M., Herring, A. H., Baird, D. D., Hartmann, K. E., & Hoppin, J. A. (2012). Consumer product exposures associated with urinary phthalate levels in pregnant women. Journal of Exposure Science & Environmental Epidemiology, 22(5), 468–475. doi:10.1038/jes.2012.33 PubMed doi:10.1038/jes.2012.33 PMID:22760436

Carlstedt, F., Jönsson, B., & Bornehag, C. (2013). PVC flooring is related to human uptake of phthalates in infants. Indoor Air, 23(1), 32–39. doi:10.1111/j.1600-0668.2012.00788.x PubMed doi:10.1111/j.1600-0668.2012.00788.x PMID:22563949

Centers for Disease Control and Prevention. (2018). Fourth Report on Human Exposure to Environmental Chemicals, Updated Tables. Atlanta, GA: U.S. Department of Health and Human Services, Centers for Disease Control and Prevention. Retrieved from

Clayton, J. A., & Collins, F. S. (2014). NIH to balance sex in cell and animal studies. Nature, 509(7500), 282–283. doi:10.1038/509282a PubMed doi:10.1038/509282a PMID:24834516

Colborn, T., vom Saal, F. S., & Soto, A. M. (1993). Developmental effects of endocrine-disrupting chemicals in wildlife and humans. Environmental Health Perspectives, 101(5), 378–384. doi:10.1289/ehp.93101378 PubMed doi:10.1289/ehp.93101378 PMID:8080506

Dodds, E. C., & Lawson, W. (1936). Synthetic estrogenic agents without the phenanthrene nucleus. Nature, 137(3476), 996–996. doi:10.1038/137996a0 doi:10.1038/137996a0

Dodson, R. E., Nishioka, M., Standley, L. J., Perovich, L. J., Brody, J. G., & Rudel, R. A. (2012). Endocrine disruptors and asthma-associated chemicals in consumer products. Environmental Health Perspectives, 120(7), 935–943. doi:10.1289/ehp.1104052 PubMed doi:10.1289/ehp.1104052 PMID:22398195

Duty, S. M., Ackerman, R. M., Calafat, A. M., & Hauser, R. (2005). Personal care product use predicts urinary concentrations of some phthalate monoesters. Environmental Health Perspectives, 113(11), 1530–1535. doi:10.1289/ehp.8083 PubMed doi:10.1289/ehp.8083 PMID:16263507

Food and Drug Administration. (2000). Guidance for Industry and Other Stakeholders Toxicological Principles for the Safety Assessment of Food Ingredients. Redbook, 1-5.

Food and Drug Administration. (2007) Guidance for Industry and Other Stakeholders Toxicological Principles for the Safety Assessment of Food Ingredients. Redbook. Retrieved from https://www.fda.gov/Food/GuidanceRegulation/GuidanceDocuments RegulatoryInformation/IngredientsAdditivesGRAS-Packaging/ ucm2006826.htm

Gore, A. C., Chappell, V. A., Fenton, S. E., Flaws, J. A., Nadal, A., Prins, G. S., Toppari, J., & Zoeller, R. T. (2015). Executive summary to EDC-2: The Endocrine Society's Second Scientific Statement on endocrine-disrupting chemicals. Endocr. Rev. 36, 593. E1–E150.

Graham, P. R. (1973). Phthalate ester plasticizers–why and how they are used. Environmental Health Perspectives, 3, 3–12. PubMed PMID:4712540

Gray, L. E., Ostby, J., Furr, J., Price, M., Veeramachaneni, D. N., & Parks, L. (2000). Perinatal exposure to the phthalates DEHP, BBP, and DINP, but not DEP, DMP, or DOTP, alters sexual differentiation of the male rat. Toxicological Sciences, 58(2), 350–365. doi:10.1093/toxsci/58.2.350 PubMed doi:10.1093/toxsci/58.2.350 PMID:11099647

Gross, C., & Colony, J. (1972). An Etiological Study of Phthalate Self-Contamination of Spacecraft and Contamination from Their Earthly Environs. Retrieved from

Guo, H., Han, B., Qin, L., Li, B., You, H., Yang, J., . . . Yang, X. (2012). Pulmonary toxicity and adjuvant effect of di-(2-exylhexyl) phthalate in ovalbumin-immunized BALB/c mice. PLoS One, 7(6), e39008. doi:10.1371/journal.pone.0039008 PubMed doi:10.1371/journal.pone.0039008 PMID:22701742

Han, Y., Wang, X., Chen, G., Xu, G., Liu, X., Zhu, W., . . . Miao, J. (2014). Di-(2-ethylhexyl) phthalate adjuvantly induces imbalanced humoral immunity in ovalbumin-sensitized BALB/c mice ascribing to T follicular helper cells hyperfunction. Toxicology, 324, 88–97. doi:10.1016/j.tox.2014.07.011 PubMed doi:10.1016/j.tox.2014.07.011 PMID:25093321

Hauser, R., & Calafat, A. M. (2005). Phthalates and human health. Occupational and Environmental Medicine, 62(11), 806–818. doi:10.1136/oem.2004.017590 PubMed doi:10.1136/oem.2004.017590 PMID:16234408

He, M., Inoue, K.-I., Yoshida, S., Tanaka, M., Takano, H., Sun, G., & Ichinose, T. (2013). Effects of airway exposure to di-(2-ethylhexyl) phthalate on allergic rhinitis. Immunopharmacology and Immunotoxicology, 35(3), 390–395. doi:10.3109/08923973.2013.787432 PubMed doi:10.3109/08923973.2013.787432 PMID:23672524

Heindel, J. J., & Vandenberg, L. N. (2015). Developmental origins of health and disease: A paradigm for understanding disease etiology and prevention. Current Opinion in Pediatrics, 27(2), 248–253. doi:10.1097/MOP.0000000000000191 PubMed doi:10.1097/MOP.0000000000000191 PMID:25635586

Heindel, J. J., Newbold, R. R., Bucher, J. R., Camacho, L., Delclos, K. B., Lewis, S. M., . . . Schug, T. T. (2015). NIEHS/FDA CLARITYBPA research program update. Reproductive Toxicology (Elmsford, N.Y.), 58, 33–44. doi:10.1016/j.reprotox.2015.07.075 PubMed doi:10.1016/j.reprotox.2015.07.075 PMID:26232693

Heudorf, U., Mersch-Sundermann, V., & Angerer, J. (2007). Phthalates: Toxicology and exposure. International Journal of Hygiene and Environmental Health, 210(5), 623–634. doi:10.1016/j.ijheh.2007.07.011 PubMed doi:10.1016/j.ijheh.2007.07.011 PMID:17889607

Hine, C. H., Kodama, J. K., Anderson, H. H., Simonson, D. W., & Wellington, J. S. (1958). The toxicology of epoxy resins. Arch. Indust. Heal., 17, 129–144. PubMed PMID:13497307

Hiroi, H., Tsutsumi, O., Momoeda, M., Takai, Y., Osuga, Y., & Taketani, Y. (1999). Differential interactions of bisphenol A and 17 beta-estradiol with estrogen receptor alpha (ERalpha) and ERbeta. Endocrine Journal, 46(6), 773–778. doi:10.1507/endocrj.46.773 PubMed doi:10.1507/endocrj.46.773 PMID:10724352

Hormann, A. M., vom Saal, F. S., Nagel, S. C., Stahlhut, R. W., Moyer, C. L., Ellersieck, M. R., . . . Taylor, J. A. (2014). Holding thermal receipt paper and eating food after using hand sanitizer results in high serum bioactive and urine total levels of bisphenol A (BPA). PLoS One, 9(10), e110509. doi:10.1371/journal.pone.0110509 PubMed doi:10.1371/journal.pone.0110509 PMID:25337790

Jaeger, R. J., & Rubin, R. J. (1970). Plasticizers from plastic devices: Extraction, metabolism, and accumulation by biological systems. Science, 170(3956), 460–462. doi:10.1126/science.170.3956.460 PubMed doi:10.1126cience.170.3956.460 PMID:5460077

Just, A. C., Miller, R. L., Perzanowski, M. S., Rundle, A. G., Chen, Q., Jung, K. H., . . . Whyatt, R. M. (2015). Vinyl flooring in the home is associated with children's airborne butylbenzyl phthalate and urinary metabolite concentrations. Journal of Exposure Science & Environmental Epidemiology, 25(6), 574–579. doi:10.1038/jes.2015.4 PubMed doi:10.1038/jes.2015.4 PMID:25690585

Kim, K., Park, H., Yang, W., & Lee, J. H. (2011). Urinary concentrations of bisphenol A and triclosan and associations with demographic factors in the Korean population. Environmental Research, 111(8), 1280–1285. doi:10.1016/j.envres.2011.09.003 PubMed doi:10.1016/j.envres.2011.09.003 PMID:21925656

Koch, H. M., Bolt, H. M., & Angerer, J. (2004). Di(2-ethylhexyl)phthalate (DEHP) metabolites in human urine and serum after a single oral dose of deuterium-labelled DEHP. Archives of Toxicology, 78(3), 123–130. doi:10.1007/s00204-003-0522-3 PubMed doi:10.100700204-003-0522-3 PMID:14576974

Koch, H. M., Bolt, H. M., Preuss, R., & Angerer, J. (2005). New metabolites of di(2-ethylhexyl)phthalate (DEHP) in human urine and serum after single oral doses of deuteriumlabelled DEHP. Archives of Toxicology, 79(7), 367–376. doi:10.1007/s00204-004-0642-4 PubMed doi:10.100700204-004-0642-4 PMID:15700144

Koch, H. M., Lorber, M., Christensen, K. L. Y., Pälmke, C., Koslitz, S., & Brüning, T. (2013). Identifying sources of phthalate exposure with human biomonitoring: Results of a 48h fasting study with urine collection and personal activity patterns. International Journal of Hygiene and Environmental Health, 216(6), 672–681. doi:10.1016/j.ijheh.2012.12.002 PubMed doi:10.1016/j.ijheh.2012.12.002 PMID:23333758

Kolarik, B., Naydenov, K., Larsson, M., Bornehag, C.-G., & Sundell, J. (2008). The association between phthalates in dust and allergic diseases among Bulgarian children. Environmental Health Perspectives, 116(1), 98–103. doi:10.1289/ehp.10498 PubMed doi:10.1289/ehp.10498 PMID:18197306

Konieczna, A., Rutkowska, A., & Rachon, D. (2015). Health risk of exposure to Bisphenol A (BPA). Roczniki Panstwowego Zakladu Higieny, 66(1), 5–11. PubMed PMID:25813067

Krewski, D., ... (2010). Toxicity testing in the 21st century: A vision and a strategy. J. Toxicol. Environ. Heal. B. Critical Review, 13, 51–138. PubMed PMID:20574894

Krishnan, A., Stathis, P., Permuth, S. F., Tokes, L., & Feldman, D. (1993). Bisphenol-A: An estrogenic substance is released from polycarbonate flasks during autoclaving. Endocrinology, 132(6), 2279–2286. doi:10.1210/endo.132.6.8504731 PubMed doi:10.1210/endo.132.6.8504731 PMID:8504731

Kuhn, T. S. (1970). The structure of scientific revolutions (2nd ed.). The University of Chicago Press.

Kuiper, G. G., Lemmen, J. G., Carlsson, B., Corton, J. C., Safe, S. H., van der Saag, P. T., . . . Gustafsson, J.-Å. (1998). Interaction of estrogenic chemicals and phytoestrogens with estrogen receptor beta. Endocrinology, 139(10), 4252–4263. doi:10.1210/endo.139.10.6216 PubMed doi:10.1210/endo.139.10.6216 PMID:9751507

Kuo, C. H., Hsieh, C.-C., Kuo, H.-F., Huang, M.-Y., Yang, S.-N., Chen, L.-C., . . . Hung, C.-H. (2013). Phthalates suppress type I interferon in human plasmacytoid dendritic cells via epigenetic regulation. Allergy, 68(7), 870–879. doi:10.1111/all.12162 PubMed doi:10.1111/all.12162 PMID:23738920

La Kind, J. S., & Naiman, D. Q. (2011). Daily intake of bisphenol A and potential sources of exposure: 2005-2006 National Health and Nutrition Examination Survey. Journal of Exposure Science & Environmental Epidemiology, 21(3), 272–279. doi:10.1038/jes.2010.9 PubMed doi:10.1038/jes.2010.9 PMID:20237498

Li, J., Li, L., Zuo, H., Ke, C., Yan, B., Wen, H., . . . Yang, X. (2014). T-helper type-2 contact hypersensitivity of Balb/c mice aggravated by dibutyl phthalate via long-term dermal exposure. PLoS One, 9(2), e87887. doi:10.1371/journal.pone.0087887 PubMed doi:10.1371/journal.pone.0087887 PMID:24498391

Li, L. X., Chen, L., Meng, X.-Z., Chen, B.-H., Chen, S.-Q., Zhao, Y., . . . Zhang, Y.-H. (2013). Exposure levels of environmental endocrine disruptors in mother-newborn pairs in China and their placental transfer characteristics. PLoS One, 8(5), e62526. doi:10.1371/journal.pone.0062526 PubMed doi:10.1371/journal.pone.0062526 PMID:23667484

Marcel, Y. L., & Noel, S. P. (1970). A plasticizer in lipid extracts of human blood. Chemistry and Physics of Lipids, 4(3), 418–419. doi:10.1016/0009-3084(70)90040-X PubMed doi:10.1016/0009-3084(70)90040-X PMID:5511751

Marx, J. L. (1972). Phthalic acid esters – biological impact uncertain. Science, 178(4056), 46–47. doi:10.1126/science.178.4056.46 PubMed doi:10.1126cience.178.4056.46 PMID:5070514

Matthews, J. B., Twomey, K., & Zacharewski, T. R. (2001). In vitro and in vivo interactions of bisphenol A and its metabolite, bisphenol A glucuronide, with estrogen receptors alpha and beta. Chemical Research in Toxicology, 14(2), 149–157. doi:10.1021/tx0001833 PubMed doi:10.1021/tx0001833 PMID:11258963

Michalowicz, J. (2014). Bisphenol A--sources, toxicity and biotransformation. Environmental Toxicology and Pharmacology, 37(2), 738–758. doi:10.1016/j.etap.2014.02.003 PubMed doi:10.1016/j.etap.2014.02.003 PMID:24632011

Myers, J. P., vom Saal, F. S., Akingbemi, B. T., Arizono, K., Belcher, S., Colborn, T., . . . Zoeller, R. T. (2009). Why public health agencies cannot depend on good laboratory practices as a criterion for selecting data: The case of bisphenol A. Environmental Health Perspectives, 117(3), 309–315. doi:10.1289/ehp.0800173 PubMed doi:10.1289/ehp.0800173 PMID:19337501

Nakajima, Y., Goldblum, R. M., & Midoro-Horiuti, T. (2012). Fetal exposure to bisphenol A as a risk factor for the development of childhood asthma: An animal model study. [Excellent animal model of BPA exposure.]. Environmental Health, 11(1), 8. doi:10.1186/1476-069X-11-8 PubMed doi:10.1186/1476-069X-11-8 PMID:22353195

National Toxicology Program. (2018). Draft NTP Research Report on the CLARITY-BPA Core Study: A Perinatal and Chronic Extended-Dose-Range Study of Bisphenol A in Rats. Retrieved from https://ntp.niehs.nih.gov/ntp/about_ntp/rrprp/2018/april/rr09peerdraft.pdf

Nishioka, J., Iwahara, C., Kawasaki, M., Yoshizaki, F., Nakayama, H., Takamori, K., . . . Iwabuchi, K. (2012). Di-(2-ethylhexyl) phthalate induces production of inflammatory molecules in human macrophages. Inflammation Research, 61(1), 69–78. doi:10.1007/s00011-011-0390-x PubMed doi:10.100700011-011-0390-x PMID:22005928

North, M. L., Takaro, T. K., Diamond, M. L., & Ellis, A. K. (2014). Effects of phthalates on the development and expression of allergic disease and asthma. Annals of Allergy, Asthma & Immunology, 112(6), 496–502. doi:10.1016/j.anai.2014.03.013 PubMed doi:10.1016/j.anai.2014.03.013 PMID:24726194

NTP. (1982). Carcinogenesis bioassay of bisphenol A. Natl. Toxicol. Prgram Tech. Rep. 2015, 1–116.

O'Brien, E., Bergin, I. L., Dolinoy, D. C., Zaslona, Z., Little, R. J. A., Tao, Y., . . . Mancuso, P. (2014). Perinatal bisphenol A exposure beginning before gestation enhances allergen sensitization, but not pulmonary inflammation, in adult mice. Journal of Developmental Origins of Health and Disease, 5(2), 121–131. doi:10.1017/S204017441400004X PubMed doi:10.1017/S204017441400004X PMID:24847698

Ochiai, S., ... (2014). CD326(lo)CD103(lo)CD11b(lo) dermal dendritic cells are activated by thymic stromal lymphopoietin during contact sensitization in mice. Journal of Immunology (Baltimore, Md.: 1950), 193(5), 2504–2511. doi:10.4049/jimmunol.1400536 PubMed doi:10.4049/jimmunol.1400536 PMID:25057004

Olsén, L., Lampa, E., Birkholz, D. A., Lind, L., & Lind, P. M. (2012). Circulating levels of bisphenol A (BPA) and phthalates in an elderly population in Sweden, based on the Prospective Investigation of the Vasculature in Uppsala Seniors (PIVUS). Ecotoxicology and Environmental Safety, 75(0), 242–248. doi:10.1016/j.ecoenv.2011.09.004 PubMed doi:10.1016/j.ecoenv.2011.09.004 PMID:21955883

Patel, S., Brehm, E., Gao, L., Rattan, S., Ziv-Gal, A., & Flaws, J. A. (2017). Bisphenol A exposure, ovarian follicle numbers, and female sex steroid hormone levels: Results from a CLARITYBPA study. Endocrinology, 158(6), 1727–1738. doi:10.1210/en.2016-1887 PubMed doi:10.1210/en.2016-1887 PMID:28324068

Petzold, S., Averbeck, M., Simon, J. C., Lehmann, I., & Polte, T. (2014). Lifetime-dependent effects of bisphenol A on asthma development in an experimental mouse model. PLoS One, 9(6), e100468. doi:10.1371/journal.pone.0100468 PubMed doi:10.1371/journal.pone.0100468 PMID:24950052

Richter, C. A., Taylor, J. A., Ruhlen, R. L., Welshons, W. V., & vom Saal, F. S. (2007). Estradiol and Bisphenol A stimulate androgen receptor and estrogen receptor gene expression in fetal mouse prostate mesenchyme cells. Environmental Health Perspectives, 115(6), 902–908. doi:10.1289/ehp.9804 PubMed doi:10.1289/ehp.9804 PMID:17589598

Ritter, S. (2011). BPA Is Indispensible For Making Plastics. Chemical and Engineering News, 89. Retrieved from https://pubs.acs.org/cen/coverstory/ 89/8923cover4.html

Rochester, J. R., & Bolden, A. L. (2015). Bisphenol S and F: A systematic review and comparison of the hormonal activity of bisphenol A substitutes. Environmental Health Perspectives, 123(7), 643–650. doi:10.1289/ehp.1408989 PubMed doi:10.1289/ehp.1408989 PMID:25775505

Rosenfeld, C. S. (2015). Bisphenol A and phthalate endocrine disruption of parental and social behaviors. Frontiers in Neuroscience, 9, 57. doi:10.3389/fnins.2015.00057 PubMed doi:10.3389/fnins.2015.00057 PMID:25784850

Rudel, R. A., Gray, J. M., Engel, C. L., Rawsthorne, T. W., Dodson, R. E., Ackerman, J. M., . . . Brody, J. G. (2011). Food packaging and bisphenol A and bis(2-ethyhexyl) phthalate exposure: Findings from a dietary intervention. Environmental Health Perspectives, 119(7), 914–920. doi:10.1289/ehp.1003170 PubMed doi:10.1289/ehp.1003170 PMID:21450549

Schug, T. T., Heindel, J. J., Camacho, L., Delclos, K. B., Howard, P., Johnson, A. F., . . . Bucher, J. R. (2013). A new approach to synergize academic and guideline-compliant research: The CLARITY-BPA research program. Reproductive Toxicology (Elmsford, N.Y.), 40, 35–40. doi:10.1016/j.reprotox.2013.05.010 PubMed doi:10.1016/j.reprotox.2013.05.010 PMID:23747832

Shaffer, C. B., Carpenter, C. P., & Smyth Jr., H. F. (1945). Acute and subacute toxicity of di (2- ethylhexyl) phthalate with note upon its metabolism. The Journal of Industrial Hygiene and Toxicology, 27(5), 130–135.

Shigeno, T., Katakuse, M., Fujita, T., Mukoyama, Y., & Watanabe, H. (2009). Phthalate ester-induced thymic stromal lymphopoietin mediates allergic dermatitis in mice. Immunology, 128(1Suppl), e849–e857. doi:10.1111/j.1365-2567.2009.03094.x PubMed doi:10.1111/j.1365-2567.2009.03094.x PMID:19740346

Shin, I. S., Lee, M.-Y., Cho, E.-S., Choi, E., Son, H.-Y., & Lee, K.-Y. (2014). Effects of maternal exposure to di(2-ethylhexyl)phthalate (DEHP) during pregnancy on susceptibility to neonatal asthma. Toxicology and Applied Pharmacology, 274(3), 402–407. doi:10.1016/j.taap.2013.12.009 PubMed doi:10.1016/j.taap.2013.12.009 PMID:24370437

Stahlhut, R. W., Welshons, W. V., & Swan, S. H. (2009). Bisphenol A data in NHANES suggest longer than expected half-life, substantial nonfood exposure, or both. Environmental Health Perspectives, 117(5), 784–789. doi:10.1289/ehp.0800376 PubMed doi:10.1289/ehp.0800376 PMID:19479022

Tepper, L. B. (1973). Phthalic acid esters – An overview. Environmental Health Perspectives, 3, 179–182. PubMed PMID:4704568

Teuten, E. L., Saquing, J. M., Knappe, D. R. U., Barlaz, M. A., Jonsson, S., Bjo¨rn, A., . . . Ochi, D. (2009). Transport and release of chemicals from plastics to the environment and to wildlife. Philos. Trans. R. Soc. B Biol. Sci., 364, 2027–2045. PubMed PMID:19528054

Thornton, J., Lewis, J., Lebrun, C. M., & Licskai, C. J. (2012). Clinical characteristics of women with menstrual-linked asthma. Respiratory Medicine, 106(9), 1236–1243. doi:10.1016/j.rmed.2012.05.003 PubMed doi:10.1016/j.rmed.2012.05.003 PMID:22703945

Tian, X., Takamoto, M., & Sugane, K. (2003). Bisphenol A promotes IL-4 production by Th2 cells. International Archives of Allergy and Immunology, 132(3), 240–247. doi:10.1159/000074305 PubMed doi:10.1159/000074305 PMID:14646385

Tickner, J. (2011). Phthalates and Their Alternatives: Health and Environmental Concerns. Lowell Center for Sustainable Production. Retrieved from https://www.uml.edu/docs/Phthalate%20and%20their%20 Alternatives_tcm18-229903.pdf

Uemura, Y., Liu, T.-Y., Narita, Y., Suzuki, M., & Matsushita, S. (2008). 17 Beta-estradiol (E2) plus tumor necrosis factor-alpha induces a distorted maturation of human monocyte-derived dendritic cells and promotes their capacity to initiate T-helper 2 responses. Human Immunology, 69(3), 149–157. doi:10.1016/j.humimm.2008.01.017 PubMed doi:10.1016/j.humimm.2008.01.017 PMID:18396206

United States Government Accountability Office. (1979). Operations of the National Cancer Institute's Carcinogenesis Programs, HRD-79-51. Retrieved from http://www.gao.gov/products/HRD-79-51

Vandenberg, L. N., Chahoud, I., Heindel, J. J., Padmanabhan, V., Paumgartten, F. J. R., & Schoenfelder, G. (2010). Urinary, circulating, and tissue biomonitoring studies indicate widespread exposure to bisphenol A. Environmental Health Perspectives, 118(8), 1055–1070. doi:10.1289/ehp.0901716 PubMed doi:10.1289/ehp.0901716 PMID:20338858

Vandenberg, L. N., Colborn, T., Hayes, T. B., Heindel, J. J., Jacobs, D. R., Jr., Lee, D.-H., . . . Myers, J. P. (2012). Hormones and endocrinedisrupting chemicals: Low-dose effects and nonmonotonic dose responses. Endocrine Reviews, 33(3), 1–378. doi:10.1210/er.2011-1050 PubMed doi:10.1210/er.2011-1050 PMID:22419778

Vandenberg, L. N., Colborn, T., Hayes, T. B., Heindel, J. J., Jacobs, D. R., Jr., Lee, D.-H., . . . Zoeller, R. T. (2013). Regulatory decisions on endocrine disrupting chemicals should be based on the principles of endocrinology. Reproductive Toxicology (Elmsford, N.Y.), 38, 1–15. doi:10.1016/j.reprotox.2013.02.002 PubMed doi:10.1016/j.reprotox.2013.02.002 PMID:23411111

Vandenberg, L. N., Hauser, R., Marcus, M., Olea, N., & Welshons, W. V. (2007). Human exposure to bisphenol A (BPA). Reproductive Toxicology (Elmsford, N.Y.), 24(2), 139–177. doi:10.1016/j.reprotox.2007.07.010 PubMed doi:10.1016/j.reprotox.2007.07.010 PMID:17825522

Vandenberg, L. N., Maffini, M. V., Sonnenschein, C., Rubin, B. S., & Soto, A. M. (2009). Bisphenol-A and the great divide: A review of controversies in the field of endocrine disruption. Endocrine Reviews, 30(1), 75–95. doi:10.1210/er.2008-0021 PubMed doi:10.1210/er.2008-0021 PMID:19074586

Vogel, S. A. (2009). The politics of plastics: The making and unmaking of bisphenol A 'safety'. American Journal of Public Health, 99(S3), S559–S566. doi:10.2105/AJPH.2008.159228 PubMed doi:10.2105/AJPH.2008.159228 PMID:19890158

Vom Saal, F. S. (2018). Commentary: FDA Statement on BPA's Safety Is Premature. Environ. Heal. News. Retrieved from https://www.ehn.org/ fda-flawed-statement-science-bpa-2542621453.html

Welshons, W. V., Nagel, S. C., & vom Saal, F. S. (2006). Saal FSv. Large effects from small exposures. III. Endocrine mechanisms mediating effects of bisphenol A at levels of human exposure. Endocrinology, 147(6), s56–s69. doi:10.1210/en.2005-1159 PubMed doi:10.1210/en.2005-1159 PMID:16690810

Whyatt, R. M., Perzanowski, M. S., Just, A. C., Rundle, A. G., Donohue, K. M., Calafat, A. M., . . . Miller, R. L. (2014). Asthma in inner-city children at 5-11 years of age and prenatal exposure to phthalates: The Columbia Center for Children's Environmental Health Cohort. Environmental Health Perspectives, 122(10), 1141–1146. doi:10.1289/ehp.1307670 PubMed doi:10.1289/ehp.1307670 PMID:25230320

Wormuth, M., Scheringer, M., Vollenweider, M., & Hungerbuhler, K. (2006). What are the sources of exposure to eight frequently used phthalic acid esters in Europeans. Risk Analysis, 26(3), 803–824. doi:10.1111/j.1539-6924.2006.00770.x PubMed doi:10.1111/j.1539-6924.2006.00770.x PMID:16834635

Chapter 14
Bisphenol A and Phthalates Exhibit Similar Toxicogenomics and Health Effects

Sumaya Hassan
https://orcid.org/0000-0002-9658-6936
University of Kashmir, India

Rohaya Ali
University of Kashmir, India

Durdana Shah
University of Kashmir, India

Nasreena Sajjad
University of Kashmir, India

Jasfeeda Qadir
University of Kashmir, India

ABSTRACT

Bisphenol A and phthalates are most frequently detected organic pollutants found in our surroundings because of their regular use as plasticizers in daily use polymeric products. BPA is used in manufacturing baby feeding bottles, water pipes, canned food linings, and food packaging materials. Phthalates are used in polyvinyl chloride products including clothing, toys, medical devices, and food packaging. These chemicals are not bound to the matrix and leach out into the surroundings on slight change in the environment, like alteration in pH, temperature, and pressure. Humans are continuously exposed to these chemicals through skin contact, inhalation, or ingestion when the leachates enter food, drinks, air, water, or soil. The Comparative Toxicogenomics Database (CTD) revealed that Bisphenol A has 1932 interactions with genes/proteins and few frequently used phthalates (DEHP, MEHP, DBP, BBP, and MBP) showed 484 gene/protein interactions. Similar toxicogenomics and adverse effects of Bisphenol A and phthalates on human health are attributed to their 89 common interacting genes/proteins.

DOI: 10.4018/978-1-5225-9452-9.ch014

INTRODUCTION

Plastic Pollution

Plastics, being essential materials in modern civilization, are used widely, almost everywhere in the world. Plastics and many products manufactured from them promote risks to human health and environment (Thompson et al., 2009). Plastics contain many hazardous substances including Bisphenol A, pthalates, brominated flame retardants and poly-fluorinated chemicals, etc. that causes various human health issues like respiratory problems, liver dysfunction, vision failure, skin diseases, cancers, lungs problems, dizziness, headache, reproductive problems, birth defects, cardiovascular and gastrointestinal troubles (Proshad et al.,2018). BPA and phthalates are found in many widely used products including medical devices, perfumes, flooring materials, food packaging, toys, cosmetics, computers and CDs and hence, represent a considerable component of plastic (Meeker &Ferguson, 2012).

Bisphenol A

Bisphenol A (BPA, 2,2-bis (4-hydroxyphenyl)propane) is a monomer that was developed in 1890s as a synthetic estrogen. Later in 1930s, it was reported to have stimulatory effects on the female reproductive system of rats as that of estrone (Dodds, 1936). BPA has also been used in various consumer products, like polycarbonate plastic, PVC, dental sealants and food packaging. Humans are usually exposed to BPA through via their diet, inhalation and dermal route (Vandenberg et al., 2012). In 2008, it was estimated that 2.8 million metric tons of BPA were produced and subsequently 5.5 million metric tons were expected in 2011 (Bailin et al., 2008). BPA is an identified endocrine disruptor as it binds to estrogen receptors and hence produces estrogenic effects. Although BPA has a lower affinity for nuclear estrogen receptors as compared to 17-beta estradiol (E2) (Figure 1A), its estrogenic strength is equal to that of E2 for responses that are mediated by non-nuclear estrogen receptor (Vinas et al., 2012). BPA can also act as an anti-estrogen by blocking the estrogenic response while competing with endogenous estradiol (Richter et al., 2007; Bonefeld-Jorgensen et al., 2007). BPA directly bind to androgen receptors, and hence, possibly acts as anti-androgenic by blocking the endogenous androgen activity (Sohoni et al., 1998; Wetherill et al., 2007). BPA has also been found to bind thyroid receptors possessing both agonistic and antagonistic effects on thyroid function (Moriyama et al., 2002). BPA also interacts with CNS, pancreas and immune system (Wetherill et al., 2007). Various *in vitro*, *in vivo* and epidemiologic studies have shown that BPA is associated with several diseases, including coronary heart disease (Melzer et al., 2010), cardiovascular disease (Magliano and Lyons, 2013), diabetes (Shankar and Teppala, 2011) and obesity (Wang et al., 2012). It has also been employed as a model for determining the low dose and non-monotonic nature of hormones that regulate our endocrine system (Vandenberg et al., 2012). BPA has been reported to have significant effects at low doses, which may not be present at higher doses used in toxicology studies (Vandenberg et al., 2012). Since most of us are exposed to low doses of BPA regularly, it becomes necessary to determine the health effects of BPA on humans. There are ample studies that link BPA with various adverse health effects in mammalian and non-mammalian models (Richter et al., 2007; Bonefeld-Jorgensen et al., 2007; Saal et al., 2007; Crain et al., 2007). The results are obviously worrying as humans are ubiquitously exposed to BPA. The exposure to BPA starts

Figure 1: Structure of β-estradiol (A) and Bisphenol A (B)

A

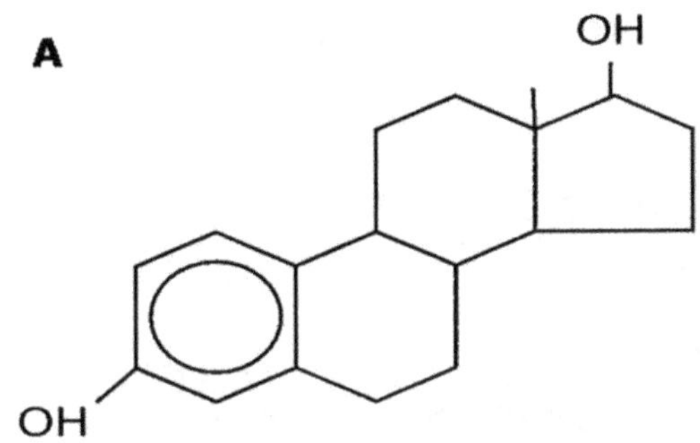

B

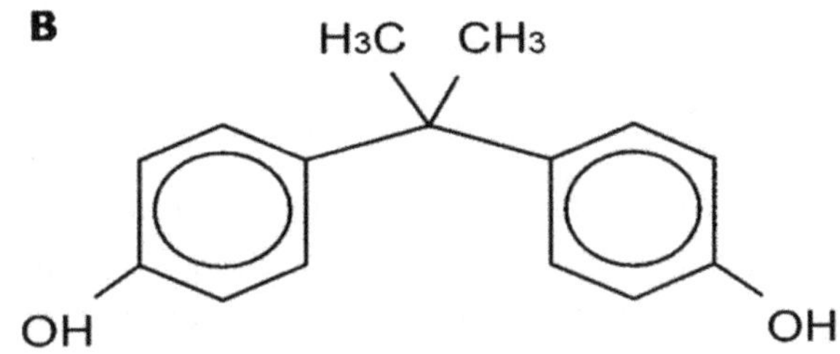

in the womb itself as it is detected in the follicular and amniotic fluid, placental tissue, cord blood and human fetal liver (Ikezuki et al., 2002; Schonfelder et al., 2002; Nahar et al., 2012). BPA is also detected in urine samples of adults and children, serum of pregnant women and breast milk (Schonfelder et al., 2002; Calafat et al., 2005; Kuruto-Niwa et al., 2007; Braun et al., 2011).

Phthalates

Phthalates or phthalic acid diesters are high volume chemicals that are being produced for the manufacture of polyvinyl chloride plastics (EPA, 2015). The first phthalate that was introduced in the world in late 1920s was Diethylhexyl phthalate (DEHP). In 1931, it was introduced as plasticizer for PVC (Kyrides, 1933). Since then, phthalates have been used in diverse fields including cosmetics and perfumes, increasing its use by humans with every passing day despite its known toxicity reported by Ferguson et al. in 1946. Phthalates are used as plasticizer that fills the lattice spaces of the polymer thereby imparting the plasticity to the plastics. The plasticity of a plastic is determined by the percentage of phthalate that has been blended in it (Josh et al., 2012). Unlike other fillers that are used in plastic manufacturing, phthalates have no chemical bonding with the plastic polymer and any minor alteration in the environment (pH, temperature and pressure), irradiation with UV, sunlight or microwave or contact with lipid or any other solvent would lead to the leaching of phthalate from the plastic polymer into the surrounding, which will eventually tell upon the human health (Benjamin et al., 2015). The leachates from the plastics enter our food, drinks, soil, water, air and blood that would pose severe damage to entire ecosystem, especially humans. Data from *in silico*, *in vitro* and *in vivo* studies on phthalates provide evidences of its hazardous effects on humans, especially by influencing the endocrine system (Latini et al., 2010; Kim and Park

Figure 2: General structure of phthalate

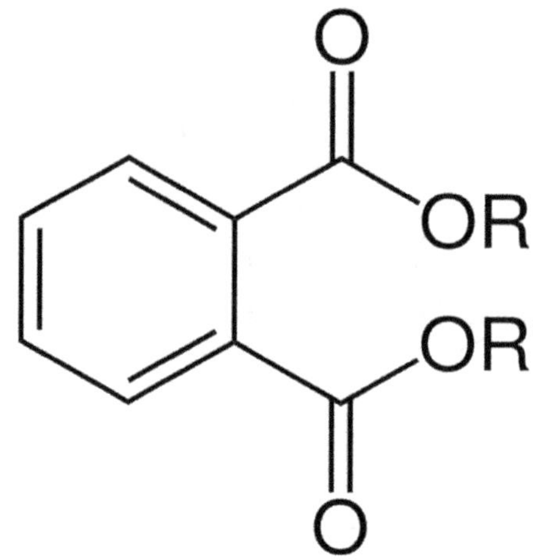

2014).Significant concentrations of phthalate esters are accumulating over time throughout the globe because of the extensive use in daily products (Gasperi et al., 2008; Rowsell et al., 2010) leading to more human exposure (Net et al., 2015). Even at very low concentration, phthalates are causative agents of mutagenicity and carcinogenicity (Caldwell, 2012; Park et al., 2012).The most remarkable effects of phthalates are observed during fetal development and reproductive differences, especially in "phthalate syndrome" (Sharpe and Skakkebaek, 2008), accompanied by insulin resistance and obesity (Halden, 2010; Latini et al., 2010; Kuo et al., 2013).

SOURCES AND ROUTE OF ENTRY OF BISPHENOL A AND PHTHALATES

BPA and Phthalates are omnipresent and hence, all the parts of human body are susceptible to their exposure. The presence of BPA and phthalates in the eatables is the major threat to human health. In additional, dermal contact, inhalation either occupational or non-occupational, non-dietary ingestions and medical exposure are also potent concerns (Kimber et al., 2010).BPA is used in the synthetic polymers including epoxy resins and polycarbonates (Flint et al., 2012). It is also used as a stabilizer and antioxidant while manufacturing vinyl chloride (Nam et al., 2010). It is also used in thermal paper production and as a result finds its way in daily use stationery like register receipts, books, newspapers, labels, faxes, ticket, mailing envelopes, toilet paper and kitchen rolls (Liao et al., 2012; Nam et al., 2010). BPA is added to the environment only because of anthropogenic activity and the addition is so much so that it is difficult to identify the most important source of the exposure.

Atmosphere

BPA and phthalates are found in the atmosphere in varying concentrations. Their presence in the atmosphere is mainly due to the industrial activity. BPA is usually found in water in low concentrations. The effluents from BPA-related factories are the major source of BPA in the waters (Lee et al., 2013). In heavily urbanized areas atmospheric fallout, sewer overflows and runoff are the major sources of

BPA (Cladiere et al., 2013). Ground waters near the plastic waste dumps contain significant higher concentration of BPA (Kawagoshi et al., 2003). BPA is also found in higher concentrations higher in leachates from landfills, industrial sewages and raw sewage sludges (Coors et al., 2003; Lee and Peart, 2000). Phthalate exposure occurs by construction materials, vehicle parts, carrying pipes, etc. Other routes include medications (medical devices and bags, tubing, implants, blood transfusion and dialysis materials and pill covers), clothing, ornaments, etc.

Food and Drinking Water

Food remains the most important source of BPA to general population. The presence of BPA in food containers makes it readily available for human exposure. It is literally considered we consume BPA each day with food and such exposure is increasing with each passing day. Vandenberg et al. (2007) estimated that the BPA exposure to human alimentary canal was 0.48 to 1.6 µg/kg/body weight/day.BPA is also found in significant amounts in fish (Munguıa-Lopez et al., 2005), meat products (Shao et al., 2007), cereals (Niu et al., 2012) and fruits and vegetables (Yoshida et al., 2001). Tinned food contains more BPA concentration than fresh food (Yonekubo et al., 2008).Canned vegetables and fruits and canned seafood also contain significantly high amounts of BPA (Cunha et al., 2012; Cunha and Fernandes, 2013). Higher BPA concentration is usually found in bottled water. Colin et al. (2013) found that BPA is present in considerable amounts in water stored in PC bottles. Much higher concentrations were found in freshly manufactured bottles. Phthalate exposure via food is carried out by food casings, wrappers, washing sink, bottles, microwaving, cooking aids, infant formulae and milk, liquors, carbonated drinks, toys, denture materials, etc.

Dust

Humans are exposed to BPA and phthalates through respiration and skin contact as these are present in the atmospheric dust. The exposure of BPA from dust has been found be of same order of magnitude that causes health effects in laboratory test animals (Loganathan and Kannan,2011). The current mean BPA concentration found in doors is twice higher than found decades ago because of increased use of products containing BPA. Geens et al. (2009) found that office dust contains more BPA than home dust. BPA present in the dust can penetrate through skin or inhaled through lungs but still the exposure through food and water remains the considerably alarming (Geens et al., 2009).Significant amounts of phthalates are also detected in dust (Bornehag et al., 2005; Nagorka et al., 2010). Inhalation of phthalates occurs via vapors, fragrance, cosmetics (creams, shampoos, nail polish, deodorants, hair dyes).

The first country ever to ban BPA was Canada (Morrissey, 2008). It banned the use of BPA in baby bottles and replaced it by bisphenol S (BPS). The European Commission has also restricted the use of BPA in infant feeding bottles since 2011. BPS is being used in place of BPA in the manufacture of these items (Barroso, 2011). Food and Drug Administration has also banned the use of BPA in baby formula packaging. Various countries have also set permissible exposure limit for phthalates in different consumer products. For example, the exposure limit of DEHP in drinking water has been set to a maximum of 06 µg/L in the USA (EPA, 2012) while as limits prescribed by WHO (2003) were 08 µg/L.

Toxicity Of Bisphenol A And Phthalate

BPA and phthalates are not chemically bound to the plastic polymer and can seep into the foodstuff (Talsness et al., 2009; Meeker et al., 2009). Ingestion is regarded as the chief route of BPA exposure in humans. Exposure through inhalation and absorption through skin are other possible ways (Heudorf et al., 2007). BPA is rapidly conjugated with glucuronic acid in the liver after ingestion. This conjugation is an important step for the removal and detoxification of BPA. Consequently, the half-life of BPA is short, around four hours. BPA is found in human blood and urine (Imanishi et al., 2003). The concentration of free BPA in serum after ingestion are usually found in lower ranges of 0.5-3 nM. However, higher concentrations above 100 nM have also been detected in serum samples of some highly exposed individuals (Taylor et al., 2010). BPA glucuronide is the major metabolite present in the body, which implies that only a small part of the actual body burden of BPA is measured. Additionally, a portion of absorbed non metabolized BPA is assumed to distribute to the adipose tissues, which results in the slow release of BPA into the bloodstream. BPA has been related to various health effects, such as cardiovascular disease, asthma, diabetes, allergy, etc. BPA has also been found to increase the numbers of premature deliveries and miscarriages. The effects of BPA may be due to its binding to estrogen receptors (Welshons et al., 2006; Willhite et al., 2008).

Phthalates are broadly used as plasticizers in PVC plastics, but like BPA, they can also leach into the surroundings. Phthalate exposure has been reported to cause developmental and reproductive toxicity in rodents (Singh & Li, 2011). Ingestion, inhalation and skin contact with clothing or toys are the main routes of phthalate exposure. Infants and toddlers are frequently exposed to phthalates contained in their toys. Children are more susceptible to phthalate exposure as they are in their development phase. The metabolism and removal of phthalates from body is complex (Meeker et al., 2009). Phthalates are diesters which are cleaved into their hydrolytic monoesters which can be later modified via different oxidation reactions. The hydrolytic monoesters and the oxidized metabolites bind with glucuronic acid and finally get excreted through urine. The half-life and the concentration of metabolites in the urine samples differ for various phthalates due to their structural and chain length differences. For example, 70% of DnBP (di-n-butyl phthalate) is excreted as the metabolite mono-n-butyl phthalate (MnBP) while as only 7% of DEHP (di (2-ethylhexyl) phthalate) is excreted as MEHP, its primary metabolite. Since phthalates are used in different products, hence exposure route differs between various phthalates, ages and gender groups (Stahlhut et al., 2007). Humans are highly exposed to Di-n-butyl phthalate (DnBP), benzyl butyl phthalate (BBzP), diisobutyl phthalate (DiBP) and di (2-ethylhexyl) phthalate (DEHP) through ingestion. It has been found that phthalate exposure in rodents is associated with adverse effects on kidney and liver as well as the reproductive system. The effect was observed to differ between different phthalates (Kamrin 2009). Other health conditions like diabetes, obesity and asthma have also been associated with elevated levels of phthalate metabolites in urine. Phthalate metabolites are believed to activate the peroxisome proliferator-activated receptor (PPAR`s) family of nuclear receptors which regulate insulin metabolism, lipid storage and inflammation. Hence, phthalate-induced effects are often suggested as a PPAR's mechanism (Kimber et al., 2010).

Toxicogenomics Of Bpa

The impact of environmental chemicals on human health is analyzed by the Comparative Toxicogenomics Database (CTD; http://ctd.mdibl.org) (Davis et al., 2009). The biocurators at CTD curate toxicogenomic data of 116,000 interactions between 3900 chemicals and 13,300 genes/proteins from over 270 species, 5900 gene/protein-disease direct relationships and 2500 chemical-disease direct relationships.

With the aim of understanding the probable adverse affects of BPA on human health, the curated genes/proteins interactions of BPA were obtained from CTD. The BPA toxicogenomic profile provided by Singh &Li (2012) showed that 1932 curated BPA-gene/protein interactions were reported from CTD, among which 1232 interactions were found to be unique. The most frequent curated genes/proteins were ESR1 and ESR2 having 120 and 33 interactions, respectively. Furthermore, S100G had 21 and LHB had 18 interactions in rodents but none in humans, while as TFF1 was found to have 11 interactions in humans and none in rodents.

The Gene Ontology, pathways, processes and networks of these 1232 unique genes/proteins analyzed with Meta-Core Analytical Suite revealed that 7 of the top 10 GO molecular functions were associated with protein/receptor binding. 7 and 6 of the top 20 Gene Go pathway maps of were involved in development and immune response, respectively and 6 of the top 10 GO processes of the top 33 genes/proteins were involved in cardiac cell differentiation and heart growth. The toxicity profile of 1232 unique genes/proteins interacting with BPA analyzed with IPA TOX Functions showed that the top three categories were cardiotoxicity, hepatotoxicity and nephrotoxicity. The Gene Go diseases analyzed with MetaCore by biomarkers revealed that 8 of top 20 diseases were related to neoplasms.

Toxicogenomics Of Phthalates

The toxicogenomic study of phthalates was carried out by Singh &Li (2011). The CTD data revealed 256 and 189 phthalate-gene/protein interactions for DEHP/MEHP and DBP/BBP/MBP respectively. DEHP and MEHP were grouped together because the former is metabolized to MEHP were thus combined as a group. Likewise, DBP, BBP and MBP were kept together because DBP and BBP are metabolized to MBP. The two groups of DEHP/MEHP and DBP/BBP/MBP were found to have 249 unique genes/protein interactions while 46 among these interactions were shared by both.

DEHP/MEHP had five interactions with all three PPARA, PPARG and PPARD, while as DBP/BBP/MBP had just one interaction with all these isotopes. PPARs are known to play significant role in lipid and carbohydrate metabolism and lead to the manifestation of metabolic disorders including obesity, atherosclerosis and hyperlipidemia (Desvergne et al., 2009) and provide evidence in support of phthalates exposure leading to cardiovascular diseases and metabolic disorders. DEHP/MEHP had no interaction with AR while as DBP/BBP/MBP had nine interactions with AR. Though, these phthalates do not directly interact with the androgen receptor, but rather disrupt synthesis of testosterone in rat fetal testis (Thompson et al., 2005). DEHP/MEHP were found to have only two interactions with ESR1 (Estrogen receptor 1) where as DBP/BBP/MBP had eleven interactions. Furthermore, DEHP/MEHP and DBP/BBP/MBP were also found to interact with human VEGFA (vascular endothelial growth factor A). The pathways and networks of top 34 genes/proteins were similar to 249 unique genes/proteins interacting with phthalates DEHP/MEHP and DBP/BBP/MBP and hence, these genes/proteins may be used as molecular biomarkers for determining phthalate toxicity. The GO molecular functions of 249 unique phthalate genes/proteins interactions studied by MetaCore and Pathway Studio and the top 20 functions were associated with various receptor activities. Most of the Gene Go pathways and process networks of these 249 unique phthalate interacting genes/proteins were very similar to the top 34 unique genes/proteins with three and more curated phthalate interactions which suggest that these 34 unique genes/proteins symbolize by and large the biology of all 249 genes/proteins reacting to phthalate exposure.

The toxicity of 249 unique genes/proteins interactions were analyzed with IPA Tox Functions and the analysis showed that cardiotoxicity, hepatotoxicity and nephrotoxicity were top three categories. The MetaCore analysis of the curated interactions of these 249 unique genes/proteins revealed their association with 1437 Gene Go diseases with the top diseases including cardiovascular, liver, urologic, endocrine and genital diseases.

Comparative Toxigonenomics Of Bpa And Phthalates

The comparative toxicogenomic study of BPA and phthalates was studied by Singh &Li (2012). The GeneGo pathway maps, GO processes, toxicities and GeneGo diseases related to 1232 unique genes/proteins interacting with BPA were compared with 265 unique genes/proteins interacting with Phthalates using MetaCore. The results revealed that the top ten GeneGo pathway maps with maximum probabilities were obtained from the 89 common genes/proteins interacting with both BPA and Phthalates. Taking into consideration the GO processes, all top ten BPA and Phthalate-specific GO processes were similar to those of 89 common genes/proteins. The toxicities of 1232 BPA-interacting genes/proteins and 265 Phthalate-interacting genes/proteins were compared by IPA TOX Functions and it was found that their top three categories including, cardiotoxicity, hepatotoxicity and nephrotoxicity were very similar. Ten top most GeneGo diseases related to BPA and Phthalate specific genes/proteins interactions were similar to 89 common genes/proteins interactions of both BPA and Phthalates, even though five among the top 10 BPA-specific GeneGo diseases were having higher probabilities and all top 10 Phthalate-specific GeneGo diseases were found to have much lower probabilities, indicating that these 89 common genes/proteins interactions might act as a useful biomarkers for identifying exposure to BPA and phthalates.

MetaCore was used to analyse the GeneGo toxicity network of these 89 common genes/proteins interactions of BPA and phthalates. The analysis revealed that five among the top 10 GeneGo toxicity networks were associated with inflammation. Six of the top 10 GeneGo diseases were found to be urogenitial, prostatic, male genital, female genital, endometrial and breast neoplasms. Further analysis with IPA revealed that cancer, developmental disorder and reproductive diseases were top three categories of diseases associated with these 89 common genes/proteins interactions.

BPA and phthalates were found to interact with ESR1 and ESR2 (Singh &Li, 2012); Singh &Li, 2011) and this finding is in supports of both BPA and phthalatesbeing considered as endocrine disruptors. Furthermore, both have been associated with developmental and reproductive disorders (Meeker et al., 2009; Talsness et al., 2009).

Hepatotoxicity was found to be among top three toxic categories by biomarkers of BPA and Phthalates. BPA and Phthalates are having weak estrogenic characteristics which could be attributed to their weak carcinogenic nature and hence their exposure could increase the susceptibility for developing cancers (Cavalieri & Rogan, 2010; Soto & Sonnenschein, 2010). 5/6 of top 10 GeneGo diseases by biomarkers of BPA and Phthalates were shown to be associated with prostatic, genital, endometrial and breast neoplasms (Singh &Li, 2012). BPA and phthalates having estrogenic characters and since estrogen is also known modulate the immune system (Dietert et al., 2010), five of the top 10 GeneGo toxicity networks of 89 common genes/proteins interacting with both BPA and PAEs were involved in inflammation.

HEALTH EFFECTS OF BISPHENOL A AND PHTHALATES

Effects on Reproductive health

It is believed that chemicals present in our environment impair human reproduction and BPA has been shown to affect many endpoints of reproduction (Mantovani, 2006; Wetherill et al., 2007). In patients undergoing infertility treatments, including IVF, poor ovarian response and hence decreased IVF success has been associated with increased total urinary BPA (Mok-Lin et al., 2010). Another study on a population of women from the MGH Fertility Center, found that higher urinary BPA was significantly correlated with lower serum E2 and oocyte yield. Furthermore, higher urinary BPA corresponded to reduced maturation of the oocytes (Ehrlich et al., 2012). Phthalates also affect the reproductive health of females like BPA. The occurrence of phthalates in the body has been associated with delayed onset of pubarche in young females (Frederiksen et al., 2012), decreased oocyte yield (Hauser et al., 2015), low gestational age of fetus (Latini et al., 2003), endometriosis (Upson et al., 2013), increased incidences of birth loss (Mu et al., 2015; Hauser et al., 2015) and infertility (Du et al., 2016). A study carried by Frederiksen et al. (2012) demonstrated that the high first morning urinary content of DEHP, DINP, MBP and MBzP metabolites in young females was positively correlated with less advanced pubertal development. Elevated levels of MEHP and MBP metabolites were also found in urine and follicular fluid of infertile women in China (Du et al., 2016).

BPA has been found to affect male reproduction as well. Studies carried out by Li et al. (2010a, 2010b) on men working in BPA manufacturing companies revealed that the workers had significantly lower sexual function, including sexual desire, erectile function, orgasmic function and overall contentment with sex life. The reduced sexual function by BPA was seen to be dose-dependent (Li et al., 2010b). However additional studies on men with environmental, but not occupational, exposure to BPA also showed decreased sexual function in case of sexual desire and overall satisfaction with sex life (Li et al., 2010a). It is important to note here that BPA has a negative impact on male sexual function even when the exposure is low, as in case of environmental exposure. One of the major affects of phthalate toxicity on male reproductive system is the "phthalate syndrome" also known as "testicular dysgenesis syndrome" which is characterized by hypospadias, cryptorchidism, reduced anogenital distance, undescended testes, low sperm count and quality and increase in sterility (Sharpe et al., 2008; Swan, 2008). Anogenital distance is the distance between anus and genitalia. It is one of the major markers of phthalate toxicity in humans (Swan et al., 2005; Marsee et al., 2006; Sharpe and Skakkebaek, 2008). It is caused due to the prenatal exposure of fetus to various phthalates inside the womb (Swan et al., 2005). Male sterility has been linked with quality of semen including sperm count, motility and morphology. Studies carried out for MBP and MBzP toxicity in subfertile married males revealed that their concentration was positively associated with spermatotoxicity (Duty et al., 2003; Hauser et al., 2006).

Effects on Endocrine System

BPA exposure in adults and neonates has been found to alter the endogenous sex hormone concentrations, including androgens, estrogens and gonadotropins, in addition to sex hormone binding globulin. FSH (Follicle-stimulating hormone) has been studied to decrease significantly in subjects exposed to occupational bisphenol A diglycidyl ether (BADGE) (Hanaoka et al., 2002). Urinary BPA was also measured to be higher in these workers.BPA exposure has been found to disturb function of endocrine system (Flint et al., 2012). It behaves similarly to natural estrogen. In addition to nuclear ERα and ERβ, BPA can bind to receptors outside the nucleus, even at very low concentrations (ranging from pico to nanomolar) and exert multitude effects on physiological functions of cells (Wetherill et al., 2007). Furthermore, most of the estrogenic activities are exerted by BPA metabolites rather than BPA itself (Alonso-Magdalena et al., 2012). Exposure of BPA to growing mice and rats was found to alter the structure and functions of their brains via affecting neurohormone receptors. Reproductive organ development, sperm production and testosterone secretion was also affected in these animals (Richter et al., 2007). This outcome was attributed to the effect of BPA on brain-gonads-pituitary gland axis function. BPA exposure also affects the thyroid functions by altering thyroid specific transcriptional factors in zebra fish and CV-1 cells derived from *Cercopithecus aethiopis* monkey kidneys (Gentilcore et al., 2013; Sheng et al., 2012). A study on Chinese population carried by Wang et al. (2013) revealed that elevated urinary BPA levels were associated with an increased level of free tri-iodothyronine and a decreased concentration of TSH (thyroid-stiumlating hormone).

Phthalates chiefly act as hormone sensitizers by interrupting with their normal physiological mechanisms. The longer the biological half-life of phthalates, the greater are its impact on health. The effect of various phthalates is because of their binding to hormone receptors as in case of DEHP where all its three stereo forms are able to bind to progesterone receptor and potentially compete with the original substrate (Sheikh, 2016). Phthalates and their monoesters have been found to have strong interaction with various receptors including human peroxisome proliferator-activated receptor α,β or γ subtypes (PPARs), pregnane-X-receptor (PXR), retinoid X receptors (RXRα,β,γ), estrogens and ketosteroid than their natural agonists (Josh et al., 2014a, 2014b, 2015 and 2016). DEHP was also found to interact with hRXR more strongly than its natural ligands (Josh et al., 2014b). The unfavorable effects of phthalates in endocrine disruption activities, developmental and reproductive toxicities may be attributed to their interruption of hypothalamic–pituitary–gonad/thyroid axis (Boas et al., 2010).

Effects on Obesity

Researchers have proven that chemical compounds that disrupt endocrine balance may also contribute to obesity. BPA and phthalates are known endocrine disruptors and both tend to exert their effect on the fat tissues that have alpha and beta receptors. Obesity is one of the most studied health condition in response to BPA. A study carried on non-PCOS women by Takeuchi et al. (2004) revealed that elevated BPA levels were associated with increased BMI. Furthermore, the obese controls were found to have higher serum BPA concentrations as compared to non-obese controls. Carwile and Michels (2011) suggested from the data of NHANES 2003-2006 participants, that higher urinary BPA had a significant association with higher BMI and waist circumference, indicating its association with general as well as central obesity. BPA affects the activity of aromatase, lipoprotein lipase, lipogenesis regulators and fat tissue hormones (lectin and adiponectin), critical for maintaining proper body weight (Saal et al., 2012).

Various *in vitro* and *in vivo* studies have suggested that phthalates have significant effect on the development of obesity. Exposure to phthalates is considered as a key contributor to obesity, independent of physical activity and diet (Swan, 2008; Desvergne et al., 2009). Different phthalates have different obesity related outcomes on various age groups and sex (Buser et al., 2014; Zhang et al., 2014). Low molecular weight phthalate metabolites including MnBP, MiBP and MEP, have been significantly associated with children and adolescent obesity in males while high molecular weight phthalate metabolites like MECPP, MEOHP, MEHHP, MEHP, MCNP, MBzP and MCOP were seen to show significant association with obesity in all adults (Buser et al., 2014).

Effects on Diabetes

Type-2 diabetes and BPA have been correlated in various human studies. Lang et al. (2008) carried out the first study regarding the association of BPA with diabetes in humans. In this study the elevated urinary BPA was found to be significantly associated with increased diagnosis of type-2 diabetes (Lang et al., 2008). An *in vivo* study conducted by Liu et al. (2013) on pregnant mice revealed that administration of BPA during pregnancy resulted in glucose intolerance and decreased insulin secretion in the off springs. This effect of BPA was assumed to be due to the metabolic disorders relevant to glucose homeostasis. Another study by Shankar and Teppala (2011) suggested the association between urinary BPA concentration and diabetes mellitus in the NHANES in 2003-2008. The positive association between elevated BPA level and diabetes was independent of race, age, gender and body mass index. Another study by Hong et al. (2009) on adult Korean population found significant correlation between increased insulin resistance and elevated urinary BPA. Wang et al. (2012) suggested that high urinary BPA levels were significantly associated with insulin resistance in Chinese population. PCOS women who had serum BPA levels more than 0.45 ng/ml also had severe insulin resistance (Tarantino et al., 2012).

Phthalates are believed to increase diabetes risk by activating PPARs (Casals-Casas and Desvergne 2011; Josh et al, 2014b), as these are the main regulators of lipid and glucose metabolism (Evans et al., 2004). Various epidemiological studies also revealed the presence various phthalates and their metabolites in urine and blood samples of diabetic patients (Svensson, et al., 2011; Lind et al., 2012; Dirinck et al., 2014; Attina and Trasande, 2015). In these studies DEHP and its metabolites including, MEHP, 2cx-MEXP, 5oxo-MEHP, 5OH-MEHP and 5cx-MEHP, were found to be the common factor, followed by MBP, MEP and MBzP. DHEP metabolites were also found to be significantly elevated in the urine samples of subjects studied by Svensson et al. (2011).

Epigenetics Modulation by BPA and Phthalates

The epigenetic modulations mediated by endocrine disruption chemicals may alter the inherited epigenetic memory by altering the gene expression (Rajesh and Balasubramanian, 2014).Epigenetic changes developed by BPA exposure have been studied to cause immediate or long term effects (Yamaguchi et al., 2005; Baccarelli et al., 2009). During hypermethylation of DNA the methyl groups are added to cytosines at CpG islands, that project from the DNA backbone into the major groove, thereby inhibiting the transcription of genes. Higher free serum BPA levels have been associated with low methylation at TSP50_P137 CpG location in the promoter site of TSP50 in IVF patients studied by Bloom et al. (2011a, 2011b) (Hanna et al., 2012). Similar epigenetic effect is found in patients suffering from breast cancer (Fernandez et al., 2012). Higher urinary BPA levels were significantly linked with increased expression of ERα and ERβ in adult males (Melzer et al., 2011). These alterations represent the platform for carrying out the estrogenic activity of BPA. Yang et al. (2006) found positive association of BPA with increased sister chromatid exchange (SCE) in lymphocytes, which is considered chromosome stability marker while determining the effects of any carcinogen or mutagen (Sonoda et al., 1999). Neonatal BPA exposure in rats is also found to change the promoter methylation and hence, expression of nucleosome binding protein-1 and hippocalcin-like 1 genes. It also leads to hypermethylation of promoter regions of estrogen receptor in rat testis, which indicates that a possible mechanism of BPA effects on fertility and spermatogenesis (Prins et al., 2008; Tang et al., 2012).

Toxicogenomic effect of phthalates is attributed to their binding to histone tails of DNA, thereby altering the availability of genes to be expressed (Wu et al., 2010; Manikkam et al., 2013). Exposure of pregnant Wistar rats to DEHP impaired glucose homeostasis and insulin signaling in the offsprings. The effect was due to the hypermethylation at the promoter region of Glut4 which caused its down regulation. The gestational phthalate exposure predisposes the offspring to glucometabolic dysfunctions during adulthood because of the genetic effect (Rajesh and Balasubramanian, 2014). Maternal exposure of DEHP in mice leads to testicular dysfunction by down regulating of insulin like hormone-3, which is essential for testosterone synthesis (Wu et al., 2010). Epigenetic transgenerational inheritance in rats due to DEHP and DBP exposure influences the onset of ovarian disease, testicular dysfunction and obesity (Manikkam et al., 2013). Prenatal exposure of phthalates including DEHP in humans was found to demethylate the paternally expressed Igf2 and maternally expressed H19 genes, which play critical role in the embryonic and placental growth (LaRocca et al., 2014).

CONCLUSION

Plastics are extensively used in present life. Their unbound chemicals BPA and phthalates can leach from plastic containers into foods and beverages. The worldwide production of BPA and phthalates is rising exponentially because of extensive use of plastic in modern life. BPA is used in hard, clear plastic, like baby bottles. Phthalates help make plastic, like pacifiers, flexible. Various scientific evidences suggest that BPA and phthalates are associated with a wide range of health issues, including hormonal and developmental problems. Infants and young children are potentially at high risk, as they are in their developmental years. Both BPA and phthalates disrupt the endocrine system, including reproductive hormones, thyroid functioning, glucose homeostasis, etc. The epigenetic modifications brought about by BPA and phthalates are regarded as main culprit to their effects on health. Furthermore, the toxicogenomic profile of both BPA and phthalates revealed that they have 89 common genes/proteins interactions, which attributes to their similar toxicogenomics.

The growing awareness and toxicological effects of these chemicals has led to the remarkable concern regarding their elimination from the environment. Since the past decade, researchers are examining the association between BPA and phthalates and the development of health effects. Though BPA and phthalates affect most of the biotic and abiotic components of ecosystem, humans represent the most affected victim. It is evident from various epidemiologic studies that humans are ubiquitously exposed to these chemicals because of their use in daily use products. The need of the hour is to define the mechanism of action of these chemicals and the doses at which their effects are caused. Additionally, the identification of the most susceptible populations should also be done, so as to minimize their effects by taking necessary measures.

Figure 3: Epigenetic modifications by BPA and phthalates

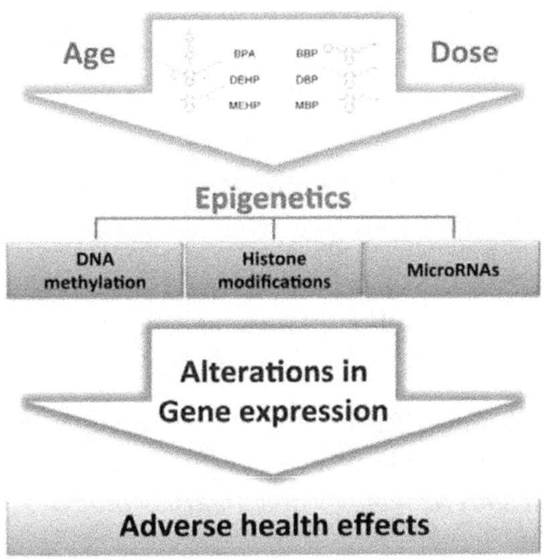

SUGGESTIONS AND RECOMMENDATIONS

Taking into consideration the significant toxicity of BPA and phthalates, it is the need of the hour to minimize their use on daily basis. There is still much to investigate about the mechanistic pathways and consequences of BPA and phthalate exposure on human health that can later help us in identifying the suitable substitutes. The potential risks and sources of exposure should be properly addressed to the masses. The Food Safety Authority should determine safe and limited doses of BPA and phthalates exposure that is only possible when extensive studies on the helath implications of BPA and phthalates is carried out.

REFERENCES

Alonso-Magdalena, P., Ropero, A., Rosiano, S., Garcia-Arevalo, M., Ripolli, C., Fuentes, E., ... Nadal, A. (2012). Bisphenol-A acts as a potent estrogen via non-classical estrogentriggered pathways. *Molecular and Cellular Endocrinology*, *355*(2), 201–207. doi:10.1016/j.mce.2011.12.012 PMID:22227557

Attina, T. M., & Trasande, L. (2015). Association of exposure to di-2-ethylhexylphthalate replacements with Increased insulin resistance in adolescents from NHANES 2009–2012. *The Journal of Clinical Endocrinology and Metabolism*, *100*(7), 2640–2650. doi:10.1210/jc.2015-1686 PMID:25993640

Baccarelli, A., Wright, R. O., Bollati, V., Tarantini, L., Litonjua, A. A., Suh, H. H., ... Schwartz, J. (2009). Rapid DNA methylation changes after exposure to traffic particles. *American Journal of Respiratory and Critical Care Medicine*, *179*(7), 572–578. doi:10.1164/rccm.200807-1097OC PMID:19136372

Bailin, P.D., Byrne, M., Lewis, S., & Liroff, R. (2008). Public awareness drives market for safer alternatives:bisphenol A market analysis report. *Investor Environmental Health Network,* 1-37.

Barroso, M. (2011). Commission Directive 2011/8/EU of 28 January 2011 Amending Directive2002/72/EC as Regards the Restriction of Use of Bisphenol A in Plastic Infant Feeding Bottles (Text with EEA relevance).

Benjamin, S., Pradeep, S., Josh, M. S., Kumar, S., & Masai, E. (2015). A monograph on the remediation of hazardous phthalates. *Journal of Hazardous Materials*, *298*(15), 58–72. doi:10.1016/j.jhazmat.2015.05.004 PMID:26004054

Bloom, M. S., Kim, D., VomSaal, F. S., Taylor, J. A., Cheng, G., Lamb, J. D., & Fujimoto, V. Y. (2011a). Bisphenol A exposure reduces the estradiol response to gonadotropin stimulation during *in vitro* fertilization. *Fertility and Sterility*, *96*(3), 672–7.e2. doi:10.1016/j.fertnstert.2011.06.063 PMID:21813122

Bloom, M. S., VomSaal, F. S., Kim, D., Taylor, J. A., Lamb, J. D., & Fujimoto, V. Y. (2011b). Serum unconjugated bisphenol A concentrations in men may influence embryo quality indicators during in vitrofertilization. *Environmental Toxicology and Pharmacology*, *32*(2), 319–323. doi:10.1016/j.etap.2011.06.003 PMID:21843814

Boas, M., Frederiksen, H., Feldt-Rasmussen, U., Skakkebæk, N. E., Hegedus, L., Hilsted, L., ... Main, K. M. (2010). Childhood exposure to phthalates: Associations with thyroid function, insulinlike growth factor I and growth. *Environmental Health Perspectives*, *118*(10), 1458–1464. doi:10.1289/ehp.0901331 PMID:20621847

Bonefeld-Jorgensen, E. C., Long, M., Hofmeister, M. V., & Vinggaard, A. M. (2007). Endocrine-disrupting potential of bisphenol A, bisphenol A dimethacrylate, 4-n-nonylphenol, and 4-n-octylphenol *in vitro*: New data and a brief review. *Environmental Health Perspectives*, *115*(1), 69–76. doi:10.1289/ehp.9368 PMID:18174953

Bornehag, C. G., Lundgren, B., Weschler, C. J., Sigsgaard, T., Hagerhed-Engman, L., & Sundell, J. (2005). Phthalates in indoor dust and their association with building characteristics. *Environmental Health Perspectives*, *113*(10), 1399–1404. doi:10.1289/ehp.7809 PMID:16203254

Braun, J. M., Kalkbrenner, A. E., Calafat, A. M., Yolton, K., Ye, X., Dietrich, K. N., & Lanphear, B. P. (2011). Impact ofearly-life bisphenol A exposure on behavior and executive function in children. *Pediatrics*, *128*(5), 873–882. doi:10.1542/peds.2011-1335 PMID:22025598

Buser, M. C., Murray, H. E., & Scinicariello, F. (2014). Age and sex differences in childhood and adulthood obesity association with phthalates: Analyses of NHANES 2007–2010. *International Journal of Hygiene and Environmental Health*, *217*(6), 687–694. doi:10.1016/j.ijheh.2014.02.005 PMID:24657244

Calafat, A. M., Kuklenyik, Z., Reidy, J. A., Caudill, S. P., Ekong, J., & Needham, L. L. (2005). Urinary concentrations of bisphenol A and 4-nonylphenol in a human reference population. *Environmental Health Perspectives*, *113*(4), 391–395. doi:10.1289/ehp.7534 PMID:15811827

Caldwell, J. C. (2012). DEHP: Genotoxicity and potential carcinogenic mechanisms—a review. *Mutation Research/Reviews in Mutation Research*, *751*(2), 82–157. doi:10.1016/j.mrrev.2012.03.001 PMID:22484601

Carwile, J.L., & Michels, K.B. (2011). Urinary bisphenol A and obesity: NHANES 2003-2006. *Environmental Research, 111*(6), 825-30. doi: : 21676388. doi:10.1016/j.envres.2011.05.014PMID

Casals-Casas, C., & Desvergne, B. (2011). Endocrine disruptors: From endocrine to metabolic disruption. *Annual Review of Physiology*, *73*(1), 135–162. doi:10.1146/annurev-physiol-012110-142200 PMID:21054169

Cavalieri, E. L., & Rogan, E. G. (2010). Is bisphenol A a weak carcinogen like the natural estrogens and diethylstilbestrol? *International Union of Biochemistry and Molecular Biology Life*, *62*(10), 746–751. doi:10.1002/iub.376 PMID:20945454

Cladiere, M., Gasperi, J., Lorgeoux, C., Bonhomme, C., Rocher, V., & Tassin, B. (2013). Alkylphenolic compounds and bisphenol A contamination within heavily urbanized area: Case study of Paris. *Environmental Science and Pollution Research International*, *20*(5), 2973–2983. doi:10.100711356-012-1220-6 PMID:23054786

Colin, A., Bach, C., Rosin, Ch., Munoz, J.-F., & Dauchy, X. (2013). Is drinking water a major route of human exposure toalkylphenol and bisphenol contaminants in France? *Archives of Environmental Contamination and Toxicology*, *66*(1), 86–99. doi:10.100700244-013-9942-0 PMID:23921451

Coors, A., Jones, P., Giesy, J., & Ratte, H. (2003). Removal of estrogenic activity from municipal waste landfill leachate assessed with a bioassay based on reporter gene expression. *Environmental Science & Technology*, *37*(15), 3430–3434. doi:10.1021/es0300158 PMID:12966991

Crain, D. A., Eriksen, M., Iguchi, T., Jobling, S., Laufer, H., LeBlanc, G. A., & Guillette, L. J. Jr. (2007). An ecological assessment of bisphenol-A: Evidence from comparative biology. *Reproductive Toxicology (Elmsford, N.Y.)*, *24*(2), 225–239. doi:10.1016/j.reprotox.2007.05.008 PMID:17604601

Cunha, S., Cunha, C., Ferreira, A., & Fernandes, J. (2012). Determination of bisphenol A and bisphenol B in canned seafood combining QuEChERS extraction with dispersive liquid-liquid microextraction followed by gaschromatography-mass spectrometry. *Analytical and Bioanalytical Chemistry*, *404*(8), 2453–2463. doi:10.100700216-012-6389-5 PMID:22995997

Cunha, S., & Fernandes, J. (2013). Assessement of bisphenol A and bisphenol B in canned vegetables and fruits by gaschromatography-mass spectrometry after QuEChERS and dispersive liquid-liquid microextraction. *Food Control*, *33*(2), 549–555. doi:10.1016/j.foodcont.2013.03.028

Davis, A. P., Murphy, C. G., Saraceni-Richards, C. A., Rosenstein, M. C., Wiegers, T. C., & Mattingly, C. J. (2009). Comparative Toxicogenomics Database: A knowledgebase and discovery tool for chemical–gene–disease networks. *Nucleic Acids Research*, *37*(Database), 786–792. doi:10.1093/nar/gkn580 PMID:18782832

Desvergne, B., Feige, J. N., & Casals-Casas, C. (2009). PPAR-mediated activity of phthalates: A link to the obesity epidemic? *Molecular and Cellular Endocrinology*, *304*(1-2), 43–48. doi:10.1016/j.mce.2009.02.017 PMID:19433246

Dietert, R. R., DeWitt, J. C., Germolec, D. R., & Zelikoff, J. T. (2010). Breaking patterns of environmentally influenced disease for health risk reduction: Immune perspectives. *Environmental Health Perspectives*, *118*(8), 1091–1099. doi:10.1289/ehp.1001971 PMID:20483701

Dirinck, E., Dirtu, A. C., Geens, T., Covaci, A., Van Gaal, L., & Jorens, P. G. (2015). Urinary phthalate metabolites are associated with insulin resistance in obese subjects. *Environmental Research*, *137*, 419–423. doi:10.1016/j.envres.2015.01.010 PMID:25622280

Dodds, E. C., & Lawson, W. (1936). Synthetic estrogenic agents without the phenanthrene nucleus. *Nature*, *137*(3476), 996. doi:10.1038/137996a0

Du, Y. Y., Fang, Y. L., Wang, Y. X., Zeng, Q., Guo, N., Zhao, H., & Li, Y. F. (2016). Follicular fluid and urinary concentrations of phthalate metabolites among infertile women and associations with in vitro fertilization parameters. *Reproductive Toxicology (Elmsford, N.Y.)*, *61*, 142–150. doi:10.1016/j.reprotox.2016.04.005 PMID:27067915

Duty, S. M., Silva, M. J., Barr, D. B., Brock, J. W., Ryan, L., Chen, Z., ... Hauser, R. (2003). Phthalate exposure and human semen parameters. *Epidemiology (Cambridge, Mass.)*, *14*(3), 269–277. doi:10.1097/01.EDE.0000059950.11836.16 PMID:12859026

Ehrlich, S., Williams, P. L., Missmer, S. A., Flaws, J. A., Ye, X., Calafat, A. M., & ... . (2012). Urinary bisphenolA concentrations and early reproductive health outcomes among women undergoing IVF. *HumanReproduction*, *27*(12), 2583–2592. doi:10.1093/humrep/des328

EPA. (2012). *Phthalates action plan*. Retrieved from https://www.epa.gov/sites/production/files/2015-09/documents/phthalates_actionplan_revised_2012-03-14.pdf

EPA. (2015). *Phthalates*. Retrieved from https://www.epa.gov/ace/biomonitoring-phthalates

Evans, R. M., Barish, G. D., & Wang, Y. X. (2004). PPARs and the complex journey to obesity. *Nature Medicine*, *10*(4), 355–361. doi:10.1038/nm1025 PMID:15057233

Ferguson, M. S., Graham, O. H., Bang, F. B., & Hairston, N. G. (1946). Studies on Schistosomiasis japonica. V. Protection experiments against Schistosomiasis japonica. *American Journal of Epidemiology*, *44*(3), 367–378. doi:10.1093/oxfordjournals.aje.a119103 PMID:20274589

Fernandez, S. V., Huang, Y., Snider, K. E., Zhou, Y., Pogash, T. J., & Russo, J. (2012). Expression and DNA methylation changes in human breast epithelial cells after bisphenol A exposure. *International Journal of Oncology*, *41*(1), 369–377. doi:10.3892/ijo.2012.1444 PMID:22576693

Flint, S., Markle, T., Thomson, S., & Wallace, E. (2012). Bisphenol Aexposure effects and policy; a wildlife perspective. *Journal of Environmental Management*, *104*, 19–34. doi:10.1016/j.jenvman.2012.03.021 PMID:22481365

Frederiksen, H., Sørensen, K., Mouritsen, A., Aksglaede, L., Hagen, C. P., Petersen, J. H., ... Juul, A. (2012). High urinary phthalate concentration associated with delayed pubarche in girls. *International Journal of Andrology*, *35*(3), 216–226. doi:10.1111/j.1365-2605.2012.01260.x PMID:22428786

Gasperi, J., Garnaud, S., Rocher, V., & Moilleron, R. (2008). Priority pollutants in wastewater and combined sewer overflow. *The Science of the Total Environment*, *407*(1), 263–272. doi:10.1016/j.scitotenv.2008.08.015 PMID:18814902

Geens, T., Roosens, L., Neels, H., & Covaci, A. (2009). Assessment of human exposure to bisphenol-A, triclosan andtetrabromobisphenol-A through indoor dust intake in Belgium. *Chemosphere*, *76*(6), 755–760. doi:10.1016/j.chemosphere.2009.05.024 PMID:19535125

Gentilcore, D., Porreca, I., Rizzo, F., Ganbaatar, E., Carchia, E., Mallorado, M., ... Ambrosino, C. (2013). Bisphenol Ainterferes with thyroid specific gene expression. *Toxicology*, *304*(8), 21–31. doi:10.1016/j.tox.2012.12.001 PMID:23238275

Halden, R. U. (2010). Plastics and health risks. *Annual Review of Public Health*, *31*(1), 179–194. doi:10.1146/annurev.publhealth.012809.103714 PMID:20070188

Hanaoka, T., Kawamura, N., Hara, K., & Tsugane, S. (2002). Urinary bisphenol A and plasma hormone concentrations in male workers exposed to bisphenol A diglycidyl ether and mixed organic solvents. *Occupational and Environmental Medicine*, *59*(9), 625–628. doi:10.1136/oem.59.9.625 PMID:12205237

Hanna, C. W., Bloom, M. S., Robinson, W. P., Kim, D., Parsons, P. J., vom Saal, F. S., ... Fujimoto, V. Y. (2012). DNA methylation changes in whole blood is associated with exposure to the environmental contaminants, mercury, lead, cadmium and bisphenol A, in women undergoing ovarian stimulation for IVF. *Human Reproduction (Oxford, England)*, *27*(5), 1401–1410. doi:10.1093/humrep/des038 PMID:22381621

Hauser, R., Gaskins, A. J., Souter, I., Smith, K. W., Dodge, L. E., Ehrlich, S., ... Williams, P. L. (2015). Urinary phthalate metabolite concentrations and reproductive outcomes among women undergoing in vitro fertilization: Results from the EARTH study. *Environmental Health Perspectives*, *124*(6), 831–839. doi:10.1289/ehp.1509760 PMID:26545148

Hauser, R., Meeker, J. D., Duty, S., Silva, M. J., & Calafat, A. M. (2006). Altered semen quality in relation to urinary concentrations of phthalate monoester and oxidative metabolites. *Epidemiology (Cambridge, Mass.)*, *17*(6), 682–691. doi:10.1097/01.ede.0000235996.89953.d7 PMID:17003688

Heudorf, U., Mersch-Sundermann, V., & Angerer, J. (2007). Phthalates: Toxicology and exposure. *International Journal ofHygiene and Environmental Health*, *210*(5), 623–634. doi:10.1016/j.ijheh.2007.07.011 PMID:17889607

Hong, Y. C., Park, E. Y., Park, M. S., Ko, J. A., Oh, S. Y., Kim, H., ... Ha, E.-H. (2009). Community level exposure to chemicals and oxidative stress in adult population. *Toxicology Letters*, *184*(2), 139–144. doi:10.1016/j.toxlet.2008.11.001 PMID:19049859

Ikezuki, Y., Tsutsumi, O., Takai, Y., Kamei, Y., & Taketani, Y. (2002). Determination of bisphenol A concentrations in human biological fluids reveals significant early prenatal exposure. *Human Reproduction (Oxford, England)*, *17*(11), 2839–2841. doi:10.1093/humrep/17.11.2839 PMID:12407035

Imanishi, S., Manabe, N., Nishizawa, H., Morita, M., Sugimoto, M., Iwahori, M., & Miyamoto, H. (2003). Effects of oral exposure of bisphenol A on mRNA expression of nuclear receptors in murine placentae assessed by DNA microarray. *The Journal ofReproduction and Development*, *49*(5), 329–336. doi:10.1262/jrd.49.329 PMID:14967926

Josh, M. S., Pradeep, S., Adarsh, V. K., Vijayalekshmi Amma, K. S., Sudha Devi, R., Balachandran, S., ... Benjamin, S. (2014a). *In silico* evidences for the binding of phthalates onto human estrogen receptor α, β subtypes and human estrogen-related receptor γ. *Molecular Simulation*, *40*(5), 408–417. doi:10.1080/08927022.2013.814131

Josh, M. S., Pradeep, S., Balachandran, S., Devi, R. S., Amma, K. V., & Benjamin, S. (2012). Temperatureand solvent-dependent migrations of di (2-ethylhexyl) phthalate, the hazardous plasticizer from commercial PVC blood storage bag. *Journal of Polymer Research*, *19*(7), 1–9. doi:10.100710965-012-9915-4

Josh, M. S., Pradeep, S., Balan, A. K., Sreejith, M. N., & Benjamin, S. (2016). Accessing the molecular interactions of phthalates and their primary metabolites with the human pregnane X receptor using in silico profiling. *Journal of Applied Toxicology*, *36*(12), 1599–1604. doi:10.1002/jat.3321 PMID:27071811

Josh, M. S., Pradeep, S., Vijayalekshmi Amma, K. S., Balachandran, S., Abdul-Jaleel, U. C., Mukesh, D., ... Sailas, B. (2014b). Phthalates efficiently bind to human peroxisome proliferator activated receptor and retinoid X receptor α, β, γ subtypes: An *in silico* approach. *Journal of Applied Toxicology*, *34*(7), 754–765. doi:10.1002/jat.2902 PMID:23843199

Josh, M. S., Pradeep, S., Vijayalekshmy Amma, K. S., Sudha Devi, R., Balachandran, S., Sreejith, M. N., & Benjamin, S. (2015). Human ketosteroid receptors interact with hazardous phthalate plasticizers and their metabolites: An *in silico* study. *Journal of Applied Toxicology*, *36*(6), 836–843. doi:10.1002/jat.3221 PMID:26304264

Kamrin, M. A. (2009). Phthalate risks, phthalate regulation, and public health: A review. *Journal of Toxicology and Environmental Health. Part B, Critical Reviews*, *12*(2), 157–174. doi:10.1080/10937400902729226 PMID:19235623

Kawagoshi, Y., Fujita, Y., Kishi, I., & Fukunaga, I. (2003). Estrogenic chemicals and estrogenic activity in leachate from municipal waste landfill determined by yeast two-hybrid assay. *Journal of Environmental Monitoring*, *5*(2), 269–274. doi:10.1039/b210962j PMID:12729267

Kim, S. H., & Park, M. J. (2014). Phthalate exposure and childhood obesity. *Annals of Pediatric Endocrinology & Metabolism*, *19*(2), 69–75. doi:10.6065/apem.2014.19.2.69 PMID:25077088

Kimber, I., & Dearman, R. J. (2010). An assessment of the ability of phthalates to influence immune and allergic responses. *Toxicology*, *271*(3), 73–82. doi:10.1016/j.tox.2010.03.020 PMID:20371260

Kuo, C. C., Moon, K., Thayer, K. A., & Navas-Acien, A. (2013). Environmental chemicals and type 2 diabetes: An updated systematic review of the epidemiologic evidence. *Current Diabetes Reports*, *13*(6), 831–849. doi:10.100711892-013-0432-6 PMID:24114039

Kuruto-Niwa, R., Tateoka, Y., Usuki, Y., & Nozawa, R. (2007). Measurement of bisphenol A concentrations in human colostrum. *Chemosphere*, *66*(6), 1160–1164. doi:10.1016/j.chemosphere.2006.06.073 PMID:16904728

Kyrides, L. P. (1933). U.S. Pat. No. 1,923,938.

Lang, I. A., Galloway, T. S., Scarlett, A., Henley, W. E., Depledge, M., Wallace, R. B., & ... . (2008). Association of urinary bisphenol A concentration with medical disorders and laboratory abnormalities in adults. *Journal of the American Medical Association, 300*(11), 1303–1310. doi:10.1001/jama.300.11.1303 PMID:18799442

LaRocca, J., Binder, A. M., McElrath, T. F., & Michels, K. B. (2014). The impact of first trimester phthalate and phenol exposure on IGF2/H19 genomic imprinting and birth outcomes. *Environmental Research, 133*, 396–406. doi:10.1016/j.envres.2014.04.032 PMID:24972507

Latini, G., De Felice, C., Presta, G., Del Vecchio, A., Paris, I., Ruggieri, F., & Mazzeo, P. (2003). In utero exposure to di-(2-ethylhexyl) phthalate and duration of human pregnancy. *Environmental Health Perspectives, 111*(14), 1783–1785. doi:10.1289/ehp.6202 PMID:14594632

Latini, G., Knipp, G., Mantovani, A., Marcovecchio, M. L., Chiarelli, F., & Soder, O. (2010). Endocrine disruptors and human health. *Mini-Reviews in Medicinal Chemistry, 10*(9), 846–855. doi:10.2174/138955710791608271 PMID:20482499

Lee, Ch.-Ch., Jiang, L.-Y., Kuo, Y.-L., Hsieh, Ch., Chen, C. S., & Tien, C.-J. (2013). The potential role of water quality parameters on occurrence of nonylphenol and bisphenol A and identificationof their discharge sources in the river ecosystems. *Chemosphere, 91*(7), 904–911. doi:10.1016/j.chemosphere.2013.02.006 PMID:23473432

Lee, H., & Peart, T. (2000). Bisphenol A contamination in Canadian municipal and industrial wastewater and sludge samples. *Water Quality Research Journal of Canada, 35*(2), 283–298. doi:10.2166/wqrj.2000.018

Li, D. K., Zhou, Z., Miao, M., He, Y., Qing, D., Wu, T., ... Yuan, W. (2010a). Relationship between urine bisphenol-A level and declining male sexual function. *Journal of Andrology, 31*(5), 500–506. doi:10.2164/jandrol.110.010413 PMID:20467048

Li, D. K., Zhou, Z., Qing, D., He, Y., Wu, T., Miao, M., ... Yuan, W. (2010b). Occupational exposure to bisphenol-A (BPA) and the risk of self-reported male sexual dysfunction. *Human Reproduction (Oxford, England), 25*(2), 519–527. doi:10.1093/humrep/dep381 PMID:19906654

Liao, Ch., Liu, F., & Kannan, K. (2012). Bisphenol S, a new bisphenol analogue in paper products and currency bills and its association with bisphenol A residues. *Environmental Science & Technology, 46*(12), 6515–6522. doi:10.1021/es300876n PMID:22591511

Lind, P. M., Zethelius, B., & Lind, L. (2012). Circulating levels of phthalate metabolites are associated with prevalent diabetes in the elderly. *Diabetes Care, 35*(7), 1519-1524. doi:10.2337/dc11-2396

Liu, J., Yu, P., Qian, W., Li, Y., Zhao, J., Huan, F., ... Xiao, H. (2013). Perinatal bisphenol A exposure and adult glucose homeostasis: Identifying critical windows of exposure. *PLoS One, 8*(5), e64143. doi:10.1371/journal.pone.0064143 PMID:23675523

Loganathan, S., & Kannan, K. (2011). Occurrence of bisphenol A in indoor dust from two locations in the Eastern United States and implications for human exposures. *Archives of Environmental Contamination and Toxicology, 61*(1), 68–73. doi:10.100700244-010-9634-y PMID:21221962

Magliano, D. J., & Lyons, J. G. (2013). Bisphenol A and diabetes, insulin resistance, cardiovascular disease and obesity: Controversy in a (plastic) cup? *The Journal of Clinical Endocrinology and Metabolism*, *98*(2), 502–504. doi:10.1210/jc.2012-3058 PMID:23264398

Manikkam, M., Tracey, R., Guerrero-Bosagna, C., & Skinner, M. K. (2013). Plastics derived endocrine disruptors (BPA, DEHP and DBP) induce epigenetic transgenerational inheritance of obesity, reproductive disease and sperm epimutations. *PLoS One*, *8*(1), e55387. doi:10.1371/journal.pone.0055387 PMID:23359474

Mantovani, A. (2006). Risk assessment of endocrine disrupters: The role of toxicological studies. *Annals of the New York Academy of Sciences*, *1076*(1), 239–252. doi:10.1196/annals.1371.063 PMID:17119206

Marsee, K., Woodruff, T. J., Axelrad, D. A., Calafat, A. M., & Swan, S. H. (2006). Estimated daily phthalate exposures in a population of mothers of male infants exhibiting reduced anogenital distance. *Environmental Health Perspectives*, *114*(6), 805–809. doi:10.1289/ehp.8663 PMID:16759976

Meeker, J. D., & Ferguson, K. K. (2012). Dioxins and health: including other persistent organic pollutantsand endocrine disruptors. In *Phthalates: human exposure and related health effects*. Hoboken, NJ: Wiley.

Meeker, J. D., Sathyanarayana, S., & Swan, S. H. (2009). Phthalates and other additives in plastics: Human exposure and associated health outcomes. *Philosophical Transactions of the Royal Society of London. Series B, Biological Sciences*, *364*(1526), 2097–2113. doi:10.1098/rstb.2008.0268 PMID:19528058

Melzer, D., Rice, N. E., Lewis, C., Henley, W. E., & Galloway, T. S. (2010). Association of urinary bisphenol a concentration with heart disease: Evidence from NHANES 2003/06. *PLoS One*, *5*(1), e8673. doi:10.1371/journal.pone.0008673 PMID:20084273

Mok-Lin, E., Ehrlich, S., Williams, P. L., Petrozza, J., Wright, D. L., Calafat, A. M., ... Hauser, R. (2010). Urinary bisphenol A concentrations and ovarian response among women undergoing IVF. *International Journal of Andrology*, *33*(2), 385–393. doi:10.1111/j.1365-2605.2009.01014.x PMID:20002217

Moriyama, K., Tagami, T., Akamizu, T., Usui, T., Saijo, M., Kanamoto, N., ... Nakao, K. (2002). Thyroid hormone action is disrupted by bisphenol A as an antagonist. *TheJournal of Clinical Endocrinology and Metabolism*, *87*(11), 5185–5190. doi:10.1210/jc.2002-020209 PMID:12414890

Morrissey, S. (2008).. . *Chemical and Engineering News*.

Mu, D., Gao, F., Fan, Z., Shen, H., Peng, H., & Hu, J. (2015). Levels of Phthalate Metabolites in Urine of Pregnant Women and Risk of Clinical Pregnancy Loss. *Environmental Science & Technology*, *49*(17), 10651–10657. doi:10.1021/acs.est.5b02617 PMID:26251123

Munguıa-Lopez, E., Gerardo-Lugo, S., Peralta, E., Bolumen, S., & Soto-Valdez, H. (2005). Migration of bisphenol A (BPA) from can coatings into a fatty-food stimulant and tuna fish. *Food Additives and Contaminants*, *22*(9), 892–898. doi:10.1080/02652030500163674 PMID:16192075

Nagorka, R., Conrad, A., Scheller, C., Sussenbach, B., & Moriske, H. J. (2010). Plasticizers and flame retardants in household dust — part 1: Phthalates. Gefahrstoffe — Reinhalt. *Luft*, *70*(3), 70–76.

Nahar, M. S., Liao, C., Kannan, K., & Dolinoy, D. C. (2012). Fetal Liver Bisphenol A Concentrations and Biotransformation Gene Expression Reveal Variable Exposure and Altered Capacity for Metabolism in Humans. *Journal of Biochemical and Molecular Toxicology*, *27*(2), 116–123. doi:10.1002/jbt.21459 PMID:23208979

Nam, S., Seo, Y., & Kim, M. (2010). Bisphenol A migration from polycarbonate baby bottle with repeated use. *Chemosphere*, *79*(9), 949–952. doi:10.1016/j.chemosphere.2010.02.049 PMID:20334893

Net, S., Rabodonirina, S., Ben Sghaier, R., Dumoulin, D., Chbib, C., Tlili, I., & … . (2015). Distribution of phthalates, pesticides and drug residues in the dissolved, particulate and sedimentary phases from transboundary rivers (France–Belgium). *The Science of the Total Environment*, *521-522*, 152–159. doi:10.1016/j.scitotenv.2015.03.087 PMID:25829293

Niu, Y., Zhang, J., Wu, Y., & Shao, B. (2012). Analysis of bisphenol A and alkylphenols in cereals by automated on-line solid-phase extraction and liquid chromatography tandem massspectrometry. *Journal of Agricultural and Food Chemistry*, *60*(24), 6116–6122. doi:10.1021/jf301401k PMID:22646661

Park, M. A., Hwang, K. A., Lee, H. R., Yi, B. R., Jeung, E. B., & Choi, K. C. (2012). Cell growth of BG-1 ovarian cancer cells is promoted by di-n-butyl phthalate and hexabromocyclododecane via upregulation of the cyclin D and cyclin-dependent kinase-4 genes. *Molecular Medicine Reports*, *5*(3), 761–766. doi:10.3892/mmr.2011.712 PMID:22179484

Prins, G. S., Tang, W. Y., Belmonte, J., & Ho, S. M. (2008). Developmental exposure to bisphenol a increases prostate cancer susceptibility in adult rats: Epigenetic mode of action is implicated. *Fertility and Sterility*, *89*(2Suppl), e41. doi:10.1016/j.fertnstert.2007.12.023 PMID:18308059

Proshad, R., Kormoker, T., Islam, M. S., Haque, M. S., Rahman, M. M., & Mithu, M. M. R. (2018). Toxic effects of plastic on human health and environment: A consequences of health risk assessment in Bangladesh. *International Journal of Health*, *6*(1), 1–5. doi:10.14419/ijh.v6i1.8655

Rajesh, P., & Balasubramanian, K. (2014). Phthalate exposure in utero causes epigenetic changes and impairs insulin signalling. *Journal of Endocrinology, 223*(1), 47-66. doi:10.1530/JOE-14-0111

Richter, C., Birnbaum, L., Farabollini, F., Newbold, R., Rubin, B., Talsness, C., ... Saal, F. (2007). *In vivo* effects of bisphenol A in laboratory rodent studies. *Reproductive Toxicology (Elmsford, N.Y.)*, *24*(2), 199–224. doi:10.1016/j.reprotox.2007.06.004 PMID:17683900

Rowsell, V. F., Tangney, P., Hunt, C., & Voulvoulis, N. (2010). Estimating levels of micro pollutants in municipal waste water. *Water, Air, and Soil Pollution*, *206*(1–4), 357–368. doi:10.100711270-009-0112-y

Saal, F., Nagel, S., Coe, B., Angle, B., & Taylor, J. (2012). The estrogenicendocrine disrupting chemical bisphenol A (BPA) and obesity. *Molecular and Cellular Endocrinology*, *354*(1-2), 74–84. doi:10.1016/j.mce.2012.01.001 PMID:22249005

Saal, F. S., Akingbemi, B. T., Belcher, S. M., Birnbaum, L. S., Crain, D. A., Eriksen, M., & … . (2007). Chapel Hill bisphenol A expert panel consensus statement: Integration of mechanisms, effects in animals and potential to impact human health at current levels of exposure. *Reproductive Toxicology (Elmsford, N.Y.)*, *24*(2), 131–138. doi:10.1016/j.reprotox.2007.07.005 PMID:17768031

Schonfelder, G., Wittfoht, W., Hopp, H., Talsness, C. E., Paul, M., & Chahoud, I. (2002). Parent bisphenol A accumulation in the human maternal-fetal-placental unit. *Environmental Health Perspectives*, *110*(11), A703–A707. doi:10.1289/ehp.021100703 PMID:12417499

Shankar, A., & Teppala, S. (2011). Relationship between urinary bisphenol A levels and diabetes mellitus. *The Journal of Clinical Endocrinology and Metabolism*, *96*(12), 3822–3826. doi:10.1210/jc.2011-1682 PMID:21956417

Shankar, A., & Teppala, S. (2011). Relationship between urinary bisphenol A levels and diabetes mellitus. *The Journal of Clinical Endocrinology and Metabolism*, *96*(12), 3822–3826. doi:10.1210/jc.2011-1682 PMID:21956417

Shao, B., Han, H., Li, D., Ma, Y., Tu, X., & Wu, Y. (2007). Analysis ofalkylphenol and bisphenol A in meat by accelerated solvent extraction and liquid chromatography with tandem massspectrometry. *Food Chemistry*, *105*(3), 1236–1241. doi:10.1016/j.foodchem.2007.02.040

Sharpe, R. M., & Skakkebaek, N. E. (2008). Testicular dysgenesis syndrome: Mechanstic insights and potential new downstream effects. *Fertility and Sterility*, *89*(2), 33–38. doi:10.1016/j.fertnstert.2007.12.026 PMID:18308057

Sheikh, I. A. (2016). Stereoselectivity and the potential endocrine disrupting activity of di-(2-ethylhexyl) phthalate (DEHP) against human progesterone receptor: A computational perspective. *Journal of Applied Toxicology*, *36*(5), 741–747. doi:10.1002/jat.3302 PMID:26879776

Sheng, Z. G., Tang, Y., Liu, Y. X., Yuan, Y., Zhao, B. Q., Chao, X. J., & Zhu, B. Z. (2012). Low concentrations of bisphenol a suppressthyroid hormone receptor transcription through anongenomic mechanism. *Toxicology and Applied Pharmacology*, *259*(1), 133–142. doi:10.1016/j.taap.2011.12.018 PMID:22227104

Singh, S., & Shoei-Lung, L. S. (2011). Phthalates: Toxicogenomics and inferred human diseases. *Genomics*, *97*(3), 148–157. doi:10.1016/j.ygeno.2010.11.008 PMID:21156202

Singh, S., & Shoei-Lung, L. S. (2012). Bisphenol A and phthalates exhibit similar toxicogenomics and health effects. *Gene*, *494*(1), 85–91. doi:10.1016/j.gene.2011.11.035 PMID:22173104

Sonoda, E., Sasaki, M. S., Morrison, C., Yamaguchi-Iwai, Y., Takata, M., & Takeda, S. (1999). Sister chromatid exchanges are mediated by homologous recombination in vertebrate cells. *Molecular and Cellular Biology*, *19*(7), 5166–5169. doi:10.1128/MCB.19.7.5166 PMID:10373565

Soto, A. M., & Sonnenschein, C. (2010). Environmental causes of cancer: Endocrine disruptors as carcinogens. *Nature Reviews. Endocrinology*, *6*(7), 363–370. doi:10.1038/nrendo.2010.87 PMID:20498677

Stahlhut, R. W., Van Wijngaarden, E., Dye, T. D., Cook, S., & Swan, S. H. (2007). Concentrations of urinary phthalate metabolites are associated with increased waist circumference and insulin resistance in adult U.S. males. *Environmental Health Perspectives*, *115*(5), 876–882. doi:10.1289/ehp.9882 PMID:17589594

Svensson, K., Hernández-Ramírez, R. U., Burguete-García, A., Cebrián, M. E., Calafat, A. M., Needham, L., ... López-Carrillo, L. (2011). Phthalate exposure associated with self-reported diabetes among Mexican women. *Environmental Research*, *111*(6), 792–796. doi:10.1016/j.envres.2011.05.015 PMID:21696718

Swan, S. H. (2008). Environmental phthalate exposure in relation to reproductive outcomes and other health endpoints in humans. *Environmental Research, 108*(2), 177–184. doi:10.1016/j.envres.2008.08.007 PMID:18949837

Swan, S. H., Main, K. M., Liu, F., Stewart, S. L., Kruse, R. L., Calafat, A. M., ... Teague, J. L. (2005). Decrease in anogenital distance among male infants with prenatal phthalate exposure. *Environmental Health Perspectives, 113*(8), 1056–1061. doi:10.1289/ehp.8100 PMID:16079079

Takeuchi, T., Tsutsumi, O., Ikezuki, Y., Takai, Y., & Taketani, Y. (2004). Positive relationship between androgen and the endocrine disruptor, bisphenol A, in normal women and women with ovarian dysfunction. *Endocrine Journal, 51*(2), 165–169. doi:10.1507/endocrj.51.165 PMID:15118266

Talsness, C. E., Andrade, A. J., Kuriyama, S. N., Taylor, J. A., & vom Saal, F. S. (2009). Components of plastic: Experimental studies in animals and relevance for human health. *Philosophical Transactions of the Royal Society of London. Series B, Biological Sciences, 364*(1526), 2079–2096. doi:10.1098/rstb.2008.0281 PMID:19528057

Tang, W. Y., Morey, L. M., Cheung, Y. Y., Birch, L., Prins, G. S., & Ho, S. M. (2010). Neonatal exposure to estradiol/bisphenol A alters promoter methylation and expression of *Nsbp1* and *Hpcal1* genes and transcriptional programs of Dnmt3a/b and Mbd2/4 in the rat prostate gland throughout life. *Endocrinology, 153*(1), 42–55. doi:10.1210/en.2011-1308 PMID:22109888

Tarantino, G., Valentino, R., Di Somma, C., D'Esposito, V., Passaretti, F., Pizza, G., & ... . (2012). Bisphenol A in Polycystic Ovary Syndrome and its Association with Liver-Spleen Axis. *Horumon To Rinsho, 78*(3), 447–453. doi:10.1111/j.1365-2265.2012.04500.x PMID:22805002

Taylor, J. A., Vom Saal, F. S., Welshons, W. V., Drury, B., Rottinghaus, G., Hunt, P. A., ... VandeVoort, C. A. (2010). Similarity of bisphenol A pharmacokinetics in rhesus monkeys and mice: Relevance for human exposure. *Environmental Health Perspectives, 119*(4), 422–430. doi:10.1289/ehp.1002514 PMID:20855240

Thompson, C. J., Ross, S. M., Hensley, J., Liu, K., Heinze, S. C., Young, S. S., & Gaido, K. W. (2005). Differential steroidogenic gene expression in the fetal adrenal gland versus the testis and rapid and dynamic response of the fetal testis to di(n-butyl) phthalate. *Biology of Reproduction, 73*(5), 908–917. doi:10.1095/biolreprod.105.042382 PMID:15987825

Thompson, R. C., Moore, C. J., vom Saal, F. S., & Swan, S. H. (2009). Plastics, the environment and human health: Current consensus and future trends. *Philosophical Transactions of the Royal Society of London. Series B, Biological Sciences, 364*(1526), 2153–2166. doi:10.1098/rstb.2009.0053 PMID:19528062

Upson, K., Sathyanarayana, S., De Roos, A. J., Thompson, M. L., Scholes, D., Dills, R., & Holt, V. L. (2013). Phthalates and risk of endometriosis. *Environmental Research, 126*, 91–97. doi:10.1016/j.envres.2013.07.003 PMID:23890968

Vandenberg, L., Hauser, R., Marcus, M., Olea, N., & Welshons, W. (2007). Human exposure to bisphenol A (BPA). *Reproductive Toxicology (Elmsford, N.Y.), 24*(2), 139–177. doi:10.1016/j.reprotox.2007.07.010 PMID:17825522

Vandenberg, L. N., Colborn, T., Hayes, T. B., Heindel, J. J., Jacobs, D. R. Jr, Lee, D. H., ... Myers, J. P. (2012). Hormonesand endocrine-disrupting chemicals: Low-dose effects and nonmonotonic dose responses. *Endocrine Reviews*, *33*(3), 378–455. doi:10.1210/er.2011-1050 PMID:22419778

Vinas, R., Jeng, Y. J., & Watson, C. S. (2012). Non-genomic effects of xenoestrogen mixtures. *International Journal of Environmental Research and Public Health*, *9*(8), 2694–2714. doi:10.3390/ijerph9082694 PMID:23066391

Wang, T., Li, M., Chen, B., Xu, M., Xu, Y., Huang, Y., ... Ning, G. (2012). Urinary bisphenol A (BPA) concentration associates with obesity and insulin resistance. *The Journal of Clinical Endocrinology and Metabolism*, *97*(2), E223–E227. doi:10.1210/jc.2011-1989 PMID:22090277

Wang, T., Lu, J., Xu, M., Xu, Y., Li, M., Liu, Y., ... Ning, G. (2013). Urinary bisphenol Aconcentration and thyroid function in Chinese adults. *Epidemiology (Cambridge, Mass.)*, *24*(2), 295–302. doi:10.1097/EDE.0b013e318280e02f PMID:23337242

Welshons, W. V., Nagel, S. C., & Vomsaal, F. S. (2006). Large effects fromsmall exposures. III. Endocrine mechanisms mediating effects of bisphenol A at levels of human exposure. *Endocrinology*, *147*(6), 56–69. doi:10.1210/en.2005-1159 PMID:16690810

Wetherill, Y., Akingbemi, B., Kanno, J., McLachlan, J., Nadal, A., Sonnenschein, C., ... Belcher, S. (2007). In vitro molecular mechanisms of bisphenol A action. *Reproductive Toxicology (Elmsford, N.Y.)*, *24*(2), 178–198. doi:10.1016/j.reprotox.2007.05.010 PMID:17628395

WHO. (2003). Retrieved from http://www.who.int/water_sanitation_health/dwq/chemicals/di2ethylhexyphthalate.pdf

Willhite, C. C., Ball, G. L., & McLellan, C. J. (2008). Derivation of a bisphenol A oral reference dose (RfD) and drinking-water equivalent concentration. *Journal of Toxicology and Environmental Health*, *11*(2), 69–146. doi:10.1080/10937400701724303 PMID:18188738

Wu, S., Zhu, J., Li, Y., Lin, T., Gan, L., Yuan, X., ... Wei, G. (2010). Dynamic effect of di-2- (ethylhexyl) phthalate on testicular toxicity: Epigenetic changes and their impact on gene expression. *International Journal of Toxicology*, *29*(2), 193–200. doi:10.1177/1091581809355488 PMID:20335514

Yamaguchi, A., Ishibashi, H., Kohra, S., Arizono, K., & Tominaga, N. (2005). Short-term effects of endocrine-disrupting chemicals on the expression of estrogen-responsive genes in male medaka (Oryzias latipes*). Aquatic Toxicology (Amsterdam, Netherlands)*, *72*(3), 239–249. doi:10.1016/j.aquatox.2004.12.011 PMID:15820104

Yang, M., Kim, S. Y., Chang, S. S., Lee, I. S., & Kawamoto, T. (2006). Urinary concentrations of bisphenol A in relation to biomarkers of sensitivity and effect and endocrine-related health effects. *Environmental and Molecular Mutagenesis*, *47*(8), 571–578. doi:10.1002/em.20230 PMID:16795089

Yonekubo, J., Hayakawa, K., & Sajiki, J. (2008). Concentrations of bisphenol A, bisphenol A diglycidyl ether, and their derivatives in canned foods in Japanese markets. *Journal of Agricultural and Food Chemistry*, *56*(6), 2041–2047. doi:10.1021/jf073106n PMID:18284199

Yoshida, T., Horie, M., Hoshino, Y., Nakazawa, H., Horie, M., & Nakazawa, H. (2001). Determination of bisphenol A in canned vegetables and fruitby high performance liquid chromatography. *Food Additives and Contaminants*, *18*(1), 69–75. doi:10.1080/026520301446412 PMID:11212549

Zhang, Y., Meng, X., Chen, L., Li, D., Zhao, L., Zhao, Y., ... Shi, H. (2014). Age and sex-specific relationships between phthalate exposures and obesity in Chinese children at puberty. *PLoS One*, *9*(8), e104852. doi:10.1371/journal.pone.0104852 PMID:25121758

KEY TERMS AND DEFINITIONS

Comparative Toxicogenomics Database: The Comparative Toxicogenomics Database (CTD) is a research tool that provides curated scientific data describing the relationship between various chemicals, genes/proteins, diseases, phenotypes, pathways, and interaction components.

Gene Ontology: Gene ontology (GO) is a bioinformatics tool used to unify the representation of gene/gene product attributes across all the species.

Plasticizers: Plasticizers are the chemical additives thatincrease the elasticity of plastic. Plasticizers tend to soften the plastic in order to make it more flexible and bendable.

Epigenetic Modifications: Epigenetic modifications alter the genomic expression and its effects without altering the actual DNA sequence. These include DNA methylation, histone modification and microRNA-mediated genetic silencing.

Chapter 15
Environmental Phthalate Exposure in Relation to Reproductive Outcomes and Other Health Endpoints in Humans

Irfan Ashraf Badroo
Sant Gadge Baba Amravati University, India

Zainab Kalimuddin Ali
Sant Gadge Baba Amravati University, India

Ashiq Hussain Khanday
Sant Gadge Baba Amravati University, India

Suriya Ashraf Badroo
Barkatuallah University, India

ABSTRACT

Phthalates are a group of manmade chemicals which may be regarded as heroes having profound application in industries belongs to dieters of 1, 2-benzenedicarboxylic acid (phthalic acid). They are mainly used as plasticizer. Phthalates may be of high and low molecular weight, and have find their existence in the manufacturing of various products that are of daily use to humans and pose threat to non-occupational humans besides of those working in the industries where phthalate based products are manufactured. Phthalates are now widely used and therefore it is difficult to avoid their exposure; thus, its adverse effects are very certain. The literature present revealed that phthalate exposure has made alteration both to females and males, like reproductive alterations: including damaging the sperm quality, semen concentration and sperm DNA, breast cancer in females, AGD, endocrine disruption. The phthalate exposure has been shown to alter the behavior, which is an indication of nervous system damage. Phthalate exposure has been revealed to affect the respiration. Phthalate after exposure has been found to get metabolized in various end points and their detection by various techniques has made an insight towards understanding the mechanism of phthalates toxicity. Phthalates both of low and high molecular weight have found their way to fauna and created a mess with the physiology of animals or humans. Thus, precaution is better, as said prevention is better than cure. The suggestive remedy for phthalate exposure is to make less use of products that contain phthalate material, more importantly

DOI: 10.4018/978-1-5225-9452-9.ch015

during pregnancy and developmental stage of infants. Utmost care has been taken in regard to the literature cited. The data included in this chapter has been taken from those research articles with indexing of Science Citation Index Expanded, Scopus as for authenticity, and also using the Web of Science Database, which provides interactive citation.

INTRODUCTION

Phthalates (common name) are group of manmade chemicals regarded as heroes which have profound application in industries, medical, automotive and consumer product industries (US Department of Health and Human Services Centers for Disease Control and Prevention, 2013) belongs to dieters of 1, 2-benzenedicarboxylic acid (phthalic acid). They are mainly used as plasticizer to impart flexibility to polyvinylchloride (PVC) (ATSDR, 1995; ATSDR, 1997; ATSDR, 2001; ATSDR, 2002). Phthalates being the family of industrial compounds have found its use in various products like perfumes, lotions, cosmetics, paints, medical devices, pharmaceuticals, flooring and wall coverings, food contact applications, and medical devices etc. (ATSDR, 1995; ATSDR, 1997; ATSDR, 2001; ATSDR, 2002; Blount *et al.*, 2000; Blount, 2000; CERHR, 2000; NTP-CERHR, 2000; Hauser *et al.*, 2004).

Phthalates may be of high molecular weight and of low molecular weight, which have found their existence in the manufacture of various products that are of daily use to humans and pose threat to non-occupational humans besides those working in the industries where phthalate based products are manufactured. Phthalates are now widely used and therefore it is difficult to avoid the exposure, thus its adverse effects are probably very certain.

Di (2-ethylhexyl) phthalate (DEHP), di-isononyl phthalate (DiNP), di-n-octyl phthalate (DnOP), butyl benzyl phthalate (BBzP) are some examples of high molecular weight phthalates that are used as plasticizers in polyvinyl chloride (ATSDR, 1997: David *et al.*, 2001; ATSDR, 2002; Wormuth *et al.*, 2006; Cao, 2010; USEPA, Zota *et al.*, 2014). Low molecular weight phthalates like diethyl phthalate (DEP) and dibutyl phthalate (DBP) have found their use as a solvent in daily usage products like perfumes, lotions, cosmetics, scent, to hold colour for personal care products (Duty *et al.* 2005; Sathyanarayana, 2008) and as plasticizers for making varnishes, lacquers etc., (ATSDR, 1995: ATSDR, 2001; David *et al.*,2001).

Phthalate use has now become so abundant that it is very difficult to get rid of. Usage of it in daily products has led to an alarming condition and has resulted in various abnormalities both in animals and human beings. On investigation in laboratory animals Phthalates are now known to be carcinogenic causing injury of various vital organs like liver, testes and may cause malformations, reproductive toxicity, anti-androgenic activity and even fetal death (ATSDR, 1995; ATSDR, 1997; ATSDR, 2001; ATSDR, 2002; ATSDR, 2002, Valles *et al.*, 2003), while in humans carcinogenicity of phthalates is uncertain (IARC, 2000; Klaunig *et al.*, 2003; Latini *et al.*, 2004; Wilson *et al.*, 2004). With regard to some of its products it has been held responsible for causing male reproductive deformities, thus is reproductive toxicant (Gray *et al.*, 2000; Parks *et al.*, 2000; Ema, 2001).

Phthalates have also been involved in interfering the function of endocrine system (Damstra *et al.*, 2004; Sharpe and Irvine, 2004; Latini *et al.*, 2004), which are responsible for growth and sexual development of both males and females (Sharpe, 2001; Lovekamp-Swan and Davis, 2003). There is increasing evidence to indicate that environmental exposure to phthalates is associated with adverse effects on human fecundity (Swan, 2008; Meeker *et al.*, 2009).

EXPOSURE OF PHTHALATES

As Phthalates are being extensively used in many frequently used products, hence found easily their way to humans. The route of exposure are many and effects are quite obvious. Humans in their lives have high chances of phthalate exposure through inhalation, ingestion and through dermal exposure (Adibi *et al.*, 2003; Latini *et al.*, 2003a,b).

EXPOSURE THROUGH ORAL ROUTE

For phthalates being mainly used as plasticizers such as DEPH, exposure through oral route predominates, (Huber *et al.*, 1996; Doull *et al.*, 1999; Silva *et al.*, 2003). Phthalates have low volatility and their presence in indoor air (Adibi *et al.*, 2003; Rudel *et al.*, 2003; Bornehag *et al.*, 2005; Kolarik *et al.*, 2008) and house dust (Rudel *et al.*, 2003) is reported. Oral exposure is one of the main route, it may be via food, water and other liquids and in children's it may be through mouthing of toys and teethers. While inhalation can also act as a source of exposure as phthalates are volatile and sources may be PVC, nail polish, hair spray, and other phthalate-containing products. Maternal exposure to fetus may also happen via: tubing used in neonatal intensive care nurseries, as phthalates have been found to cross placenta and their presence has been reported in amniotic fluid and may cause developmental abnormalities (Latini *et al.*, 2003).

EXPOSURE THROUGH DERMAL CONTACT

Dermal contact of diethyl phthalate (DEP) via; cosmetics and other personal care products has also been reported (ATSDR, 1995, 1997, 2001, 2002; Wormuth *et al.*, 2006; Bradley *et al.*, 2013). Large scale use of phthalates in medical devices mostly PVC devices may also contribute to its exposure (FDA, 2001; ATSDR, 2002; Shea, 2003). However, the relative contribution from the various sources and routes of exposure to phthalates is unknown (Wormuth *et al.*, 2006)

EXPOSURE THROUGH DIET

Koch *et al.*, (2013) in their investigation found that diet is the main source of phthalate (DEHP, DiNP and DiDP) exposure, while nonfood exposure of phthalates (DMP, DEP, DiBP, DnBP and BBzP) was reported. Same report of phthalates (DMP, DEP, DnBP, DiBP and DnOP) exposure was reported by (Colacino *et al.*, 2010; Trasande *et al.*, 2013). Various daily usage items used in packaging food were found to be responsible for migration of phthalates in food. These materials (lid gaskets, food-packaging films, gloves) are used in preparation of food and thus contaminate it (Cao, 2010; Indirect Food Additives, 2014). While foods high in fat have been found to be contaminated with high molecular Phthalates like DEPH (Cao, 2010). A large investigation of food monitoring survey in North America, Asia and Europe was reviewed and found varied food phthalate concentrations (Wormuth, *et al.*, 2006; Cao *et al.*, 2008; Montouri *et al.*, 2008; Poças *et al.*, 2010; Fierens *et al.*, 2012; Martine *et al.*, 2013; Schecter, 2013).

DEPH was found in beef in United States and Canada (Schecter *et al.*, 2013; Page and Lacroix, 1995). Pageand Lacroix, 1995 also repoted that oils and fats including butter, margarine, cooking oils and animal fats such as lard were contaminated with DEHP, DnBP and BBzP. Whilst, low dairy products: yogurt, milk, eggs, grain, pasta, noodles, rice, fruits and vegetables found in jars were significantly contaminated with phthalates . Drinking water was also seen to have been contaminated with phthalates (DEPH) of highest concentration (Wormuth *et al.*, 2006).

Phthalate contamination in food products is certain as their use in food additives has been approved (US FDA, 2000, 2003).DEPH is most prevalent in food among the phthalates (Hannas *et al.*, 2011) and is seen to cause developmental abnormalities in early life stages (Swan, 2008).

MARKERS OF PHTHALATES

Phthalates after its exposure are rapidly metabolised with elimination half-lives of less than 24 hours (Koch *et al.*, 2005). After metabolism it is excreted in urine and faeces (ATSDR, 1997; ATSDR, 20002; ATSDR, 1995; ATSDR, 2001). While in humans urine is preferred matrix for determination (Calafat and McKee, 2006). The same statement has been supported by Teitelbaum *et al.*, (2008) who mentioned that single spot urine sample is sufficient for phthalate determination. While according to Needham *et al.*, (2005) saliva, sweat, milk and the storage matrices of fat (generally adipose tissue) and bone can also be preferred to monitor for phthalate exposure .

Phthalates after exposure undergo biotransformation phases and are metabolized further. Low molecular weight phthalates (for example, DEP) metabolism ends with the hydrolytic monoester, (Albro and Moore, 1974; ATSDR, 2001). While high molecular weight phthalates are first metabolized to their respective hydrolytic monoesters then after enzymatic oxidation yield oxidative metabolites. (Albro *et al.*, 1973; Albro and Thomson, 1973; Albro and lavenhar, 1989; McKee *et al.*, 2002). This transformation is regarded as phase I biotransformation in both cases of low and high molecular weight phthalates. After the first phase transformation, they can be excreted in urine or through faeces without undergoing any further change or they can under go another phase transformation called phase II biotransformation to produce glucuronide conjugates with increased water solubility and therefore increased urinary excretion. (ATSDR, 2002). The metabolism of some higher molecular weight phthalates (for example, DEHP, DiNP, di- isodecyl phthalate DiDP) and their oxidative products has been found in urine (McKee *et al.*, 2002; Koch *et al.*, 2004). In case of humans for these phthalates mono (2-ethyl-5-oxohexyl) phthalate (MEOHP), mono (2-ethyl-5-hydroxyhexyl) phthalate (MEHHP) and mono (2-ethylhexyl) phthalate (MEHP), are excreted in glucuronidated form (Kato *et al.*, 2004), while as monoethyl phthalate (MEP), the hydrolytic monoester of DEP, is mostly excreted in its free form (Silva *et al.*, 2003).

Phthalates are metabolised into various end products, thus sole biomarkers can be misleading. There are two ways to check or determine the phthalates exposure either by ambient monitoring or biological monitoring. Biological monitoring cannot justify the route of exposure (Weiss and Angerer, 2002; Wittassek and Angerer 2008).

Various methods have been framed to determine the phthalate in body fluids after their metabolism (Dirven *et al.*, 1993; Niino *et al.*, 2002; Koch *et al.*, 2003, Paris *et al.*, 2003; Silva *et al.*, 2003; Barr *et al.*, 2003; Kato *et al.*, 2004; 2004; Calafat *et al.*, 2004; Holm *et al.*, 2004; Preuss *et al.*, 2005). While for its determination in environment various studied has also been done (Otake *et al.*, 2001;Suzuki *et al.*, 2001; Vikelsoe *et al.*, 2002; Mihovec-Grdic *et al.*, 2002; Lin *et al.*, 2003; Psillakis *et al.*, 2004). Urinary phthalate monoester metabolites as biomarkers are being considers as an approach to detect phthalate exposure (Dirven *et al.*, 1993; Blount *et al.*, 2000).In case of rodents oxidative phthalate monoesters are major metabolites detected in urine after metabolism of DiNP and DnOP, like DEHP. (ATSDR, 1997; Albro, 1974; McKee *et al.*, 2002; Silva *et al.*, 2005). The aqueous solubility of the phthalate metabolites is major factor in case of humans to mark the percentage of free monoester excretion (Kato *et al.*, 2004; Silva *et al.*, 2003). In case of humans more precisely, the shorter-chain-length dialkyl phthalates (e.g. DEP and DBP) are predominantly metabolized by ester hydrolysis to the simple monoester phthalates, which are excreted in the urine, usually after glucuronidation. The longer-chain-length dialkyl phthalates, including DEHP, DnOP and DiNP, are similarly hydrolyzed to their respective monoester phthalates, but extensively further metabolized by oxidation of their alkyl side chain

DETECTION OF PHTHALATES

Phthalate monoesters are considered as biologically active molecules thus have an advantage. Chromatography technique has been used to measure the phthalate monoesters in urine, serum, breast milk, saliva, ovarian follicular fluid, seminal plasma, and amniotic fluid. High performance liquid chromatography (HPLC) is most common (Blount *et al.*, 2000; Kato *et al.*, 2003a; Holm *et al.*, 2004; Takatori *et al.*, 2004). Phthalate monoesters are converted to volatile derivatives and then measured by Gas chromatography (Alzaga *et al.*, 2003). While trace levels of phthalate monoesters in biological matrices has been measured using isotope dilution HPLC coupled with tandem mass spectrometry (MS/MS) (Blount*et al.*, 2000; Silva *et al.*, 2003; Kato *et al* 2003a; Kato *et al.*, 2003b; Koch *et al.*, 2003, 2004; Takatori *et al.*, 2004; Calafat *et al.*, 2004; Silva *et al.*, 2004; Kato *et al.*, 2005; Preuss *et al.*, 2005). The recent availability of sensitive, specific, and economical assays make such measures practicable for epidemiological studies (Silva *et al.*, 2007).

FEMALE ABNORMALITIES

Breast Cancer, Cryptorchidism Anomalies in Pregnancy, Endocrine Disruptive and Anogenital Distance in Females

Phthalates serum level was held responsible for premature development of breast (thelarche) in young girls (Colon *et al.*, 2000). Phthalate metabolite level is linked to endometrioses a rear condition seen in females (Silva *et al.*, 2005). Breast cancer has also been linked to urinary concentration of phthalate metabolites (Lopez-Carillo *et al.*, 2010). Diethyl phthalate, the parent compound of MEP may be associated with increased risk of breast cancer (López-Carrillo *et al.*, 2010). Cryptorchidism a condition seen in males found its relation to phthalate exposure while breast feeding (Main *et al.*, 2006). AGD in females is also linked to phthalate exposure (Phillip *et al.*, 1996; Callegari *et al.*, 1987).Female exposure to monoethyl phthalate (MEP) was associated with longer time to pregnancy (Thomsen *et al.*, 2016) while DEHP was responsible for shorter time to pregnancy (Specht *et al.*, 2015) and its metabolites showed lower reproducibility. Phthalate in men and pregnant women has been reported to interfere with thyroid function (Meeker *et al.*, 2007; Huang *et al.*, 2007).

In animal studies phthalate esters are not found to be estrogenic (Zacharewski *et al.*, 1998). However, DEHP and its metabolite MEHP are toxic to ovary of mature rats (Davis *et al.*, 1994a,b; Lovekamp *et al.*, 2001). Hypoestrogenic, hypoprogestinic, anovulatory cycles were also reported in adult female rats when exposed to DEHP and MEHP (Lovekamp *et al.*, 2001). Harris *et al.*, (1997) reported Butyl benzyl phthalate (BBzP), di-n-butyl phthalate (DBP), di isobutyl phthalate (DIBP), di ethyl phthalate (DEP) and di-isononyl phthalate (DINP) are responsible for weak estrogenic activity *in vitro*, while DBP and DEHP were not shown to be estrogenic. (Gray *et al.*, 1984). The insight related to animal toxicity discussed above can also be seen in humans.

MALE ABNORMALITIES

Liver was also seen found to be the affected with chances at histological level and was even found to be carcinogenic when exposure was due to some phthalates (for example, DEHP and DiNP) (ATSDR, 1997 McKee *et al.*, 2002), while in case of humans these effects are un settled as of metabolic differences among species (Melnick, 2001; Doull *et al.*, 1999; IARC, 2000; Klaunig *et al.*, 2003)

Phthalate (DBP) dose during gestation was found to be responsible for reproductive tract developmental anomalies in rats (Mylchreest *et al.*, 1998; Mylchreest *et al.*, 1999; Mylchreest *et al.*, 2000). This could also be the case with humans; therefore, necessary measures and the human examination in the similar regard are of prime importance.

Hypospadias, Cryptorchidism, and Anogenital Distance and Gynecomastia

In humans androgen receptor bfunction was affected by (DBP, BBzP, DEHP, and DINP) (Foster *et al.*, 2001).Phthalates have been found to cause hypospadias, cryptorchidism, and anogenital distance in males when exposure was from maternal route (Van Tongeren *et al.*, 2002; Salazar- Martinez *et al.*, 2004; Morales-Suarez-Varela *et al.,* 2011). Same study of anogenital distance was reported by Swan *et al.*, (2005). Anogenital distance was also confirmed, while phthalate exposure on animals was investigated (Parks *et al.*, 2000; Barlow and Foster, 2003; Tyl *et al.*, 2004). Gynecomastia is linked to phthalate exposure (Durmaz *et al.,* 2010). In rodents Di (2-ethylhexyl) phthalate (DEHP), di-n-butyl phthalate (DBP), benzyl butyl phthalate (BzBP), di-isononyl phthalate (DINP) and BzBP was found to be responsible for causing abnormalities in reproductive tract (Parks *et al.*, 2000; Akingbemi *et al.*, 2004; Borch *et al.*, 2005; Foster, 2006; Gray *et al.*, 2000). Testosterone reduction by leydig cells and insulin-like growth factor-3 (Insl-3) after phthalate (DBP, DEHP and BzBP) exposure cause "phthalate syndrome" which may result in anogenital distance include hypospadias, cryptorchidism and malformations of the epididymis, vas deferens, seminal vesicles, and prostate (Foster, 2006; Welsh *et al.*, 2008; Wirth *et al.*, 2008; Pant *et al.*, 2008).

Testicular Toxicity

Testicular toxicity has been seen in case of rats and the level of toxicity was depend on side chain length of phthalates (Foster *et al.*, 1980; Gray *et al.*, 1984; Gray *et al.*, 2000). DBP, BBzP, DEHP exposure from teenage to adulthood in experimental animals reported testicular toxicity (Parks *et al.*, 2000; Srivastava *et al.*, 1990), although mature animals were more resistant and were less effected than puberty age animals

(Higuchi *et al.*, 2003). The toxicity was of germ cell loss thus effecting spermatogenesis (Li *et al.*, 2003). However species response was varied with low response in marmosets than in rodents. (Kurata *et al.*, 1998). Hardell *et al.*, (1997) reported phthalates have potential of causing testicular cancer. Decreased semen quality a marker of testicular toxicity was reported in association of phthalate exposure in adult men by (Joensen *et al.*, 2012). Histological changes were predominant in seminiferous tubules when exposed to DEHP, DBP and the main urinary metabolite, MBP (Gangolli, 1982).

Sperm Damage

While phthalate exposure has been found to alter the sperm DNA, semen characteristics and reproductive hormones (Akingbemi *et al.*, 2001; Duty *et al.*, 2003, 2005). Phthalate exposure was found to alter the serum level of FSH, LH, SHBG, testosterone, and inhibin-B thus depicting relationship of urinary level of phthalate with that of serum hormones (Duty *et al.*, 2005). Ge *et al.*, (2007) reported that low dose of phthalates increase the testosterone production either by increasing the leydig cell number (Foster *et al.*, 2001) or by increasing the testosterone production, while higher dose in rats had the opposite effect inhibiting the testosterone level. However, the other studies reported low protein level in fetal leydig cells and had an impact on cholesterol and steroid synthesis (Borch *et al.*, 2006). In case of female rats it induces a syndrome resembling to testicular dysgenesis in the rat male offspring (Foster *et al.*, 2001, Fisher *et al.*, 2003).Comet assay was performed on sperm DNA and it was found that phthalates (MEP and MEHP) have the potential to damage the DNA (Duty *et al.,* 2003; Hauser *et al.*, 2007). Semen characteristics, sperm DNA damage, and serum reproductive hormones in men attending an infertility clinic were found to have exposure of phthalates (Duty *et al.*, 2003a, b). Phthalates have proved to have potential to cause reproduction and development anomalies in humans (NTP-CERHR, 2000)

Semen Quality

Relationship between sperm concentration and DBP concentration in cellular fraction of ejaculation was seen as reported by (Murature *et al.*, 1987). In the same vein a case reported from India Rozati *et al.*, (2002) found poor semen quality among the studied men which were found to have concentration of some mixtures of phthalates (DMP, DEP, DBP, BBzP, DEHP, and DnOP) in seminal plasma, with affected sperm DNA. Congruence reports of low semen quality by phthalate exposure was reported by (Murature *et al.*, 1987; Rozati *et al.*, 2002; Duty *et al.*, 2003; Duty *et al.*, 2004; Hauser *et al.*, 2006, 2007; Pant *et al.*, 2008; Wirth *et al.*, 2008; Herr *et al.*, 2009; Han *et al.*, 2009; Liu *et al.*, 2012). Industrial chemicals containing phthalates (Sharpe and Skakkebaek, 1993) have found to decline the sperm counts in developing countries (Swan *et al.*, 2000; Gangolli, 1982).

Studies on humans revealed that phthalates led to decreased sperm quality (Duty *et al.*, 2003a, b, 2005a, b; Hauser *et al.*, 2004, 2006; Kamrin, 2009) and have negative effects on children's health (Sathy-anarayana *et al.*, 2008), further reducing birth weight (Wolff *et al.*, 2008) and finally makes reproductive development anomalies (Lottrup *et al.*, 2006).

PHTHALATE EXPOSURE AFFECTING NERVOUS SYSTEM

Phthalate exposure was seen to disrupt the nervous system thus affecting behaviour among the studied boys and girls, and the behaviour alteration was of opposite pattern among them suggesting sex-specific effects of phthalates (Engel *et al.* 2009). Urinary phthalate concentration particularly LMW phthalate was found to be responsible with behavioural alterations like conduct problems, attention problems, and depression clinical scales, as well externalizing problems and behavioral symptoms index (BSI) (Engel *et al.,* 2010). While relationship of higher LMW Prenatal urinary phthalate concentrations was linked to Social Responsiveness Scale (SRS) measurements, positively with poorer scores on social cognition, social communication, and social awareness (Miodovnik *et al.,* 2011).

RESPIRATION RELATED ABNORMALITIES

Phthalate presence has been reported in house hold items and indoor air (Rudel *et al.*, 2003), thus phthalates acts as allergens or may play a role as adjuvant (Oie *et al.*, 1997; Jaakkola *et al.*, 1999). Phthalates have been related to asthma and allergy (Jaakkola *et al.,* 1999; Jaakkola *et al.*, 2000; Ponsonby *et al.*, 2003; Bornehag*et al.*, 2004; Kolarik *et al.*, 2008). Some other researchers have examined and related the use of PVC and phthalates in house dust to asthma and allergy (Jaakkola *et al.*, 1999; Jaakkola *et al.*, 2000; Bornehag *et al.*, 2004). BzBP and DEHP were also found to be associated with allergic like symptoms (Bornehag *et al.*, 2004; Kolarik *et al.*, 2008). PVC based products may cause air way inflammation and result in bronchial obstruction and asthma. MEHP is among the examples causing bronchial hypersensitivity in rats, (Doelman *et al.*, 1990), the reason may be it is similar to prostaglandins, potent mediators of inflammation. (Oie et al., 1997). Preterm infants were at high risk of bronchial asthma when exposed to PVC tubing materials (Shneider *et al.*, 1989). An investigation conducted on 2568 Finnish children aged 1–7 years by Jaakkola *et al.*, (2000) revealed the relationship between the presence of plastic wall materials in the home and respiratory health. An association was seen between the phthalate monoesters levels in urine with various pulmonary function parameters (forced vital capacity, forced expiratory volume, peak expiratory flow, and maximum mid-expiratory flow) (Hoppin and Ulmer, 2004).

CONCLUSION

As we have come to know that phthalates are being widely used in the daily use products and it is very difficult to stay out of their reach. Therefore, it is very necessary that everyone should have knowledge of their deleterious effects on humans (infants as well as adults). It is suggested that everyone should minimize the use of daily products which contains phthalates and try to keep these products out of the reach of kids.

ABBREVIATIONS

BBzP = Butyl benzyl phthalate
DBP = di-n-butyl phthalate
DEHP = Di (2-ethylhexyl) phthalate
DEP = diethyl phthalate
DiBP = di isobutyl phthalate
DiDP = di- isodecyl phthalate
DINP = di-isononyl phthalate
DMP = dimethyl phthalate
DnOP = di-n-octyl phthalate
FSH = Follicle stimulating hormone
LH = luteinizing hormone
LMW = LMW low molecular weight
MEHHP = mono (2-ethyl-5-hydroxyhexyl) phthalate
MEHP = mono (2-ethylhexyl) phthalate
MEOHP = Mono (2-ethyl-5-oxohexyl) phthalate
MEP = MEP monoethyl phthalate
PVC = polyvinylchloride
SHBG = SHBG sex-hormone binding globulin

REFERENCES

Adibi, J. J., Perera, F. P., Jedrychowski, W., Camann, D. E., Barr, D., Jacek, R., & Whyatt, R. M. (2003). Prenatal exposures to phthalates among women in New York City and Krakow, Poland. *Environmental Health Perspectives*, *111*(14), 1719–1722. doi:10.1289/ehp.6235 PMID:14594621

Adibi, J. J., Whyatt, R. M., Williams, P. L., Calafat, A. M., Camann, D., Herrick, R., ... Hauser, R. (2008). Characterization of phthalate exposure among pregnant women assessed by repeat air and urine samples. *Environmental Health Perspectives*, *116*(4), 467–473. doi:10.1289/ehp.10749 PMID:18414628

Akingbemi, B. T., Ge, R., Klinefelter, G. R., Zirkin, B. R., & Hardy, M. P. (2004). Phthalate-induced Leydig cell hyperplasia is associated with multiple endocrine disturbances. *Proceedings of the National Academy of Sciences of the United States of America*, *101*(3), 775–780. doi:10.1073/pnas.0305977101 PMID:14715905

Akingbemi, B. T., Youker, R. T., Sottas, C. M., Ge, R., Katz, E., Klinefelter, G. R., ... Hardy, M. P. (2001). Modulation of rat Leydig cell steroidogenic function by di (2-ethylhexyl) phthalate. *Biology of Reproduction*, *65*(4), 1252–1259. doi:10.1095/biolreprod65.4.1252 PMID:11566751

Albro, P. W., & Lavenhar, S. R. (1989). Metabolism of di(2-ethylhexyl)phthalate. *Drug Metabolism Reviews*, *21*(1), 13–34. doi:10.3109/03602538909029953 PMID:2696633

Albro, P. W., & Moore, B. (1974). Identification of the metabolites of simple phthalate diesters in rat urine. *Journal of Chromatography. A*, *94*, 209–218. doi:10.1016/S0021-9673(01)92368-4 PMID:4844611

Albro, P. W., & Thomas, R. O. (1973). Enzymatic hydrolysis of di-(2-ethylhexyl) phthalate by lipases. *BiochimicaetBiophysica Acta (BBA)- Lipids and Lipid Metabolism*, *306*(3), 380–390. doi:10.1016/0005-2760(73)90176-8

Alzaga, R., Peña, A., & Bayona, J. M. (2003). Determination of phthalic monoesters in aqueous and urine samples by solid-phase microextraction–diazomethane on-fibrederivatization–gas chromatography–mass spectrometry. *Journal of Separation Science*, *26*(1-2), 87–96. doi:10.1002/jssc.200390020

ATSDR. (1995). Toxicological profile for diethylphthalate, U.S. Department of Health and Human Services, Public Health Service, Agency for Toxic Substances and Disease Registry.

ATSDR. (1997). Toxicological profile for di-n-octylphthalate. U.S. Department of Health and Human Services, Public HealthS ervice, Agency for Toxic Substances and Disease Registry.

ATSDR. (2001). Toxicological profile for di-n-butyl phthalate. Agency for Toxic Substances and Disease Registry, Public Health Service Atlanta, Department of Health and Human Services.

ATSDR. (2002). Toxicological profile for di(2-ethylhexyl)phthalate (DEHP). U.S. Department of Health and Human Services, Public Health Service, Agency for Toxic Substances and Disease Registry.

Barlow, N. J., & Foster, P. M. (2003). Pathogenesis of male reproductive tract lesions from gestation through adulthood following in utero exposure to di (n-butyl) phthalate. *Toxicologic Pathology*, *31*(4), 397–410. PMID:12851105

Barr, D. B., Silva, M. J., Kato, K., Reidy, J. A., Malek, N. A., Hurtz, D., ... Calafat, A. M. (2003). Assessing human exposure to phthalates using monoesters and their oxidized metabolites as biomarkers. *Environmental Health Perspectives*, *111*(9), 1148–1151. doi:10.1289/ehp.6074 PMID:12842765

Blount, B. C., Milgram, K. E., Silva, M. J., Malek, N. A., Reidy, J. A., Needham, L. L., & Brock, J. W. (2000). Quantitative detection of eight phthalate metabolites in human urine using HPLC– APCI-MS/MS. *Analytical Chemistry*, *72*(17), 4127–4134. doi:10.1021/ac000422r PMID:10994974

Blount, B. C., Silva, M. J., Caudill, S. P., Needham, L. L., Pirkle, J. L., Sampson, E. J., ... Brock, J. W. (2000). Levels of seven urinary phthalate metabolites in a human reference population. *Environmental Health Perspectives*, *108*(10), 979–982. doi:10.1289/ehp.00108979 PMID:11049818

Borch, J., Axelstad, M., Vinggaard, A. M., & Dalgaard, M. (2006). Diisobutyl phthalate has comparable anti-androgenic effects to di-n-butyl phthalate in fetal rat testis. *Toxicology Letters*, *163*(3), 183–190. doi:10.1016/j.toxlet.2005.10.020 PMID:16458459

Borch, J., Dalgaard, M., & Ladefoged, O. (2005). Early testicular effects in rats perinatally exposed to DEHP in combination with DEHA—Apoptosis assessment and immunohistochemical studies. *Reproductive Toxicology (Elmsford, N.Y.)*, *19*(4), 517–525. doi:10.1016/j.reprotox.2004.11.004 PMID:15749266

Bornehag, C. G., Sundell, J., Weschler, C. J., Sigsgaard, T., Lundgren, B., Hasselgren, M., & Hägerhed-Engman, L. (2004). The association between asthma and allergic symptoms in children and phthalates in house dust: A nested case–control study. *Environmental Health Perspectives, 112*(14), 1393–1397. doi:10.1289/ehp.7187 PMID:15471731

Bornehag, C. G., Sundell, J., Weschler, C. J., Sigsgaard, T., Lundgren, B., Hasselgren, M., & Hägerhed-Engman, L. (2004). The association between asthma and allergic symptoms in children and phthalates in house dust: A nested case–control study. *Environmental Health Perspectives, 112*(14), 1393–1397. doi:10.1289/ehp.7187 PMID:15471731

Bradley, E. L., Burden, R. A., Bentayeb, K., Driffield, M., Harmer, N., Mortimer, D. N., & Castle, L. (2013). Exposure to phthalic acid, phthalate diesters and phthalate monoesters from foodstuffs: UK total diet study results. *Food Additives & Contaminants: Part A, 30*(4), 735–742. doi:10.1080/19440049.2013.781684 PMID:23641808

Calafat, A. M., & McKee, R. H. (2006). Integrating biomonitoring exposure data into the risk assessment process: Phthalates [diethyl phthalate and di (2-ethylhexyl) phthalate] as a case study. *Environmental Health Perspectives, 114*(11), 1783–1789. doi:10.1289/ehp.9059 PMID:17107868

Calafat, A. M., Slakman, A. R., Silva, M. J., Herbert, A. R., & Needham, L. L. (2004). Automated solid phase extraction and quantitative analysis of human milk for 13 phthalate metabolites. *Journal of Chromatography. B, Analytical Technologies in the Biomedical and Life Sciences, 805*(1), 49–56. doi:10.1016/j.jchromb.2004.02.006 PMID:15113539

Callegari, C., Everett, S., Ross, M., & Brasel, J. A. (1987). Anogenital ratio: Measure of fetal virilization in premature and full-term newborn infants. *The Journal of Pediatrics, 111*(2), 240–243. doi:10.1016/S0022-3476(87)80075-6 PMID:3612396

Cao, X. L. (2008). Determination of phthalates and adipate in bottled water by headspace solid-phase microextraction and gas chromatography/mass spectrometry. *Journal of Chromatography. A, 1178*(1-2), 231–238. doi:10.1016/j.chroma.2007.11.095 PMID:18082753

Cao, X. L. (2010). Phthalate esters in foods: Sources, occurrence, and analytical methods. *Comprehensive Reviews in Food Science and Food Safety, 9*(1), 21–43. doi:10.1111/j.1541-4337.2009.00093.x

CDC. (2003). Second national report on human exposure to environmental chemicals. US Department of Health and Human Services, Centers for Disease Control and Prevention, National Center for Environmental Health, Division of Laboratory Sciences.

CDC. (2005). Third national report on human exposure to environmental chemicals. US Department of Health and Human Services, Centers for Disease Control and Prevention, National Center for Environmental Health, Division of Laboratory Sciences.

Center for the Evaluation of Risks to Human Reproduction (CERHR). (2000). *NTP-CERHR Expert Panel Report on Di(2-ethyl- hexyl) Phthalate*. Alexandria, VA: Science International, Inc.

Colacino, J. A., Harris, T. R., & Schecter, A. (2010). Dietary intake is associated with phthalate body burden in a nationally representative sample. *Environmental Health Perspectives, 118*(7), 998–1003. doi:10.1289/ehp.0901712 PMID:20392686

Colón, I., Caro, D., Bourdony, C. J., & Rosario, O. (2000). Identification of phthalate esters in the serum of young Puerto Rican girls with premature breast development. *Environmental Health Perspectives, 108*(9), 895. PMID:11017896

Damstra, T., Barlow, S., Bergman, A., Kavlock, R., & Van Der Kraak, G. (Eds.). (2004). *Global assessment of the state of the science of endocrine disruptors.* International Programme on Chemical Safety. Retrieved from http://ehp.niehs.nih.gov/who/

David, R. M., McKee, R. H., Butala, J. H., Barter, R. A., &Kayser, M. (2001). Esters of Aromatic Mono-, Di-, and Tricarboxylic Acids, Aromatic Diacids and Di-, Tri-, OrPolyalcohols. *Patty's Toxicology.*

Davis, B. J., Maronpot, R. R., & Heindel, J. J. (1994). Di-(2-ethylhexyl) phthalate suppresses estradiol and ovulation in cycling rats. *Toxicology and Applied Pharmacology, 128*(2), 216–223. doi:10.1006/taap.1994.1200 PMID:7940536

Davis, B. J., Weaver, R., Gaines, L. J., & Heindel, J. J. (1994). Mono-(2-ethylhexyl) phthalate suppresses estradiol production independent of FSH-cAMP stimulation in rat granulosa cells. *Toxicology and Applied Pharmacology, 128*(2), 224–228. doi:10.1006/taap.1994.1201 PMID:7940537

Dirven, H. A. A. M., Van Den Broek, P. H. H., & Jongeneelen, F. J. (1993). Determination of four metabolites of the plasticizer di (2-ethylhexyl) phthalate in human urine samples. *International Archives of Occupational and Environmental Health, 64*(8), 555–560. doi:10.1007/BF00517700 PMID:8314613

Doelman, C. J. A., Borm, P. J. A., & Bast, A. (1990). Plasticizers and bronchial hyper reactivity. *Lancet, 335*(8691), 725. doi:10.1016/0140-6736(90)90839-W PMID:1969080

Doull, J., Cattley, R., Elcombe, C., Lake, B. G., Swenberg, J., Wilkinson, C., ... Van Gemert, M. (1999). A cancer risk assessment of di (2-ethylhexyl) phthalate: Application of the new US EPA Risk Assessment Guidelines. *Regulatory Toxicology and Pharmacology, 29*(3), 327–357. doi:10.1006/rtph.1999.1296 PMID:10388618

Durmaz, E., Özmert, E. N., Erkekoğlu, P., Giray, B., Derman, O., Hıncal, F., & Yurdakök, K. (2010). Plasma phthalate levels in pubertal gynecomastia. *Pediatrics, 125*(1), e122–e129. doi:10.1542/peds.2009-0724 PMID:20008419

Duty, S. M., Ackerman, R. M., Calafat, A. M., & Hauser, R. (2005). Personal care product use predicts urinary concentrations of some phthalate monoesters. *Environmental Health Perspectives, 113*(11), 1530–1535. doi:10.1289/ehp.8083 PMID:16263507

Duty, S. M., Calafat, A. M., Silva, M. J., Brock, J. W., Ryan, L., Chen, Z., ... Hauser, R. (2004). The relationship between environmental exposure to phthalates and computer-aided sperm analysis motion parameters. *Journal of Andrology, 25*(2), 293–302. doi:10.1002/j.1939-4640.2004.tb02790.x PMID:14760016

Duty, S. M., Calafat, A. M., Silva, M. J., Ryan, L., & Hauser, R. (2005). Phthalate exposure and reproductive hormones in adult men. *Human Reproduction (Oxford, England), 20*(3), 604–610. doi:10.1093/humrep/deh656 PMID:15591081

Duty, S. M., Silva, M. J., Barr, D. B., Brock, J. W., Ryan, L., Chen, Z., ... Hauser, R. (2003). Phthalate exposure and human semen parameters. *Epidemiology (Cambridge, Mass.)*, *14*(3), 269–277. doi:10.1097/01.EDE.0000059950.11836.16 PMID:12859026

Duty, S. M., Singh, N. P., Silva, M. J., Barr, D. B., Brock, J. W., Ryan, L., ... Hauser, R. (2003). The relationship between environmental exposures to phthalates and DNA damage in human sperm using the neutral comet assay. *Environmental Health Perspectives*, *111*(9), 1164–1169. doi:10.1289/ehp.5756 PMID:12842768

Ema, M., & Miyawaki, E. (2001). Effects of monobutyl phthalate on reproductive function in pregnant and pseudopregnant rats. *Reproductive Toxicology (Elmsford, N.Y.)*, *15*(3), 261–267. doi:10.1016/S0890-6238(01)00131-9 PMID:11390170

Engel, S. M., Miodovnik, A., Canfield, R. L., Zhu, C., Silva, M. J., Calafat, A. M., & Wolff, M. S. (2010). Prenatal phthalate exposure is associated with childhood behavior and executive functioning. *Environmental Health Perspectives*, *118*(4), 565–571. doi:10.1289/ehp.0901470 PMID:20106747

Engel, S. M., Zhu, C., Berkowitz, G. S., Calafat, A. M., Silva, M. J., Miodovnik, A., & Wolff, M. S. (2009). Prenatal phthalate exposure and performance on the Neonatal Behavioral Assessment Scale in a multiethnic birth cohort. *Neurotoxicology*, *30*(4), 522–528. doi:10.1016/j.neuro.2009.04.001 PMID:19375452

Fierens, T., Servaes, K., Van Holderbeke, M., Geerts, L., De Henauw, S., Sioen, I., & Vanermen, G. (2012). Analysis of phthalates in food products and packaging materials sold on the Belgian market. *Food and Chemical Toxicology*, *50*(7), 2575–2583. doi:10.1016/j.fct.2012.04.029 PMID:22554646

Fierens, T., Vanermen, G., Van Holderbeke, M., De Henauw, S., & Sioen, I. (2012). Effect of cooking at home on the levels of eight phthalates in foods. *Food and Chemical Toxicology*, *50*(12), 4428–4435. doi:10.1016/j.fct.2012.09.004 PMID:22985986

Fisher, J. S., Macpherson, S., Marchetti, N., & Sharpe, R. M. (2003). Human 'testicular dysgenesis syndrome': A possible model using in-utero exposure of the rat to dibutyl phthalate. *Human Reproduction (Oxford, England)*, *18*(7), 1383–1394. doi:10.1093/humrep/deg273 PMID:12832361

Food, U. S., & Adminstration, D. (2001). *Safety Assessment of Di (2-ethylhexyl) phthalate (DEHP) Released from PVC Medical Devices*. Rockville, MD: Center for Devices and Radiological Health, US Food and Drug Administration.

Foster, P. M. (2006). Disruption of reproductive development in male rat offspring following in utero exposure to phthalate esters. *International Journal of Andrology*, *29*(1), 140–147. doi:10.1111/j.1365-2605.2005.00563.x PMID:16102138

Foster, P. M., Thomas, L. V., Cook, M. W., & Gangolli, S. D. (1980). Study of the testicular effects and changes in zinc excretion produced by some n-alkyl phthalates in the rat. *Toxicology and Applied Pharmacology*, *54*(3), 392–398. doi:10.1016/0041-008X(80)90165-9 PMID:7394794

Foster, P. M. D., Mylchreest, E., Gaido, K. W., & Sar, M. (2001). Effects of phthalate esters on the developing reproductive tract of male rats. *APMIS*, *109*(S103), S272–S277. doi:10.1111/j.1600-0463.2001.tb05776.x PMID:11392369

Gangolli, S. D. (1982). Testicular effects of phthalate esters. *Environmental Health Perspectives*, *45*, 77–84. doi:10.1289/ehp.824577 PMID:6754364

Ge, R. S., Chen, G. R., Tanrikut, C., & Hardy, M. P. (2007). Phthalate ester toxicity in Leydig cells: Developmental timing and dosage considerations. *Reproductive Toxicology (Elmsford, N.Y.)*, *23*(3), 366–373. doi:10.1016/j.reprotox.2006.12.006 PMID:17258888

Gray, L. E. Jr, Ostby, J., Furr, J., Price, M., Veeramachaneni, D. R., & Parks, L. (2000). Perinatal exposure to the phthalates DEHP, BBP, and DINP, but not DEP, DMP, or DOTP, alters sexual differentiation of the male rat. *Toxicological Sciences*, *58*(2), 350–365. doi:10.1093/toxsci/58.2.350 PMID:11099647

Gray, T. J. B., & Beamand, J. A. (1984). Effect of some phthalate esters and other testicular toxins on primary cultures of testicular cells. *Food and Chemical Toxicology*, *22*(2), 123–131. doi:10.1016/0278-6915(84)90092-9 PMID:6538161

Guo, Y., Zhang, Z., Liu, L., Li, Y., Ren, N., & Kannan, K. (2012). Occurrence and profiles of phthalates in foodstuffs from China and their implications for human exposure. *Journal of Agricultural and Food Chemistry*, *60*(27), 6913–6919. doi:10.1021/jf3021128 PMID:22703192

Han, S. W., Lee, H., Han, S. Y., Lim, D. S., Jung, K. K., Kwack, S. J., ... Lee, B. M. (2009). An exposure assessment of di-(2-ethylhexyl) phthalate (DEHP) and di-n-butyl phthalate (DBP) in human semen. *Journal of Toxicology and Environmental Health. Part A.*, *72*(21-22), 1463–1469. doi:10.1080/15287390903212972 PMID:20077219

Hannas, B. R., Lambright, C. S., Furr, J., Howdeshell, K. L., Wilson, V. S., & Gray, L. E. Jr. (2011). Dose-response assessment of fetal testosterone production and gene expression levels in rat testes following in utero exposure to diethylhexyl phthalate, diisobutyl phthalate, diisoheptyl phthalate, and diisononyl phthalate. *Toxicological Sciences*, *123*(1), 206–216. doi:10.1093/toxsci/kfr146 PMID:21633115

Hansen, J. (1999). Risk for testicular cancer after occupational exposure to plastics. *International Journal of Cancer*, *82*(6), 911–912. doi:10.1002/(SICI)1097-0215(19990909)82:6<911::AID-IJC23>3.0.CO;2-O PMID:10446462

Hardell, L., Ohlson, C. G., & Fredrikson, M. (1997). Occupational exposure to polyvinyl chloride as a risk factor for testicular cancer evaluated in a case-control study. *International Journal of Cancer*, *73*(6), 828–830. doi:10.1002/(SICI)1097-0215(19971210)73:6<828::AID-IJC10>3.0.CO;2-0 PMID:9399660

Harris, C., Henttu, P., Parker, M. G., & Sumpter, J. P. (1997). The estrogenicexposures are not associated with testicular toxicity.4activity of phthalate esters in vitro. *Environmental Health Perspectives*, *105*, 802–811. doi:10.1289/ehp.97105802 PMID:9347895

Hauser, R., Duty, S., Godfrey-Bailey, L., & Calafat, A. M. (2004). Medications as a source of human exposure to phthalates. *Environmental Health Perspectives*, *112*(6), 751–753. doi:10.1289/ehp.6804 PMID:15121520

Hauser, R., Meeker, J. D., Duty, S., Silva, M. J., & Calafat, A. M. (2006). Altered semen quality in relation to urinary concentrations of phthalate monoester and oxidative metabolites. *Epidemiology (Cambridge, Mass.)*, *17*(6), 682–691. doi:10.1097/01.ede.0000235996.89953.d7 PMID:17003688

Hauser, R., Meeker, J. D., Singh, N. P., Silva, M. J., Ryan, L., Duty, S., & Calafat, A. M. (2006). DNA damage in human sperm is related to urinary levels of phthalate monoester and oxidative metabolites. *Human Reproduction (Oxford, England)*, *22*(3), 688–695. doi:10.1093/humrep/del428 PMID:17090632

Hauser, R., Meeker, J. D., Singh, N. P., Silva, M. J., Ryan, L., Duty, S., & Calafat, A. M. (2007). DNA damage in human sperm is related to urinary levels of phthalate monoester and oxidative metabolites. *Human Reproduction (Oxford, England)*, *22*(3), 688–695. doi:10.1093/humrep/del428 PMID:17090632

Herr, C., zurNieden, A., Koch, H. M., Schuppe, H. C., Fieber, C., Angerer, J., ... Stilianakis, N. I. (2009). Urinary di (2-ethylhexyl) phthalate (DEHP)—Metabolites and male human markers of reproductive function. *International Journal of Hygiene and Environmental Health*, *212*(6), 648–653. doi:10.1016/j.ijheh.2009.08.001 PMID:19733116

Higuchi, T. T., Palmer, J. S., Gray, L. E. Jr, & Veeramachaneni, D. R. (2003). Effects of dibutyl phthalate in male rabbits following in utero, adolescent, or postpubertal exposure. *Toxicological Sciences*, *72*(2), 301–313. doi:10.1093/toxsci/kfg036 PMID:12655036

Holm, A., Solbu, K., Molander, P., Lundanes, E., & Greibrokk, T. (2004). Sensitive biomonitoring of phthalate metabolites in human urine using packed capillary column switching liquid chromatography coupled to electrospray ionization ion-trap mass spectrometry. *Analytical and Bioanalytical Chemistry*, *378*(7), 1762–1768. doi:10.100700216-003-2488-7 PMID:14758462

Hoppin, J. A., Ulmer, R., & London, S. J. (2004). Phthalate exposure and pulmonary function. *Environmental Health Perspectives*, *112*(5), 571–574. doi:10.1289/ehp.6564 PMID:15064163

Huang, P. C., Kuo, P. L., Chou, Y. Y., Lin, S. J., & Lee, C. C. (2009). Association between prenatal exposure to phthalates and the health of newborns. *Environment International*, *35*(1), 14–20. doi:10.1016/j.envint.2008.05.012 PMID:18640725

Huang, P. C., Kuo, P. L., Guo, Y. L., Liao, P. C., & Lee, C. C. (2007). Associations between urinary phthalate monoesters and thyroid hormones in pregnant women. *Human Reproduction (Oxford, England)*, *22*(10), 2715–2722. doi:10.1093/humrep/dem205 PMID:17704099

Huber, W. W., Grasl-Kraupp, B., & Schulte-Hermann, R. (1996). Hepatocarcinogenic potential of di (2-ethylhexyl) phthalate in rodents and its implications on human risk. *Critical Reviews in Toxicology*, *26*(4), 365–481. doi:10.3109/10408449609048302 PMID:8817083

IARC. (2000). *IARC monographs on the evaluation of carcinogenic risks to humans*. Lyon7 Some Industrial Chemicals.

Jaakkola, J. J., Oie, L., Nafstad, P., Botten, G., Samuelsen, S. O., & Magnus, P. (1999). Interior surface materials in the home and the development of bronchial obstruction in young children in Oslo, Norway. *American Journal of Public Health*, *89*(2), 188–192. doi:10.2105/AJPH.89.2.188 PMID:9949747

Jaakkola, J. J., Oie, L., Nafstad, P., Botten, G., Samuelsen, S. O., & Magnus, P. (1999). Interior surface materials in the home and the development of bronchial obstruction in young children in Oslo, Norway. *American Journal of Public Health*, *89*(2), 188–192. doi:10.2105/AJPH.89.2.188 PMID:9949747

Jaakkola, J. J., Parise, H., Kislitsin, V., Lebedeva, N. I., & Spengler, J. D. (2004). Asthma, wheezing, and allergies in Russian schoolchildren in relation to new surface materials in the home. *American Journal of Public Health, 94*(4), 560–562. doi:10.2105/AJPH.94.4.560 PMID:15054004

Jaakkola, J. J., Verkasalo, P. K., & Jaakkola, N. (2000). Plastic wall materials in the home and respiratory health in young children. *American Journal of Public Health, 90*(5), 797–799. doi:10.2105/AJPH.90.5.797 PMID:10800434

Joensen, U. N., Frederiksen, H., Jensen, M. B., Lauritsen, M. P., Olesen, I. A., Lassen, T. H., ... Jørgensen, N. (2012). Phthalate excretion pattern and testicular function: A study of 881 healthy Danish men. *Environmental Health Perspectives, 120*(10), 1397–1403. doi:10.1289/ehp.1205113 PMID:22832070

Kamrin, M. A. (2009). Phthalate risks, phthalate regulation, and public health: A review. *Journal of Toxicology and Environmental Health. Part B, 12*(2), 157–174.

Kato, K., Shoda, S., Takahashi, M., Doi, N., Yoshimura, Y., & Nakazawa, H. (2003). Determination of three phthalate metabolites in human urine using on-line solid-phase extraction–liquid chromatography–tandem mass spectrometry. *Journal of Chromatography. B, Analytical Technologies in the Biomedical and Life Sciences, 788*(2), 407–411. doi:10.1016/S1570-0232(03)00041-2 PMID:12705982

Kato, K., Silva, M. J., Brock, J. W., Reidy, J. A., Malek, N. A., Hodge, C. C., ... Barr, D. B. (2003). Quantitative detection of nine phthalate metabolites in human serum using reversed-phase high-performance liquid chromatography-electrospray ionization-tandem mass spectrometry. *Journal of Analytical Toxicology, 27*(5), 284–289. doi:10.1093/jat/27.5.284 PMID:12908941

Kato, K., Silva, M. J., Needham, L. L., & Calafat, A. M. (2005). Determination of 16 phthalate metabolites in urine using automated sample preparation and on-line preconcentration/high-performance liquid chromatography/tandem mass spectrometry. *Analytical Chemistry, 77*(9), 2985–2991. doi:10.1021/ac0481248 PMID:15859620

Kato, K., Silva, M. J., Reidy, J. A., Hurtz, D. III, Malek, N. A., Needham, L. L., ... Calafat, A. M. (2004). Mono(2-Ethyl-5-Hydro- xyhexyl) phthalate and Mono(2-Ethyl-5-Oxohexyl) phtha- late as biomarkers for human exposure assessment to Di(2-Ethylhexyl) phthalate. *Environmental Health Perspectives, 112*(3), 327–330. doi:10.1289/ehp.6663 PMID:14998748

Kato, K., Yamauchi, T., Higashiyama, K., & Nakazawa, H. (2003). High Throughput Analysis of Di-(2-Ethylhexyl) phthalate Metabolites in Urine for Exposure Assessment. *Journal of Liquid Chromatography & Related Technologies, 26*(13), 2167–2176. doi:10.1081/JLC-120022401

Klaunig, J. E., Babich, M. A., Baetcke, K. P., Cook, J. C., Corton, J. C., David, R. M., ... Roberts, R. A. (2003). PPARα agonist-induced rodent tumors: Modes of action and human relevance. *Critical Reviews in Toxicology, 33*(6), 655–780. doi:10.1080/713608372 PMID:14727734

Klaunig, J. E., Babich, M. A., Baetcke, K. P., Cook, J. C., Corton, J. C., David, R. M., ... Roberts, R. A. (2003). PPARα agonist-induced rodent tumors: Modes of action and human relevance. *Critical Reviews in Toxicology, 33*(6), 655–780. doi:10.1080/713608372 PMID:14727734

Koch, H. M., Bolt, H. M., & Angerer, J. (2004). Di (2-ethylhexyl) phthalate (DEHP) metabolites in human urine and serum after a single oral dose of deuterium-labelled DEHP. *Archives of Toxicology*, *78*(3), 123–130. doi:10.100700204-003-0522-3 PMID:14576974

Koch, H. M., Bolt, H. M., Preuss, R., & Angerer, J. (2005). New metabolites of di (2-ethylhexyl) phthalate (DEHP) in human urine and serum after single oral doses of deuterium-labelled DEHP. *Archives of Toxicology*, *79*(7), 367–376. doi:10.100700204-004-0642-4 PMID:15700144

Koch, H. M., Drexler, H., & Angerer, J. (2003). An estimation of the daily intake of di (2-ethylhexyl) phthalate (DEHP) and other phthalates in the general population. *International Journal of Hygiene and Environmental Health*, *206*(2), 77–83. doi:10.1078/1438-4639-00205 PMID:12708228

Koch, H. M., Drexler, H., & Angerer, J. (2004). Internal exposure of nursery-school children and their parents and teachers to di (2-ethylhexyl) phthalate (DEHP). *International Journal of Hygiene and Environmental Health*, *207*(1), 15–22. doi:10.1078/1438-4639-00270 PMID:14762970

Koch, H. M., Gonzalez-Reche, L. M., & Angerer, J. (2003). On-line clean-up by multidimensional liquid chromatography–electrospray ionization tandem mass spectrometry for high throughput quantification of primary and secondary phthalate metabolites in human urine. *Journal of Chromatography. B, Analytical Technologies in the Biomedical and Life Sciences*, *784*(1), 169–182. doi:10.1016/S1570-0232(02)00785-7 PMID:12504195

Koch, H. M., Lorber, M., Christensen, K. L., Pälmke, C., Koslitz, S., & Brüning, T. (2013). Identifying sources of phthalate exposure with human biomonitoring: Results of a 48 h fasting study with urine collection and personal activity patterns. *International Journal of Hygiene and Environmental Health*, *216*(6), 672–681. doi:10.1016/j.ijheh.2012.12.002 PMID:23333758

Koch, H. M., Rossbach, B., Drexler, H., & Angerer, J. (2003). Internal exposure of the general population to DEHP and other phthalates—Determination of secondary and primary phthalate monoester metabolites in urine. *Environmental Research*, *93*(2), 177–185. doi:10.1016/S0013-9351(03)00083-5 PMID:12963402

Kolarik, B., Naydenov, K., Larsson, M., Bornehag, C. G., & Sundell, J. (2007). The association between phthalates in dust and allergic diseases among Bulgarian children. *Environmental Health Perspectives*, *116*(1), 98–103. doi:10.1289/ehp.10498 PMID:18197306

Kolarik, B., Naydenov, K., Larsson, M., Bornehag, C. G., & Sundell, J. (2008). The association between phthalates in dust and allergic diseases among Bulgarian children. *Environmental Health Perspectives*, *116*(1), 98–103. doi:10.1289/ehp.10498 PMID:18197306

Kurata, Y., Kidachi, F., Yokoyama, M., Toyota, N., Tsuchitani, M., & Katoh, M. (1998). Subchronic toxicity of di (2-ethylhexyl) phthalate in common marmosets: Lack of hepatic peroxisome proliferation, testicular atrophy, or pancreatic acinar cell hyperplasia. *Toxicological Sciences*, *42*(1), 49–56. PMID:9538047

Latini, G., De Felice, C., Presta, G., Del Vecchio, A., Paris, I., Ruggieri, F., & Mazzeo, P. (2003). Exposure to di (2-ethylhexyl) phthalate in humans during pregnancy. *Neonatology*, *83*(1), 22–24. doi:10.1159/000067012 PMID:12566679

Latini, G., De Felice, C., Presta, G., Del Vecchio, A., Paris, I., Ruggieri, F., & Mazzeo, P. (2003). In utero exposure to di-(2-ethylhexyl) phthalate and duration of human pregnancy. *Environmental Health Perspectives*, *111*(14), 1783–1785. doi:10.1289/ehp.6202 PMID:14594632

Latini, G., Gallo, F., & De Felice, C. (2004). Birth characteristics and hepatoblastoma risk in young children. *Cancer: Interdisciplinary International Journal of the American Cancer Society*, *101*(1), 210–210. doi:10.1002/cncr.20357 PMID:15222013

Latini, G., Verrotti, A., & De Felice, C. (2004). Di-2-ethylhexyl phthalate and endocrine disruption: A review. *Current Drug Targets. Immune, Endocrine and Metabolic Disorders*, *4*(1), 37–40. doi:10.2174/1568008043340017 PMID:15032624

Li, H., & Kim, K. H. (2003). Effects of mono-(2-ethylhexyl) phthalate on fetal and neonatal rat testis organ cultures. *Biology of Reproduction*, *69*(6), 1964–1972. doi:10.1095/biolreprod.103.018895 PMID:12904314

Lin, Z. P., Ikonomou, M. G., Jing, H., Mackintosh, C., & Gobas, F. A. (2003). Determination of phthalate ester congeners and mixtures by LC/ESI-MS in sediments and biota of an urbanized marine inlet. *Environmental Science & Technology*, *37*(10), 2100–2108. doi:10.1021/es026361r PMID:12785513

Liu, L., Bao, H., Liu, F., Zhang, J., & Shen, H. (2012). Phthalates exposure of Chinese reproductive age couples and its effect on male semen quality, a primary study. *Environment International*, *42*, 78–83. doi:10.1016/j.envint.2011.04.005 PMID:21524797

López-Carrillo, L., Hernández-Ramírez, R. U., Calafat, A. M., Torres-Sánchez, L., Galván-Portillo, M., Needham, L. L., & Cebrián, M. E. (2009). Exposure to phthalates and breast cancer risk in northern Mexico. *Environmental Health Perspectives*, *118*(4), 539–544. doi:10.1289/ehp.0901091 PMID:20368132

López-Carrillo, L., Hernández-Ramírez, R. U., Calafat, A. M., Torres-Sánchez, L., Galván-Portillo, M., Needham, L. L., ... Cebrián, M. E. (2010). Ex- posure to phthalates and breast cancer risk in Northen Mexico. *Environmental Health Perspectives*, *118*(4), 539–544. doi:10.1289/ehp.0901091 PMID:20368132

Lottrup, G., Andersson, A. M., Leffers, H., Mortensen, G. K., Toppari, J., Skakkebaek, N. E., & Main, K. M. (2006). Possible impact of phthalates on infant reproductive health. *International Journal of Andrology*, *29*(1), 172–180. doi:10.1111/j.1365-2605.2005.00642.x PMID:16466537

Louis, G. M. B., Sundaram, R., Sweeney, A. M., Schisterman, E. F., Maisog, J., & Kannan, K. (2014). Urinary bisphenol A, phthalates, and couple fecundity: The Longitudinal Investigation of Fertility and the Environment (LIFE) Study. *Fertility and Sterility*, *101*(5), 1359–1366. doi:10.1016/j.fertnstert.2014.01.022 PMID:24534276

Lovekamp, T. N., & Davis, B. J. (2001). Mono-(2-ethylhexyl) phthalate suppresses aromatase transcript levels and estradiol production in cultured rat granulosa cells. *Toxicology and Applied Pharmacology*, *172*(3), 217–224. doi:10.1006/taap.2001.9156 PMID:11312650

Lovekamp-Swan, T., & Davis, B. J. (2003). Mechanisms of phthalate ester toxicity in the female reproductive system. *Environmental Health Perspectives*, *111*(2), 139–145. doi:10.1289/ehp.5658 PMID:12573895

Main, K. M., Mortensen, G. K., Kaleva, M. M., Boisen, K. A., Damgaard, I. N., Chellakooty, M., ... Skakkebaek, N. E. (2006). Human breast milk contamination with phthalates and alterations of endogenous reproductive hormones in infants three months of age. *Environmental Health Perspectives*, *114*(2), 270–276. doi:10.1289/ehp.8075 PMID:16451866

Martine, B., Cendrine, D., Fabrice, A., & Marc, C. (2013). Assessment of adult human exposure to phthalate esters in the urban centre of Paris (France). *Bulletin of Environmental Contamination and Toxicology*, *90*(1), 91–96. doi:10.100700128-012-0859-5 PMID:23090363

McKee, R. H., El-Hawari, M., Stoltz, M., Pallas, F., & Lington, A. W. (2002). Absorption, disposition and metabolism of di-isononyl phthalate (DINP) in F-344 rats. *Journal of Applied Toxicology: An International Journal*, *22*(5), 293–302. doi:10.1002/jat.861 PMID:12355558

Meeker, J. D., Calafat, A. M., & Hauser, R. (2007). Di (2-ethylhexyl) phthalate metabolites may alter thyroid hormone levels in men. *Environmental Health Perspectives*, *115*(7), 1029–1034. doi:10.1289/ehp.9852 PMID:17637918

Meeker, J. D., Calafat, A. M., & Hauser, R. (2009). Urinary metabolites of di (2-ethylhexyl) phthalate are associated with decreased steroid hormone levels in adult men. *Journal of Andrology*, *30*(3), 287–297. doi:10.2164/jandrol.108.006403 PMID:19059903

Melnick, R. L. (2001). Is peroxisome proliferation an obligatory precursor step in the carcinogenicity of di (2-ethylhexyl) phthalate (DEHP)? *Environmental Health Perspectives*, *109*(5), 437–442. doi:10.1289/ehp.01109437 PMID:11401753

Mihovec-Grdiæ, M., Šmit, Z., Puntariæ, D., & Bošnir, J. (2002). Phthalates in underground waters of the Zagreb area. *Croatian Medical Journal*, *43*(4), 493–497. PMID:12187530

Miodovnik, A., Engel, S. M., Zhu, C., Ye, X., Soorya, L. V., Silva, M. J., ... Wolff, M. S. (2011). Endocrine disruptors and childhood social impairment. *Neurotoxicology*, *32*(2), 261–267. doi:10.1016/j.neuro.2010.12.009 PMID:21182865

Montuori, P., Jover, E., Morgantini, M., Bayona, J. M., & Triassi, M. (2008). Assessing human exposure to phthalic acid and phthalate esters from mineral water stored in polyethylene terephthalate and glass bottles. *Food Additives and Contaminants*, *25*(4), 511–518. doi:10.1080/02652030701551800 PMID:18348049

Morales-Suárez-Varela, M. M., Toft, G. V., Jensen, M. S., Ramlau-Hansen, C., Kaerlev, L., Thulstrup, A. M., ... Bonde, J. P. (2011). Parental occupational exposure to endocrine disrupting chemicals and male genital malformations: A study in the Danish National Birth Cohort study. *Environmental Health*, *10*(1), 3. doi:10.1186/1476-069X-10-3 PMID:21235764

Murature, D. A., Tang, S. Y., Steinhardt, G., & Dougherty, R. C. (1987). Phthalate esters and semen quality parameters. *Biomedical & Environmental Mass Spectrometry*, *14*(8), 473–477. doi:10.1002/bms.1200140815 PMID:2957007

Murature, D. A., Tang, S. Y., Steinhardt, G., & Dougherty, R. C. (1987). Phthalate esters and semen quality parameters. *Biomedical & Environmental Mass Spectrometry*, *14*(8), 473–477. doi:10.1002/bms.1200140815 PMID:2957007

Mylchreest, E., Cattley, R. C., & Foster, P. M. (1998). Male reproductive tract malformations in rats following gestational and lactational exposure to di (n-butyl) phthalate: An antiandrogenic mechanism? *Toxicological Sciences*, *43*(1), 47–60. doi:10.1093/toxsci/43.1.47 PMID:9629619

Mylchreest, E., Sar, M., Cattley, R. C., & Foster, P. M. (1999). Disruption of androgen-regulated male reproductive development by di (n-butyl) phthalate during late gestation in rats is different from flutamide. *Toxicology and Applied Pharmacology*, *156*(2), 81–95. doi:10.1006/taap.1999.8643 PMID:10198273

Mylchreest, E., Wallace, D. G., Cattley, R. C., & Foster, P. M. (2000). Dose-dependent alterations in androgen-regulated male reproductive development in rats exposed to di (n-butyl) phthalate during late gestation. *Toxicological Sciences*, *55*(1), 143–151. doi:10.1093/toxsci/55.1.143 PMID:10788569

National Toxicology Program, Center for the Evaluation of Risks to Human Reproduction. NTP-CERHR Expert Panel Report on Di(2-Ethylhexyl) Phthalate. (2000). Available at: http://cerhr.niehs.nih.gov/news/index.html

National Toxicology Program, Center for the Evaluation of Risks to Human Reproduction (NTP-CERHR): Monograph on the Potential Human Reproductive and Developmental Effects of Butyl Benzyl Phthalate (BBP). (2003). NIH Publication No. 03–4487.

Needham, L. L., Patterson, D. G. Jr, Barr, D. B., Grainger, J., & Calafat, A. M. (2005). Uses of speciation techniques in biomonitoring for assessing human exposure to organic environmental chemi- cals. *Analytical and Bioanalytical Chemistry*, *381*(2), 397–404. doi:10.100700216-004-2975-5 PMID:15616776

Niino, T., Ishibashi, T., Itho, T., Sakai, S., Ishiwata, H., Yamada, T., & Onodera, S. (2002). Simultaneous determination of phthalate di-and monoesters in poly (vinylchloride) products and human saliva by gas chromatography–mass spectrometry. *Journal of Chromatography. B, Analytical Technologies in the Biomedical and Life Sciences*, *780*(1), 35–44. doi:10.1016/S1570-0232(02)00413-0 PMID:12383478

Oie, L., Hersoug, L. G., & Madsen, J. O. (1997). Residential exposure to plasticizers and its possible role in the pathogenesis of asthma. *Environmental Health Perspectives*, *105*(9), 972–978. doi:10.1289/ehp.97105972 PMID:9374082

Øie, L., Nafstad, P., Botten, G., Magnus, P., & Jaakkola, J. J. (1999). Ventilation in homes and bronchial obstruction in young children. *Epidemiology (Cambridge, Mass.)*, *10*(3), 294–299. doi:10.1097/00001648-199905000-00018 PMID:10230841

Otake, T., Yoshinaga, J., & Yanagisawa, Y. (2001). Analysis of organic esters of plasticizer in indoor air by GC– MS and GC– FPD. *Environmental Science & Technology*, *35*(15), 3099–3102. doi:10.1021/es001914o PMID:11505983

Page, B. D., & Lacroix, G. M. (1992). Studies into the transfer and migration of phthalate esters from aluminium foil-paper laminates to butter and margarine. *Food Additives and Contaminants*, *9*(3), 197–212. doi:10.1080/02652039209374064 PMID:1397395

Page, B. D., & Lacroix, G. M. (1995). The occurrence of phthalate ester and di-2-ethylhexyl adipate plasticizers in Canadian packaging and food sampled in 1985–1989: A survey. *Food Additives and Contaminants*, *12*(1), 129–151. doi:10.1080/02652039509374287 PMID:7758627

Pan, G., Hanaoka, T., Yoshimura, M., Zhang, S., Wang, P., Tsukino, H., ... Takahashi, K. (2006). Decreased serum free testosterone in workers exposed to high levels of di-n-butyl phthalate (DBP) and di-2-ethylhexyl phthalate (DEHP): A cross-sectional study in China. *Environmental Health Perspectives*, *114*(11), 1643–1648. doi:10.1289/ehp.9016 PMID:17107847

Pant, N., Shukla, M., Patel, D. K., Shukla, Y., Mathur, N., Gupta, Y. K., & Saxena, D. K. (2008). Correlation of phthalate exposures with semen quality. *Toxicology and Applied Pharmacology*, *231*(1), 112–116. doi:10.1016/j.taap.2008.04.001 PMID:18513777

Paris, I., Ruggieri, F., Mazzeo, P., & Carlucci, G. (2003). Simultaneous determination of di (2-ethylhexyl) phthalate and mono (2-ethylhexyl) phthalate in human plasma by high-performance liquid chromatography. *Analytical Letters*, *36*(12), 2649–2658. doi:10.1081/AL-120024639

Parks, L. G., Ostby, J. S., Lambright, C. R., Abbott, B. D., Klinefelter, G. R., Barlow, N. J., & Gray, L. E. Jr. (2000). The plasticizer diethylhexyl phthalate induces malformations by decreasing fetal testosterone synthesis during sexual differentiation in the male rat. *Toxicological Sciences*, *58*(2), 339–349. doi:10.1093/toxsci/58.2.339 PMID:11099646

Petersen, J. H., & Jensen, L. K. (2010). Phthalates and food-contact materials: Enforcing the 2008 European Union plastics legislation. *Food Additives and Contaminants*, *27*(11), 1608–1616. doi:10.1080/19440049.2010.501825 PMID:20737341

Phillip, M., De, C. B., Pilpel, D., Karplus, M., & Sofer, S. (1996). Clitoral and penile sizes of full term newborns in two different ethnic groups. *Journal of pediatric endocrinology & metabolism. Journal of Pediatric Endocrinology & Metabolism*, *9*(2), 175–179. PMID:8887140

Poças, M. F., Oliveira, J. C., Pereira, J. R., & Hogg, T. (2010). Consumer exposure to phthalates from paper packaging: An integrated approach. *Food Additives and Contaminants*, *27*(10), 1451–1459. doi:10.1080/19440049.2010.490790 PMID:20597021

Ponsonby, A. L., Dwyer, T., Kemp, A., Cochrane, J., Couper, D., & Carmichael, A. (2003). Synthetic bedding and wheeze in childhood. *Epidemiology (Cambridge, Mass.)*, *14*(1), 37–44. doi:10.1097/00001648-200301000-00012 PMID:12500044

Preuss, R., Koch, H. M., & Angerer, J. (2005). Biological monitoring of the five major metabolites of di-(2-ethylhexyl) phthalate (DEHP) in human urine using column-switching liquid chromatography–tandem mass spectrometry. *Journal of Chromatography. B, Analytical Technologies in the Biomedical and Life Sciences*, *816*(1-2), 269–280. doi:10.1016/j.jchromb.2004.11.048 PMID:15664359

Psillakis, E., Mantzavinos, D., & Kalogerakis, N. (2004). Monitoring the sonochemical degradation of phthalate esters in water using solid-phase microextraction. *Chemosphere*, *54*(7), 849–857. doi:10.1016/j.chemosphere.2003.09.039 PMID:14637342

Qiao, L., Zheng, L., & Cai, D. (2007). Study on the di-n-butyl phthalate and di-2-ethylhexyl phthalate level of girl serum related with precocious puberty in Shanghai. *Wei sheng yanjiu=. Wei Sheng Yen Chiu*, *36*(1), 93–95. PMID:17424861

Rozati, R., Reddy, P. P., Reddanna, P. A., & Mujtaba, R. (2002). Role of environmental estrogens in the deterioration of male factor fertility. *Fertility and Sterility*, *78*(6), 1187–1194. doi:10.1016/S0015-0282(02)04389-3 PMID:12477510

Rudel, R., Camann, D., Spengler, J. D., Barr, D., & Brody, J. G. (2003, March). Household exposure to phthalates, pesticides, alkylphenols, pbdes, and other endocrine active compounds. In Toxicological Sciences (Vol. 72, pp. 184-184). Oxford Univ Press.

Rudel, R. A., Camann, D. E., Spengler, J. D., Korn, L. R., & Brody, J. G. (2003). Phthalates, alkylphenols, pesticides, polybrominated diphenyl ethers, and other endocrine-disrupting compounds in indoor air and dust. *Environmental Science & Technology*, *37*(20), 4543–4553. doi:10.1021/es0264596 PMID:14594359

Salazar-Martinez, E., Romano-Riquer, P., Yanez-Marquez, E., Longnecker, M. P., & Hernandez-Avila, M. (2004). Anogenital distance in human male and female newborns: A descriptive, cross-sectional study. *Environmental Health*, *3*(1), 8. doi:10.1186/1476-069X-3-8 PMID:15363098

Sathyanarayana, S. (2008). Phthalates and children's health. *Current Problems in Pediatric and Adolescent Health Care*, *2*(38), 34–49. doi:10.1016/j.cppeds.2007.11.001 PMID:18237855

Sathyanarayana, S., Karr, C. J., Lozano, P., Brown, E., Calafat, A. M., Liu, F., & Swan, S. H. (2008). Baby care products: Possible sources of infant phthalate exposure. *Pediatrics*, *121*(2), e260–e268. doi:10.1542/peds.2006-3766 PMID:18245401

Schecter, A., Lorber, M., Guo, Y., Wu, Q., Yun, S. H., Kannan, K., ... Colacino, J. A. (2013). Phthalate concentrations and dietary exposure from food purchased in New York State. *Environmental Health Perspectives*, *121*(4), 473–479. doi:10.1289/ehp.1206367 PMID:23461894

Sharpe, R. M. (2001). Hormones and testis development and the possible adverse effects of environmental chemicals. *Toxicology Letters*, *120*(1-3), 221–232. doi:10.1016/S0378-4274(01)00298-3 PMID:11323180

Sharpe, R. M., & Irvine, D. S. (2004). How strong is the evidence of a link between environmental chemicals and adverse effects on human reproductive health? *BMJ (Clinical Research Ed.)*, *328*(7437), 447–451. doi:10.1136/bmj.328.7437.447 PMID:14976101

Sharpe, R. M., & Skakkebaek, N. E. (1993). Are oestrogens involved in falling sperm counts and disorders of the male reproductive tract? *Lancet*, *341*(8857), 1392–1396. doi:10.1016/0140-6736(93)90953-E PMID:8098802

Shea, K. M. (2003). Pediatric exposure and potential toxicity of phthalate plasticizers. *Pediatrics*, *111*(6), 1467–1474. doi:10.1542/peds.111.6.1467 PMID:12777573

Shneider, B., Schena, J., Truog, R., Jacobson, M., & Kevy, S. (1989). Exposure to di (2-ethylhexyl) phthalate in infants receiving extracorporeal membrane oxygenation. *The New England Journal of Medicine*, *320*(23), 1563–1563. doi:10.1056/NEJM198906083202322 PMID:2725593

Silva, M. J., Barr, D. B., Reidy, J. A., Kato, K., Malek, N. A., Hodge, C. C., ... Brock, J. W. (2003). Glucuronidation patterns of common urinary and serum monoester phthalate metabolites. *Archives of Toxicology*, *77*(10), 561–567. doi:10.100700204-003-0486-3 PMID:14574443

Silva, M. J., Kato, K., Gray, E. L., Wolf, C., Needham, L. L., & Calafat, A. M. (2005). Urinary metabolites of di-n-octyl phthalate in rats. *Toxicology*, *210*(2-3), 123–133. doi:10.1016/j.tox.2005.01.012 PMID:15840426

Silva, M. J., Malek, N. A., Hodge, C. C., Reidy, J. A., Kato, K., Barr, D. B., ... Brock, J. W. (2003). Improved quantitative detection of 11 urinary phthalate metabolites in humans using liquid chromatography–atmospheric pressure chemical ionization tandem mass spectrometry. *Journal of Chromatography. B, Analytical Technologies in the Biomedical and Life Sciences*, *789*(2), 393–404. doi:10.1016/S1570-0232(03)00164-8 PMID:12742130

Silva, M. J., Samandar, E., Preau, J. L. Jr, Reidy, J. A., Needham, L. L., & Calafat, A. M. (2007). Quantification of 22 phthalate metabolites in human urine. *Journal of Chromatography. B, Analytical Technologies in the Biomedical and Life Sciences*, *860*(1), 106–112. doi:10.1016/j.jchromb.2007.10.023 PMID:17997365

Silva, M. J., Slakman, A. R., Reidy, J. A., Preau, J. L. Jr, Herbert, A. R., Samandar, E., ... Calafat, A. M. (2004). Analysis of human urine for fifteen phthalate metabolites using automated solid-phase extraction. *Journal of Chromatography. B, Analytical Technologies in the Biomedical and Life Sciences*, *805*(1), 161–167. doi:10.1016/j.jchromb.2004.02.038 PMID:15113553

Specht, I. O., Bonde, J. P., Toft, G., Lindh, C. H., Jönsson, B. A., & Jørgensen, K. T. (2015). Serum phthalate levels and time to pregnancy in couples from Greenland, Poland and Ukraine. *PLoS One*, *10*(3), e0120070. doi:10.1371/journal.pone.0120070 PMID:25786246

Srivastava, S. P., Srivastava, S., Saxena, D. K., Chandra, S. V., & Seth, P. K. (1990). Testicular effects of di-n-butyl phthalate (DBP): Biochemical and histopathological alterations. *Archives of Toxicology*, *64*(2), 148–152. doi:10.1007/BF01974401 PMID:2350234

Stahlhut, R. W., van Wijngaarden, E., Dye, T. D., Cook, S., & Swan, S. H. (2007). Concentrations of urinary phthalate metabolites are associated with increased waist circumference and insulin resistance in adult US males. *Environmental Health Perspectives*, *115*(6), 876–882. doi:10.1289/ehp.9882 PMID:17589594

Suzuki, T., Yaguchi, K., Suzuki, S., & Suga, T. (2001). Monitoring of phthalic acid monoesters in river water by solid-phase extraction and GC-MS determination. *Environmental Science & Technology*, *35*(18), 3757–3763. doi:10.1021/es001860i PMID:11783656

Swan, S. H. (2008). Environmental phthalate exposure in relation to reproductive outcomes and other health endpoints in humans. *Environmental Research*, *108*(2), 177–184. doi:10.1016/j.envres.2008.08.007 PMID:18949837

Swan, S. H., Elkin, E. P., & Fenster, L. (2000). The question of declining sperm density revisited: An analysis of 101 studies published 1934-1996. *Environmental Health Perspectives*, *108*(10), 961–966. doi:10.1289/ehp.00108961 PMID:11049816

Swan, S. H., Main, K. M., Liu, F., Stewart, S. L., Kruse, R. L., Calafat, A. M., ... Teague, J. L. (2005). Decrease in anogenital distance among male infants with prenatal phthalate exposure. *Environmental Health Perspectives*, *113*(8), 1056–1061. doi:10.1289/ehp.8100 PMID:16079079

Takatori, S., Kitagawa, Y., Kitagawa, M., Nakazawa, H., & Hori, S. (2004). Determination of di (2-ethylhexyl) phthalate and mono (2-ethylhexyl) phthalate in human serum using liquid chromatography-tandem mass spectrometry. *Journal of Chromatography. B, Analytical Technologies in the Biomedical and Life Sciences*, *804*(2), 397–401. doi:10.1016/j.jchromb.2004.01.056 PMID:15081935

Teitelbaum, S. L., Britton, J. A., Calafat, A. M., Ye, X., Silva, M. J., Reidy, J. A., ... Wolff, M. S. (2008). Temporal variability in urinary concentrations of phthalate metabolites, phytoestrogens and phenols among minority children in the United States. *Environmental Research*, *106*(2), 257–269. doi:10.1016/j.envres.2007.09.010 PMID:17976571

Trasande, L., Sathyanarayana, S., Messito, M. J., Gross, R. S., Attina, T. M., & Mendelsohn, A. L. (2013). Phthalates and the diets of US children and adolescents. *Environmental Research*, *126*, 84–90. doi:10.1016/j.envres.2013.07.007 PMID:24041780

Tyl, R. W., Myers, C. B., Marr, M. C., Fail, P. A., Seely, J. C., Brine, D. R., ... Butala, J. H. (2004). Reproductive toxicity evaluation of dietary butyl benzyl phthalate (BBP) in rats. *Reproductive Toxicology (Elmsford, N.Y.)*, *18*(2), 241–264. doi:10.1016/j.reprotox.2003.10.006 PMID:15019722

United States Environmental Protection Agency (USEPA). (n.d.). *Phthalates action plan summary*. Retrieved from http://www.epa.gov/oppt/existingchemicals/pubs/ actionplans/phthalates.html

US Department of Health and Human Services Centers for Disease Control and Prevention. (2013). *Fourth national report on human exposure to environmental chemicals*. Atlanta, GA: Author.

US FDA. (2000). *Contaminates: Action Levels for Poisonous or Deleterious Substances in Human Food and Animal Feed*. Author.

US FDA. (2003). *Labeling & Nutrition: Interim Procedures for Qualified Health Claims in the Labeling of Conventional Human Food and Human Dietary Supplements*. Author.

Valles, E. G., Laughter, A. R., & Dunn, C. S. (2003). Role of the perox- isome proliferator-activated receptor alpha in responses to diisononyl phthalate. *Toxicology*, *191*(2–3), 211–225. doi:10.1016/S0300-483X(03)00260-9 PMID:12965124

Van Tongeren, M., Nieuwenhuijsen, M. J., Gardiner, K., Armstrong, B., Vrijheid, M., Dolk, H., & Botting, B. (2002). A job–exposure matrix for potential endocrine-disrupting chemicals developed for a study into the association between maternal occupational exposure and hypospadias. *The Annals of Occupational Hygiene*, *46*(5), 465–477. PMID:12176761

Vikelsøe, J., Thomsen, M., & Carlsen, L. (2002). Phthalates and nonylphenols in profiles of differently dressed soils. *The Science of the Total Environment*, *296*(1-3), 105–116. doi:10.1016/S0048-9697(02)00063-3 PMID:12398330

Weiss, T., & Angerer, J. (2002). Simultaneous determination of various aromatic amines and metabolites of aromatic nitro compounds in urine for low level exposure using gas chromatography–mass spectrometry. *Journal of Chromatography. B, Analytical Technologies in the Biomedical and Life Sciences*, *778*(1-2), 179–192. doi:10.1016/S0378-4347(01)00542-4 PMID:12376125

Welsh, M., Saunders, P. T., Fisken, M., Scott, H. M., Hutchison, G. R., Smith, L. B., & Sharpe, R. M. (2008). Identification in rats of a programming window for reproductive tract masculinization, disruption of which leads to hypospadias and cryptorchidism. *The Journal of Clinical Investigation*, *118*(4), 1479–1490. doi:10.1172/JCI34241 PMID:18340380

Wilson, V. S., Lambright, C., Furr, J., Ostby, J., Wood, C., Held, G., & Gray, L. E. Jr. (2004). Phthalate ester-induced gubernacular lesions are associated with reduced insl3 gene expression in the fetal rat testis. *Toxicology Letters*, *146*(3), 207–215. doi:10.1016/j.toxlet.2003.09.012 PMID:14687758

Wirth, J. J., Rossano, M. G., Potter, R., Puscheck, E., Daly, D. C., Paneth, N., ... Diamond, M. P. (2008). A pilot study associating urinary concentrations of phthalate metabolites and semen quality. *Systems Biology in Reproductive Medicine*, *54*(3), 143–154. doi:10.1080/19396360802055921 PMID:18570050

Wittassek, M., & Angerer, J. (2008). Phthalates: Metabolism and exposure. *International Journal of Andrology*, *31*(2), 131–138. doi:10.1111/j.1365-2605.2007.00837.x PMID:18070048

Wittassek, M., Koch, H. M., Angerer, J., & Brüning, T. (2011). Assessing exposure to phthalates–the human biomonitoring approach. *Molecular Nutrition & Food Research*, *55*(1), 7–31. doi:10.1002/mnfr.201000121 PMID:20564479

Wolf, C., Lambright, C., Mann, P., Price, M., Cooper, R. L., Ostby, J., & Gray, L. E. Jr. (1999). Administration of potentially antiandrogenic pesticides (procymidone, linuron, iprodione, chlozolinate, p, p′-DDE, and ketoconazole) and toxic substances (dibutyl-and diethylhexyl phthalate, PCB 169, and ethane dimethanesulphonate) during sexual differentiation produces diverse profiles of reproductive malformations in the male rat. *Toxicology and Industrial Health*, *15*(1-2), 94–118. doi:10.1177/074823379901500109 PMID:10188194

Wolff, M. S., Engel, S. M., Berkowitz, G. S., Ye, X., Silva, M. J., Zhu, C., ... Calafat, A. M. (2008). Prenatal phenol and phthalate exposures and birth outcomes. *Environmental Health Perspectives*, *116*(8), 1092–1097. doi:10.1289/ehp.11007 PMID:18709157

Wormuth, M., Scheringer, M., Vollenweider, M., & Hungerbühler, K. (2006). What are the sources of exposure to eight frequently used phthalic acid esters in Europeans? *Risk Analysis*, *26*(3), 803–824. doi:10.1111/j.1539-6924.2006.00770.x PMID:16834635

Zacharewski, T. R., Meek, M. D., Clemons, J. H., Wu, Z. F., Fielden, M. R., & Matthews, J. B. (1998). Examination of the in vitro and in vitro estrogenic activities of eight commercial phthalate esters. *Toxicological Sciences*, *46*(2), 282–293. PMID:10048131

Zota, A. R., Calafat, A. M., & Woodruff, T. J. (2014). Temporal trends in phthalate exposures: Findings from the National Health and Nutrition Examination Survey, 2001–2010. *Environmental Health Perspectives*, *122*(3), 235–241. doi:10.1289/ehp.1306681 PMID:24425099

ADDITIONAL READING

Erkekoglu, P., & Kocer-Gumusel, B. (2016). Environmental effects of endocrine-disrupting chemicals: A special focus on phthalates and bisphenol A. In *Environmental Health Risk-Hazardous Factors to Living Species*. IntechOpen.

Ferguson, K. K., McElrath, T. F., & Meeker, J. D. (2014). Environmental phthalate exposure and preterm birth. *JAMA Pediatrics*, *168*(1), 61–67.

Moreno, M. (2014). Phthalate Exposure and Health Risks. *JAMA Pediatrics*, *168*(1), 96–96.

National Research Council. (2009). *Phthalates and cumulative risk assessment: the tasks ahead*. National Academies Press.

Suzuki, Y., Niwa, M., Yoshinaga, J., Mizumoto, Y., Serizawa, S., & Shiraishi, H. (2010). Prenatal exposure to phthalate esters and PAHs and birth outcomes. *Environment International*, *36*(7), 699–704.

Yan, X., Calafat, A., Lashley, S., Smulian, J., Ananth, C., Barr, D., ... Robson, M. G. (2009). Phthalates biomarker identification and exposure estimates in a population of pregnant women. *Human and Ecological Risk Assessment*, *15*(3), 565–578.

KEY TERMS AND DEFINITIONS

Chromatography: is a laboratory technique for the separation of a mixture.

Hypoestrogenic: refers to a lower than normal level of estrogen, the primary sex hormone in women.

Hypospadias: (hi-poe-SPAY-dee-us) is a birth defect (congenital condition) in which the opening of the urethra is on the underside of the penis instead of at the tip.

Cryptorchidism: is the absence of one or both testes from the scrotum.

Gynecomastia: is a condition that makes breast tissue swell in boys and men.

Phthalate syndrome: In tests of lab rats, chemicals called phthalates, which are widely used in plastic and personal care products, cause several reproductive abnormalities that scientists have dubbed "testicular dysgenesis syndrome" or "phthalate syndrome."

Puberty: is the time in life when a boy or girl becomes sexually mature.

Chapter 16
Environmental Phthalate Exposure in Relation to Reproductive Outcomes and Other Health Endpoints in Humans

Sameena
P. M. B. Gujarati Science College, India

Riyes Un Aziz
Government Holkar College, India

Aubid Bashir
Barkatullah University, India

ABSTRACT

Phthalates are the class of chemicals that exhibit numerous adverse effects to health. These non-persistent chemicals are produced in high volume annually and are used in a wide array of industrial consumer products. The overall exposure of phthalates to humans is via ingestion of contaminated food from wrapped materials or dermally via consumer care products. Pthalates are anti-androgenic compounds, so for this reason, they obtrude with the expression of testosterone by manipulating gene expression of proteins and enzymes involved in production of testosterone. The primarily exposure of Pthalates during fetal development stage results in number of harmful effects in male offspring in humans, like abnormalities of the sperm-producing organs, abnormal development of penile, hypospadias, reduced anogenital distance, as well as a risk for prostate cancer and cryptorchidism. The purpose of this chapter was to review the environmental impact of phthalate exposure in relation to reproductive behavior and other health problems in humans.

DOI: 10.4018/978-1-5225-9452-9.ch016

INTRODUCTION

The advancement of civilization resulted in foundation of new and progressive technologies, consumer products and goods whose manufacture needs new raw materials and chemical compounds. Most of the compounds among them are long-lasting and are not degraded after releasing in to the environment. They get deposited in the food chain and are then migrated across countries or even continents (Ziolkowska and Wyszkowska, 2010). Environmental pollutants affect soil properties (Wyszkowska and Wyszkowski, 2002; Wyszkowski and Sivitskaya, 2012) and exert a generally negative influence on flora, fauna and other forms of life (Ziolkowska and Wyszkowska, 2010; Wyszkowska and Wyszkowski, 2009). They can result in the endocrinological and reproductive problems. Selected chemical substances have androgen synthesis (Adamsson *et al.,* 2009). Phthalates, or esters of phthalic acid, are environmental pollutants (Grynkiewicz, 2011). Those leading plasticizers are added to polyvinyl chloride in order to enhance its hardness and flexibility. Phthalates are used almost in every industry, and they can be found in construction materials, food packaging, pharmaceuticals, varnish, cosmetics, printing inks, latex paint, medical products clothing,, such as intravenous cannulas, and insecticides (Koniecki *et al.,* 2011; Fierens *et al.*, 2012).

The aim of this study was to differentiate phthalates, to find out the sources of phthalate pollution in the environment, and to describe their affect on living organisms.

MODE OF ACTION, MECHANISM OF ACTION AND COMMON ADVERSE OUTCOMES (NATIONAL RESEARCH COUNCIL, 2008)

Mode of action and mechanism of action are terms that are often used in risk assessment and usually used interchangeably. Both these terms refer to the bio-logic pathway to some final health outcome; the difference between the terms is the level of detail used to describe the pathway. Typically, mode of action is used to describe the key events along the pathway and mechanism of action is used to describe the pathway at the molecular level, Although the committee identifies the distinction and does not want to contribute to over confusion regarding the use of the terms, mechanism of action is used in this report to explain the biologic pathway.

Currently, the concentrate in cumulative risk assessment has been on those chemical compounds that have common mechanisms of action. As described below in greater detail, the committee finds that the concentration in cumulative risk assessment must be on the health outcomes and not on the pathways that lead to them, whether defined as modes of action or as mechanisms of action. Several pathways can result to a common outcome, and a focus on only an accurate pathway can lead to limit an approach in conducting a cumulative risk assessment. Accordingly, the chemicals that should be considered for cumulative risk assessment must be ones that cause the same types of health outcomes or the same health outcomes such as specific effects on development of male reproductive system not ones that cause the health issues only by a specific pathway. The committee refers to the health outcomes of interest as common adverse outcomes.

CHARACTERISTICS OF PTHALATES

Phthalates are esters of phthalic acid, also known as esters of benzene-1, 2-dicarboxylic acid are man-made chemicals widely used in industry and commerce. This particular group of manufactured chemicals compounds has a broad spectrum of industrial applications and these chemicals ultimately appear extensively in food processing, consumer products, as well as in medical applications. Phthalates have a benzene ring with two functional (ester) groups. Their solubility in water decreases with an increase in the length of the carbon chain. Phthalates are colorless and odorless oily liquids characterized by limited solubility in water, satisfactory solubility in most organic solvents, high boiling point or molecular weight, low volatility. The esterification reaction to phthalic acid with various alcohols results in the production of the compounds. The amplest use of phthalates in many consumer and personal-care products result in expansive non occupational exposure to humans through several routes (Hauser *et al.*, 2007).

Phthalates are broadly divided into two basic categories; "High molecular-weight phthalates (HMWPs) eg, di2-ethylhexylphthalate (DEHP) and butyl benzyl phthalate (BBzP) include carbon side chains more than 6 (Bradlee and Thomas, 2003), are commonly used in building products, flooring and wall coverings, food packaging and processing materials, and medical devices. Low molecular weight phthalates (LMWPs)" which include carbon chain less than 6, eg, diethyl phthalate (DEP), benzyl butyl phthalate (BBzP), and diisobutyl phthalate (DiBP) are widely used in a variety of cosmetic and personal-hygiene products, toys, childcare products, fragrances as scent stabilizers, varnishes and lacquers (Jurica *et al.*, 2016).

The most widely used phthalates are di(2-ethylhexyl) phthalate (DEHP), diisodecyl phthalate (DIDP), diisononyl phthalate (DINP) and di-n-butyl phthalate (DBP) (Peijnenburg *et al.*, 2008). Di (2-ethylhexyl) phthalate (DEHP): DEHP is also known as dioctyl phthalate (DOP) it is produced by the esterification reaction of 2-ethylhexanol with phthalic anhydride (Ventrice *et al.,* 2013). This is the most common member of the class of phthalates, frequently used in construction materials, consumer goods, and electronics, medical such as infusion fluid containers, surgical drains, intravenous cannulas, blood storage and blood transfusion equipment (Heudorf *et al.,* 2007). According to Lyche, phthalates are ubiquitous contaminants in the environments found in drinking water at the concentration of 0.16-170 μg · dm –3,, in sediments, at 0.0003-218 mg kg –1, indoor air at 20-240 ng · m–3, atmospheric air at <0.4-65 ng · m–3,, dust at 2.38-4.1 g · kg –1, soil at 0.03-1280 mg · kg –1 and wastewater at 0.0004-58.3 g · kg –1. DEHP is characterized by high levels of reproductive toxicity, developmental toxicity and it can also cause reduced fertility, and may damage the neonates.

Diisodecyl Phthalate (DIDP): DIDP is mainly added to polyvinyl chloride (PVC). It can be found in various PVC products, including cable jackets, roofing panels flooring, wall panels, sealants and interior car parts (Risk Assessment Report, (2003) and Kransler *et al.,* (2013).

Diisononyl Phthalate (DINP): DINP is an organic substance. About 95% of globally manufactured DINP is primarily used as PVC plasticizer. It is found in electronics and home appliances footwear, lubricants, paper products inks, pigments flooring, coatings, sealants, varnish and paint (Hays *et al.,* 2011). DINP is a major plasticizer used in children's toys. DINP is obtained by the esterification reaction of phthalic anhydride with isononyl alcohol (Risk Assessment Report, 2003)

Di-n-butyl Phthalate (DBP): DBP is mainly used as a plasticizer for nitrocellulose, polyvinyl chloride and polyvinyl acetate, in coatings, in adhesives and in miscellaneous applications. DBP is obtained by the esterification reaction of phthalic anhydride with n-butanol in the presence of concentrated sulfuric

Table 1. Phthalate parent compounds and their metabolites

Phthalate name	Abbreviation	Urinary metabolite	Abbreviation
Dimethyl phthalate	DMP	Mono-n-methyl phthalate	MnMP
Diethyl phthalate	DEP	Mono-ethyl phthalate	MEP
Di-isobutyl phthalate	DiBP	Mono-isobutyl phthalate	MiBP
Di-n-butyl phthalate	DnBP	Mono-n-butyl phthalate	MnBP
Di-n-octyl phthalate	DnOP	Mono-(3-carboxypropyl) phthalate	MCPP
Di-isononyl phthalate	DiNP	Mono-carboxyoctyl phthalate	MCOP
Di-isodecyl phthalate	DiDP	Mono-carboxynonyl phthalate	MCNP
Benzylbutyl phthalate	BzBP	Mono-benzyl phthalate	MBzP
Di-2-ethylhexyl phthalate	DEHP	Mono-2-ethylhexyl phthalate	MEHP
		Mono-(2-ethyl-5-hydroxyhexyl) phthalate	MEHHP
		Mono-(2-ethyl-5-oxohexyl) phthalate	MEOHP
		Mono-(2-ethyl-5-carboxypentyl) phthalate	MECPP

acid. It dissolves easily in most organic solvents, including acetone, diethyl ether, ethanol and benzene (Pałaszewska *et al.,* 2012)

Global assessment of phthalate production in the environment is estimated at 5 million Mg per year, of which more than 60% is used by the processing industries of Japan, North America and Europe (Fierens *et al.,* 2012) When used as plasticizers, phthalates do not bind chemically with the material to which they are added to and are easily released in to the air, water, food and soil. Phthalates are of lipophilic nature, thus are readily dissolved and accumulated in lipids (Fierens *et al.,* 2012 and Heudorf *et al.,* 2007.) The phthalates are not chemically bound in the polymers and hence are leached into the environment from the product and are ubiquitously found in, air, water, soils, and dust. The migration of phthalates occurs during all the stages of life cycle of a product from production, through use, to disposal and the phthalates are thereby ubiquitous in the environment.

STRUCTURE OF PHTHALATES

The viscosity and plasticizer effectiveness of phthalates are because of their chemical structures. Phthalates constitute a broad chemical family comprised of a benzene ring, two carbonyl groups, and two alcohol groups to produce a diester structure. Common branched phthalates such as DINP DBP, DEHP, and BBP feature branched-chain alcohol moieties of 6 to 13 carbons. The linear phthalates contain linear alcohol groups and include short chain phthalates such as DMP and DEP, and other phthalates with chain lengths of 7 to 11 carbons are used to impart increased flexibility at lower temperatures. The benzene ring based structure of phthalates leads to decrease their viscosity level but also makes them harder to degrade. Phthalates move rapidly through the PVC polymer resulting in increased flexibility, softness, and elongation. Since they are not chemically connected to the PVC, and are fairly released in air, water, blood, saliva, since phthalates are highly lipophilic (fat soluble) and get accumulated more readily into lipid-containing solutions. Based on the circumstances of use, 2% - 50% of the phthalate content can emerge from products over their life cycle.

SOURCES OF PHTHALATES IN THE ENVIRONMENT

Phthalates are ubiquitous in household environments in both house dust and indoor air (Rudel *et al.*, 2003). Phthalate levels measured in indoor air are typically many times higher than in outdoor air. People are exposed to phthalates through inhalation and dermal absorption of indoor air. They have also been measured in variety of sources like foodstuff, drinking water and milk. However, the specific share from the various sources and phthalate exposure routes is unknown (Wormuth *et al.*, 2006).

High molecular weight phthalates, such as di(2-ethylhexyl) phthalate [DEHP], di-isononyl phthalate [DiNP], di-n-octyl phthalate [DnoP] are chiefly used as plasticizers to soften polyvinyl chloride (PVC) products which are widely used in personal care products food-containing materials, building materials, cosmetics, medical equipments(ATSDR, 2002). Highest exposure to DEHP can occur in the working environment (e.g. during the manufacture and processing of DEHP or DEHP containing products), during consumer use of these products, or through environmental media (food, air, water, dust). The use of DEHP in consumer products to which children are exposed e.g. toys, bath books, food packaging, and medical devices such as blood, intravenous tubing and nutrient bags are of great concern because of the increased vulnerability of general public

Lower molecular weight phthalates, including di-n-butyl phthalate (DnBP) and diethyl phthalate (DEP), are used personal-care products (e.g. perfumes, lotions, and cosmetics), as solvents and plasticizers for cellulose acetate, in the manufacture of lacquers, varnishes and coatings of drugs (ATSDR, 1995; ATSDR,2001), including those used to make time-release in some pharmaceutical products (Hauser, 2004). DEP (urinary metabolite MEP) levels measured in population samples are found in major quantity than those of DBP and DEHP (CDC, 2003; CDC, 2005). DEP has been found commonly in a large number of cosmetics and personal care products as shampoos, body washes conditioners, shaving gels, hair styling gels, deodorants and lotions and, in adults (Duty, 2005a) and youngsters (Sathyanarayana, 2008) associated with the use of such products

ROUTES OF EXPOSURE TO PHTHALATES

Humans are exposed to phthalates by several routes, and the most likely route varies by phthalate. Exposures can be oral (e.g. DEHP via phthalate-contaminated food, water and other liquids) or dermal (e.g. DEP, via cosmetics and other personal care products) and in infants and toddlers through frequent mouthing of toys) or can also be via inhalational exposure (FDA, 2001).Phthalates exposure to neonates occurs through the placenta or breast-feeding. Breast milk is known to contain detectable amounts of phthalates, particularly the most hydrophobic compounds, DINP and DEHP (Calafat *et al.*, 2004). Parenteral exposure from phthalate containing products and medical devices also lead to higher phthalate exposures mainly Di (2-ethylhexyl) phthalate (DEHP) to hospitalized populations (ATSDR, 2002; Green *et al.*, 2005). Phthalates are readily absorbed into the human blood stream or body fluids and are converted quickly into their respective primary and secondary metabolites. Unlike some other chemicals, they tend to excrete out of the body quickly through fecal matter and urine and. Phthalates can interact and associate with each other and hence enhance the toxicity.

PHTHALATE TOXICITY

Phthalate exposure in human beings is associated with potential disturbance in the development and function of reproductive organs through endocrine disruption, delays in fertility, impairment in fetal development, Sertoli cell dysfunction, and hormonal disruption in Leydig's cells, testicular effects increased risk of allergies, toxicity to kidneys, asthma, and cancer. The current tolerable daily intake (TDI) values for BBP, DBP and DEHP established by the EU Scientific Committee for Toxicity, Ecotoxicity and the Environment (CSTEE) is 37 μg/kg body weight/day based on available studies of reproductive toxicity, since wide spread exposure and reproductive toxicity seem to have greater relevance for humans beings than the proliferation of peroxisome in laboratory animal (rat) liver causing cancer (EFSA, 2003,2005; EU Scientific committee, 2017). One must be fully conscious that phthalate levels determined in the general public are far below the threshold levels at which the first toxic effects were detected in laboratory animals (Koch *et al.*, 2004; Duty *et al.,* 2003). However, because of the multiple contributing sources and routes of human exposure to different chemical classes (e.g. polybrominated diphenyl ethers, polychlorinated biphenyls, currently used pesticides– pyrethroids and organophosphates, bisphenol A, and phthalates) it is of great challenge to recognize which chemical or metabolite is responsible for adverse health outcomes (Robinson and Miller, 2015).

PHTHALATES ARE TOXIC TO MULTIPLE ORGAN SYSTEMS IN HUMANS AND ANIMAL MODELS

Phthalates are a class of chemicals that cause adverse health effects to multiple organ systems in humans and animal models. It is well known that phthalates are anti-androgenic compounds: that is, they alter the expression of the male sex hormone testosterone by reducing the expression or function of genes of enzymes and proteins involved in testosterone secretion. This may result in reduced fertility in males, and the production of non fertile sperm, as well as profound effects on the development of sexual organs during prenatal development. Male sex hormone, testosterone is important during fetal development in mammals, for the development of male reproductive organs. Exposure to phthalates during this critical period results in constellation of effects in male neonates in animal models, including abnormal development penis, abnormalities of the sperm-producing structures, cryptorchidism (undescended testes), reduced anogenital distance (AGD) (a marker of feminization), retained nipples and hypospadias (urethral opening on the underside of the penis instead of the tip) Similar effects have been observed in human studies associated with fetal or infant exposure to phthalates. Decreased anogenital distance and penile size is associated with poor semen quality in young men (Mendiola *et al.,* 2011), as well as higher risk for prostate cancer (Castano-Vinyals *et al.,* 2012). Effects on sexual development in both boys and girls are associated with phthalate exposure during childhood. Reproductive effects such as increased rates of miscarriage and decreased gestational age have also been observed in human studies.

A serious issue is the potential for phthalate exposure to affect intellectual development and other aspects of behavior. Prenatal phthalate exposure in humans is directly correlated with poorer cognitive performance during childhood, poorer psychomotor development during infancy and poorer social behavior. Prenatal exposure to phthalates is associated with a reduced masculine play behavior in boys during childhood. Phthalate exposure during childhood is significantly associated with decreased IQ and vocabulary scores, and learning disabilities and mental disorders, impulsivity, autism spectrum disorder and attention deficit hyperactivity disorder (ADHD) behaviors. Experimental animal studies also documented that phthalate exposure during early life can alter brain neurochemistry and induces abnormal behavioral presentations. Possible mechanisms include maternal thyroid dysfunction during pregnancy; interference with receptors on cells that are involved in various processes during early fetal development; interference with calcium signaling (functionally essential for communication between nerve cells); and interference with normal lipid metabolism, which is crucial for normal functioning and development of brain (Miodovnik *et al.,* 2014). Phthalates also affect normal immune system function by producing and secreting potent inflammatory factors in intact animals in vitro (tissue culture or cell) systems. Prenatal and postnatal exposure to phthalate is strongly linked with an enhancement in allergic responses like increase in asthma, congestion, breathlessness, wheezing, and eczema in children, and an increase in inflammatory response in both children and adults.

Phthalate exposure is strongly correlated with overweight/obesity in both children and adults, as well as an increase in elevated fasting glucose and insulin levels in adults. Phthalate exposure also alters thyroid hormone levels; increased risk of cardiovascular disease increased blood pressure, and increased risk for fibroids and endometriosis.

EVALUATING HUMAN EXPOSURE TO PHTHALATES

Because of the universal nature of environmental phthalate exposure, conventional epidemiological exposure estimation data (questionnaire information, environmental monitoring medical records, etc.) are of confined utility in assessing individual exposure. Instead, biomarkers of exposure are prominent. Urine is the preferred matrix as biomarker for phthalate determination in humans (Calafat and McKee, 2006). As a result of quick metabolism, metabolite levels in urine are typically higher, and are therefore more accurately biomonitored than levels of the total phthalate compound found in other media. Use of metabolites as biomarkers is preferred, because the possibility of accidental contamination during collection, storage and evaluation is greatly reduced. Phthalates or their metabolites have also been detected in many body fluids or secretions, including; urine, plasma, saliva, serum, breast milk, amniotic fluid, me conium and placenta. Phthalate exposures that occur during prenatal development are more likely to result in profound and permanent damaging effects on development than postnatal exposures, conducting such studies in human populations is of great challenge. First, in order to determine exposure precisely during fetal development, it is necessary to carefully monitor the assays by using archived samples from women during pregnancy. Second, such studies need reliable assessment of the offspring of those pregnancies. While this is considerably easy while prenatal stage, in order to examine associated outcomes occurring in postnatal life such as decreased semen quality, impaired fertility- it is essential to follow the pregnancy cohort for decades. The latest availability of various sensitive, specific, and economical assays makes such measures more functional for epidemiological studies (Silva *et al.,* 2007). Moreover, international quality control programs for phthalate metabolite measurements in human samples leads to the enhancement of comparability of results across laboratories worldwide.

Phthalates are quickly metabolized and excreted from the body, with the elimination half-lives less than 24 hours (Koch *et al.,* 2005). Most recent studies have examined the variability of urinary phthalate metabolites within-person (Hoppin *et al.,* 2004) and found that the Pearson correlation coefficient in phthalate or phthalate metabolite concentration in women's samples measured on two consecutive days ranged from 0.5 for mBzP to 0.8 for mBP and concluded that exposure may be adequately stable to assign an exposure level in spite of their short half-lives, based on a single sample. Accordingly,(Hauser, 2004) demonstrated that despite high day-to-day and month-to-month variability in men's individual urinary phthalate metabolite concentrations, a single spot urine sample sufficiently represented average concentration over 3 months period (Teitelbaum *et al.,* 2008) examined that sources of variability in biomarkers of environmental exposures in minority children, including phthalates, and found that a single urine sample is reasonable predictive of exposure over a 6-month interval to authorize its use as an exposure estimate in environmental epidemiology studies The data published on levels of phthalate metabolites in a large population-based sample of the US population over 6 years of age by Centers for Disease Control and Prevention (CDC) (CDC, 2003; CDC, 2005) revealed that widespread nature of phthalate metabolites and variation in measurements by sex ethnicity, age and sex. Wormuth (2006) concluded that phthalate metabolite levels estimated in a European population and estimates of exposure to DEHP and DBP in neonates are about one order of magnitude greater than those in adults. Furthermore, levels of methylbutylphthalate (MBP), monomethylphthalate (MMP) and methyleth-ylphthalate (MEP), in newborns, are directly related to the number of baby care products (creams, powders and lotions) used by their mothers (Sathyanarayana, 2008).

HUMAN FETAL OR INFANT PHTHALATE EXPOSURE AND ASSOCIATED HEALTH OUTCOMES

There were few studies conducted on environmental phthalate exposure associated with human health outcomes prior to 2000.

Evidence for the "Phthalate Syndrome" in Human

Over the past ten years, various experimental studies on rodents reported that several phthalates (most notably, BzBP, DBP and DEHP), disrupt the androgen-signaling pathway in males, causes male reproductive tract abnormalities when administered at the critical window for the development of the reproductive tract (Gray, 2000, Akingbemi, 2004, Foster, 2006). Lee and Koo (2007) the anti-androgenic effects of seven phthalates (DEHP and its metabolite, mono-2-ethyhexyl phthalate (MEHP), BzBP, DBP as well as di-n-heptyl phthalate (DnHP), di-isodecyl phthalate (DIDP), di-isononyl phthalate (DINP), were demonstrated by the Hershberger assay in castrated male SD rats, consequently this anti-androgenic action during prenatal period causes interference with the normal development of reproductive system, most notably results in reduced anogenital distance (AGD). Anogenital distance is the distance between the anus and external genetalia in newborn rodent pups. AGD is used as a sensitive biomarker of prenatal exposure to anti-androgens, including phthalates, flutamide and vinclozilin. Only a single human study had examined AGD in human males (Salazar-Martinez, 2004), although two other studies had examined AGD in female infants prior to 2005 (Callegari, 1987, Phillip *et al.,* 1996). These studies examined the possible sexual dimorphism of AGD in humans, consistent with rodent studies. However, these studies did not address the relationship of AGD to chemical exposure.

Numerous animal studies have reported that DBP, BzBP and DEHP induces marked reductions in testicular testosterone (T) production in neonates and reduces the expression of insulin-like growth factor-3 (Insl-3),exert diverging effects on male reproductive organs which, in addition to shortened AGD, other abnormalities include cryptorchidism, hypospadias, low sperm counts and malformations of the prostate, epididymis,, seminal vesicles, vas deferens and; altered hormone levels together they comprise the "phthalate syndrome" (Foster, 2006; Welsh, 2008).

While a variety of anti-androgens alter anogenital distance AGD in rodents, most are androgen receptor (AR) antagonists. The syndrome induced by the AR-antagonists differs from that induced by the phthalates, which suppress fetal testosterone and Insl-3 synthesis (Wilson *et al.,* 2008, Wilson, 2004). A variety of potentially anti-androgens including linuron (L), procymidone (P), linuron (L), p,p -DDE and flutamide (F) were tested. P, L, and p,p -DDE produced F-like profiles, that include reduced AGD but were different from those produced by DEHP and DBP (Gray, 2000). Thus, detection of male genital defects with reduced anogenital distance (AGD) appears to signal prenatal anti-androgen exposure, but it quiet necessary to broaden up the knowledge of the complete profile of genital dysmorphology and to focus a potential etiologic agent.

Phthalates in Relation to Genital Development in Human Infants

Study population by Shanna and swan (2008)—The SFF (Study for Future Families) is a multi-center pregnancy cohort study in which Shanna and swan (2008) collected and stored serum and urine samples obtained in mid pregnancy. The collection and availability of serum and urine samples, permitted them to link phthalate exposure in prenatal to outcomes in the children born to couples registered in SFF. Hence, Shanna and Swan (2008) started the Study of Phthalates in Pregnant Women and Children (PPWC) in order to observe genital parameters and AGD in human infants in relation to exposure of pthalates to their mother's. Shanna and swan (2008) provided evidence that a human analogue of the "phthalate syndrome" may be observed in male infants.

Infant Measurement (Shanna and Swan, 2008)

Shanna and Swan (2008) carried out the male infant examination included a detailed description of the scrotum and testes, measurement of the penis, AGD and location of testes. All measurements including AGD as well as penile size was done with a precision calipers. AGD (In males) is the distance (mm) from the center of the anus to the cephalad (towards the head) base of the penis, while AGD (female) is the distance (in mm) from the center of the anus to the cephalad base of the clitoris. Examiners studied also testicular descent, which was grouped as "incomplete" if one or both testicles were observed not to be "normal retractile" or "normal". Moreover, penile width and length were observed. Neither the support staff nor the pediatric physicians had any knowledge of level of phthalate concentration in the mother.

Phthalate measurements (Shanna and Swan, 2008) initially as SFF was not, designed to study biomarkers of prenatal exposure, urine collection was begun midway through the assessment only (but rather semen quality across four areas of the US). There were at least 106 pairs of mother-son with both boy's genital measurements and prenatal phthalate concentration. The concentrations of phthalate metabolite were examined in samples of urine provided at the time of pregnancy (mean 28.6 week of pregnancy, as measured from the last menstrual period), by a sensitive method that includes the enzymatic deconjugation of the phthalate metabolites from their glucuronidated form, automated on-line solid-phase extraction, separation with HPLC (high performance liquid chromatography), and observation by isotope-dilution tandem mass spectrometry (Silva, 2007).

Reproductive and Developmental Toxicity (Shanna and Swan, 2008)

Phthalates having a long alkyl side-chain in the ortho position have a strong potential for developmental and reproductive toxic effects in humans. These include (in the order of their toxic potential) DEHP>DBP>BBP as well as diisobutyl phthalate (DiBP), di-n-hexyl phthalate (DnHP), and diisononyl phthalate (DiNP) (Lyche, 2011; Fabjan *et al.,* 2006). Matsumoto *et al.,* (2008) reported a relationship between shorter duration of pregnancy and higher DEHP serum levels. The other reproductive effects such as decreased semen quality and cryptorchidism could be due to the ability of phthalate monoesters to cross the placental barrier and enter the umbilical cord blood of the foetus (Mose *et al.,* 2007).

Most of the studies (Swan *et al.,* 2010; Duty, 2003; Bornehag *et al.,* 2015; Hauser *et al.,* 2007) have provided evidence that changes in male reproductive parameters, such as anogenital distance (AGD, a biomarker of prenatal androgen exposure in male newborns), decreased reproductive hormone levels and DNA sperm damage could be associated with environmental exposure to phthalates. More recent studies with uncertain results suggest for further research of the effects of adult exposure to phthalates on male reproductive endpoints at ambient levels (Sharpe, 2001; Thurston *et al.,* 2016). whereas, studies on animals to the effects of phthalates on female reproductive endpoints (ovary weight, serum oestradiol levels) recommend that exposure to higher levels than ambient ones is essential to induce relevant changes (Kamrin, 2009). Although higher concentration of di-n-octyl phthalate (DOP), DBP, BBP and DEHP levels were observed in the blood of women with endometriosis (Cobellis, 2003; Reddy *et al.,* 2006), the problems in immune system functioning also lead the development of endometriosis (Matsumoto *et al.,* 2008). Several studies report phthalates as hormone disruptors (Lopez carrillo *et al.,* 2010; De coster and Larebeke, 2012), which means that they are able to interfere with the endocrine system responsible for development and growth and ultimately cause feminization of males, called as the "phthalate syndrome" (Wilson, 2008) and typical reduced male behavior in boys (Lovekamp and Davis, 2003; Sharpe *et al.,* 2008). The other syndrome associated to phthalate exposure is the TDS (testicular dysgenesis syndrome), which may involve hypospadias, cryptorchidism, higher incidence of prostate cancer and lower sperm count (Sharpe *et al.,* 2008). Exposure to phthalates in utero may affect production of hormone and formation of testis and later in life cause problems in the reproductive function (Lopez carillo *et al.,* 2010; Latini *et al.,* 2006). Environmental phthalates are able to cross the placental barrier from mother to foetus blood and are excreted in mother's breast milk (Latini, 2003; Calafat *et al.,* 2004; Kavlock *et al.,* 2006). Pthalates metabolites were examined in infants' urine also (Latini *et al.,* 2006). A Danish-Finish cohort study observed that elevated concentrations of DBP metabolites in mother's milk correlated inversely with free serum testosterone levels in three month-old male newborn (Main *et al.,* 2006). Adibi *et al.* (2010) examined intrauterine exposure to phthalates and resulted that urinary levels of phthalate metabolites correlated inversely with trophoblast differentiation gene expression, which is important for development of human placenta. There was no correlation found with the expression of genes characteristic for Steroidogenesis metabolite levels [monoisobutyl phthalate (MiBP), monomethyl phthalate (MMP)and monoethyl phthalate (MEP)] in infants and correlated them with the baby cosmetics that are used in daily basis (shampoo, infant powder and lotions). They recommended that exposure of phthalate can be minimized by lowering the use of childcare products. Most countries for example, European Parliament and the European Commission have set the MAC (maximum allowed concentrations) of phthalates in children's items for relaxation, toys, pacifiers and food, because of these toxic effects, especially on developing organisms like children (Regulations EC, 2017). Stalhnut *et al.* (2007) regarding endocrine disruption studied that least levels of testosterone in adult men exposed to phthalates were related with insulin resistance and obesity. Phthalates may also affect immune functions, thyroid signaling and metabolic homeostasis (Jaakkola and Knight, 2008; Meeker *et al.,* 2007). High concentrations of DEHP metabolite such as mono-(2-ethylhexyl) phthalate (MEHP) in urine are related with lower thyroid stimulating hormone levels and thyroid hormone (Meeker *et al.,* 2007). Urinary DBP metabolite such as monobutyl phthalate (MBP) in some pregnant women correlated inversely with levels of thyroxin (Haung *et al.,* 2009). People especially children who ate food having DEHP had low levels of TSH (thyroid stimulating hormone) in serum (Wu MT *et al.,* 2013). The thyroid hormone is one of the important hormones for the development and growth of the reproductive system. Its deficiency during fetal/prenatal or postnatal development leads to neurological disorders and brain damage.

Phthalates and Gestational Age at Delivery (Shanna and Swan, 2008)

Latini (2003) measured serum MEHP and DEHP in the cord blood of 84 infants and observed concentrations in relation to gestational age (which was not defined). MEHP and DEHP were present each in 65 of 84 (77.4%) of the examined samples. Infants in which MEHP was observed in cord blood were grouped as "MEHP-positive" (with a definition similar for DEHP). MEHP positive newborn infants showed a lower gestational age significantly when compared with MEHP negative infants (38.16 ± 2.34 vs. 39.35 ± 1.35; $t = -2.163$, $p = 0.033$). There was no relationship found for DEHP and no significant relations were observed between either MEHP or DEHP and birth weight. Colon *et al.* (2000) compared serum levels of phthalates in 35 pediatric controls (median age of 46 months) with forty one Puerto Rican girls (median age of 20 months) with premature thelarche (premature breast development). The highest differences between controls and cases were between serum DEHP concentration in controls and cases; 70 and 450 mg/ml, respectively ($p < 0.05$). There are various concerns involving several aspects of the study design (McKee, 2004) like the fact that exposure was measured concurrent with diagnosis, the large age difference between cases and controls, and potential sample contamination.

Phthalates in Relation to Allergy, Asthma and Respiratory Function

A number of experiments have observed allergy, asthma and respiratory function in children in relation to the use of phthalates in house dust and PVC containing products or articles in the home (Bornehag *et al.,* 2004; Jaakkola, 1999; Jaakkola, 2000) although none has used biomarkers to define exposure. 2 cross-sectional studies had provided relationship between house dust levels of DEHP and BzBP and allergic symptoms (Bornehag *et al.,* 2004; Kolarik *et al.,* 2008).

SUMMARY OF HEALTH OUTCOMES IN ADULTS (SHANNA AND SWAN (2008)

Phthalates in relation to sex hormones in males and semen quality — Most of the researchers published a series of experiments that reported serum reproductive hormones in men attending an infertility clinic, urinary phthalate levels, sperm DNA damage and semen characteristics (Duty, 2005; Duty, 2003a; Duty, 2003b; Hauser *et al.,* 2004). There were dose dependent relationships of low sperm concentration with MBP (smoking status (1.0, 3.1, 2.5, 3.3; P for trend= 0.04), adjusted for age, motility (1.0, 1.5, 1.5, 1.8; P for trend = 0.04), abstinence time, and and odds ratio per quartile. There was higher evidence of an association between the low sperm concentration and highest MBzP quartile (1.0, 1.1, 1.1,1.9; P for trend = 0.13). DEHP, MEP or the MMP metabolites was having no relationship with these semen parameters. These results completely differed from those recorded by Jonsson (2005), who did not recorded any relationship between phthalate exposure and semen quality in a study of young healthy military recruits. A small study in Shanghai (Zhang, 2006) observed concentration of 3 phthalates (DBP, DEP and DEHP) in semen samples. No relationship was seen with sperm concentration. DEHP was correlated significantly to "rate of malformation" (presumably impaired morphology). All three phthalates (DBP, DEP and DEHP) were positively related with sample liquefaction time.

Phthalates in Relation to Metabolism and Thyroid Function in Adults

There are certain human studies of phthalate effects in adults other than studies of male reproduction function.

Only a single study till date has been examined markers of metabolic syndrome in relation to phthalate exposure. Stahlhut *et al.* (2007) examined phthalate exposure and its relation with insulin resistance and abdominal obesity in adult male participants in the National Health and Nutrition Examination Survey (NHANES) 1999–2002. They kept six phthalate metabolites as predictors of HOMA (a measure of insulin resistance) and waist circumference using multiple linear regression, adjusted for urine creatinine, age, fat, race/ethnicity, physical activity level, serum cotinine, and total calorie consumption. Three with elevated HOMA (MBP, MBzP, and MEP) and four metabolites were associated significantly with increased waist circumference (MEHHP, MBzP, MEP and MEOHP).

Meeker *et al.* (2007) recorded urinary concentrations of phthalate monoester metabolites and MEHP in 408 male partners in couples that were sub fertile and resulted that in adult men, Urinary MEHP concentrations may be associated with altered free T3 or/and total T4 levels. Moreover, they saw an inverse association between free T4 and T3 serum levels and MEHP urinary concentrations. The inverse association between free T4 remained and MEHP when adjusting for oxidative metabolite concentrations, which simultaneously reported a positive association with free T4.

RESPIRATORY TOXICITY

Exposure of humans to phthalates during childhood (as well as in the neonatal and foetal period) is often related with impaired lung function, allergies in children, asthma in adults and risk of bronchial obstruction (Jaakkola and Knight, 2008; Hoppin *et al.,* 2004). The lungs of newly born rats exposed to DEHP exhibit histological changes similar to those studied in the lungs of children with a chronic lung disease particularly of preterm infants known as broncho pulmonary dysplasia, (Magliozzi *et al.,* 2003). Asthma, rhinitis and Wheezing in children could be associated with increased concentrations of DEHP and BBP in house dust (Bornehag and Nanberg, 2010; Bornehag *et al.,* 2004; Kolarik *et al.*, 2008). Hoping *et al* (2004) studied the relation between four pulmonary function parameters in the Third National Health and Nutrition Examination Survey (NHANES, 1988–1994) and phthalate exposure. After controlling for smoking, race, height, age and body mass index, there was an inverse relation between three measures of pulmonary function (PEF,FVC, FEV1) and MBP and elevated concentration of MEP was associated with lower FEV1 and FVC values in men. No consistent associations were found with other phthalate metabolites and in females (Hoppin *et al.,* 2004).

DNA DAMAGE AND CARCINOGENESIS

Hauser *et al.*, (2007); Hauser (2008) reported that DEP and DEHP levels are correlated with DNA damage in sperm in exposed humans. Lopez-Carrillo *et al.,* (2010) provided a possible connection between exposure to DEP through a personal care products and cosmetics with an elevated risk of breast cancer, which is related to demethylating DEP the estrogen receptor complex. IARC (The International Agency for Research on Cancer) has provided evidence that DEHP cannot be grouped as human carcinogen because DEHP stimulates liver tumors in rodents by a process activating PPARα that is not found in humans (Klaunig *et al.,* 2003; Guyton *et al.,* 2009). Moreover, as there are no availability of data for DEHP carcinogenicity in humans but there is more evidence of DEHP carcinogenicity in experimental animals, it has been grouped as possibly carcinogenic to humans (Group 2B) (IARC, 2013).

PHTHALATE MIGRATION AND REGULATIONS

Research gives evidence that phthalates are able to migrate to bottled and tap water (Bosnir *et al.*, 2007; Kereszles *et al.*, 2013; IARC, 2013; Khedr, 2013) and alcoholic and soft drinks (Jurica *et al.,* 2016; Bosnir *et al.,* 2007; Chatonnet *et al.,* 2014; March and Cerda, 2015, Wang *et al.,* 2015). Migration of phthalates from plastic packaging to soft drinks is 5 to 40 times more than migration to mineral water (Bosnir *et al.,* 2007). One of the reasons for this higher concentration may be due to the difference in pH: more than 5 in all mineral waters and less than 3 in soft drinks. The MACs of the several common phthalate DEHP in drinking water set by the US EPA and World Health Organization (WHO) are 6 µg L-1 and 8 µg L-1 respectively (US EPA, 2017; WHO, 2017). One of the key acts to mention here is that under the European Regulation (EC) No. 1907/2006 (REACH) and its amendments (until February 2017) (Regulation EC, 2017). It mentions that DIBP, DBP, BBP and DEHP should not be used in any of the childcare products, toys and matrices in specific, from 21 February 2015 (so called "sunset date") due to the evidence of strong toxic effects on reproduction. More particularly, childcare products and toys containing phthalates in a concentration higher than 0.1% of the plasticized material weight must not be marketed. Other phthalates, namely diisodecyl phthalate (DIDP), DOP, and DINP have only been banned in childcare products and toys that children can put in the mouth (Regulation EC, 2017). The tolerable daily intake (TDI) set by the European Food Safety Authority (EFSA) is 500 µg kg-1 bw for BBP (EFSA, 2003-2005), 150 µg kg-1 bw for DINP and DIDP (EFSA, 2003-2005), 50 µg kg-1 bw for DEHP (EFSA, 2003-2005) and 10 µg kg-1 bw for DBP (EFSA, 2003-2005). With EU Regulation No. 10/2011 EC of 14 January 2011 (EU, 2017), the EU has established the so-called SML (specific migration limits) in plastics likely to come into contact with beverages and food. SML (specific migration limits) is the MAC of a given substance released from a article or material into food stimulants or food. For BBP 30.0 mg kg-1 food, for DEHP 1.5 mg kg-1 food and for DBP it is 0.3 mg kg-1 food. DIBP is not permitted in food contact articles. This EU regulation indirectly limits the maximum concentrations of those substances that are undesirable in alcoholic beverages. In some countries, producers of spirits are not required to observe phthalates in alcoholic beverages, but in some MACs are prescribed. Let us take the example of Slovakian Regulations on the General Code for Contaminants and Groceries in Food define the MAC for phthalates as a sum of DBP and DEHP, which is 2 mg kg-1 in alcoholic beverages, fruits, flour, leaved vegetables and 0.7 mg kg-1 in the potatoes and root vegetables (Vinos, 2004).

Magnitude and Time Course

For assessing the overall human exposure to phthalates, two methods have been adopted. One is modeling approach method of exposures based on environmental phthalate behavioral assessments and measurements. The second is biomonitoring of phthalate metabolite or phthalate levels in human fluids especially body fluids like urine and calculating exposures based on these analyses.

Modeling Exposures Using Data From Environmental Analysis and Behaviors

One of the important approaches I.e. modeling approach is examined by combining information on: (1) human behaviors, e.g., the amount of food ingested, the characteristics and duration of toy behavior etc. Based on this information, total exposure through all routes of exposure and the amount of exposure level through each route may be calculated and (2) the levels of phthalates in the environment, e.g., consumer products, food, air, toys, water etc. The accuracy of the resulting value is based upon knowledge of: (1) behaviors, such as frequency of ingestion and amount of food of each type ingested (2) the concentrations of each phthalate in each of the sources and how these levels vary over location and time and (3) all significant sources of each phthalates. Because of the complication in collecting such data on phthalates from the multiplicity of possible sources, uncertainties in level of exposure values derived from this methodology are significant. Moreover, as phthalates are present everywhere, contamination of samples or products from environmental sources may be a serious problem and may lead to large overestimates of exposures. While keeping in mind these difficulties, the modeling approach does have the benefit of giving data for all age groups like infant, children, adults etc. on the apportionment of exposure among sources and on the duration and timing of exposures information that is generally not available from biomonitoring.

Estimating Exposures Based on Biomonitoring Data

The other most important exposure assessment methodology is biomonitoring, which gives direct ways to measure the amount of each phthalate metabolite or phthalate in human body fluids like blood, urine and tissues. These body fluid or tissue levels must be translated then into exposures. This translation needs knowledge of the relation- ship between the amounts of parent metabolites or compounds found in the body fluids or tissues and the magnitude of the phthalate exposure. In the past seven or eight years, several biomonitoring measurements concentrated on phthalate metabolites rather than their parent compounds or metabolite. As there are large significant gaps in knowledge regarding the fate and metabolism of phthalates, it is hard here to mention that which metabolite is the most appropriate or accurate analyte. Since each of metabolite may have a significant impact on the exposure estimate, literature exposure values may significantly vary when they are based on various metabolites (Calafat and McKee, 2006). Another important cause of uncertainty is that the conversion from body fluid concentrations to levels of exposure is based on collected data from adults and it is not even clear how much applicable these data are to other age groups, especially children and infants.

RECOMMENDATIONS FOR EFFECTIVE CONTROL OF PHTHALATE EXPOSURE

As the frequency and quantity of phthalates exposure to human is often unknown, research should concentrate on the routes and sources and try to answer the basic question that at which level the phthalates are hazardous for health of human and other living creatures. It is certainly important to biologically monitor phthalates concentrations by determining their metabolites in body fluids, principally in the urine. Their MACs should be monitored in alcoholic beverages, drinking water and food. In order to avoid economic losses in markets with defined MACs, the producers of food products and alcoholic beverages should introduce phthalate monitoring through product safety systems and internal quality management. Moreover, exposure of phthalates could further be lowered by introducing and finding alternative, plasticizers and phthalate-free materials into the production of consumer products or parts used in beverage and food processing and storage.

CONCLUSION

Phthalates, the esters and salts of phthalic acid, are universal in the environment. They are used as plasticizers during the making of food packaging, adhesives, paint, and cosmetics and PVC. The manufactured compounds are present in every home and they have the ability to easily migrate to the environment and make environment polluted. Phthalates are found everywhere especially in air, soil, treated effluents, water, land filled waste and plants. Moreover, they do not bind themselves permanently with the products to which they are added. Phthalates create a risk of exposure for living organism especially to humans and are rapidly released into the environment. They are represented by reproductive toxicity in animals and humans; they are able to cause reproductive problems and infertility in males. Phthalates are considered more toxic to young children, which are much more vulnerable to phthalate exposure, including fetal life. Phthalates are very difficult to eliminate from our daily surroundings as they are used in numerous industries.

REFERENCES

Adamsson, A., Salonen, V., Paranko, J., & Toppari, J. (2009). Effects of maternal exposure to diisononylphthalate (DINP) and 1, 1-dichloro-2, 2-bis (p-chlorophenyl) ethylene (p,p′ -DDE)on steroidogenesis is the fetal rat testis and adrenal gland. *Reproductive Toxicology (Elmsford, N.Y.)*, *28*(1), 66–74. doi:10.1016/j.reprotox.2009.03.002 PMID:19490997

Adibi, J. J., Whyatt, R. M., Hauser, R., Bhat, H. K., Davis, B. J., Calafat, A. M., ... Williams, P. L. (2010). Transcriptional biomarkers of steroidogenesis and trophoblast differentiation in the placenta in relation to prenatal phthalate exposure. *Environmental Health Perspectives*, *118*(2), 291–296. doi:10.1289/ehp.0900788 PMID:20123604

Akingbemi, B. T., Ge, R., Klinefelter, G. R., Zirkin, B. R., & Hardy, M. P. (2004). Phthalate-induced Leydig Cell Hyperplasia is Associated with Multiple Endocrine Disturbances. *Proceedings of the National Academy of Sciences of the United States of America*, *101*(3), 775–780. doi:10.1073/pnas.0305977101 PMID:14715905

ATSDR. (1995) Agency for Toxic Substances and Disease Registry. Atlanta, GA: Division of Toxicology.

ATSDR. (2001). Agency for Toxic Substances and Disease Registry. Atlanta, GA: Division of Toxicology.

ATSDR. (2002) Agency for Toxic Substances and Disease Registry. Atlanta, GA: Division of Toxicology.

ATSDR. (2002). *Toxicological profile for di(2-ethylhexyl)phthalate (DEHP)*. Atlanta, GA: Agency for Toxic Substances and Disease Registry.

Bornehag, C. G., Carlstedt, F., Jönsson, B. A., Lindh, C. H., Jensen, T. K., Bodin, A., ... Swan, S. H. (2015). Prenatal phthalate exposures and anogenital distance in Swedish boys. *Environmental Health Perspectives*, *123*(1), 101–107. doi:10.1289/ehp.1408163 PMID:25353625

Bornehag, C. G., & Nanberg, E. (2010). Phthalate exposure and asthma in children. *International Journal of Andrology*, *33*, 333–345.

Bornehag, C. G., Sundell, J., Weschler, C. J., Sigsgaard, T., Lundgren, B., Hasselgren, M., & Hägerhed-Engman, L. (2004). The association between asthma and allergic symptoms in children and phthalates in house dust: A nested case-control study. *Environmental Health Perspectives*, *112*(14), 1393–1397. doi:10.1289/ehp.7187 PMID:15471731

Bošnir, J., Puntarić, D., Galić, A., Škes, I., Dijanić, T., Klarić, M., ... Šmit, Z. (2007). Migration of phthalates from plastic containers into soft drinks and mineral water. *Food Technology and Biotechnology*, *45*, 91–95.

Calafat, A. M., & McKee, R. H. (2006). Integrating biomonitoring exposure data into the risk assessment process: Phthalates [diethyl phthalate and di(2-ethylhexyl) phthalate] as a case study. *Environmental Health Perspectives*, *114*(11), 1783–1789. doi:10.1289/ehp.9059 PMID:17107868

Calafat, A. M., Slakman, A. R., Silva, M. J., Herbert, A. R., & Needham, L. L. (2004). Automated solid phase extraction and quantitative analysis of human milk for 13 phthalate metabolites. *Journal of Chromatography. B, Analytical Technologies in the Biomedical and Life Sciences*, *805*(1), 49–56. doi:10.1016/j.jchromb.2004.02.006 PMID:15113539

Calafat, A. M., Slakman, A. R., Silva, M. J., Herbert, A. R., & Needham, L. L. (2004). Automated solid phase extraction and quantitative analysis of human milk for 13 phthalate metabolites. *Journal of Chromatography. B, Analytical Technologies in the Biomedical and Life Sciences*, *805*(1), 49–56. doi:10.1016/j.jchromb.2004.02.006 PMID:15113539

Callegari, C., Everett, S., Ross, M., & Brasel, J. A. (1987). Anogenital ratio: Measure of fetal virilization in premature and full-term newborninfants. *The Journal of Pediatrics*, *111*(2), 240–243. doi:10.1016/S0022-3476(87)80075-6 PMID:3612396

Cao, X. L. (2008). Determination of phthalates and adipate in bottled water by headspace solid-phase microextraction and gas chromatography/mass spectrometry. *Journal of Chromatography. A*, *1178*(1-2), 231–238. doi:10.1016/j.chroma.2007.11.095 PMID:18082753

Castaño-Vinyals, G., Carrasco, E., Lorente, J. A., Sabaté, Y., Cirac-Claveras, J., Pollán, M., & Kogevinas, M. (2012). Anogenital distance and the risk of prostate cancer. *BJU International*, *110*(11b), E707–E710. doi:10.1111/j.1464-410X.2012.11516.x PMID:22984847

CDC. (2003). Second national report on human exposure to environmental chemicals. Atlanta, GA: National Center for Environmental Health, Division of Laboratory Sciences.

CDC. (2005). Third national report on human exposure to environmental chemicals. Atlanta, GA: National Center for Environmental Health, Division of Laboratory Sciences.

Chatonnet, P., Boutou, S., & Plana, A. (2014). Contamination of wines andspirits by phthalates: Types of contaminants present, contamination sources and means of prevention. *Food Addit. Contam. Part A*, *31*(9), 1605–1615. doi:10.1080/19440049.2014.941947 PMID:25099435

Cobellis, L. (2003). High plasma concentrations of di-(2-ethylhexyl)-phthalate in women with endometriosis. *Human Reproduction (Oxford, England)*, *18*(7), 1512–1515. doi:10.1093/humrep/deg254 PMID:12832380

Colon, I. (2000). Identification of phthalate esters in the serum of young Puerto Rican girls with premature breast development. *Environmental Health Perspectives*, *108*, 895–900. PMID:11017896

De Coster, S., & van Larebeke, N. (2012). Endocrine-disrupting chemicals: Associated disorders and mechanisms of action. *Journal of Environmental and Public Health*. PMID:22991565

Duty, S. M., Ackerman, R. M., Calafat, A. M., & Hauser, R. (2005a). Personal care product use predicts urinary concentrations of some phthalate monoesters. *Environmental Health Perspectives*, *113*(11), 1530–1535. doi:10.1289/ehp.8083 PMID:16263507

Duty, S. M., Silva, M. J., Barr, D. B., Brock, J. W., Ryan, L., Chen, Z., ... Hauser, R. (2003a). Phthalate exposure and human semen parameters. *Epidemiology (Cambridge, Mass.)*, *14*(3), 269–277. doi:10.1097/01.EDE.0000059950.11836.16 PMID:12859026

Duty, S. M., Singh, N. P., Silva, M. J., Barr, D. B., Brock, J. W., Ryan, L., ... Hauser, R. (2003). The relationship between environmental exposures to phthalates and DNA damage in human sperm using the neutral comet assay. *Environmental Health Perspectives*, *111*(9), 1164–1169. doi:10.1289/ehp.5756 PMID:12842768

Duty, S. M., Singh, N. P., Silva, M. J., Barr, D. B., Brock, J. W., Ryan, L., ... Hauser, R. (2003b). The relationship between environmental exposures to phthalates and DNA damage in human sperm using the neutral comet assay. *Environmental Health Perspectives*, *111*(9), 1164–1169. doi:10.1289/ehp.5756 PMID:12842768

EU Scientific Committee on Toxicity Ecotoxicity and the Environment (CSTEE). (2017). *Opinion on phthalate migration from soft PVC toys and child-care articles*. Brussels: Author.

European Commission. (2011). *Commission Regulation (EU) No 10/2011 of 14 January 2011 on Plastic materials and articles intended to come into contact with food*. Author.

European Food Safety Authority (EFSA). (2003a). *Opinion of the Scientific Panel on food additives, flavourings, processing aids and materials in contact with food (AFC) related to Butylbenzylphthalate (BBP) for use in food contact materials*. Author.

European Food Safety Authority (EFSA). (2003b). *Opinion of the scientific panel on food additives, flavouring, processing aids and material in contact with food on a request from the Commission related to di-isodecylphthalate (DIDP) for use in food contact materials*. Author.

European Food Safety Authority (EFSA). (2005a). *Opinion of the Scientific Panel on food additives, flavourings, processing aids and material in contact with food (AFC) related to di-Butylphthalate (DBP) for use in food contact materials*. Author.

European Food Safety Authority (EFSA). (2005b). *Opinion of the Scientific Panel on food additives, flavourings, processing aids and materials in contact with food (AFC) related to Bis(2-ethylhexyl)phthalate (DEHP) for use in food contact materials*. Author.

European Food Safety Authority (EFSA). (2005c). *Opinion of the scientific panel on food additives, flavouring, processing aids and material in contact with food on a request from the Commission related to di-isononylphthalate (DINP) for use in food contact materials*. Author.

Fabjan, E., Hulzebos, E., Mennes, W., & Piersma, A. H. (2006). A category approach for reproductive effects of phthalates. *Critical Reviews in Toxicology*, *36*(9), 695–726. doi:10.1080/10408440600894914 PMID:17050082

FDA. (2001). Food and Drug Administration Total Diet Study; summary of residues found ordered by pesticide market baskets 91-3--99-1. Rockville, MD: Office of Plant and Dairy Foods and Beverages.

Fierens, T., Servaes, K., Van Holderbeke, M., Geerts, L., De Henauw, S., Sioen, I., & Vanermen, G. (2012). Analysis of phthalates in food products and packaging materials sold on the Belgian market. *Food and Chemical Toxicology*, *50*(7), 2575–2583. doi:10.1016/j.fct.2012.04.029 PMID:22554646

Fierens, T., Van Holderbeke, M., Willems, H., De Henauw, S., & Sioen, I. (2012). Transfer of eight phthalates through the milk chain - A case study. *Environment International*, *2013*(51), 1–7. PMID:23138015

Foster, P. M. (2006). Disruption of Reproductive Development in Male Rat Offspring Following in Utero Exposure to Phthalate Esters. *International Journal of Andrology*, *29*(1), 140–147. doi:10.1111/j.1365-2605.2005.00563.x PMID:16102138

Gray, L. E. J. R. (2000). Perinatal exposure to the phthalates DEHP, BBP, and DINP, but not DEP, DMP, or DOTP, alters sexual differentiation of the male rat. *Toxicological Sciences*, *58*(2), 350–365. doi:10.1093/toxsci/58.2.350 PMID:11099647

Green, R., Hauser, R., Calafat, A. M., Weuve, J., Schettler, T., Ringer, S., ... Hu, H. (2005). Use of di(2-ethylhexyl) phthalate-containing medical products and urinary levels of mono(2-ethylhexyl) phthalate in neonatal intensive care unit infants. *Environmental Health Perspectives*, *113*(9), 1222–1225. doi:10.1289/ehp.7932 PMID:16140631

Grynkiewicz-Bylina, B. (2011). Dangerous phthalates in children's environment. *Ecological Chemistry and Engineering. S*, *18*(4), 455–463.

Guyton, K. Z., Chiu, W. A., Bateson, T. F., Jinot, J., Siegel Scott, C., Brown, R. C., & Caldwell, J. C. (2009). A reexamination of the PPAR-alpha activation mode of action as a basis for assessing human cancer risks of environmental contaminants. *Environmental Health Perspectives*, *117*(11), 1664–1672. doi:10.1289/ehp.0900758 PMID:20049115

Hauser, R. (2008). *Urinary phthalate metabolites and semen quality:a review of a potential biomarker of susceptibility*. Academic Press.

Hauser, R., Duty, S., Godfrey-Bailey, L., & Calafat, A. M. (2004a). Medications as a source of human exposure tophthalates. *Environmental Health Perspectives*, *112*(6), 751–753. doi:10.1289/ehp.6804 PMID:15121520

Hauser, R., Meeker, J. D., Park, S., Silva, M. J., & Calafat, A. M. (2004b). Temporal variability of urinary phthalate metabolite levels in men of reproductive age. *Environmental Health Perspectives*, *112*(17), 1734–0. doi:10.1289/ehp.7212 PMID:15579421

Hauser, R., Meeker, J. D., Singh, N. P., Silva, M. J., Ryan, L., Duty, S., & Calafat, A. M. (2007). DNA damage in human sperm is related to urinary levels of phthalate monoester and oxidative metabolites. *Human Reproduction (Oxford, England)*, *22*(3), 688–695. doi:10.1093/humrep/del428 PMID:17090632

Hays, S. M., Aylward, L. L., Kirman, C. R., Krishnan, K., & Nong, A. (2011). Biomonitoring equivalents for di-isononyl phthalate (DINP). *Regulatory Toxicology and Pharmacology*, *60*(2), 181–188. doi:10.1016/j.yrtph.2011.03.013 PMID:21466828

Heudorf, U., Mersch-Sundermann, V., & Angerer, J. (2007). Phthalates: Toxicology and exposure. *International Journal of Hygiene and Environmental Health*, *210*(5), 623–634. doi:10.1016/j.ijheh.2007.07.011 PMID:17889607

Hoppin, J. A., Ulmer, R., & London, S. J. (2004). Phthalate exposure and pulmonary function. *Environmental Health Perspectives*, *112*(5), 571–574. doi:10.1289/ehp.6564 PMID:15064163

Huang, P. C., Kuo, P. L., Chou, Y. Y., Lin, S. J., & Lee, C. C. (2009). Association between prenatal exposure to phthalates and the health of newborns. *Environment International*, *35*(1), 14–20. doi:10.1016/j.envint.2008.05.012 PMID:18640725

IARC. (2013). Working Group on the Evaluation of Carcinogenic Risks to Humans. Some chemicals present in industrial and consumer products, food and drinking-water. *IARC Monographs on the Evaluation of Carcinogenic Risks to Humans*, *101*, 9–549. PMID:24772663

Jaakkola, J. J. (2000). Plastic wall materials in the home and respiratory health in young children. *American Journal of Public Health*, *90*(5), 797–799. doi:10.2105/AJPH.90.5.797 PMID:10800434

Jaakkola, J. J., Oie, L., Nafstad, P., Botten, G., Samuelsen, S. O., & Magnus, P. (1999). Interior surface materials in the home and the development of bronchial obstruction inyoung children in Oslo, Norway. *American Journal of Public Health*, *89*(2), 188–192. doi:10.2105/AJPH.89.2.188 PMID:9949747

Jaakkola, J. J. K., & Knight, T. L. (2008). The role of exposure to phthalates from polyvinyl chloride products in the development of asthma and allergies: A systematic review and meta-analysis. *Environmental Health Perspectives*, *116*(7), 845–853. doi:10.1289/ehp.10846 PMID:18629304

Jonsson, B. A. (2005). Urinary phthalate metabolites and biomarkers of reproductive function in young men. *Epidemiology (Cambridge, Mass.)*, *16*, 487–493. doi:10.1097/01.ede.0000164555.19041.01 PMID:15951666

Jurica, K., Brčić Karačonji, I., Lasić, D., Vukić Lušić, D., Anić Jurica, S., & Lušić, D. (2016). Determination of phthalates in plum spirit and their occurrence during plum spirit production. *Acta Alimentaria*, *45*(1), 141–148. doi:10.1556/066.2016.45.1.17

Kamrin, M. A. (2009). Phthalate risks, phthalate regulation, and public health: A review. *Journal of Toxicology and Environmental Health. Part B, Critical Reviews*, *12*(2), 157–174. doi:10.1080/10937400902729226 PMID:19235623

Kavlock, R., Barr, D., Boekelheide, K., Breslin, W., Breysse, P., Chapin, R., ... Williams, P. (2006). NTP-CERHR Expert Panel update on the reproductive and developmental toxicity of di(2-ethylhexyl) phthalate. *Reproductive Toxicology (Elmsford, N.Y.)*, *22*(3), 291–399. doi:10.1016/j.reprotox.2006.04.007 PMID:17068859

Keresztes, S., Tatár, E., Czégény, Z., Záray, G., & Mihucz, V. G. (2013). Study on the leaching of phthalates from polyethylene terephthalate bottles into mineral water. *The Science of the Total Environment*, *458-460*, 451–458. doi:10.1016/j.scitotenv.2013.04.056 PMID:23688967

Khedr, A. (2013). Optimized extraction method for LC-MS determination of bisphenol A, melamine and di(2-ethylhexyl) phthalate in selected soft drinks, syringes, and milk powder. *Journal of Chromatography. B, Analytical Technologies in the Biomedical and Life Sciences*, *930*, 98–103. doi:10.1016/j.jchromb.2013.04.040 PMID:23727873

Klaunig, J. E., Babich, M. A., Baetcke, K. P., Cook, J. C., Corton, J. C., David, R. M., ... Fenner-Crisp, P. A. (2003). PPARalpha agonist-induced rodent tumors: Modes of action and human relevance. *Critical Reviews in Toxicology*, *33*(6), 655–780. doi:10.1080/713608372 PMID:14727734

Koch, H. M., Drexler, H., & Angerer, J. (2004). Internal exposure of nursery-school children and their parents and teachers to di(2-ethylhexyl)phthalate (DEHP). *International Journal of Hygiene and Environmental Health, 207*(1), 15–22. doi:10.1078/1438-4639-00270 PMID:14762970

Kolarik, B., Naydenov, K., Larsson, M., Bornehag, C. G., & Sundell, J. (2008). The association between phthalates in dust and allergic diseases among Bulgarian children. *Environmental Health Perspectives, 116*(1), 98–103. doi:10.1289/ehp.10498 PMID:18197306

Kransler, K. M., Bachman, A. N., & McKee, R. H. (2013). Estimates of daily di-isodecyl phthalate (DIDP) intake calculated from urinary biomonitoring data. *Regulatory Toxicology and Pharmacology, 65*(1), 29–33. doi:10.1016/j.yrtph.2012.11.004 PMID:23174424

Latini, G., De Felice, C., Presta, G., Del Vecchio, A., Paris, I., Ruggieri, F., & Mazzeo, P. (2003). In utero exposure to di-(2-ethylhexyl)phthalate and duration of human pregnancy. *Environmental Health Perspectives, 111*(14), 1783–1785. doi:10.1289/ehp.6202 PMID:14594632

Latini, G., Del Vecchio, A., Massaro, M., Verrotti, A., & De Felice, C. (2006). *In utero exposure to phthalates and fetal development*. Academic Press.

Lee, B. M., & Koo, H. J. (2005). (DEHP) in human urine and serum after single oral doses of deuterium-labeled DEHP. *Archives of Toxicology, 79*, 367–376. doi:10.100700204-004-0642-4 PMID:15700144

López-Carrillo, L., Hernández-Ramírez, R. U., Calafat, A. M., Torres-Sánchez, L., Galván-Portillo, M., Needham, L. L., ... Cebrián, M. E. (2010). Exposure to phthalates and breast cancer risk in northern Mexico. *Environmental Health Perspectives, 118*(4), 539–544. doi:10.1289/ehp.0901091 PMID:20368132

Lovekamp-Swan, T., & Davis, B. J. (2003). Mechanisms of phthalate ester toxicity in the female reproductive system. *Environmental Health Perspectives, 111*(2), 139–145. doi:10.1289/ehp.5658 PMID:12573895

Lyche, J. L. (2011). Phthalates. In R. C. Gupta (Ed.), *Reproductive andDevelopmental Toxicology* (1st ed.; pp. 637–655). Amsterdam: Academic Press. doi:10.1016/B978-0-12-382032-7.10048-7

Magliozzi, R., Nardacci, R., Scarsella, G., Di Carlo, V., & Stefanini, S. (2013). Effects of the plasticiser DEHP on lung of newborn rats: Catalase immunocytochemistry and morphometric analysis. *Histochemistry and Cell Biology, 120*(1), 41–49. doi:10.100700418-003-0543-2 PMID:12802597

Main, K. M., Mortensen, G. K., Kaleva, M. M., Boisen, K. A., Damgaard, I. N., Chellakooty, M., ... Skakkebæk, N. E. (2006). Human breast milk contamination with phthalates and alterations of endogenous reproductive hormones in infants three months of age. *Environmental Health Perspectives, 114*(2), 270–276. doi:10.1289/ehp.8075 PMID:16451866

March, J. G., & Cerdà, V. (2015). An innovative arrangement for in-vial membrane-assisted liquid-liquid microextraction: Application to the determination of esters of phthalic acid in alcoholic beverages by gas chromatography-mass spectrometry. *Analytical and Bioanalytical Chemistry, 407*(14), 4213–4217. doi:10.100700216-015-8646-x PMID:25876533

Matsumoto, M., Hirata-Koizumi, M., & Ema, M. (2008). Potential adverse effects of phthalic acid esters on human health: A review of recent studies on reproduction. *Regulatory Toxicology and Pharmacology, 50*(1), 37–49. doi:10.1016/j.yrtph.2007.09.004 PMID:17983696

McKee, R. H. (2004). Toxicology Research Task G. Phthalate exposure and early thelarche. *Environmental Health Perspectives*, *112*(10), A541–A543. doi:10.1289/ehp.112-a541b PMID:15238295

Meeker, J. D., Calafat, A. M., & Hauser, R. (2007). Di(2-ethylhexyl) phthalate metabolites may alter thyroid hormone levels in men. *Environmental Health Perspectives*, *115*(7), 1029–1034. doi:10.1289/ehp.9852 PMID:17637918

Meeker, J. D., Calafat, A. M., & Hauser, R. (2007). Di(2-ethylhexyl) phthalate metabolites may alter thyroid hormone levels in men. *Environmental Health Perspectives*, *115*(7), 1029–1034. doi:10.1289/ehp.9852 PMID:17637918

Mendiola, J., Stahlhut, R. W., Jørgensen, N., Liu, F., & Swan, S. H. (2011). Shorter anogenital distance predicts poorer semen quality in young men in Rochester, New York. *Environmental Health Perspectives*, *119*(7), 958–963. doi:10.1289/ehp.1103421 PMID:21377950

Miodovnik, A., Edwards, A., Bellinger, D. C., & Hauser, R. (2014). Developmental neurotoxicity of ortho-phthalate diesters: Review of human and experimental evidence. *Neurotoxicol.*, *41*, 112–122. doi:10.1016/j.neuro.2014.01.007 PMID:24486776

Mose, T., Mortensen, G. K., Hedegaard, M., & Knudsen, L. E. (2007). Phthalate monoesters in perfusate from a dual placenta perfusion system, the placenta tissue and umbilical cord blood. *Reproductive Toxicology (Elmsford, N.Y.)*, *23*(1), 83–91. doi:10.1016/j.reprotox.2006.08.006 PMID:17049806

National Research Council. (2008). *Pthalates and cumulative risk assessment the task ahead. Committee on the health risk of pthalates*. National research council.

Pałaszewska-Tkacz, A., & Czerczak, S., & Dibutylu, F. (2012). (Di-n-butyl phthalate - inhaled fraction. Occupational exposure limits for phthalates). *Podstawy i Metody Oceny Środ Pracy.*, *73*(3), 37–70.

Peijnenburg, W. J. G. M., Sven, E. J., & Brian, F. (2008). Phthalates. In S. E. Jørgensen & B. D. Fath (Eds.), *Encyclopedia of Ecology*. Oxford, UK: Academic Press. doi:10.1016/B978-008045405-4.00419-5

Phillip, M. (1996). Clitoral and penile sizes of full term newborns in two different ethnic groups. *Journal of Pediatric Endocrinology & Metabolism*, *9*, 175–179. PMID:8887140

Reddy, B. S., Rozati, R., Reddy, B. V. R., & Raman, N. V. V. S. S. (2006). Association of phthalate esters with endometriosis in Indian women. *BJOG Int J Obstet Gynaecol*, *113*(5), 515–520. doi:10.1111/j.1471-0528.2006.00925.x PMID:16637895

Regulation (EC) No 1907/2006 of the European Parliament and of the Council of 18 December 2006 concerning the Registration, Evaluation, Authorisation and Restriction of Chemicals (REACH), establishing a European Chemicals Agency, amending Directive 1999/45/EC and repealing Council Regulation (EEC) No 793/93 and Commission Regulation (EC) No 1488/94 as well as Council Directive 76/769/EEC and Commission Directives 91/155/EEC, 93/67/ EEC, 93/105/EC and 2000/21/EC [displayed 8 May 2017].

Report, R. A. (2003a). 1,2-benzenedicarboxylic acid, di-C9-11-branched alkyl esters, C10-rich and di-"isodecyl" phthalate (DIDP). Institute for Health and Consumer Protection. *European Chemicals Bureau*, *36*, 234.

Report, R. A. (2003b). 1,2-benzenedicarboxylic acid, di-C8-10-branched alkyl esters, C9-rich and di-"isononyl" phthalate (DINP). Institute for Health and Consumer Protection. *European Chemicals Bureau*, *35*, 290.

Robinson, L., & Miller, R. (2015). The impact of bisphenol A and phthalates on allergy, asthma, and immune function: A review of latest findings. *Current Environmental Health Reports*, *2*(4), 379–387. doi:10.100740572-015-0066-8 PMID:26337065

Rudel, R. A., Camann, D. E., Spengler, J. D., Korn, L. R., & Brody, J. G. (2003). Phthalates, alkylphenols, pesticides, polybrominated diphenyl ethers, and other endocrine-disrupting compounds in indoor air and dust. *Environmental Science & Technology*, *37*(20), 4543–4553. doi:10.1021/es0264596 PMID:14594359

Salazar-Martinez, E., Romano-Riquer, P., Yanez-Marquez, E., Longnecker, M. P., & Hernandez-Avila, M. (2004). Anogenital distance in human male and female newborns: A descriptive, cross-sectional study. *Environmental Health*, *3*(1), 8–8. doi:10.1186/1476-069X-3-8 PMID:15363098

Sathyanarayana, S. (2008) Baby care products: possible sources of infant phthalate exposure. *Pediatrics, 121*.

Shanna, H. (2008). Environment pthalate exposure in relation to reproductive outcomes and other health endpoints in humans. *Environmental Research*, *108*(2), 177–184. doi:10.1016/j.envres.2008.08.007 PMID:18949837

Sharpe, R. M. (2001). Hormones and testis development and the possible adverse effects of environmental chemicals. *Toxicology Letters*, *120*(1-3), 221–232. doi:10.1016/S0378-4274(01)00298-3 PMID:11323180

Sharpe, R. M., & Skakkebaek, N. E. (2008). Testicular dysgenesis syndrome: Mechanistic insights and potential new downstream effects. *Fertility and Sterility*, *89*(Suppl 2), e33–e38. doi:10.1016/j.fertnstert.2007.12.026 PMID:18308057

Silva, M. J. (2007). Quantification of 22 phthalate metabolites in human urine. *Journal of Chromatography. A*, *860*, 106–112. PMID:17997365

Stahlhut, R. W., van Wijngaarden, E., Dye, T. D., Cook, S., & Swan, S. H. (2007). Concentrations of urinary phthalate metabolites are associated with increased waist circumference and insulin resistance in adult U.S. males. *Environmental Health Perspectives*, *115*(6), 876–882. doi:10.1289/ehp.9882 PMID:17589594

Swan, S., Liu, F., Hines, M., Kruse, R. L., Wang, C., Redmon, J. B., ... Weiss, B. (2010). Prenatal phthalate exposure and reduced masculine play in boys. *International Journal of Andrology*, *33*(2), 259–269. doi:10.1111/j.1365-2605.2009.01019.x PMID:19919614

Teitelbaum, S. L., Britton, J. A., Calafat, A. M., Ye, X., Silva, M. J., Reidy, J. A., ... Wolff, M. S. (2008). Temporal variability in urinary concentrations of phthalate metabolites, phytoestrogens and phenols among minority children in the United States. *Environmental Research*, *106*(2), 257–269. doi:10.1016/j.envres.2007.09.010 PMID:17976571

Thurston, S. W., Mendiola, J., Bellamy, A. R., Levine, H., Wang, C., Sparks, A., ... Swan, S. H. (2016). Phthalate exposure and semen quality in fertile US men. *Andrology*, *4*(4), 632–638. doi:10.1111/andr.12124 PMID:26601918

US Environmental Protection Agency (2012). Phthalates Action Plan, Revised 03/14/2012.

Ventrice, P., Ventrice, D., Russo, E., & De Sarro, G. (2013). Phthalates: European regulation, chemistry, pharmacokinetic and related toxicity. *Environmental Toxicology and Pharmacology*, *36*(1), 88–96. doi:10.1016/j.etap.2013.03.014 PMID:23603460

Výnos Ministerstva Pôdohospodárstva Slovenskej republiky a Ministerstva Zdravotníctva Slovenskej republiky z 15. marca 2004 No. 608/3/2004 - 100, ktorým sa vydáva hlava Potravinového Kódexu Slovenskej republiky upravujúca kontaminanty v potravinách [Slovak decree of the Ministry of Agriculture of the Slovak Republic and the Slovak Ministry of Health of 15 March 2004 No. 608/3/2004 - 100, issuing the chapter Slovak Republic Foodstuffs Code governing contaminants in food, in Slovak]. Ministerstva Pôdohospodárstva Slovenskej republiky 2004.

Wang, J., Li, X., Zhang, Q., Xiong, J., & Li, H. (2015). Determination of phthalate esters in Chinese spirits using isotope dilution gaschromatography with tandem mass spectrometry. *Journal of Separation Science*, *38*(10), 1700–1710. doi:10.1002/jssc.201401001 PMID:25755215

Welsh, M., Saunders, P. T. K., Fisken, M., Scott, H. M., Hutchison, G. R., Smith, L. B., & Sharpe, R. M. (2008). Identification in rats of a programming window for reproductive tract masculinization, disruption of which leads to hypospadias and cryptorchidism. *The Journal of Clinical Investigation*, *118*(4), 1479–1490. doi:10.1172/JCI34241 PMID:18340380

Wilson, V. S., Blystone, C. R., Hotchkiss, A. K., Rider, C. V., & Gray, L. E. (2008). Diverse mechanisms of anti-androgen action: Impact on male rat reproductive tractdevelopment. *International Journal of Andrology*, *31*(2), 178–187. doi:10.1111/j.1365-2605.2007.00861.x PMID:18315717

Wilson, V. S., Blystone, C. R., Hotchkiss, A. K., Rider, C. V., & Gray, L. E. (2008). Diverse mechanisms of anti-androgen action: Impact on male rat reproductive tract development. *International Journal of Andrology*, *31*(2), 178–187. doi:10.1111/j.1365-2605.2007.00861.x PMID:18315717

Wilson, V. S., Lambright, C., Furr, J., Ostby, J., Wood, C., Held, G., & Gray, L. E. Jr. (2004). Phthalate ester-induced gubernacular lesions are associatedwith reduced insl3 gene expression in the fetal rat testis. *Toxicology Letters*, *146*(3), 207–215. doi:10.1016/j.toxlet.2003.09.012 PMID:14687758

World Health Organization (WHO). (2017). *Guidelines for Drinking-Water Quality*. WHO.

Wormuth, M., Scheringer, M., Vollenweider, M., & Hungerbuhler, K. (2006). What are the sources of exposure to eight frequently used pthalic acid esters in Europeans. *Risk Analysis*, *26*(3), 803–824. doi:10.1111/j.1539-6924.2006.00770.x PMID:16834635

Wu, M. T., Wu, C. F., Chen, B. H., Chen, E. K., Chen, Y. L., Shiea, J., ... Wu, J. R. (2013). Intake of phthalate-tainted foods alters thyroid functions in Taiwanese children. *PLoS One*, *8*(1), e55005. doi:10.1371/journal.pone.0055005 PMID:23383031

Wyszkowska, J., & Wyszkowski, M. (2002). Effect of cadmium and magnesium on microbiological activity in soil. *Polish Journal of Environmental Studies*, *11*(5), 585–591.

Wyszkowski, M., & Sivitskaya, V. (2012). Changes in the content of organic carbon and available forms of macronutrients in soil under the influence of soil contamination with fuel oil and application of different substances. *Journal of Elementology*, *17*(1), 139–148.

Wyszkowski, M., & Wyszkowska, J. (2009). The effect of contamination with cadmium on spring barley (Hordeum vulgare L.) and its relationship with the enzymatic activity of soil. *Fresenius Environmental Bulletin*, *18*(7), 1046–1053.

Zhang, Y. H. (2006). Phthalate exposure and human semen quality in Shanghai: a cross-sectional study. *Biomedical and Environmental Sciences*, *19*, 205–209. PMID:16944777

Ziółkowska, A., & Wyszkowski, M. (2010). Toxicity of petroleum s ubstances to microorganisms and plants. *Ecological Chemistry and Engineering. S*, *17*(1), 73–82.

ADDITIONAL READING

Swan, S. H., Main, K. M., Liu, F., Stewart, S. L., Kruse, R. L., Calafat, A. M., ... Teague, J. L. (2005). the Study for Future Families Research Team. Decrease in anogenital distance among male infants with prenatal phthalate exposure. *Environmental Health Perspectives*, *113*(8), 1056–1061. doi:10.1289/ehp.8100 PMID:16079079

Talsness, C. E., Andrade, A. J. M., Kuriyama, S. N., Taylor, J. A., & vom Saal, F. S. (2009). Components of plastic: Experimental studies in animals and relevance for human health. *Philosophical Transactions of the Royal Society of London. Series B, Biological Sciences*, *364*(1526), 2079–2096. doi:10.1098/rstb.2008.0281 PMID:19528057

Wang, Y. C., Chen, H. S., Long, C. Y., Tsai, C. F., Hsieh, T. H., Hsu, C. Y., & Tsai, E. M. (2012). Possible mechanism of phthalates-induced tumorigenesis. *The Kaohsiung Journal of Medical Sciences*, *28*(7), S22–S27. doi:10.1016/j.kjms.2012.05.006 PMID:22871597

Whyatt, R. M., Liu, X., Rauh, V. A., Calafat, A. M., Just, A. C., Hoepner, L., ... Factor-Litvak, P. (2012). Maternal prenatal urinary phthalate metabolite concentrations and child mental, psychomotor,and behavioral development at 3 years of age. *Environmental Health Perspectives*, *120*(2), 290–295. doi:10.1289/ehp.1103705 PMID:21893441

KEY TERMS AND DEFINITIONS

Asthma: A condition in which a person's airways become inflamed, narrow and swell, and produce extra mucus, which makes it difficult to breathe.

Biomonitoring: It is the measurement of the body burden of toxic chemical compounds, elements, or their metabolites, in biological substances. Often, these measurements are done in blood and urine.

Cryptorchidism: It is the absence of one or both testes from the scrotum.

Pthalates: Phthalates, or phthalate esters, are esters of phthalic acid. They are mainly used as plasticizers (i.e., substances added to plastics to increase their flexibility, transparency, durability, and longevity). They are used primarily to soften polyvinyl chloride.

Steroidogenesis: It is a synthetic process that begins with cholesterol as a substrate and, through a series of enzymatic reactions, produces a wide array of bioactive interrelated signaling molecules.

Chapter 17
Environmental Phthalate Exposure in Relation to Reproduction Outcomes and Health Endpoints

Anjum Afshan
University of Kashmir, India

Md Niamat Ali
https://orcid.org/0000-0002-5128-9284
University of Kashmir, India

Farooz Ahmed Bhat
SKUAST-K, India

ABSTRACT

Environmental pollutants, like xenobiotic substances released as byproducts of anthropogenic actions, naturally lead to pollution of the environment. They negatively affect the environment through unfavorable impacts on growth, development, and reproduction of organisms including humans. One of the outstanding examples of xenobiotics is endocrine disrupting compounds (EDCs) such as phthalate esters (PEs), which have the efficacy to disturb numerous biological systems including the invertebrate, reptilian, avian, aquatic, and also the mammalian systems. Phthalates are family of xenobiotic hazardous compounds amalgamating in plastics to intensify their plasticity, flexibility, longevity, versatility, and durability. Ignoring the rising issue on the hazardous nature of various phthalates and their metabolites, ruthless usage of phthalates as plasticizer in plastics and as additives in innumerable consumer products continues due to their low eminent properties, their cost-effectiveness, and lack of suitable alternatives. Globally epidemiological human studies showed various phthalates and their metabolites ingested passively by man from the general environment, foods, drinks, breathing air, and routine household products cause various dysfunctions. This comprehensive chapter on the hazards of phthalates would benefit the general population, academia, scientists, clinicians, environmentalists, and law or policymakers to decide upon whether usage of phthalates to be continued swiftly without sufficient deceleration or regulated by law or to be phased out from earth forever.

DOI: 10.4018/978-1-5225-9452-9.ch017

INTRODUCTION

The word plastic is derived from plasticos (Greek), which means capable of sculping into different shapes. With swift advancement in technology and the geometric progression of the global population growth, plastic materials have found resourceful applications in every aspect of modern human life. A number of substances are blended in plastics at various proportions to improve their performance and reduce cost (Tokiwa et al., 2009). Phthalates are one of such organic compounds used as plasticizers. Phthalate esters (PAEs), one derivative of phthalic acid (PA), are aromatic colorless liquids with high-molecular weight, high stability, low-volatility and low-solubility in water (Chang et al., 2004; Chao et al., 2006). Phthalates are family of xenobiotic hazardous compounds amalgamating in plastics to intensify their plasticity, flexibility, longevity, versatility and durability.

Besides they are also used as lubricants, solvents, additives, softeners etc. They are present in number of day to day used products such as PVC products, building materials (paint, adhesive, wall covering), personal-care products (perfume, eye shadow, moisturizer, nail polish, deodorizer, liquid soap, and hair spray), medical devices, detergents and surfactants, packaging, children's toys, printing inks coatings, pharmaceuticals and food products, textiles, household applications such as shower curtains, floor tiles, food containers and wrappers, cleaning materials. Phthalates are bound to polymer matrix physically and hence released easily to surrounding environment directly or indirectly during manufacture, use and disposal (Cadogan et al., 1993). Phthalates are ubiquitous in environment found in atmospheric aerosols (Xie et al., 2007; Fu et al., 2009), sludge from sewage and treated waste water (Dargnat et al., 2009), River and marine waters/sediments (Xie et al.,2007; Net et al.,2014), drinking water (Gao et al., 2014). Direct release of phthalates to the atmosphere is considered to be the main mode of their entry to the environment (Staples et al., 1997; Wang et al., 2014). Once entering the environment, they pose remarkable toxicological threats to the myriad of non target organisms, discover its way to the food chain, and threaten ecological balance and biodiversity of nature.

In 1856 Caster oil was used as first plasticizer in making cellulose nitrate. Later Camphor replaced it in 1870. To combat the problem related to odorous nature of volatile Camphor, phthalates were introduced as an alternative in 1920s. Use of phthalates in industries began worldwide in 1930s. Presently the overall yearly global use of PAEs is estimated at over 30 million tons with the yearly consumption of Europealone is about 1million ton (Net et al., 2015).The production of phthalates increased from 1.8 million tons in 1975 (Peijnenburg & Struijs,2006) to more the 8 million tons in 2011 (Schreiber et al., 2011). Phthalates are extensively explored as hazardous organic pollutants and their presence in the environment can be of great threat to human beings and wildlife. Few of phthalates are suspected to be hepato-toxins, mutagens and carcinogens. As environmental adulterates, phthalates influence reproduction, harm development and induce genetic impairments in humans even at low doses, so ensuing in an increasing environmental concerns (Heudorf et al., 2007). Some phthalates have endocrine disruptive activity and their environmental behaviour has drawn significant attention because of their possible impact on ecosystem functioning in general and public health in particular. The most notable unfavorable impacts of phthalates are seen in fetal development and reproductive anomalies, especially the so-called "phthalate syndrome" (Sharpe & Skakkebaek, 2008; Le Moal et al., 2015), coupled with insulin resistance and obesity (Swan, 2008; Halden, 2010; Latini et al., 2010; Casals-Casas & Desvergne, 2011; Kuo et al., 2013; Kim & Park,2014). Thus, it is appropriate time to look into unpropitious health impacts of phthalates on humans.

Six of PAEs have been positioned in priority pollutant list of United States Environmental Protection Agency (USEPA), the European Union (EU), and in the list of priority pollutants in Chinese waters (CEC, 2007; Yuan & Graham, 2008). Due to potential risk of phthalates for human health and environment, a number of them have been incorporated in the priority pollutant list of several national and supranational federations. Section 307 of US clean water act listed di-n-butyl phthalate(DnBP), dimethyl phthalate(DMP) and diethyl phthalate(DEP) as priority pollutants (USEPA,1999).The utilization of PAEs is now an issue to stricter control and some have been interdicted or their curtailment in numerous products have been advocated.

COMMONLY USED PHTHALATES

Phthalates are formed up of dialkyl ester or alkyl and aryl esters of orthophthalic acid (1,2-dicarboxyllic acid). They are manufactured at large scale by reacting 1,2-dicarboxyllic acid with a number of alcohols ranging from methanol to tridecanol. Phthalates vary from each other in length of carbon side chain having the general chemical structure shown in Figure 1.

The molecular mass of the phthalate may vary from the shortest (dimethyl phthalate) (194.18 *Da*) to the longest ditridecyl phthalate (530.82 *Da*). Some of the commonly used phthalates and their general uses are summarized in the Table 1.

EXPOSURE ROUTES OF ENTRY

Phthalates are ubiquitous: in water, food, breast milk, breathing air, dust, soil, dress materials, dwelling house, and hospital – everywhere. Even human body has the potency for absorption of phthalates, as it can cross placenta, thereby affecting the foetus and neonates adversely. Means of entry can be through: food (casings), bottles, wrappers, microwaving, vessels and washing sink, cooking aids, spoons, *etc.*); infant formulae and milk; water and drinks (drinking, bathing, washing waters; liquors, carbonated drinks, *etc.*); inhalation (indoor air, house dust, vapors, fragrance, innumerable household materials); medications and nutritional supplements; medical devices (bags and tubing, implants, blood transfusion and dialysis materials; medical bottles, containers, pans, covers of pills); cosmetics and perfumes (creams, deodorants, moisturizers and shampoos; nail polish, lipsticks, hair dyes, *etc.*); clothing(gloves artificial leather, waterproof clothings; ornaments, toys; footwear, *etc.*); toys (mouthing, rubbing and playing, sex dolls); denture materials (denture soft lining materials, moulds, *etc.*); construction materials, vehicle parts, carrying pipes, *etc.* Exposure of humans to phthalates can occur via number of routes including

Figure 1. General chemical structure of an o-phthalate

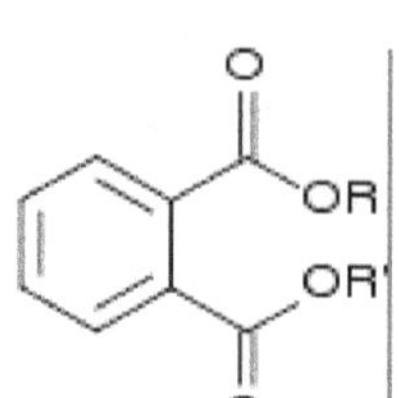

Table 1. Showing commonly used phthalates

Phthalate	Uses
DMP	Insect repellent, plastic
DEP	Shampoo, scents, soap, lotion, cosmetics, industrial solvent, medications
DBP	Adhesives, caulk, cosmetics, industrial solvent, medications
DIBP	Adhesives, caulk, cosmetics, industrial solvent
BBP	Vinyl flooring, adhesives, sealants, industrial solvent
DCHP	Stabilizer in rubber, polymers
DEHP	Soft plastic, including tubing, toys, home products, food containers, food packaging
DOP	Soft plastic
DINP	Soft plastics, replacement for DEHP

ingestion of polluted water and food, inhalation of adulterate air, consumption of certain medications and skin contact with lotions or cosmetics containing phthalates as additives (Wittassek et al., 2011). Figure 2 showing the migration of phthalates into the environment from the embodiment of plastics. Compared to adults, infants and children are more vulnerable to phthalate exposure because of their hand-to-mouth behavior. Levels of exposures of phthalates in the general population are estimated to be in the order of tens of microgram (μg)/ kilogram (kg) body weight (bw)/ day (d), *i.e.*, the standard unit (μg/kg bw/day) of expression of phthalate exposure, as in the case of any other hazardous chemicals.

RISK ASSESSMENT AND HAZARD INDEX OF PHTHALATES

On the basis of human-biomonitoring data, the risk assessment of various phthalates can be individually evaluated. Human-biomonitoring is an effective procedure used to estimate the total background exposure of phthalates. Further, based on the hazard index (HI) approach (Kortenkamp and Faust, 2010; Soeborg et al., 20102) which assumes dose addition (USEPA, 2003; USEPA, 2007) a cumulative risk assessment for various exposures to chemicals with similar toxicity has been developed for Phthalates. As defined in a National Research Council (NRC) report (2008), the HI furnishes a direct and simple procedure for relating the intake of certain of chemicals to their reference values (RfVs). The hazard quotient (HQ) is estimated as the ratio of the calculating exposure level to the RfV of corresponding chemical. The HQs are then added together to estimate the overall HI. The information received from the biomonitoring process would be a strong base for assessing the risk in the target population. Reference dose (the tolerable daily intake; TDI) of phthalate exposure (μg/kg bw/d) set by the USEPA or such safety levels set by other regulatory or scientific bodies for the common phthalates is: MMP (3500), DEP(800), DBP (100), BBP(200), DEHP metabolites (80), DINP (120) and, DnOP (3500), *i.e.*, it depicts that the least recommended TDI is for DEHP, and that the exposure of each of its metabolite (MEHP, MEHHP,

Figure 2. Showing the migration of phthalates into the environment from the embodiment of plastics

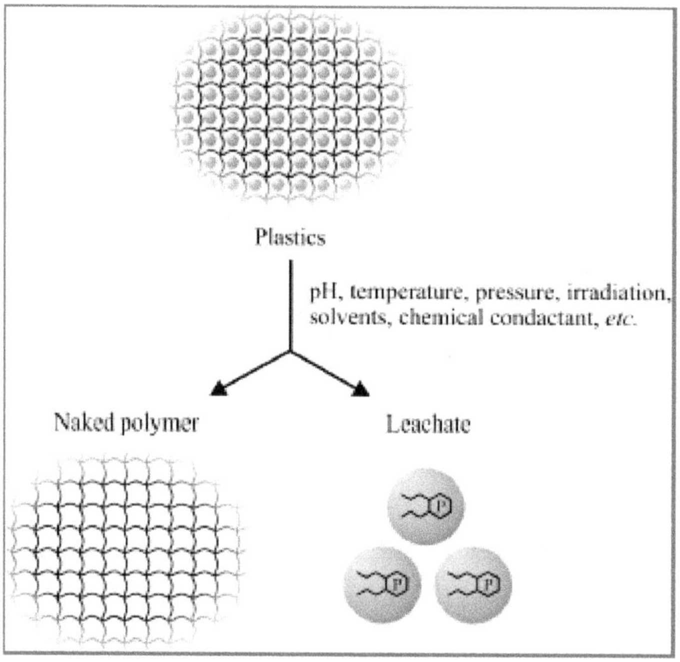

MEOHP, and MECHP) should not exceed 20 µg/kg bw/d (ACC, 2016). It depicts that it is safe if a healthy man with 75 kg body weight is exposed up to 6 mg DEHP/day; on the other hand, that he can tolerate DMP up to 263 mg/day. But, in daily life, humans capitulate to multiple phthalate exposures throughout the life, which may go beyond 1.0 g/ day or even more. And if he or she continues to expose to such high dose routinely along with other hazardous chemicals, what would be her or his eventual health outcome?

Most of human studies on phthalate ester exposure are chiefly focused on the exposure levels of various phthalates so as to compare whether the exposure level is within the limit of the permitted TDI or not. Unfortunately many studies keep mum on the comparison of their findings in terms of TDI. Urine has been considered as the chief matrix for the analysis of biomarkers (phthalates and its metabolites) (Itoh et al., 2007; Janjua et al., 2007; Wittassek et al., 2007; Berman et al., 2009; Koch et al.,2013; Tranfo et al., 2013; Kim et al., 2014; Huang et al., 2015); but a few studies clubbed the analysis of other matrices too for examining the biomarkers - those responsible for inflammation and oxidative stress(Ferguson et al., 2011), breast milk and blood serum of postpartum women (Hogberg et al., 2008;Fromme et al., 2011) or indirect sampling - evaluating the source of contamination, *e.g.*, food (Das et al.,2014).No doubt, as in all other studies; along with other phthalates, DEP, BBP and, DEHP and their primary and secondary metabolites have been the common target in biomonitoring studies. In order to establish sources of phthalate intake, Koch et al. (2013) made an interesting study in 5 middle aged youths (3female and 2 males; aged between 27 and 47 yrs), who fasted (48 h) only on glass-bottled water; and confirmed that exposure to high molecular weight phthalates like DEHP was through dietary intake, while the low molecular weight phthalates like DEP enter in to the body through non-dietary sources such as personal care products, dust, vapor and indoor air. In addition to the urinary concentrations of phthalates, Ferguson et al. (2011) examined C-reactive protein (CRP) and γ-glutamyl transferase (GGT) as additional biomarkers from the serum, and confirmed that MBzP and MiBP were notably related with CRP, while DEHP and its metabolites were related with GGT. Das et al. (2014) adopted indirect procedure for monitoring and evaluating the phthalate exposure in humans in Delhi, India; for which they examined (using GC-MS) various exposure sources (food and drinking water, indoor and outdoor air and dust), and observed that DEHP was the most abundant congener (over 70 µg/kg/d exposure), followed by DBP, DMP and BBP; and that food and drinking water contributed about 75% of these congeners. In Italy, 74 males and 83females were subjected to biomonitoring and risk assessment studies; and that MEP depicted the highest concentration in females (72.94 µg/g creatine) and males (56.35); followed by MBP (20.26), MBzP (16.44) and MEHHP (10.77) in females; while MBP (17.55), MBzP (16.44) and MEHHP (10.77) in males (Tranfo et al., 2013). In Israel, 3410 µg/L urinary DEP was detected in pregnant women living in Jerusalem, and the concentration of DEHP metabolites (ΣMEHP, MEOHP, MEHHP, MECPP) was 262µg/L (Berman et al., 2009). It is obvious that all these evaluations are made based on the level of the phthalates in the matrix examined using highly sophisticated analytical procedures capable of noticing the residual phthalate in the body at nanogram levels; consequently, the alarming signs received from these studies should be taken in to account seriously. Chang et al. (2017) assessed the daily intakes (DIs) and cumulative risk of phthalates in Taiwan's general population after the food scandal in 2011. The DIs of 6 phthalates, including di-n-butyl phthalate (DBP), di-iso-butyl phthalate (DiBP), and DEHP, was assessed using urinary phthalate metabolites. Hazard quotients of phthalates classified as influencing the reproductive (HQrep) and hepatic (HQhep) systems were assessed using cumulative approach. The creatinine-based model showed that the highest DI values in children 7-to 12- years-old were for DEHP (males: median: 4.79 µg/kg bw/d; females: median: 2.62 µg/kg bw/d). The 95th percentile (P95) of HQrep values were all >1 in the 7- to12-year-old and 18- to 40-year-old male groups. The P95 of HQhep values were all >1 in the 7- to 18-year-old male groups. Most of the HQrep was imputable to the HQs of DBP and DiBP (53.9–84.7%),and DEHP contributed most to HQhep (83.1–98.6%), which reveals that DBP, DiBP and DEHP were the chief risk of phthalate exposure for Taiwanese. Taiwan's general population is broadly exposed to DBP, DiBP and DEHP, mainly for young children. Zare et al. (2018) did a study to estimate the exposure and related health risks of phthalates, and to evaluate the health risks from integrated exposure to three of the phthalates sharing the same mode of action (anti-androgenicity) in children. They assessed the internal exposure of 56 Iranian children and adolescents aged 6 to 18 years by examining seven urinary metabolites of five phthalates. The approximated daily intake values derived from the biomonitoring data ranged from 0.01 µg/kg bw/day for butyl benzyl phthalate (BBP), to 17.85 µg/kg bw/day for di(2-ethylhexyl) phthalate (DEHP). The risk assessment depicted that not only the exposure to the individual phthalates, but also the clubbed exposure to the three anti-androgenic phthalates (DEHP, DBP, BBP) did not raise a safety concern (hazard index values averaged 0.2). The range of maximum cumulative ratio values varied from around 1 for most individuals to around 2 in some individuals, specifying that the clubbed exposures were dominated by one and in some cases by two of the three anti-androgenic phthalates, substantially dibutyl phthalate (DBP) and/or DEHP. Based on biomonitoring data, the overall clubbed exposure of Iranian children to phthalates does not raise a concern, while cutback of exposure is best focused on DEHP and DBP that showed the highest hazard quotient.

PHTHALATES AS ENDOCRINE DISRUPTING CHEMICALS, THE EDCS

Phthalates are quickly absorbed to human blood or other body fluids being chiefly lipophilic in nature and rapidly get transformed into respective primary and secondary metabolites; before excretion, few of these metabolites would falsely interact (xeno-sensing) with the endocrine molecular signaling system as ligands (agonist or antagonist or co-activator) of transcription factors inhabiting in the nucleus -resulting in unexpected health effects. It appears that phthalates chiefly act as hormone sensitizers by disrupting or impairing with the usual physiological mechanisms, which would directly reflect in the malfunction of body system - implicating strong association between EDCs and human diseases (Latini et al, 2004; Grun & Blumberg, 2009, Jugan et al, 2010; Halden, 2010; Hatch et al., 2010; Miodovnik et al., 2011; Casals-Casas & Desvergene, 2011; Maqbool et al., 2015; Benjamin et al., 2015).

Nevertheless vital share of data on the EDC nature of phthalates comes from non-human studies, evidences collected from the clinical studies during the last twenty years herald that: the increasing sex abnormalities such as endometriosis, altered reproductive development, early puberty, sex reversal and fertility issues in males and females; prevalence of various cancers, chiefly skin and breast cancer; asthma and allergy and; obesity and overweight, type II diabetes and insulin resistance; attention-deficit hyperactivity disorder; impaired neurodevelopment; mental, decreased intelligent quotient; psychomotor and behavioral issues; autism spectrum disorders, etc., are the ill-impacts of phthalates directly exhibited in humans evoked by the disabled multiple intermolecular communications.

Nevertheless numerous studies indicating the ED properties of phthalates; examination of the patterns, possible causes, and affect on health, and disease conditions (epidemiological data) are the customary formulae acquired in evaluating the untoward effects of phthalates in humans. Additional to this, progressive biological consequences of various xenobiotics in health outcome, data based on the epigenetic effects of endocrine disruptors, their concurrence with fetal programming, and their potency for unmasking cryptic genetic differences would furnish adequate proof to answer the question on: Why unparallel rise in the portion of life-style diseases like diabetes and obesity and, associated with chronic cardio-vascular diseases and cancer has appeared up at end of the last millennium and advancing at an alarming speed presently? (Schneider et al., 2014).

PHTHALATES AND EPIGENETIC MODULATION

Conventional evolutionary notion on epigenetic transgenerational phenotype chiefly depends on genetic mutation as the principal source of variance. Contrarily, EDC-mediated epigenetic modulation may reprogram the innate epigenetic imprint or epigenetic memory through altered gene expression (transcription and translation, and the expression of non coding micro RNAs) leading to epigenetic inheritance epitomized by adult onset diseases (Ayala-García et al., 2013; Rajesh & Balasubramanian, 2014). Genotoxicity of phthalates mediate through DNA methylation, demethylation and alteration of chromatin through histone at the promoter regions of imprinted genes (Figure 3).

Phthalates may attach to histone tails and result in alteration of the extent of DNA wrapped around it and the availability of genes to be activated (Wu et al., 2010; Manikkam et al., 2013). DNA methylation or demethylation, and condensation of chromatin at the promoter region of critical genes through changes in histone and phosphorylation of expressed proteins are the principal epigenetic changes imparted by phthalates. Methyl groups can tag the cytosine base during methylation. These methyl groups

Figure 3. Plausible molecular signaling mechanism vis-à-vis epigenetic modulation of phthalates and their metabolites

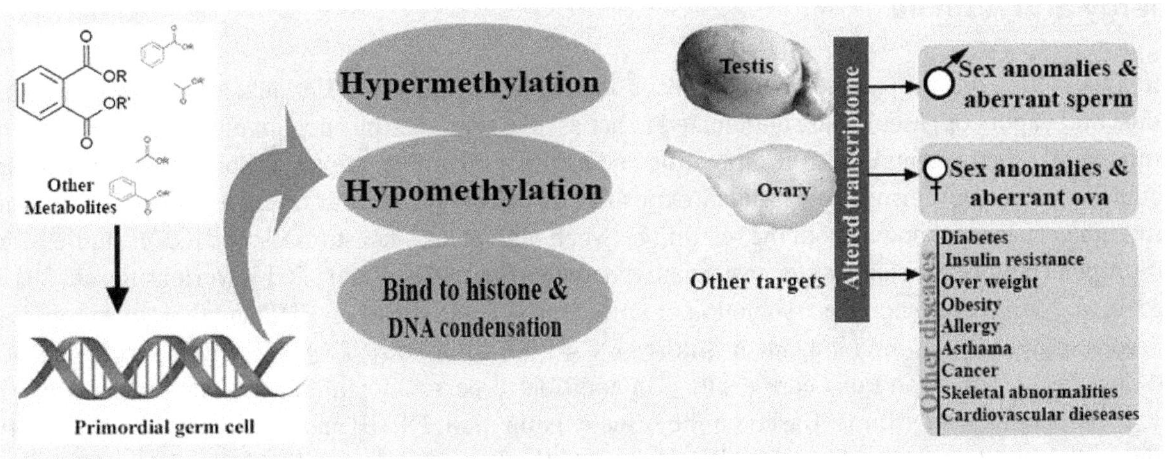

would project into the major groove of DNA and hinder transcription. The demethylation process is very important for epigenetic re-programming of genes and is also directly connected with many notable disease mechanisms such as tumor progression (Rajesh & Balasubramanian, 2014). Exposure of phthalates during gestation predisposes glucometabolic dysfunctions at adulthood in succeeding generations, by modulating the function of the critical genes (Rajesh & Balasubramanian, 2014).

Maternal exposure of DEHP in mice showed testicular dysfunction mediated through DNA hypermethylation leading to the increased expression of DNA methyl transferases for DNA Methylation and down regulation of insulin like hormone-3, a gene critical for the production of testosterone (Wu et al., 2010). DEHP and DBP were shown to heavily influence the adult onset diseases including pubertal abnormalities, ovarian disease (polycystic ovary and primary ovarian insufficiency), testis dysfunction and obesity through epigenetic transgenerational inheritance in rats (Manikkam et al., 2013). It was mediated by differential DNA methylation (epimutation) at the promoter regions of imprinting genes for epigenetic memory, especially of paternally inherited insulin like growth factor 2 receptor (Igf2r) gene and paternally-expressed gene 3 (Peg3) (Manikkam et al., 2013; Li et al., 2014). Phthalates like DBP may induce DNA hypomethylation at CpGrich region of the myc gene promoter in rat liver through the activation of peroxisome proliferator- activated receptors (PPARs), thereby promote cancer (Kostka et al.,2010). Using spermatogonial transplantation technique in mice, it was shown that DEHP decreased sperm count and its motility up to F4 generation by disrupting testicular organization and spermatogonial stem cells (Doyle et al. 2013). Sex differentiation may also be dysregulated through the hypothalamo-pituitary-gonadal axis by the epigenetic regulation of granulin and p_{130} genes (Lee et al., 2006). In humans, prenatal exposure of phthalates including DEHP heavily demethylated the paternally expressed Igf2 and maternally expressed H19 genes, which play crucial role in the embryonic and placental growth (Larocca et al., 2014).

PHTHALATES AND CHILD HEALTH

Allergy and Asthma

Allergy and lung diseases are notable health consequences of phthalates. Phthalates (mostly in the form of dust and vapors or gases) being anticipated to act as allergens and thus negatively modulating the immunological system, bringing to inflammation and asthma. Incurable chronic inflammation and asthma results from recurrent episodes of phthalate exposures that ultimately lead to severe associated symptoms. Although very less is known about the relation between phthalates and asthma, some recent studies done on European children depicted a clear association between them (Beko et al., 2013; Bertelsenet al., 2013). Beko et al. (2013) examined the association of DEP, DnBP, DiBP, BBzP, DEHP and their metabolites as allergens in inducing asthma in Danish children (N = 200, 3 to 6 yrs). They studied the urine samples, and dust in the homes and day care centers, in addition to personal examination for constructing the link of phthalates with asthma. Based on the urine examination, DEHP and its metabolites showed the highest TDI (4.42 μg/ kg bw/d), while BBzP showed the lowest exposure (0.49 μg). Regarding exposures to air and dust in the indoor environments, DEP, DiBP and DnBP accounted for approximately 100%, 50% of and 15%, respectively of the total intake; with dermal absorption (in vapor from) being the chief exposure route; and over 90% of the total intake of BBzP and DEHP was contributed by other sources than indoor air and dust. Everyday intake of DBP and DiBP from all exposure routes exceeded the TDI in 11 and 12% children (of the study population), respectively, and indoor exposures resulted in an average daily DiBP intake that exceeded the TDI in 7% children under study (Beko et al., 2013). A study was done to find out relation between exposure to phthalates in residential buildings and its health effects in children. Six phthalates were detected in the dust samples of children's bedroom. Indoor modern decoration and frequent use of household cleaning products were related to elevated phthalate levels, consequently to children's asthma and allergy. Higher levels of DEP and DBP were remarkably associated to children diagnosed with asthma (Sun et al., 2017). Table 2 demonstrates relation between phthalate exposure and adverse respiratory (allergy, asthma) outcomes children.

Diabetes, Insulin Resistance & Obesity: Association of phthalate exposure and growing prevalence of childhood insulin resistance (Trasande et al., 2013a) and obesity (Teitelbaum et al., 2012; Wang et al., 2013; Buser et al., 2014; Zhang et al., 2014; Huang et al., 2015) is one of the major concern across the globe. In one of the studies in China, exposure to phthalates was observed to be linked to increased body mass and waist circumference (WC), i.e., the direct twin indicator of obesity (Wang et al., 2013). Age and sex are intimately linked with the extent of phthalate exposure in controlling childhood obesity

Table 2. Respiratory Health outcomes in children associated with phthalate exposure

System	Timing of exposure	Sex	Outcome	Phthalate or metabolite (measured in urine unless otherwise noted)	References
Respiratory, allergy and asthma	Childhood	Males/ females	Rhinitis and eczema Asthma Wheezing, rhinitis and eczema	BBzP (in house dust) DEHP (in house dust) DEHP (in house dust)	Bornehag *et al.*, 2004 Bornehag *et al.*, 2004 Kolarik, 2008

(Buser et al., 2014; Zhang et al., 2014). Low molecular weight (MW) phthalates and their metabolites (MEP, MnBP and MiBP) were linked with obesity in adolescents and male children; while in high MW metabolites (MEHP, MECPP, MEHHP, MEOHP, MBzP, MCNP and MCOP) were found linked with elevated levels of obesity in adults. Additionally, DEHP metabolites were found notable linked with obesity in all adult females participated in the study, while its effect was found prominent only in older males (> 60 yrs) (Buser et al., 2014). Phthalates found to have prominent obesogenic impact in children and teen agers. Trasande et al. (2013b) clearly demonstrated in a cross-sectional study, completed in the USA, that the low MW phthalates - especially metabolites of DMP and DEP - are firmly linked with overweight (21%prevalence) and obesity (22%), and phthalic acid (PA) in urine and MEP, DBP and PA in serum were found associated with obesity in Korean girls (Choi et al., 2014). Swift rates of phthalate metabolism in children and adolescents than mothers and adults (Song et al., 2013) clubbed with the food style – especially fast food culture of children and adolescents (Das et al., 2014; Zota et al., 2016) would firmly affect their health outcomes.

Autism Spectrum Disorders (ASD) and Cognitive Behavior: There is a negative correlation between Phthalate exposure and the neuro and cognitive developments in children (Ejaredar et al., 2015; Huang et al., 2015). ASD or Pervasive Developmental Disorder was observed to be linked with the exposure of DEHP secondary metabolites (5-OH- and 5-oxo-MEHPs); importantly, 5-oxo-MEHP showed 91% specificity in recognizing patients with ASDs (Testa et al., 2012). In a longitudinal study (Taiwan), 430 pregnant women in their third trimester participated in the study, and their 110, 79, 76, and 73 children were followed up, i.e., the cumulated turn out at the ages of 2, 5, 8, and 11, respectively (Huang et al., 2015). The authors compared the urinary concentrations of phthalates in relation to the Bayley and IQ scores for evaluating neuro-cognitive functions and intelligence, and depicted postnatal exposure to DEHP metabolites were strongly linked with low cognitive function.

In children and adolescents, eruption of life style diseases like overweight, obesity and insulin resistance, and airway diseases like asthma must be addressed otherwise this age group unknowingly succumb to this calamity that result from the action of adults. Phthalates alone may not be responsible for this global epidemics but progressive impacts of other environmental hazardous contaminants contribute in a supplementary or complementary manner, and thus this reality should be addressed to lessen such health outcomes in children.

PHTHALATES AND MALE REPRODUCTIVE HEALTH

The "phthalate syndrome" or "Testicular Dysgenesis Syndrome" is one of the chief adverse impact of phthalate toxicity characterized by cryptorchidism, hypospadias, undescended testes, reduced anogenital distance, decrease in sperm count or its quality, increase in sterility and testicular cancer (Sharpe& Skakkebaek,2008; Swan, 2008). Anogenital distance (the distance between anus and genitalia) is taken as one of the principal markers for evaluating the effect of phthalates in human males (Swan et al., 2005; Marsee et al., 2006; Sharpe & Skakkebaek, 2008; Suzuki et al., 2012), which is under the control of dihydrotestosterone – a sex steroid hormone (androgen) in males; and that anogenital distance is the most sensitive marker for judging anti-androgenic action in toxicologic studies (Swan et al., 2005). It is found that this abnormality is affected by the prenatal exposure of fetes to various phthalates while in womb. In their pioneer study, Swan et al. (2005) analyzed the anogenital index in 134 boys (2-36 months of age), which was found significantly correlated with the penile volume and the proportion of boys within complete testicular descent. Of nine phthalate monoesters tested in the prenatal urine, concentrations of MEP, MBP, MBzP and MiBP were found inversely related to reduced anogenital distance, of which MEP showed the highest concentration (13.7 μg/mL urine), while DEHP showed no correlation with the anogenital distance (Swan et al., 2005). In a different study, in utero exposure of DBP was found critical in inducing anti-androgenic effects on the fetus (Huang et al., 2009); while a study conducted among Japanese population showed the link of DEHP with male fetal toxicity (Suzuki et al., 2012). Since they analyzed amniotic fluid and urine of mothers for the presence of MBP, MEHP,

MEP, MBzP and MMP (in addition to physical examination of neonates), Huang's in utero study (Huanget al., 2009) seems to be much noteworthy. The anti-androgenic effect of DEHP and its metabolites due to prenatal exposure cannot be ruled out (Wittassek et al., 2009), as the adverse effect of MEHP in the germ cell lineage has been demonstrated through organ culture, i.e., human testis culture in vitro (Lambrot et al., 2009). Figure 4 showed disturbed androgen action in males upon phthalate exposure.

PROBABLE MOLECULAR MECHANISM

Effect of phthalates on Hypothalamic–pituitary–gonadal axis (HPG axis) in concert might play crucial role in reproductive and immune systems (Lee et al., 2006; Pocar et al., 2011) with the involvement of multiple pathways in maintaining steroid homeostasis and biosynthesis of steroid hormones (Pocar et al., 2011). It was shown from the epidemiological and experimental animal studies that "Testicular Dysgenesis Syndrome" occurs due to impaired functions of Sertoli (inhibiting the progression of meiosis during spermatogenesis and spermeiogenesis) (Uren-Webster et al., 2010) and inhibiting testosterone production (product of Leydig cell) through the suppression of insulin-like growth factor 3 (Igf-3) (Ge et al., 2007). Leydig cell hyperplasia was observed due to enhanced expression of survival proteins like

Figure 4. Showing altered male reproductive outcomes upon phthalate exposure

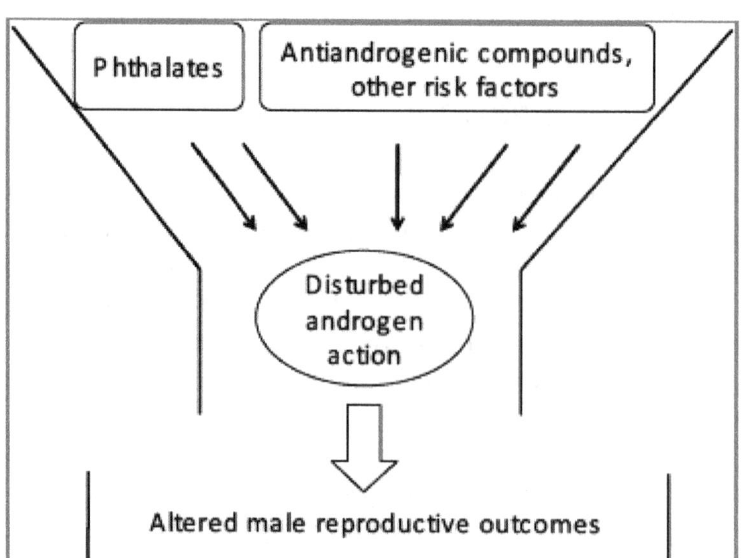

TRPM-2 and Bcl-2 and the down-regulation of c-kit receptor (crucial for testicular development and function) (Ma et al., 2006).

Figure 5 depicts probable molecular signaling mechanism elicited by phthalates and their metabolites in the male reproductive system.

Figure 5. Depicts probable molecular signaling mechanism elicited by phthalates and their metabolites in the male reproductive system

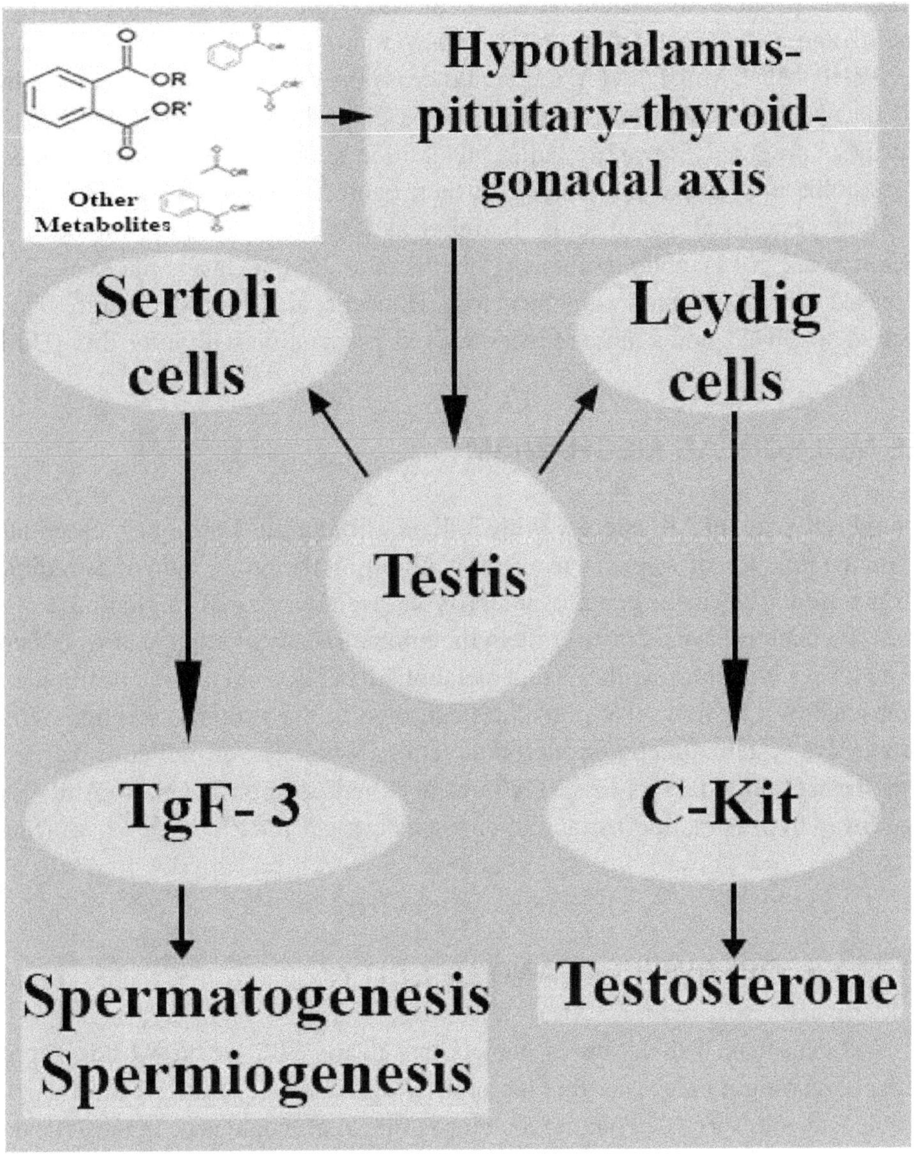

PHTHALATES AND WOMEN HEALTH

Extensive biomonitoring and risk evaluation studies in women depicts that phthalates can be detected from any fluid in women, i.e., urine, saliva, blood, cord blood; amniotic fluid, follicular fluid and milk (Silva et al., 2004; Huang et al., 2007; Berman et al., 2009; Lin S et al., 2011; Lin L-C et al., 2011; Du et al., 2016). The effect of phthalates on pregnant and breast feeding women would directly affect a new generation to come, additional to their own health; hence, this section of population should be given special attention compare to other sections of population in a different perspective.

Identification of phthalates in amniotic fluid (Huang et al., 2009; Tranfo et al., 2014), follicular fluid (Du et al., 2016), peritoneal fluid (Cobellis et al., 2003), cord blood (Latini et al., 2003; Lin S et al., 2011; LinL-C. et al., 2011), and breast milk (Hines et al., 2009; Lin S. et al., 2011) shows that phthalates can penetrate the whole body system. Huang et al. (2009) detected 85.2ng/mL MBP in utero, and warned against its anti-androgenic action on the fetus. Tranfo et al. (2014) showed that DEHP, DEP, DnBP, BBzP, MEHP, MEP, MnBP and MBzP could cross the placental barrier in their free form. Lin S. et al. (2011) detected metabolites of five commonly used phthalates (DEHP,DIBP, DnBP, BBP and DINP) in the urine of pregnant Taiwanean ladies, in addition to the presence of these phthalates in cord serum and breast milk after delivery, and urine of their babies. The presence of phthalates was found associated with low gestational age of fetus (Latini et al., 2003), delayed appearance of pubarche in girls (Frederiksen et al., 2012), endometriosis (Cobellis et al., 2003;Masuyama et al., 2003; Upson et al., 2013), increased clinical pregnancy and birth loss (Hauser et al.,2015; Mu et al., 2015), low yield of oocytes (Hauser et al., 2015), and a more recent one is its association with infertility (Du et al., 2016).

PROBABLE MOLECULAR MECHANISM

Phthalates complexed with PPAR interact with follicle stimulating hormones, essential to pubertal development and the function of women's ovaries by inhibiting the production of estradiol, i.e., by suppressing the aromatase activity in the granulosa cells through reducing cAMP signaling (Lovekamp-Swan and Davis 2003). Phthalates have a critical role in the human risk evaluation as it would concomitantly elicit multiple pathways including synthesis and metabolism of ERs and thyroid hormones (Ghisari and Bonefeld-Jorgensen2009). It shows that phthalates can modify the genomic and non-genomic activity of female reproductive system directly through interactions with ERs, or indirectly as regulators or co-activators of the transcription factors like PPARs or aryl hydrocarbon receptor (AhR), or through an independent pathway by modulating metabolic enzymes critical for ER metabolism (Shanle and Xu, 2010) (figure 6).

PHTHALATES VS. OVERWEIGHT AND OBESITY

A recent statistical data from 188 countries depicts that nearly 30% of the worlds population (~ 2.1 billion) are either overweight or obese ; this increase in world obesity rates over the last 30 years has been considerable and widespread, depicting a major public health epidemic in both the developed and the developing world (Ng et al., 2014). Among other reasons, exposure to phthalates is increasingly recognized as a major contributor (Obesogen or metabolic disruptor) to obesity, which is independent

Figure 6. Plausible molecular signaling mechanism elicited by phthalates and their metabolites in imparting dysfunctions in the female reproductive system. Abbreviations: AhR (aryl hydrocarbonreceptor), PPAR (peroxisome proliferator-activated receptor), TR (thyroid receptor), ER (estrogenreceptor) and PR (progesterone receptor).

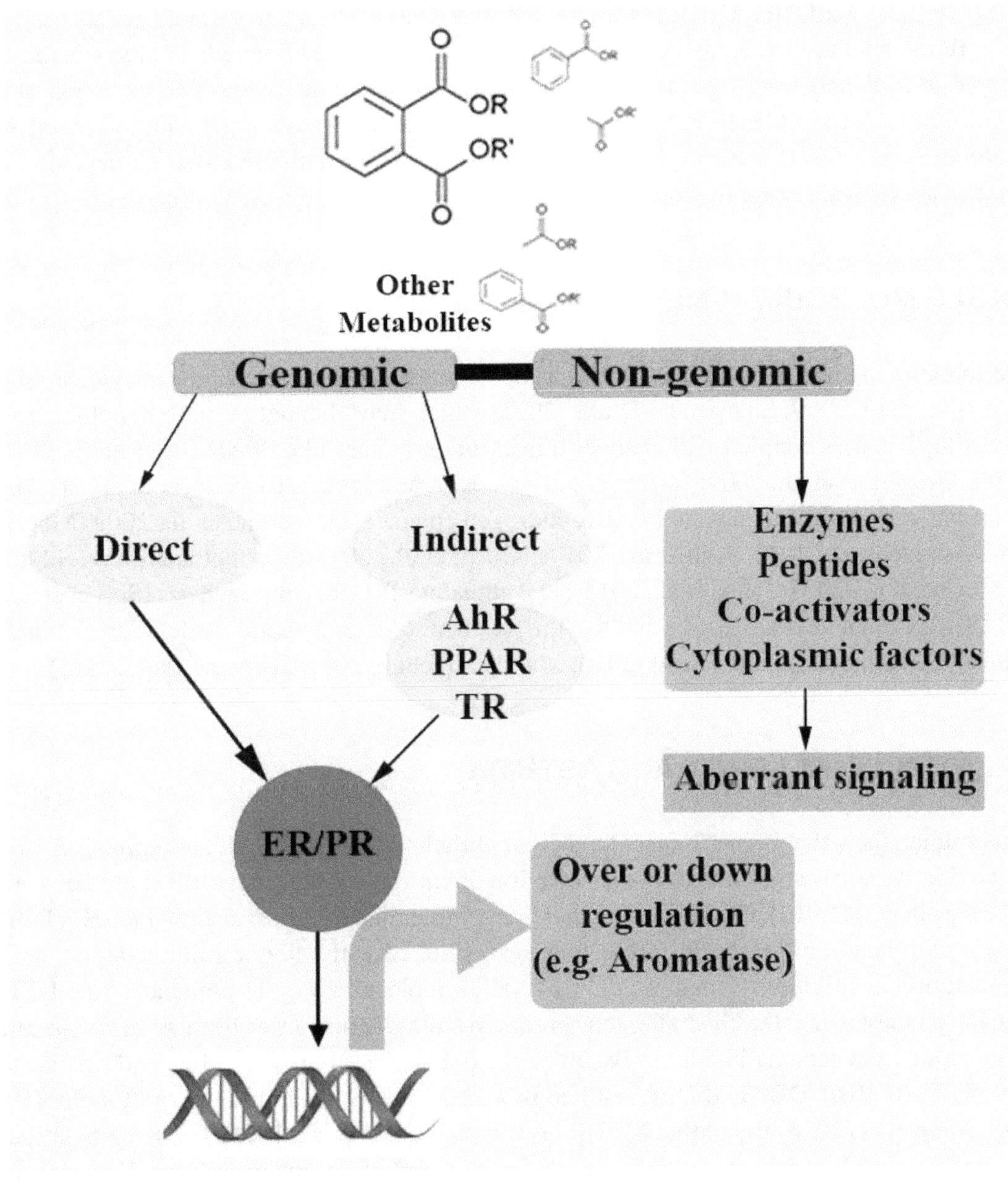

of diet and physical activity (Swan, 2008; Desvergne et al., 2009). Based on epidemiological studies, significant association has been reported for obesity with one or more phthalates (Stahlhut et al., 2007; Hatch et al., 2008; Lindet al., 2012; Dirtu et al., 2013; Buser et al., 2014). Different phthalates may act differently on age groups and sex vis-à-vis obesity outcomes (Hatch et al., 2008; Buser et al., 2014; Zhang et al., 2014). Increased association with phthalate metabolites (MEP, MEHP, MBzP, MEHHP and MEOHP) was found with obesity outcomes in the U.S. population, which was signified by notable differences by gender and age groups (Hatch et al., 2008). Low MW phthalate metabolites (MnBP, MEP and MiBP) were significantly associated with obesity in male children and adolescents; while high MW phthalate metabolites (MECPP, MEHHP, MEOHP, MEHP, MBzP, MCNP, and MCOP) along with that of DEHP (MEHHP, MEOHP, MEHP and MECPP) were significantly associated with obesity in all adults; DEHP metabolites are significantly associated with obesity in all female adults; whereas DEHP and high MW metabolites were significantly associated with obesity in males of 60 yrs of age and older (Buser et al.,2014). MBzP, MEHHP, MEOHP and MEP were found associated with increased WC and BMI (Stahlhut et al., 2007); whereas, MiBP was found associated with increased fat deposition in the subcutaneous abdominal region in women (Lind et al., 2012).

PROBABLE MOLECULAR MECHANISM

Phthalate induced overweight and obesity might be evoked by the perturbation of nuclear signaling (Grun and Blumberg, 2009; Sharpe and Drake, 2013) which may channel through hypothalamic–pituitary–gonad/thyroid axis coupled with nuclear transcription factors like PPAR (Boas et al., 2010 ; Lee et al., 2006; Desvergne et al., 2009; Josh et al., 2014a; Kim and Park., 2014; Cocci et al., 2015), which can be summarized as: (a). phthalates-PPARα-androgen channel (Desvergne et al., 2009; Mouritsen et al., 2013;Trasande et al., 2013; Josh et al., 2014a; Cocci et al., 2015); (b). phthalate-thyroid hormone channel(Meeker et al., 2007; Johns et al., 2015); (c). phthalate-PPARγ-adipogenesis (Selvin et al., 2007; Hao etal., 2012; Campioli et al., 2014); and (d). thrifty phenotype-epigenetic modulation channel (Grun and Blumberg, 2009; Sharpe and Drake, 2013; Manikkam et al., 2013: Kim and Park, 2014).

PHTHALATES VS. ALLERGY AND ASTHMA

Numerous studies show that higher molecular weight phthalates are linked with allergies and asthma by imparting oxidative stress and changes in the secretion of various cytokines (North et al., 2014; Braunet al., 2013; Hoppin et al., 2013). Children are found more vulnerable to the exposure of DEHP, BBP, DBP and DEP through household floor dust, which in turn is linked with allergic rhinitis, atopic dermatitis and conjunctivitis in children (Bamai et al., 2014). High molecular weight phthalates like DEHP and BBP or their monoesters are the chief allergens producing allergic responses like asthma, wheezing, hay fever, itchy rashes and eczema in adults (Braun et al., 2013; Hoppin et al., 2013), and that gestational exposure of DEHP, BBP, DBP and DEP resulted in allergic responses in infants and toddler (Braun et al., 2013). Wang et al.(2015) found that MEHP level in urine was related with hypo-methylation of the promoter region of TNF-α, which was accountable for the onset of asthma in children. Disregarding age, DEHP metabolites were found linked with wheeze, chest infections and bronchitis, while that of BBP metabolites imparted higher dangers of wheeze; and prenatal exposure of these two phthalates and their metabolites were also found strongly related with the risk of asthma at the age 7 years and later(Gascon et al., 2015).

PHTHALATES VS. CANCER

There is not much information (data) evidencing the association between phthalates and cancer incidence in humans. However, it is contemplated that there exists an association between human cancer (especially liver skin and gastrointestinal cancers in the general population, breast cancer in women) and endocrine disrupting chemicals (EDC) like phthalates, due of their xenoestrogenic properties (Ardies and Dees 1998; Josh et al., 2014b). One direct evidence available in literature gives possible association of urinary concentrations of phthalates with breast cancer (López-Carrillo et al., 2010).

PROBABLE MOLECULAR MECHANISM

Animal and in vitro studies showed possible mechanism of the induction of cancer by phthalates, especially hepatic and breast carcinoma. Phthalates may be transported into the cells via MDR1 channel by the transcriptional regulation of steroid and xenobiotic receptor (SXR) (Takeshita et al., 2006). Human breast cancer progression may be through the activation of PI3K/AKT signaling pathway (Chen and Chien, 2014); or through estrogen independent AhR/HDAC6/c-myc signaling pathway, mediated by cAMP-PKA-CREB1 signaling cascade (MDA-MB- 231) (Hsieh et al., 2012). It is thought that PPARα is the mediator in phthalate induced hepatic carcinoma in rodents; but studies with PPARα null mice demonstrated that hepatic carcinoma is elicited by the c-jun proto-oncogene through c-jun/c-fos/AP1 system (Ito et al., 2007); however, PPAR may act through the epigenetic modulation of c-myc gene promoter in hepatic carcinoma (Kostka et al., 2010)

RECOMMENDATIONS

In past few years, notable media and public attention has been given to the potential health risks related with phthalate exposure. These concerns have led to the US Consumer Product Safety Improvement Act (CPSIA) of 2008, which completely banned the use of BBP, DEHP, and DBP in children's toys and child care articles and placed an interim banon DnOP, DiNP, and DiDP. Regardless these measures, childhood phthalate exposure exists, likely because of the ubiquitous use of these chemicals in many consumer products. In addition, these regulations may not protect the developing fetus since they do not reduce phthalate exposures among women of child bearing age.

Presently, no evidence based methods to reduce exposures exist but many scientific and professional organizations have made recommendations to reduce exposure (Resources for health professionals, 2011). Health care providers can counsel concerned patients to avoid using personal care products that may contain DEP and DBP, particularly scented products like colognes and perfumes. There are number requirements for these products to include phthalates in their ingredient lists, which makes it difficult to reduce exposure by avoiding specific products. In order to decrease exposures to DEHP or BBP, patients can avoid using vinyl flooring and minimize dusty environments by taking shoes off at the door, keeping windowsills clean, and moping/vacuuming consistently. Avoiding processed foods, foods packaged and stored in plastics, and using non-plastic cookware and storage materials may decrease DEHP and possibly DBP exposures (Rudel., 2011; Wormuth et al., 2006). Medical providers may be able to lessen or eliminate DEHP exposure associated with certain medical procedures by using alternative products.

Until governmental regulations to limit phthalate exposure are enacted, additional research to recognize the primary sources of phthalate exposure, develop interventions to lessen exposures, and understand the health effects of early life phthalate exposure would provide patients and clinicians with strategies to diminish exposure and aid policy makers in the ongoing risk-evaluation process.

CONCLUSION

The whole globe is so prudent about the influence of phthalates on human health and environment. A specialist panel of the United Nations Environment Program constituting 16 scientists from 10 nations representing North America, Europe, Africa and Asia acknowledged the endocrine-related diseases and disorders as a blazing issue, and they called the EDCs as a "global threat" (UNEP, 2013). Previously another specialist panel of the European Environment Agency submitted that "new chemical regulation may help, but the integrated influences of chemicals remain an issue" (EEA, 2010). EPA (2015) is also much perturbed about the phthalates due to their "toxicity and the proof of extensive human and environmental exposure", and they depicted eight phthalates (DBP, DIBP, BBP, DPP, DEHP, DnOP, DINP and DIDP) as in need of instant attention.

Despite phthalates have been used on commercial scale for over 5 decades but studies have mainly been conducted on human population level within last ten years. Presently we reviewed data about human exposure pathways to the phthalates and their related health outcomes. Numerous studies evidenced that exposure to PAEs and related products should be circumvented so as to ensure human safety and environmental protection. Several scientists concluded that phthalates causes various lifestyle disorders, in addition, to reproductive abnormalities in both males and females. Scientist suggests that studies should be conducted on laboratory scale to human-population level in order to evaluate associated risk. Furthermore epidemiological studies should be conducted to improve our understanding and risk management.

REFERENCES

ACC. (2016). *Biomonitoring data.* Retrieved from https://phthalates.americanchemistry.com/

Ardies, C. M., & Dees, C. (1998). Xenoestrogens significantly enhance risk for breast cancer duringgrowth and adolescence. *Medical Hypotheses, 50*(6), 457–464. doi:10.1016/S0306-9877(98)90262-6 PMID:9710315

Ayala-García, B., López-Santibáñez Guevara, M., Marcos-Camacho, L. I., Fuentes-Farías, A. L., Meléndez-Herrera, E., & Gutiérrez-Ospina, G. (2013). Speciation, phenotypic variation andplasticity: What can endocrine disruptors tell us? *International Journal of Endocrinology*. PMID:23762055

Bamai, Y. A., Shibata, E., Saito, I., Araki, A., Kanazawa, A., Morimoto, K., ... Chikara, H. (2014). Exposure to house dust phthalates in relation to asthma and allergies in both children and adults. *The Science of the Total Environment, 485*, 153–163. doi:10.1016/j.scitotenv.2014.03.059 PMID:24704966

Bekö, G., Weschler, C. J., Langer, S., Callesen, M., Toftum, J., & Clausen, G. (2013). Children's phthalate intakes and resultant cumulative exposures estimated from urine compared with estimates from dust ingestion, inhalation and dermal absorption in their homes and day care centers. *PLoS One*, *8*(4), e62442. doi:10.1371/journal.pone.0062442 PMID:23626820

Benjamin, S., Prakasan, P., Sreedharan, S., Wright, A. D. G., & Spener, F. (2015). Pros and cons of CLA consumption: An insight from clinical evidences. *Nutrition & Metabolism*, *12*(1), 1. doi:10.1186/1743-7075-12-4 PMID:25972911

Berman, T., Hochner-Celnikier, D., Calafat, A. M., Needham, L. L., Amitai, Y., Wormser, U., & Richter, E. (2009). Phthalate exposure among pregnant women in Jerusalem, Israel: Results of a pilotstudy. *Environment International*, *35*(2), 353–357. doi:10.1016/j.envint.2008.08.010 PMID:18824263

Bertelsen, R. J., Carlsen, K. C. L., Calafat, A. M., Hoppin, J. A., Håland, G., Mowinckel, P., ... Løvik, M. (2013). Urinary biomarkers for phthalates associated with asthma in Norwegianchildren. *Environmental Health Perspectives (Online)*, *121*(2), 251–256. doi:10.1289/ehp.1205256 PMID:23164678

Boas, M., Frederiksen, H., Feldt-Rasmussen, U., Skakkebæk, N. E., Hegedus, L., Hilsted, L., ... Main, K. M. (2010). Childhood exposure to phthalates: Associations with thyroid function, insulinlike growth factor I, and growth. *Environmental Health Perspectives*, *118*(10), 1458–1464. doi:10.1289/ehp.0901331 PMID:20621847

Bornehag, C. G., Sundell, J., Weschler, C. J., Sigsgaard, T., Lundgren, B., Hasselgren, M., & Hägerhed-Engman, L. (2004). The association between asthma and allergic symptoms in children and phthalates in house dust: A nested case–control study. *Environmental Health Perspectives*, *112*(14), 1393–1397. doi:10.1289/ehp.7187 PMID:15471731

Braun, J. M., Sathyanarayana, S., & Hauser, R. (2013). Phthalate exposure and children's health. *Current Opinion in Pediatrics*, *25*(2), 247–254. doi:10.1097/MOP.0b013e32835e1eb6 PMID:23429708

Buser, M. C., Murray, H. E., & Scinicariello, F. (2014). Age and sex differences in childhood andadulthood obesity association with phthalates: Analyses of NHANES 2007–2010. *International Journal of Hygiene and Environmental Health*, *217*(6), 687–694. doi:10.1016/j.ijheh.2014.02.005 PMID:24657244

Cadogan, D., Papez, M., Poppe, A. C., Pugh, D. M., & Scheubel, J. (1994). Assessment of the release, occurrence and possible effects of plasticizers in the environment. *Progress in Rubber and Plastics Technology*, *10*(1), 1–19.

Campioli, E., Martinez-Arguelles, D. B., & Papadopoulos, V. (2014). In utero exposure to the endocrine disruptor di-(2-ethylhexyl) phthalate promotes local adipose and systemic inflammation in adult male offspring. *Nutrition & Diabetes*, *4*(5), e115. doi:10.1038/nutd.2014.13 PMID:24799162

Casals-Casas, C., & Desvergne, B. (2011). Endocrine disruptors: From endocrine to metabolic disruption. *Annual Review of Physiology*, *73*(1), 135–162. doi:10.1146/annurev-physiol-012110-142200 PMID:21054169

Chang, B. V., Yang, C. M., Cheng, C. H., & Yuan, S. Y. (2004). Biodegradation of phthalate esters by two bacteria strains. *Chemosphere*, *55*(4), 533–538. doi:10.1016/j.chemosphere.2003.11.057 PMID:15006506

Chang, J. W., Lee, C. C., Pan, W. H., Chou, W. C., Huang, H. B., Chiang, H. C., & Huang, P. C. (2017). Estimated daily intake and cumulative risk assessment of phthalates in the general Taiwanese after the 2011 DEHP food scandal. *Scientific Reports*, *7*(1), 45009. doi:10.1038rep45009 PMID:28327585

Chao, W. L., Lin, C. M., Shiung, I. I., & Kuo, Y. L. (2006). Degradation of di-butyl-phthalate by soil bacteria. *Chemosphere*, *63*(8), 1377–1383. doi:10.1016/j.chemosphere.2005.09.021 PMID:16289698

Chen, F. P., & Chien, M. H. (2014). Lower concentrations of phthalates induce proliferation in human-breast cancer cells. *Climacteric*, *17*(4), 377–384. doi:10.3109/13697137.2013.865720 PMID:24228746

Choi, J., Eom, J., Kim, J., Lee, S., & Kim, Y. (2014). Association between some endocrine-disruptingchemicals and childhood obesity in biological samples of young girls: A cross-sectional study. *Environmental Toxicology and Pharmacology*, *38*(1), 51–57. doi:10.1016/j.etap.2014.04.004 PMID:24908636

Cobellis, L., Latini, G., De Felice, C., Razzi, S., Paris, I., Ruggieri, F., ... Petraglia, F. (2003). High plasma concentrations of di-(2-ethylhexyl)-phthalate in women with endometriosis. *Human Reproduction (Oxford, England)*, *18*(7), 1512–1515. doi:10.1093/humrep/deg254 PMID:12832380

Cocci, P., Mosconi, G., Arukwe, A., Mozzicafreddo, M., Angeletti, M., Aretusi, G., & Palermo, F. A. (2015). Effects of diisodecyl phthalate on PPAR: RXR-dependent gene expression pathways inSea Bream hepatocytes. *Chemical Research in Toxicology*, *28*(5), 935–947. doi:10.1021/tx500529x PMID:25825955

Commission Staff Working Document on the Implementation of the Community Strategy for Endocrine Disrupters. (2007). *A Range of Substances Suspected of Interfering with the Hormone Systems of Humans and Wildlife; CEC.* Brussels: Commission of the European Communities.

Dargnat, C., Teil, M. J., Chevreuil, M., & Blanchard, M. (2009). Phthalate removal throughout waste-water treatment plant: Case study of Marne Aval station (France). *The Science of the Total Environment*, *407*(4), 1235–1244. doi:10.1016/j.scitotenv.2008.10.027 PMID:19036415

Das, M. T., Ghosh, P., & Thakur, I. S. (2014). Intake estimates of phthalate esters for South Delhi population based on exposure media assessment. *Environmental Pollution*, *189*, 118–125. doi:10.1016/j.envpol.2014.02.021 PMID:24657605

Desvergne, B., Feige, J. N., & Casals-Casas, C. (2009). PPAR-mediated activity of phthalates: A link to the obesity epidemic? *Molecular and Cellular Endocrinology*, *304*(1), 43–48. doi:10.1016/j.mce.2009.02.017 PMID:19433246

Dirtu, A. C., Geens, T., Dirinck, E., Malarvannan, G., Neels, H., Van Gaal, L., ... Covaci, A. (2013). Phthalate metabolites in obese individuals undergoing weight loss: Urinary levels and estimation of the phthalates daily intake. *Environment International*, *59*, 344–353. doi:10.1016/j.envint.2013.06.023 PMID:23892227

Doyle, T. J., Bowman, J. L., Windell, V. L., McLean, D. J., & Kim, K. H. (2013). Transgenerationaleffects of di-(2-ethylhexyl) phthalate on testicular germ cell associations and spermatogonial stemcells in mice. *Biology of Reproduction*, *88*(5), 112. doi:10.1095/biolreprod.112.106104 PMID:23536373

Du, Y. Y., Fang, Y. L., Wang, Y. X., Zeng, Q., Guo, N., Zhao, H., & Li, Y. F. (2016). Follicular fluid andurinary concentrations of phthalate metabolites among infertile women and associations with invitro fertilization parameters. *Reproductive Toxicology (Elmsford, N.Y.)*, *61*, 142–150. doi:10.1016/j.reprotox.2016.04.005 PMID:27067915

EEA. (2010). *The European environment — state and outlook 2010: synthesis*. Copenhagen: European EnvironmentAgency.

Ejaredar, M., Nyanza, E. C., Ten Eycke, K., & Dewey, D. (2015). Phthalate exposure and childrensneurodevelopment: A systematic review. *EnvironmentalResearch*, *142*, 51–60. doi:10.1016/j.envres.2015.06.014 PMID:26101203

EPA. (2015). *On phthalates*. Retrieved from https://www.epa.gov/assessing-and-managing-chemicals-undertsca/

Ferguson, K. K., Loch-Caruso, R., & Meeker, J. D. (2011). Urinary phthalate metabolites in relation to biomarkers of inflammation and oxidative stress: NHANES 1999–2006. *Environmental Research*, *111*(5), 718–726. doi:10.1016/j.envres.2011.02.002 PMID:21349512

Frederiksen, H., Sørensen, K., Mouritsen, A., Aksglaede, L., Hagen, C. P., Petersen, J. H., ... Juul, A. (2012). High urinary phthalate concentration associated withdelayed pubarche in girls. *International Journal of Andrology*, *35*(3), 216–226. doi:10.1111/j.1365-2605.2012.01260.x PMID:22428786

Fromme, H., Gruber, L., Seckin, E., Raab, U., Zimmermann, S., Kiranoglu, M., ... Völkel, W. (2011). Phthalates and their metabolites in breast milk—Results from the Bavarian Monitoring of Breast Milk (BAMBI). *Environment International*, *37*(4), 715–722. doi:10.1016/j.envint.2011.02.008 PMID:21406311

Fu, P., Kawamura, K., & Barrie, L. A. (2008). Photochemical and other sources of organic compounds in the Canadian high Arctic aerosol pollution during winter– spring. *Environmental Science & Technology*, *43*(2), 286–292. doi:10.1021/es803046q PMID:19238953

Gao, D., Li, Z., Wen, Z., & Ren, N. (2014). Occurrence and fate of phthalate esters in full-scale domestic wastewater treatment plants and their impact on receiving waters along the Songhua River in China. *Chemosphere*, *95*, 24–32. doi:10.1016/j.chemosphere.2013.08.009 PMID:24001662

Gascon, M., Casas, M., Morales, E., Valvi, D., Ballesteros-Gómez, A., Luque, N., ... Sunyer, J. (2015). Prenatal exposure to bisphenol A and phthalatesand childhood respiratory tract infections and allergy. *The Journal of Allergy and Clinical Immunology*, *135*(2), 370–378. doi:10.1016/j.jaci.2014.09.030 PMID:25445825

Ge, R. S., Chen, G. R., Tanrikut, C., & Hardy, M. P. (2007). Phthalate ester toxicity in Leydig cells:developmental timing and dosage considerations. *Reproductive Toxicology (Elmsford, N.Y.)*, *23*(3), 366–373. doi:10.1016/j.reprotox.2006.12.006 PMID:17258888

Ghisari, M., & Bonefeld-Jorgensen, E. C. (2009). Effects of plasticizers and their mixtures on estrogen receptor and thyroid hormone functions. *Toxicology Letters*, *189*(1), 67–77. doi:10.1016/j.toxlet.2009.05.004 PMID:19463926

Grun, F., & Blumberg, B. (2009). Minireview: The case for obesogens. *Molecular Endocrinology (Baltimore, Md.)*, *23*(8), 1127–1134. doi:10.1210/me.2008-0485 PMID:19372238

Halden, R. U. (2010). Plastics and health risks. *Annual Review of Public Health*, *31*(1), 179–194. doi:10.1146/annurev.publhealth.012809.103714 PMID:20070188

Hao, C., Cheng, X., Xia, H., & Ma, X. (2012). The endocrine disruptor mono-(2-ethylhexyl) phthalate promotes adipocyte differentiation and induces obesity in mice. *Bioscience Reports*, *32*(6), 619–629. doi:10.1042/BSR20120042 PMID:22953781

Hatch, E. E., Nelson, J. W., Qureshi, M. M., Weinberg, J., Moore, L. L., Singer, M., & Webster, T. F. (2008). Association of urinary phthalate metabolite concentrations with body mass index and waist circumference: A cross-sectional study of NHANES data, 1999–2002. *Environmental Health*, *7*(27), 1–15. PMID:18522739

Hatch, E. E., Nelson, J. W., Stahlhut, R. W., & Webster, T. F. (2010). Association of endocrine disruptorsand obesity: Perspectives from epidemiological studies. *International Journal of Andrology*, *33*(2), 324–332. doi:10.1111/j.1365-2605.2009.01035.x PMID:20113374

Hauser, R., Gaskins, A. J., Souter, I., Smith, K. W., Dodge, L. E., Ehrlich, S., ... Williams, P. L. (2015). Urinary phthalate metabolite concentrations and reproductive outcomes among women undergoing *in vitro* fertilization: Results from the EARTH study. *Environmental Health Perspectives*. PMID:26545148

Heudorf, U., Mersch-Sundermann, V., & Angerer, J. (2007). Phthalates: Toxicology and exposure. *International Journal of Hygiene and Environmental Health*, *210*(5), 623–634. doi:10.1016/j.ijheh.2007.07.011 PMID:17889607

Hines, E. P., Calafat, A. M., Silva, M. J., Mendola, P., & Fenton, S. E. (2009). Concentrations ofphthalate metabolites in milk, urine, saliva, and serum of lactating North Carolina women. *Environmental Health Perspectives*, *117*(1), 86–92. doi:10.1289/ehp.11610 PMID:19165392

Högberg, J., Hanberg, A., Berglund, M., Skerfving, S., Remberger, M., Calafat, A. M., ... Håkansson, H. (2008). Phthalate diesters and their metabolites in human breast milk, blood or serum, and urine as biomarkers of exposure in vulnerable populations. *Environmental Health Perspectives*, *116*(3), 334–339. doi:10.1289/ehp.10788 PMID:18335100

Hoppin, J. A., Jaramillo, R., London, S. J., Bertelsen, R. J., Salo, P. M., Sandler, D. P., & Zeldin, D. C. (2013). Phthalate exposure and allergy in the US population: Results from NHANES 2005-2006. *Environmental Health Perspectives (Online)*, *121*(10), 1129–1134. doi:10.1289/ehp.1206211 PMID:23799650

Hsieh, T. H., Tsai, C. F., Hsu, C. Y., Kuo, P. L., Lee, J. N., Chai, C. Y., ... Tsai, E. M. (2012). Phthalates induce proliferation and invasiveness of estrogen receptor-negative breast cancer through the AhR/HDAC6/c-Myc signaling pathway. *The FASEB Journal*, *26*(2), 778–787. doi:10.1096/fj.11-191742 PMID:22049059

Huang, H. B., Chen, H. Y., Su, P. H., Huang, P. C., Sun, C. W., Wang, C. J., ... Wang, S. L. (2015). Fetal and childhood exposure to phthalate diesters and cognitive function in children up to 12 years of age: Taiwanese maternal and infant cohort study. *PLoS One*, *10*(6), e0131910. doi:10.1371/journal.pone.0131910 PMID:26121592

Huang, P. C., Kuo, P. L., Chou, Y. Y., Lin, S. J., & Lee, C. C. (2009). Association between prenatalexposure to phthalates and the health of newborns. *Environment International*, *35*(1), 14–20. doi:10.1016/j.envint.2008.05.012 PMID:18640725

Huang, P. C., Kuo, P. L., Guo, Y. L., Liao, P. C., & Lee, C. C. (2007). Associations between urinary phthalate monoesters and thyroid hormones in pregnant women. *Human Reproduction (Oxford, England)*, *22*(10), 2715–2722. doi:10.1093/humrep/dem205 PMID:17704099

Ito, Y., Yamanoshita, O., Asaeda, N., Tagawa, Y., Lee, C. H., Aoyama, T., ... Nakajima, T. (2007). Di (2-ethylhexyl) phthalate induces hepatictumorigenesis through a peroxisome proliferator-activated receptor-α independentPathway. *Journal of Occupational Health*, *49*(3), 172–182. doi:10.1539/joh.49.172 PMID:17575397

Itoh, H., Yoshida, K., & Masunaga, S. (2007). Quantitative identification of unknown exposure pathways of phthalates based on measuring their metabolites in human urine. *Environmental Science & Technology*, *41*(13), 4542–4547. doi:10.1021/es062926y PMID:17695894

Janjua, N. R., Mortensen, G. K., Andersson, A. M., Kongshoj, B., Skakkebæk, N. E., & Wulf, H. C. (2007). Systemic uptake of diethyl phthalate, dibutyl phthalate, and butyl paraben following whole-body topical application and reproductive and thyroid hormone levels in humans. *Environmental Science & Technology*, *41*(15), 5564–5570. doi:10.1021/es0628755 PMID:17822133

Johns, L. E., Ferguson, K. K., Soldin, O. P., Cantonwine, D. E., Rivera-González, L. O., Del Toro, L. V. A., ... Meeker, J. D. (2015). Urinary phthalate metabolites in relation to maternal serum thyroid and sex hormone levels during pregnancy: A longitudinal analysis. *Reproductive Biology and Endocrinology*, *13*(1), 1. doi:10.1186/1477-7827-13-4 PMID:25596636

Josh, M. S. (2014a). Phthalates efficiently bind to human peroxisome proliferator activated receptor and retinoid X receptor α, β, γ subtypes: An in silico approach. *Journal of Applied Toxicology*, *34*(7), 754–765. doi:10.1002/jat.2902 PMID:23843199

Josh, M. S., Pradeep, S., Adarsh, V. K., Vijayalekshmi Amma, K. S., Sudha Devi, R., Balachandran, S., ... Benjamin, S. (2014b). In silico evidences for the binding ofphthalates onto human estrogen receptor α, β subtypes and human estrogen-related receptor γ. *Molecular Simulation*, *40*(5), 408–417. doi:10.1080/08927022.2013.814131

Jugan, M. L., Levi, Y., & Blondeau, J. P. (2010). Endocrine disruptors and thyroid hormone physiology. *Biochemical Pharmacology*, *79*(7), 939–947. doi:10.1016/j.bcp.2009.11.006 PMID:19913515

Kim, S. H., & Park, M. J. (2014). Phthalate exposure and childhood obesity. *Annals of Pediatric Endocrinology & Metabolism*, *19*(2), 69–75. doi:10.6065/apem.2014.19.2.69 PMID:25077088

Koch, H. M., Lorber, M., Christensen, K. L., Pälmke, C., Koslitz, S., & Brüning, T. (2013). Identifying sources of phthalate exposure with human biomonitoring: Results of a 48h fasting study with urine collection and personal activity patterns. *International Journal of Hygiene and Environmental Health*, *216*(6), 672–681. doi:10.1016/j.ijheh.2012.12.002 PMID:23333758

Kolarik, B., Naydenov, K., Larsson, M., Bornehag, C. G., & Sundell, J. (2007). The association between phthalates in dust and allergic diseases among Bulgarian children. *Environmental Health Perspectives, 116*(1), 98–103. doi:10.1289/ehp.10498 PMID:18197306

Kortenkamp, A., & Faust, M. (2010). Combined exposures to anti-androgenic chemicals: Steps towards cumulative risk assessment. *International Journal of Andrology, 33*(2), 463–474. doi:10.1111/j.1365-2605.2009.01047.x PMID:20487045

Kostka, G., Urbanek-Olejnik, K., & Wiadrowska, B. (2010). Di-butyl phthalate—Induced hypomethylation of the c-myc gene in ratliver. *Toxicology and Industrial Health, 26*(7), 407–416. doi:10.1177/0748233710369124 PMID:20504828

Kuo, C. C., Moon, K., Thayer, K. A., & Navas-Acien, A. (2013). Environmental chemicals and type 2diabetes: An updated systematic review of the epidemiologic evidence. *Current Diabetes Reports, 13*(6), 831–849. doi:10.100711892-013-0432-6 PMID:24114039

Lambrot, R., Muczynski, V., Lécureuil, C., Angenard, G., Coffigny, H., Pairault, C., ... Rouiller-Fabre, V. (2009). Phthalates impair germ cell development inthe human fetal testis in vitro without change in testosterone production. *Environmental Health Perspectives, 117*(1), 32–37. doi:10.1289/ehp.11146 PMID:19165384

LaRocca, J., Binder, A. M., McElrath, T. F., & Michels, K. B. (2014). The impact of first trimester-phthalate and phenol exposure on IGF2/H19 genomic imprinting and birth outcomes. *Environmental Research, 133*, 396–406. doi:10.1016/j.envres.2014.04.032 PMID:24972507

Larsen, S. T., Hansen, J. S., Hansen, E. W., Clausen, P. A., & Nielsen, G. D. (2007). Airway inflammation and adjuvant effect after repeated airborneexposures to di-(2-ethylhexyl) phthalate and ovalbumin in BALB/c mice. *Toxicology, 235*(1), 119–129. doi:10.1016/j.tox.2007.03.010 PMID:17462807

Latini, G., De Felice, C., Presta, G., Del Vecchio, A., Paris, I., Ruggieri, F., & Mazzeo, P. (2003). In uteroexposure to di-(2-ethylhexyl) phthalate and duration of human pregnancy. *Environmental Health Perspectives, 111*(14), 1783–1785. doi:10.1289/ehp.6202 PMID:14594632

Latini, G., Knipp, G., Mantovani, A., Marcovecchio, M. L., Chiarelli, F., & Soder, O. (2010). Endocrine disruptors and human health. *Mini-Reviews in Medicinal Chemistry, 10*(9), 846–855. doi:10.2174/138955710791608271 PMID:20482499

Latini, G., Verrotti, A., & De Felice, C. (2004). Di-2-ethylhexyl phthalate and endocrine disruption: Areview. *Current Drug Targets. Immune, Endocrine and Metabolic Disorders, 4*(1), 37–40. doi:10.2174/1568008043340017 PMID:15032624

Le Moal, J., Sharpe, R. M., Jφrgensen, N., Levine, H., Jurewicz, J., Mendiola, J., … Toppari, J. (2015). Toward a multi-country monitoring system of reproductive health in the context of endocrine disrupting chemical exposure. *The European Journal of Public Health.*

Lee, H. C., Yamanouchi, K., & Nishihara, M. (2006). Effects of perinatal exposure to phthalate/Adipateesters on hypothalamic gene expression and sexual behavior in rats. *Journal of Reproduction and Development, 52*(3), 343-352.

Li, L., Zhang, T., Qin, X. S., Ge, W., Ma, H. G., Sun, L. L., ... Shen, W. (2014). Exposure to diethylhexyl phthalate (DEHP) results in a heritable modification of imprint genes DNA methylation in mouse oocytes. *Molecular Biology Reports*, *41*(3), 1227–1235. doi:10.100711033-013-2967-7 PMID:24390239

Lin, L. C., Wang, S. L., Chang, Y. C., Huang, P. C., Cheng, J. T., Su, P. H., & Liao, P. C. (2011). Associations between maternal phthalate exposure and cord sex hormones in human infants. *Chemosphere*, *83*(8), 1192–1199. doi:10.1016/j.chemosphere.2010.12.079 PMID:21272909

Lin, S., Ku, H. Y., Su, P. H., Chen, J. W., Huang, P. C., Angerer, J., & Wang, S. L. (2011). Phthalateexposure in pregnant women and their children in central Taiwan. *Chemosphere*, *82*(7), 947–955. doi:10.1016/j.chemosphere.2010.10.073 PMID:21075419

Lind, P. M., Roos, V., Ronn, M., Johansson, L., Ahlstrom, H., Kullberg, J., & Lind, L. (2012). Serumconcentrations of phthalate metabolites are related to abdominal fat distribution two years later in elderly women. *Environmental Health*, *11*(21), 10–1186. PMID:22472124

López-Carrillo, L., Hernández-Ramírez, R. U., Calafat, A. M., Torres-Sánchez, L., Galván-Portillo, M., Needham, L. L., ... Cebrián, M. E. (2010). Exposure to phthalates and breastcancer risk in northern Mexico. *Environmental Health Perspectives*, *118*(4), 539–544. doi:10.1289/ehp.0901091 PMID:20368132

Lovekamp-Swan, T., & Davis, B. J. (2003). Mechanisms of phthalate ester toxicity in the femalereproductive system. *Environmental Health Perspectives*, *111*(2), 139–145. doi:10.1289/ehp.5658 PMID:12573895

Ma, M., Kondo, T., Ban, S., Umemura, T., Kurahashi, N., Takeda, M., & Kishi, R. (2006). Exposure ofprepubertal female rats to inhaled di (2-ethylhexyl) phthalate affects the onset of puberty andpost-pubertal reproductive functions. *Toxicological Sciences*, *93*(1), 164–171. doi:10.1093/toxsci/kfl036 PMID:16763069

Manikkam, M., Tracey, R., Guerrero-Bosagna, C., & Skinner, M. K. (2013). Plastics derived endocrinedisruptors (BPA, DEHP and DBP) induce epigenetic transgenerational inheritance of obesity,reproductive disease and sperm epimutations. *PLoS One*, *8*(1), e55387. doi:10.1371/journal.pone.0055387 PMID:23359474

Maqbool, F., Mostafalou, S., Bahadar, H., & Abdollahi, M. (2015). Review of endocrine disordersassociated with environmental toxicants and possible involved mechanisms. *Life Sciences*. PMID:26497928

Marsee, K., Woodruff, T. J., Axelrad, D. A., Calafat, A. M., & Swan, S. H. (2006). Estimated dailyphthalate exposures in a population of mothers of male infants exhibiting reduced anogenital distance. *Environmental Health Perspectives*, *114*(6), 805–809. doi:10.1289/ehp.8663 PMID:16759976

Masuyama, H., Hiramatsu, Y., Kodama, J. I., & Kudo, T. (2003). Expression and potential roles ofpregnane X receptor in endometrial cancer. *The Journal of Clinical Endocrinology and Metabolism*, *88*(9), 4446–4454. doi:10.1210/jc.2003-030203 PMID:12970323

Meeker, J. D., Calafat, A. M., & Hauser, R. (2007). Di (2-ethylhexyl) phthalate metabolites may alter thyroid hormone levels in men. *Environmental Health Perspectives*, *115*(7), 1029–1034. doi:10.1289/ehp.9852 PMID:17637918

Miodovnik, A., Engel, S. M., Zhu, C., Ye, X., Soorya, L. V., Silva, M. J., ... Wolff, M. S. (2011). Endocrine disruptors and childhood social impairment. *Neurotoxicology*, *32*(2), 261–267. doi:10.1016/j.neuro.2010.12.009 PMID:21182865

Mu, D., Gao, F., Fan, Z., Shen, H., Peng, H., & Hu, J. (2015). Levels of Phthalate Metabolites in Urine ofPregnant Women and Risk of Clinical Pregnancy Loss. *Environmental Science & Technology*, *49*(17), 10651–10657. doi:10.1021/acs.est.5b02617 PMID:26251123

Net, S., Dumoulin, D., El-Osmani, R., Rabodonirina, S., & Ouddane, B. (2014). Case study of PAHs, Me-PAHs, PCBs, phthalates and pesticides contamination in the Somme River water, France. *International Journal of Environmental of Research*, *8*(4), 1159–1170.

Net, S., Sempere, R., Delmont, A., Paluselli, A., & Ouddane, B. (2015). Occurrence, fate, behavior and ecotoxicological state of phthalates in different environmental matrices. *Environmental Science & Technology*, *49*(7), 4019–4035. doi:10.1021/es505233b PMID:25730609

Ng, M., Fleming, T., Robinson, M., Thomson, B., Graetz, N., Margono, C., ... Abraham, J. P. (2014). Global, regional, and national prevalence ofoverweight and obesity in children and adults during 1980–2013: A systematic analysis for theGlobal Burden of Disease Study 2013. *Lancet*, *384*(9945), 766–781. doi:10.1016/S0140-6736(14)60460-8 PMID:24880830

North, M. L., Takaro, T. K., Diamond, M. L., & Ellis, A. K. (2014). Effects of phthalates on thedevelopment and expression of allergic disease and asthma. *Annals of Allergy, Asthma & Immunology*, *112*(6), 496–502. doi:10.1016/j.anai.2014.03.013 PMID:24726194

Peijnenburg, W. J., & Struijs, J. (2006). Occurrence of phthalate esters in the environment of the Netherlands. *Ecotoxicology and Environmental Safety*, *63*(2), 204–215. doi:10.1016/j.ecoenv.2005.07.023 PMID:16168482

Pocar, P., Fiandanese, N., Secchi, C., Berrini, A., Fischer, B., Schmidt, J. S., ... Borromeo, V. (2011). Exposure to di (2-ethyl-hexyl) phthalate (DEHP) in utero and during lactation causeslong-term pituitary-gonadal axis disruption in male and female mouseoffspring. *Endocrinology*, *153*(2), 937–948. doi:10.1210/en.2011-1450 PMID:22147016

Rajesh, P., & Balasubramanian, K. (2014). Phthalate exposure in utero causes epigenetic changes andimpairs insulin signalling. *The Journal of Endocrinology*, *223*(1), 47–66. doi:10.1530/JOE-14-0111 PMID:25232145

Resources for health professionals. (2011). Retrieved from http://www.aoec.org/pehsu/training.html

Rudel, R. A., Gray, J. M., Engel, C. L., Rawsthorne, T. W., Dodson, R. E., Ackerman, J. M., & Brody, J. G. (2011). Food packaging and bisphenol A and bis (2-ethyhexyl) phthalate exposure: Findings from a dietary intervention. *Environmental Health Perspectives*, *119*(7), 914–920. doi:10.1289/ehp.1003170 PMID:21450549

Schneider, J. E., Brozek, J. M., & Keen-Rhinehart, E. (2014). Our stolen figures: the interface of sexualdifferentiation, endocrine disruptors, maternal programming, and energy balance. *Hormones and Behavior, 66*(1), 104-119.

Schreiber, A., Fu, F., Yang, O., Wan, E., Gu, E., & Le Blanc, Y. (2011). Increasing Selectivity and Confidence in Detection When Analyzing Phthalates by LC–MS/MS. *AB Sciex (AN 3690411–01).*

Selvin, E., Feinleib, M., Zhang, L., Rohrmann, S., Rifai, N., Nelson, W. G., ... Platz, E. A. (2007). Androgens and diabetes in men results from the Third National Health and Nutrition Examination Survey (NHANES III). *Diabetes Care, 30*(2), 234–238. doi:10.2337/dc06-1579 PMID:17259487

Shanle, E. K., & Xu, W. (2010). *Endocrine disrupting chemicals targeting estrogen receptor signaling*. Academic Press.

Sharpe, R. M., & Drake, A. J. (2013). Obesogens and obesity—An alternative view? *Obesity (Silver Spring, Md.), 21*(6), 1081–1083. doi:10.1002/oby.20373 PMID:23512350

Sharpe, R. M., & Skakkebaek, N. E. (2008). Testicular dysgenesis syndrome: Mechanistic insights and potential new downstream effects. *Fertility and Sterility, 89*(2), e33–e38. doi:10.1016/j.fertnstert.2007.12.026 PMID:18308057

Silva, M. J., Reidy, J. A., Herbert, A. R., Preau, J. L., Needham, L. L., & Calafat, A. M. (2004). Detection of phthalate metabolites in human amniotic fluid. *Bulletin of Environmental Contamination and Toxicology, 72*(6), 1226-1231.

Soeborg, T., Frederiksen, H., & Andersson, A. M. (2012). Cumulative risk assessment of phthalate exposure of Danish children and adolescents using the hazard index approach. *International Journal of Andrology, 35*(3), 245–252. doi:10.1111/j.1365-2605.2011.01240.x PMID:22320716

Song, Y., Hauser, R., Hu, F. B., Franke, A. A., Liu, S., & Sun, Q. (2014). Urinary concentrations ofbisphenol A and phthalate metabolites and weight change: A prospective investigation in USwomen. *International Journal of Obesity, 38*(12), 1532–1537. doi:10.1038/ijo.2014.63 PMID:24722546

Stahlhut, R. W., van Wijngaarden, E., Dye, T. D., Cook, S., & Swan, S. H. (2007). Concentrations ofurinary phthalate metabolites are associated with increased waist circumference and insulin resistance in adult US males. *Environmental Health Perspectives, 115*(6), 876–882. doi:10.1289/ehp.9882 PMID:17589594

Staples, C. A., Peterson, D. R., Parkerton, T. F., & Adams, W. J. (1997). The environmental fate of phthalate esters: A literature review. *Chemosphere, 35*(4), 667–749. doi:10.1016/S0045-6535(97)00195-1

Sun, Y., Zhang, Q., Hou, J., Wang, P., & Sundell, J. (2017). Exposure of phthalates in residential buildings and its health effects. *Procedia Engineering, 205*, 1901–1904. doi:10.1016/j.proeng.2017.10.286

Suzuki, Y., Yoshinaga, J., Mizumoto, Y., Serizawa, S., & Shiraishi, H. (2012). Foetal exposure tophthalate esters and anogenital distance in male newborns. *International Journal of Andrology, 35*(3), 236–244. doi:10.1111/j.1365-2605.2011.01190.x PMID:21696396

Swan, S. H. (2008). Environmental phthalate exposure in relation to reproductive outcomes and otherhealth endpoints in humans. *Environmental Research, 108*(2), 177–184. doi:10.1016/j.envres.2008.08.007 PMID:18949837

Swan, S. H., Main, K. M., Liu, F., Stewart, S. L., Kruse, R. L., Calafat, A. M., ... Teague, J. L. (2005). Decrease in anogenital distance among mal infants with prenatal phthalate exposure. *Environmental Health Perspectives, 113*(8), 1056–1061. doi:10.1289/ehp.8100 PMID:16079079

Takeshita, A., Inagaki, K., Igarashi-Migitaka, J., Ozawa, Y., & Koibuchi, N. (2006). Th endocrinedisrupting chemical, diethylhexyl phthalate, activates MDR1 gene expression in human colon cancer LS174T cells. *The Journal of Endocrinology*, *190*(3), 897–902. doi:10.1677/joe.1.06664 PMID:17003290

Teitelbaum, S. L., Mervish, N., Moshier, E. L., Vangeepuram, N., Galvez, M. P., Calafat, A. M., ... Wolff, M. S. (2012). Associations between phthalate metabolite urinaryconcentrations and body size measures in New York City children. *Environmental Research*, *112*, 186–193. doi:10.1016/j.envres.2011.12.006 PMID:22222007

Testa, C., Nuti, F., Hayek, J., De Felice, C., Chelli, M., Rovero, P., ... Papini, A. M. (2012). Di-(2-ethylhexyl) phthalate and autism spectrum disorders. *ASN Neuro*, *4*(4), AN20120015. doi:10.1042/AN20120015 PMID:22537663

Tokiwa, Y., Calabia, B., Ugwu, C., & Aiba, S. (2009). Biodegradability of plastics. *International Journal of Molecular Sciences*, *10*(9), 3722–3742. doi:10.3390/ijms10093722 PMID:19865515

Tranfo, G., Papaleo, B., Caporossi, L., Capanna, S., De Rosa, M., Pigini, D., ... Paci, E. (2013). Urinary metabolite concentrations of phthalate metabolites in Central Italy healthyvolunteers determined by a validated HPLC/MS/MS analytical method. *International Journal of Hygiene and Environmental Health*, *216*(4), 481–485. doi:10.1016/j.ijheh.2012.11.003 PMID:23270838

Trasande, L., Attina, T. M., Sathyanarayana, S., Spanier, A. J., & Blustein, J. (2013b). Race/ethnicity specific associations of urinary phthalates with childhood body mass in a nationally representative sample. *Environmental Health Perspectives*, *121*(4), 501–506. doi:10.1289/ehp.1205526 PMID:23428635

Trasande, L., Spanier, A. J., Sathyanarayana, S., Attina, T. M., & Blustein, J. (2013a). Urinary phthalates and increased insulin resistance in adolescents. *Pediatrics*, *132*(3), e646–e655. doi:10.1542/peds.2012-4022 PMID:23958772

UNEP. (2013). Retrieved from http://www.unep.org/Documents.Multilingual/Default.asp?

Upson, K., Sathyanarayana, S., De Roos, A. J., Thompson, M. L., Scholes, D., Dills, R., & Holt, V. L. (2013). Phthalates and risk of endometriosis. *Environmental Research*, *126*, 91–97. doi:10.1016/j.envres.2013.07.003 PMID:23890968

Uren-Webster, T. M., Lewis, C., Filby, A. L., Paull, G. C., & Santos, E. M. (2010). Mechanisms of toxicity of di (2-ethylhexyl) phthalate on the reproductive health of male zebra fish. *AquaticToxicology*, *99*(3), 360–369. PMID:20561692

US Environmental Protection Agency. (1999). *Introduction to Water Policy Standards*. Washington, DC: Office of Water.

U.S. Environmental Protection Agency. (2003). Framework for Cumulative Risk Assessment. U.S. Environmental Protection Agency, Office of Research and Development, National Center for Environmental Assessment, Washington Office, Washington, DC. EPA/600/P-02/001F.

U.S. Environmental Protection Agency. (2007). Concepts, Methods, and Data Sources for Cumulative Health Risk Assessment of Multiple Chemicals, Exposures and Effects: A Resource Document (Final Report). U.S. Environmental Protection Agency, Washington, DC. EPA/600/R-06/013F.

Wang, H., Zhou, Y., Tang, C., He, Y., Wu, J., Chen, Y., & Jiang, Q. (2013). Urinary phthalate metabolites are associated with body mass index and waist circumference in Chinese schoolchildren. *PLoS One*, *8*(2), e56800. doi:10.1371/journal.pone.0056800 PMID:23437242

Wang, I. J., Karmaus, W. J., Chen, S. L., Holloway, J. W., & Ewart, S. (2015). Effects of phthalate exposure on asthma may be mediated through alterations in DNA methylation. *Clinical Epigenetics*, *7*(1), 1. doi:10.118613148-015-0060-x PMID:25960783

Wang, X., Tao, W., Xu, Y., Feng, J., & Wang, F. (2014). Indoor phthalate concentration and exposure in residential and office buildings in Xi'an, China. *Atmospheric Environment*, *87*, 146–152. doi:10.1016/j.atmosenv.2014.01.018

Wittassek, M., Angerer, J., Kolossa-Gehring, M., Schäfer, S. D., Klockenbusch, W., Dobler, L., ... Wiesmüller, G. A. (2009). Fetal exposure to phthalates–a pilot study. *International Journal of Hygiene and Environmental Health*, *212*(5), 492–498. doi:10.1016/j.ijheh.2009.04.001 PMID:19423389

Wittassek, M., Koch, H. M., Angerer, J., & Brüning, T. (2011). Assessing exposure to phthalates–the human biomonitoring approach. *Molecular Nutrition & Food Research*, *55*(1), 7–31. doi:10.1002/mnfr.201000121 PMID:20564479

Wittassek, M., Wiesmüller, G. A., Koch, H. M., Eckard, R., Dobler, L., Müller, J., ... Schlüter, C. (2007). Internal phthalate exposure over the last two decades–a retrospective humanbiomonitoring study. *International Journal of Hygiene and Environmental Health*, *210*(3), 319–333. doi:10.1016/j.ijheh.2007.01.037 PMID:17400024

Wormuth, M., Scheringer, M., Vollenweider, M., & Hungerbühler, K. (2006). What are the sources of exposure to eight frequently used phthalic acid esters in Europeans? *Risk Analysis*, *26*(3), 803–824. doi:10.1111/j.1539-6924.2006.00770.x PMID:16834635

Wu, S., Zhu, J., Li, Y., Lin, T., Gan, L., Yuan, X., ... Wei, G. (2010). Dynamic effect of di-2-(ethylhexyl) phthalate on testicular toxicity: Epigenetic changes and their impact on geneexpression. *International Journal of Toxicology*, *29*(2), 193–200. doi:10.1177/1091581809355488 PMID:20335514

Xie, Z., Ebinghaus, R., Temme, C., Lohmann, R., Caba, A., & Ruck, W. (2007). Occurrence and air–sea exchange of phthalates in the Arctic. *Environmental Science & Technology*, *41*(13), 4555–4560. doi:10.1021/es0630240 PMID:17695896

Yuan, B. L., Li, X. Z., & Graham, N. (2008). Aqueous oxidation of dimethyl phthalate in a Fe (VI)-TiO2-UV reaction system. *Water Research*, *42*(6-7), 1413–1420. doi:10.1016/j.watres.2007.10.010 PMID:17977571

Zare Jeddi, M., Eshaghi Gorji, M., Rietjens, I., Louisse, J., Bruinen de Bruin, Y., & Liska, R. (2018). Biomonitoring and subsequent risk assessment of combined exposure to phthalates in Iranian children and adolescents. *International Journal of Environmental Research and Public Health*, *15*(11), 2336. doi:10.3390/ijerph15112336 PMID:30360526

Zhang, Y., Meng, X., Chen, L., Li, D., Zhao, L., Zhao, Y., ... Shi, H. (2014). Age and sex-specific relationships between phthalate exposures and obesity in Chinese children at puberty. *PLoS One*, *9*(8), e104852. doi:10.1371/journal.pone.0104852 PMID:25121758

Zhang, Y., Meng, X., Chen, L., Li, D., Zhao, L., Zhao, Y., ... Shi, H. (2014). Age and sex-specific relationships between phthalate exposures and obesity in Chinese children at puberty. *PLoS One*, *9*(8), e104852. doi:10.1371/journal.pone.0104852 PMID:25121758

Zota, A. R., Phillips, C. A., & Mitro, S. D. (2016). *Recent Fast Food Consumption and Bisphenol A andPhthalates Exposures among the US Population in NHANES, 2003–2010*. Environmental Health-Perspective.

ADDITIONAL READING

Desvergne, B., Feige, J. N., & Casals-Casas, C. (2009). PPAR-mediated activity of phthalates: A link to the obesity epidemic? *Molecular and Cellular Endocrinology*, *304*(1), 43–48. doi:10.1016/j.mce.2009.02.017 PMID:19433246

Swan, S. H. (2008). Environmental phthalate exposure in relation to reproductive outcomes and other health endpoints in humans. *Environmental Research*, *108*(2), 177–184. doi:10.1016/j.envres.2008.08.007 PMID:18949837

Wang, I. J., Karmaus, W. J., Chen, S. L., Holloway, J. W., & Ewart, S. (2015). Effects of phthalate exposure on asthma may be mediated through alterations in DNA methylation. *Clinical Epigenetics*, *7*(1), 1. doi:10.118613148-015-0060-x PMID:25960783

Wu, S., Zhu, J., Li, Y., Lin, T., Gan, L., Yuan, X., ... Wei, G. (2010). Dynamic effect of di-2-(ethylhexyl) phthalate on testicular toxicity: Epigenetic changes and their impact on gene expression. *International Journal of Toxicology*, *29*(2), 193–200. doi:10.1177/1091581809355488 PMID:20335514

Zhang, Y., Meng, X., Chen, L., Li, D., Zhao, L., Zhao, Y., ... Shi, H. (2014). Age and sex-specific relationships between phthalate exposures and obesity in Chinese children at puberty. *PLoS One*, *9*(8), e104852. doi:10.1371/journal.pone.0104852 PMID:25121758

KEY TERMS AND DEFINITIONS

Allergy: A damaging immune response by a body to a substance, especially a particular food, pollen, fur, or dust, to which it has become hypersensitive.

Asthma: A respiratory condition marked by attacks of spasm in the bronchi of the lungs, causing difficulty in breathing.

Anthropogenic: Changes in nature originating by human activity.

Bioaccumulation: The accumulation of toxic substances in various tissue or organ of the living organism.

Biomonitoring: It is the measurement of the body burden of toxic chemical compounds, elements, or their metabolites.

Cancer: Group of diseases involving abnormal cell growth with the potential to invade or spread to other parts of the body.

Endocrine Disruptors: Chemicals that interfere with endocrine (or hormone) systems at certain doses.

Epidemiology: The branch of medicine that deals with the incidence, distribution, and possible control of disease and other factors relating to health.

Genotoxicity: It describes the property of chemical agents that damages the genetic information within a cell causing mutations, which may lead to cancer.

Obesity: The state of being grossly fat or overweight.

Phthalates: Esters of phthalic acid mainly used as plasticizers.

Plastic: A synthetic material made from wide range of organic polymers such as polyethylene, PVC, nylon, etc., that can be molded into shape while soft, and then set into a rigid or slightly elastic form.

Plasticizer: Substances added to plastic to increase their flexibility, longevity, durability, and transparency.

Toxicity: It is a degree to which a chemical substance or a particular mixture of substances can damage an organism.

Chapter 18
Polyhydroxyalkanoates:
An Indispensable Alternative

Javid A. Malik
Guru Ghasidas University, India

Monika Bhadauria
Guru Ghasidas University, India

ABSTRACT

Human dependence on number of chemicals or chemical derivatives has increased alarmingly. Among the commodity chemicals, plastics are becoming independent for our modern lifestyle, as the usage of plastics is increasing worryingly. However, these synthetic plastics are extremely persistent in nature and accumulate in the environment, thereby leading to serious ecological problems. So, to build our economy sustainably, a need of replacement is necessary. Biomaterials in terms of bioplastics are an anticipated option, being synthesized and catabolized by different organisms with myriad biotechnological applications. Polyhydroxyalkanoates (PHAs) are among such biodegradable bioplastics, which are considered as an effective alternative for conventional plastics due to their similar mechanical properties of plastics. A range of microbes under different nutrient and environmental conditions produce PHAs significantly with the help of enzymes. PHA synthases encoded by phaC genes are the key enzymes that polymerize PHA monomers. Four major classes of PHA synthases can be distinguished based on their primary structures, as well as the number of subunits and substrate specificity. PHAs can also be produced from renewable feedstock under, unlike the petrochemically derived plastics that are produced by fractional distillation of depleting fossil fuels. Polyhydroxybutyrate (PHB) is the simplest yet best known polyester of PHAs, as the PHB derived bioplastics are heat tolerant, thus used to make heat tolerant and clear packaging film. They have several medical applications such as drug delivery, suture, scaffold and heart valves, tissue engineering, targeted drug delivery, and agricultural fields. Genetic modification (GM) may be necessary to achieve adequate yields. The selections of suitable bacterial strains, inexpensive carbon sources, efficient fermentation, and recovery processes are also some aspects important aspects taken into consideration for the commercialization of PHA. PHA producers have been reported to reside at various ecological niches with few among them also produce some byproducts like extracellular polymeric substances, rhamnolipids and biohydrogen gas. So, the metabolic engineering thereafter promises to bring a feasible solution for the production of "green plastic" in order to preserve petroleum reserves and diminish the escalating human and animal health concerns environmental implications.

DOI: 10.4018/978-1-5225-9452-9.ch018

INTRODUCTION

In the today's world it is generally unquestionable that alternatives for innumerable fossil-resource based products such as plastics are needed in our society. Plastics, a group of non-natural polymeric materials, are presently produced at growing quantities, currently exceeding 300 Mt per year. Especially in strongly emerging economies, such as in China, India, Brazil and many other countries, plastic production and consumption is increasing almost exponentially. Plastics find their in almost every aspect as human beings have relied upon them mostly. Plastics are very much advantageous as their structure can be chemically manipulated to have a wide range of strengths and shapes. Plastics can be easily moulded into almost any desired shape including fibres and thin films. Their molecular weights range from 50,000 to 1,000,000Da (Madison and Huisman, 1999). The synthetic polyethylene, polystyrene and polyvinyl chloride are mostly used in the plastics manufacture. They are popular as disposal goods and as packaging materials, owing to their high chemical resistance and more or less elastic nature. Other molecular components can be incorporated into these structures, resulting in inorganic polymers thus dictating altered properties and creating a seemingly limitless variety of useful end-products. Not surprisingly, petroleum-derived plastics are ubiquitous in the modern world globally; plastic production in 2011 reached 280 million tons (Plastics Europe, 2013)

They are one of the greatest inventions and have been developed into an indispensable commodity for mankind. Petroleum use trends suggest that plastic is not only a huge industry nationally and globally, but also an integral part of modern society (U.S. Department of Energy, 2013).In 2006, petroleum-based products were responsible for 390 million tons of CO_2 emissions (Snell & Peoples, 2009). Furthermore, 1.8 tons of oil create one ton of plastic and 1.9 tons of CO_2 (Snell & Peoples, 2009). Activities related to extracting petroleum directly disrupts many natural habitats; this loss of habitat cascades to affect humans and animals via loss of biodiversity, spread of pathogens, and changing climate that will most noticeably affect food production (Butt *et al.*, 2013). These concerns are not simply restricted to the changing environment.

The difficulty posing in disposal of plastics is what makes them undesirable. Plastics being xenobiotic are recalcitrant to microbial degradation (Flechter, 1993). In the recent years, there has been increasing public concern over the harmful effects of petrochemical-derived plastic materials in the environment. This has prompted many countries to start developing biodegradable plastic. According to an estimate, more than 100 million tonnes of plastics are produced every year. Forty percent of the 75 billion pounds of plastics produced every year is discarded into landfills. Several hundred thousand tonnes of plastics are discarded into marine environments every year and accumulate in oceanic regions. Incineration has been one of the options in dealing with non-degradable plastics, but besides being expensive it is also dangerous. Emission of some harmful chemicals like hydrogen chloride and hydrogen cyanide during incineration occurs (Johnstone, 1990). Recycling also poses difficulties as in sorting the wide variety of plastics and there are also changes in the plastic material due to which its further application range is limited (Johnstone, 1990; Flechter, 1993). Subsequent to the above mentioned limitations, replacement of non-biodegradable by degradable plastics is of major interest both to decision-makers and the plastic industry (Song et al., 1999).

As the natural environment is continuously polluted by these hazardous plastics, the development and production of environmental-conserved biodegradable plastics are rapidly expanding in order to trim down our reliance on synthetic plastics

SOLUTION FOR PLASTICS

Human beings have relied largely on chemicals derived from fossil carbon. Due to the unsustainable nature of petroleum and coal, it is essential to develop better alternatives to produce chemicals from renewable sources. The implementation of biological processing in industrial scale may help to reduce the undesirable damage to the environment caused by the massive scale productions from the current fossil fuel based chemical industry.

The difficulty posing in disposal of plastics is what makes them undesirable. Plastics being xenobiotic are recalcitrant to microbial degradation (Flechter, 1993). In the recent years, there has been increasing public concern over the harmful effects of petrochemical-derived plastic materials in the environment. This has prompted many countries to start developing biodegradable plastic. According to an estimate, more than 100 million tonnes of plastics are produced every year. Forty percent of the 75 billion pounds of plastics produced every year is discarded into landfills. Several hundred thousand tonnes of plastics are discarded into marine environments every year and accumulate in oceanic regions.

To overcome the detrimental effects of the "Plastic Age" in which we live today, it will be essential to finally switch from these petrol-based plastics to bio-inspired alternatives. Most especially, these alternatives are expected to be based on renewable carbon feed stocks, which after their expiry shall undergo biodegradation and composting. Due to the concerns over the climate change, limitation of the fossil carbon source and environmental mitigation, there are renewed interests in bioplastics. There are mainly three types of bioplastics in the commercial scale of production.

1. Plastics derived from fossil carbon source but biodegradable, and.
2. Plastics derived from polymers converted from biomass and biodegradable, and
3. Plastics derived from polymers converted from biomass but not biodegradable.

BIOPLASTICS

A much attention on the renewable bioproduct industry is focused specifically on fuel alternatives. This is obvious as the diminishing fossil fuels supply nearly 80% of the global energy demands, and the current demand will increase by 56% by 2040 (U.S. Energy Information Administration, 2013).

Biopolymers or organic plastics are a form of plastics derived from renewable biomass sources such as vegetable oil, starch, proteins etc, unlike fossil fuel plastics which are derived from petroleum. Biopolymers play an important role in sustainable development by providing the dual advantages of conservation of fossil resources and reduction in CO_2 emissions. The possible sources range from different types biomass including proteins, lipids and polysaccharides (e.g. starch and cellulose based biopolymers). (Figure1)Others include bio-based polymers obtained from bio-derived monomers, e.g. from corn. This is the case for biopolyesters such as polylactic acid (PLA), until recently the most widely available biopolymer on the market. In contrast, polyhydroxyalkanoates (PHAs) are biogenic polyesters that can be naturally accumulated in microbial cultures.

Since the idea of biodegradable, bio-based compounds was identified years ago, the science of biodegradable plastics is relatively new (Lemoigne, 1926). Rather than petroleum sources, biopolymers are typically derived from plant and/or microorganisms. Upon degradation, the biopolymers evolve in oxygen, CO_2, and organic matter, with the released energy harnessed by the microorganisms by which

Figure 1. Different classes of polymers which are biobased and biodegradable

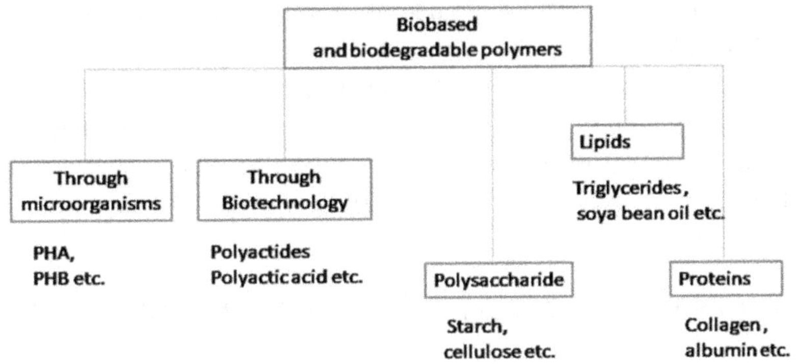

they were degraded. Thus biodegradation process differs from degradation. A complete biodegradation includes some key requirements:

- The material upon degradation must release CO_2, water, and biomass as products through microbial assimilation.
- Another key requirement is the percentage of carbon converted to CO_2. In this regard, a homopolymer, upon biodegradation releases CO_2 equal to 60% of the carbon within the product; while as for blends such as heteropolymers and copolymers, requirements are stricter, as this conversion must reach 90% (Biodegradable Products Institute, 2012).
- This conversion must occur in less than 180 days at the same rate as natural materials, and within 365 days for a radiolabeled polymer (Narayan, 2006).

Furthermore, this must occur in all soil, marine/ocean, compost, aerobic or anaerobic environments, and leave no fragments or residue (Snell & Peoples, 2009; BASF, 2010).

The United States Environmental Protection Agency (EPA) defines the term "biodegrade" as "[to] decompose into more elementary compounds by the action of living organisms, especially microbes such as bacteria" (2010). It is also important to distinguish biodegradable and compostable. The compostable products are made-up of compounds that break down over a very short period (typically, 8 weeks) and the degradation rate matches that of paper (BASF, 2010). Bioplastics are a preferred alternative to petroleum plastics in the context of sustainable plastic products. Yet, it is crucial to understand both pros and cons of bioplastics before an intentional shift in their favour can begin.

There are some concerns with bioplastics. The first and foremost is the influence on the degree to which a material is considered biodegradable. For instance, the degree to which the plastic in the final product is crystallized will affect its biodegradation. The degree of biodegradability will decrease with increasing crystallinity (molecular order) of the plastic structure (Tokiwa *et al.*, 2009). Biodegradation also depends on the surface area, as reduced surface area will also restrict the ability of a microbe to access the entire quantity of the biodegradable plastic (Tokiwa *et al.*, 2009). Furthermore, environmental temperature, pH, moisture, oxygen, nutrient content, and composition also influence the overall process.

Like petroleum-based products, there are also several variations of biodegradable plastics available. The variations are characterized by their method of biodegradation which results from their molecular composition (Reddy *et al.* 2003). One type includes ultraviolet light-sensitive groups developed as a photodegradable compound where the degradation process is initiated by sunlight to transform waste into a structure more acquiescent to microbial degradation. Another type is semi-biodegradable which are blends of starch-petroleum plastics, with the starch component intended to be targeted by soil microbes. However it results in undegraded residual petroleum particles being released by those organisms. An attractive option, specifically with regards to a landfill, is a naturally-occurring fermentation product that can be targeted in its entirety (rather than only the connecting bits) by a microbe. Such compounds are aliphatic polyesters, polysaccharides, polylactides and polyhydroxyalkanoates.

CONVERTING POLYETHYLENE TO POLYHYDROXYALKANOATES

Polyethylene is a non-degradable polymer and thus to convert it to a biodegradable polymer. Pyrolysis or thermal treatment of polyethylene to produce saturated and unsaturated hydrocarbons is the first step in the conversion process. The thermal treatment of polyethylene in the absence of air (pyrolysis) generated a complex mixture of low molecular weight paraffins with carbon chain lengths from C8 to C32 (polyethylene pyrolysis wax). These resultant smaller molecules then act as substrates for microbial fermentation. Several bacterial strains were able to grow and produce PHA from this PE pyrolysis wax. The addition of biosurfactant allowed for enhanced bacterial growth and PHA accumulation of the tested strains. Even some strains were only capable of growth and PHA accumulation in the presence of the biosurfactant. The carbon in the polyethylene pyrolysis products can be utilised to build a new carbon polymer by the microorganisms inside their cells. The resulting polymer made by the microorganisms is a biodegradable polymer. PHB is one of those polymers which has generally a much higher molecular weight than medium-chain-length PHA and is thus a stronger polymer as the molecular weight bestows greater strength to the polymer.

A vast number of industry patent applications relating to PHA production and applications are prevailing, witnessing that an ample number of chemical and biotechnology industries are keenly aware of the potential of PHA. The first identified PHA i.e., PHB (Lemoigne, 1926), has received the great attention in terms of industrial scale production. PHAs are majority commodity plastic used for bottles, surface coatings and in medicine. A specific subset of PHAs can be used as elastomers, pressure-sensitive adhesives and plastic coatings (Reddy et al., 2003).

POLYHYDROXYALKANOATES

Polyhydroxyalkanoate (PHA) is an ideal biodegradable biopolymer. Presence of a derivative of PHA was first reported in the bacterium *Bacillus megaterium* (Lemoigne, 1926) which received little attention until several decades then (Williamson & Wilkinson, 1958). Later studies have found that bacteria could naturally degrade PHA; thus, the particular biopolymer was identified early as an ideal alternative source of bioplastic (Chowdhury, 1963). PHA possesses specific qualities as such they are naturally synthesized, easy to recover, and produced from low-cost feedstocks. PHA is a naturally occurring versatile, lipid-like water-insoluble molecule that has been found in more than 75 genera of prokaryotes and archaea (Reddy, 2003; Rehm, 2003; Huang & Reusch, 1996). PHA acts as an intracellular, granular energy storage reserve inside the living cell; its synthesis and accumulation is elicited by unfavourable growth conditions by PHA synthases.

This polyester consists of 103-104 monomer subunits arranged linearly and alkyl groups are found in the R-position of the C-3 carbon and range from 1-14 carbons in length (Rehm, 2003). Its candidature as a petroleum substitute attributes to its physical and chemical similarities, but in contrast to the petroleum hydrocarbon subunit PHA is derived from an ester group

Poly-3-hydroxybutyrate (PHB) discovered first in bacteria by Lemoigne in 1925, is a homo polymer of 3-hydroxybutyrate and is the most widespread and best characterized member of the polyhydroxy-alkanoate family. Microbial biosynthesis of PHB starts with the condensation of two molecules of acetyl-CoA to give acetoacetyl-CoA, which is subsequently reduced to hydroxybutyryl-CoA. This latter compound is then used as a monomer to polymerize PHB. Biologically produced, polyhydroxybutyrate (PHB) is a semicrystalline isotactic stereo regular polymer with 100% R configuration that allows a high level of degradability (Noda et al., 1999). Other members of family are Polyhydroxy-Valerate (PHV) and PHBV.It is accumulated in intracellular granules by a wide variety of Gram-positive and Gram-negative organisms under conditions of a nutrient limitation other than the carbon source (Dawes and Senior, 1973). The inclusion of 3-hydroxyvalerate (HV) units in PHB, results in the production of the copolymer poly(3-hydroxybutyrate-co-3-hydroxyvalerate), or else PHBV. PHBV is that kind of material that becomes tougher, more flexible, and broader to thermal processing when its molar fraction in the copolymer increases. Poly-3-hydroxybutyrate (PHB) discovered first in bacteria by Lemoigne in 1925, is a homo polymer of 3-hydroxybutyrate and is the most widespread and best characterized member of the polyhydroxy-alkanoate family. Polyhydroxyalkanoate polymers can be processed to make a variety of useful products, owing to their biodegradability and naturalness which prove quite beneficial, in particular for applications in packaging and agriculture.

After the presence of PHA is confirmed, it needs to be obtained from the organism. For that several extraction processes are used for obtaining PHA from the source. One method involves the use a solvent to extract the lipophilic PHA from the cells. Other options include solvent extraction, chemical or enzymatic treatment followed by filtration and centrifugation to collect the PHA. Most protocols are modified versions on the same basic principles (Kunasundari & Sudesh, 2011).

Now about naturally-occurring PHA, it is synthesized in selected bacteria. However unfortunately, these species have longer generation times, relatively lower growth temperatures, contain endogenous PHA-degradation pathways, and can be challenging to lyse for the purposes of extraction of compounds of interest (Reddy, 2003). This idea has prompted research in the genetics underlying PHA biosynthesis.

Genetic requirements in addition to exploiting the *phaABC* operon may be necessary in order to achieve industrial scale production of PHA, if it is to be a feasible alternative to petroleum. Genetic modifications have been attempted in altering traits in some PHA-producing plants. For example, increasing drought tolerance and biomass yield would alleviate its consumption. It maximizes the actual PHA compound of interest in the land area available. Also it could be augmented for production on a low-quality soil which typically remains absent of food or biomass crop altogether. Enhanced enzymatic activity to improve cellulose hydrolysis, have ALSO been proved beneficial (Sticklen, 2008).

PHA quantity and localization differs amongst organelles. Peroxisomes, plastids, cytosol, and mitochondria possess significant levels. However, plastid to naturally contain highest levels (van Veilen and Poirier, 2008) probably due to high acetyl-CoA and carbon content. Genetic modifications can be applied to include plastid-targeting signal into *phaABC* operon, with the purpose of upregulating their activity for most efficient accumulation of PHA (Somleva *et al.*, 2008). (McLaughlin & Kszos, 2005

Figure 2. Chemical structure of some polyhydroxyalkanoates

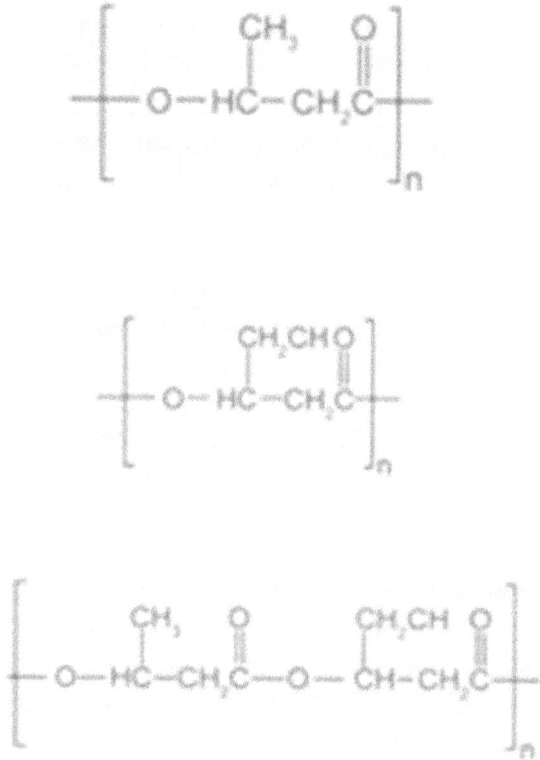

revealed that using *Agrobacterium tumefaciens,* transgenic *Panicum virgatum* 30% increase in yields than the parent plants. Biotechnological research and strain engineering has enabled the production of PHAs from cheap substrates. Continuous improvements of PHA contents within the cells and growth rates are reported on a regular basis.

PRODUCTION OF POLYHYDROXYALKANOATES

There are several ways by which PHA can be obtained and utilized. As industrial production of PHA would require a two-step process: accumulation of PHA and then followed by its extraction (Snell and Peoples, 2009). PHA is naturally occurring in over 300 bacteria as microbial aerobic fermentation product. Some other studies have shown high accumulations of PHA in organisms in symbiotic associations like in *Rhizobia spp.* (Suriyamongkol *et al.*, 2007). Suriyamongkol *et al* have also shown *Ralstonia eutropha* to contain as much as 90% dry weight of the cell as PHA (2007). Genetic modification lead increased PHA accumulation in some microorganisms; Examples include *Brassica napus* once the 12-hydroxylase promoter activity is upregulated, *Panicum virgatum* after increasing their resiliency and *Arabidopsis* which has produced the highest PHA yield of any plants designed for PHA accumulation (NewsRX, 2013; Houmiel *et al.*, 1999; Somleva*et al.*, 2008).

Numerous genes encoding enzymes involved in PHA formation and degradation have been cloned and characterized from a variety of microorganisms. Genetic studies have conferred insights into the regulation of PHA formation with respect to the growth conditions. Such studies have made clear the microbial physiology and do provide a powerful tool for designing and engineering recombinant organisms for PHA production.

The biosynthetic pathway of P(3HB) consists of three enzymatic reactions catalyzed by three different enzymes. The first reaction involves b-ketoacylCoA thiolase (encoded by phbA) and brings out the condensation of two acetyl coenzyme A (acetyl-CoA) molecules into acetoacetyl-CoA. The second reaction is the reduction of acetoacetyl-CoA to (R)-3-hydroxybutyryl-CoA by an NADPH-dependent acetoacetyl-CoA dehydrogenase (encoded by phbB). And finally in the third step, the (R)-3-hydroxybutyryl CoA monomers are polymerized into PHB by P(3HB) polymerase, encoded by phbC (Huisman et al., 1989).

Currently, economic threats hamper the broad market penetration of PHAs: production of these materials is still significantly more expensive if compared to the well-established, large-scale manufacturing of petrol-based plastics. In particular, the allocation of feed stocks needed for PHA production drastically contributes to the still high production price of these biopolyesters. So, to make PHAs competitive, they must compete with traditional plastics both in terms of material performance and in economic aspects. Quality improvement aspect of PHA-based materials is currently achieved by the selection of the microbial production strain, during the bioprocess. Further, PHAs can be processed to design products of tailored properties by blending PHAs with other biological or artificial polymeric materials, or by post-synthetic modification. Such composites and blends often constitute smart materials with tunable characteristics such as density, gas barrier properties, or degradability.

PHA Production by Recombinant Bacteria

Natural PHA-producing bacteria have a long generation time and relatively low optimal growth temperature and these are often hard to lyse. E. Bacteria like *E. Coli.* are incapable of synthesizing or degrading PHA; however it grows fast, even at high temperature and is easy to lyse. The fast growth will enable it to accumulate a large amount of polymer and the easy lysis of the cells saves the cost of the purification of the PHA granules (Wang and Bakken, 1998; Madison and Huisman, 1999). Recombinant gene technology is being intensely explored to introduce new metabolic pathways to broaden the utilizable substrate range and to enhance PHA synthesis. Some studies developed recombinant E. coli strains with the *Alcaligeneseutrophus* PHA biosynthesis genes in a stable high-copy-number plasmid and used for high PHA productivity (Zhang et al., 1994; Lee et al., 1994).

Biotechnological Production of Polyhydroxyalkanoates

The long-term impact of PHA bioplastic is attractive. No harmful effects were observed in mammals after PHA ingestion. (Forni *et al.*, 1999a; Forni *et al.*, 1999b). In microorganisms, neither the polymer nor its lytic intermediates are toxic. As Suriyamongkol *et al.* indicate, PHA depolymerase, an enzyme endogenous to many microorganisms, degrades the molecule into 3-hydroxyacid (2007). This has no effect on animals, as their systems naturally contain this molecule and thus have mechanisms for its metabolism.

There GM introduced to the host tends to render poor quality, unproductive land useable. Or it can provide an option to producer for a crop rotation while growing on a fertile land and potentially contribute agronomically in this sense. These ideas have been examined previously, and encouraging evidence exists (Huang *et al.*, 2002).

One of the most challenging aspects of implementing a biorefinery capable of PHA production is achieving an effective and appropriate infrastructure with viable economics (Wellisch *et al.* 2010). The raw products, regardless of efficiency, have no purpose without proper facilities that can utilize the materials (Wellisch *et al.,* 2010; Narayan, 2006). At present there is a huge insufficiency of these facilities, even though multiple biodegradable products are available. The infrastructure challenge has been encountered and overcome by the biofuel sector and thus could serve better for the bioplastics industry (Hannon *et al.*, 2010). Accordingly a biorefinery should be built next to existing power plants to facilitate cogeneration of various energy sources and bioproducts while approaching a complete sustainability. The cooperation of people across different sectors is critical and emphasises a crucial need for starting a completely new infrastructure, as the current landfills are so contaminated with petroleum plastic, rendering their full recovery impossible (Shivley 2006).

In spite of these challenges, several bio-based and biodegradable plastics have reached industry scale and are available to consumers. ecoflex® and ecovio® are two biodegradable plastics introduced by BASF; one is totally petroleum based, and one is a combination of petroleum and plant starch-derived (BASF, 2010).Other encouraging steps include substantial investments in Canadian bioplastic technology licensing, increased partnerships in North American bioplastic start-ups, Nestle's sugar cane-derived polyethylene packaging and growth in Europe's bioplastic packaging industry.

Metabolix®, a European-based bioscience engineering company, has successfully launched a bio-based PHA production program (Metabolix, 2013). The objectives of this platform are to optimize multi-gene expression techniques to maximize the PHB content of switch grass, camelina (high oil yields) and sugarcane (high biomass yields) (Metabolix, 2013). Another aspect related to bioplastics is simply in language which is too often overlooked. A uniform, universal set of definitions is needed to distinct between "bioplastic" (bi bopolymer), "bio-based," and "biodegradable." Different sources may assume different definitions for the various terms, however some international not-for-profit organizations exist in an effort to maintain plastic biodegradable or compostable standards conveyed by specific logos (Biodegradable Products Institute, 2012; Bureau de normalization du Québec, 2014; ASTM International, 2003).

The Definition may change under certain circumstances. For example, the degree to which bio-based acetyl cellulose is acetylated determines its susceptibility to degradation (Tokiwa *et al.*, 2009). Lastly, the conditions whose availability or non-availability to degrade the waste will determine its utility as a bio degradable compound. Before the infrastructure is established, it is beneficial to find the most ideal bio-based, biodegradable compound which must begin at the molecular level

GENETIC BASIS OF PHA FORMATION

The operon phbCAB consists of three clustered PHB biosynthetic genes phbA (for 3-ketothiolase), phbB (NADPH-dependent acetoacetyl CoAreductase), and phbC (PHB synthase) from acetyl-CoA. There is a possibility of functional constraints against co-expression of genes to be so weak that the organization of gene clusters in operon structures can be readily varied during the course of time.

Evolutionary force may have worked on the pha genes since in the first PHA produces, the PHA formation was most probably only a minor metabolic pathway, and the purpose of the pathway was different rather than synthesis of storage material (Haywood et al., 1990). However as the PHA formation became beneficial for the microbe, evolution selected PHA

BIODEGRADABILITY OF PHA

The property that distinguishes PHA from petroleum based plastics is their biodegradability. PHAs are degraded upon exposure to soil, compost, or marine sediment. Biodegradation process is dependent on various factors such as microbial activity of the environment, and the exposed surface area, moisture, temperature, pH, molecular weight (Boopathy, 2000). The nature of the monomer units also has been found to affect degradation. Microorganisms secrete enzymes that break down the polymer into its molecular building blocks, called hydroxyacids, which are utilized as a carbon source for growth. The principal enzyme for the degradation of PHB and oligomers derived from the polymer is PHB depolymerase.

PHAs are degraded upon exposure to soil, compost, or marine sediment. PHB can be biodegraded in both aerobic and anaerobic environments, without any toxic product formation (Tokiwa et al, 2009). Biodegradation depends various factors such as microbial activity, temperature, moisture, pH of the environment, and the exposed surface area, molecular weight polymer composition, nature of monomer unit and crystallinity (Boopathy, 2000).

Biodegradation of PHA under aerobic conditions results in carbon dioxide and water, whereas in anaerobic conditions the degradation products are carbon dioxide and methane. PHA are compostable over a wide range of temperatures, even at a maximum of around 60°C with moisture levels at 55%. Studies have shown that 85% of PHA were degraded in seven weeks (Flechter, 1993; Johnstone, 1990). PHA have been reported to degrade in aquatic environments (Lake Lugano, Switzerland) within 254 days even at temperatures not exceeding 6°C (Johnstone, 1990).Polhydroxyalkanotes like PHB, polypropiolactone (PPL) and PCL degraders are widely distributed in different environments (Nishida and Tokiwa, 1993; Mergaert and Swings, 1996; Suyama et al, 1998). Majority of the strains that degrade PHB belong to different taxa such as Gram negative and Gram-positive bacteria, Streptomyces and fungi (Mergaert and Swings, 1996)

PHB degrading microorganisms from Bacillus, Pseudomonas and Streptomyces species were reported for the first time by Chowdhury (Chowdhury, 1963). Since then, various PHB-degrading microrganisms have been isolated from soil (*Pseudomonas lemoigne*, *Acidovorax facealis*, *Comamonas* sp, *Aspergillus fumigates* and *Variovorax paradoxus*), activated and anaerobic sludge (*Alcaligenes faecalis*, *Illyobacter delafieldi*, *Pseudomonas*), seawater and lake water (*Comamonas testosterone*, *Pseudomonas stutzeri*) [Lee, 1996].

Microorganisms break down the polymer into its molecular building blocks, utilized as a carbon source for growth, by secreting enzymes hydroxyacids. The principal enzyme for the degradation of PHB and oligomers derived from the polymer is PHB depolymerase.

PHA has been found to be degraded by many different genera and species of bacteria and fungi, both aerobically and anaerobically (Tokiwa *et al.*, 2009). *Acidovorax faecalis, Variovorax paradoxus and Pseudomonas lemoigne* and are some of the microbes from the soil while as *Pseudomonas stutzeri is an example from aquatic* from sources, (Tokiwa *et al.*, 2009) and *Alcaligenes faecalis and Pseudomonas sp. are* from anaerobic sludge. For biodegradation, first, a degradative enzyme produced by one of these microbes must bind to the bioplastic, breaking the polymer to lower weight oligomers, dimers, monomers, and is eventually got mineralized (Tokiwa *et al.*, 2009).Composting at high temperature is one of the most promising technologies for recycling biodegradable (Tokiwa et al., 1992). Thus, those microorganisms which are capable of degrading various kinds of polyesters at high temperatures are of interest.

The microbes utilize the minerals and energy, while CO_2 and H_2O are released back -into the environment (Sudesh *et al.*, 2000). The hydrolytic cleavage action and complete degradation process of the PHA depolymerases take only 3-9 months (Suriyamongkol *et al.*, 2007).

Biodegradable plastics can be of three types; photodegradable, semi-biodegradable, and completely biodegradable. Photodegradable plastics are light sensitive so extensive ultraviolet radiation of several weeks to months can disintegrate their polymeric structure rendering them to further bacterial degradation. However, landfills tend to remainnon-degraded as they lack sunlight. Semi-biodegradable plastics are the starch-linked plastics and so once discarded into landfills, soil bacteria attack the starch and release polymer fragments that can be degraded by other bacteria. Bacteria indeed attack the starch but the polyethylene fragments remain non-degradable (Johnstone, 1990). The third type of biodegradable plastics is a rather promising new type because of its actual utilization by bacteria to form a biopolymer. Some of such kinds are polyhydroxyalkanoates (PHA), aliphatic polyesters, polylactides (PLA), polysaccharides, copolymers and/or blends of the above.

PROPERTIES AND PRACTICAL APPLICATIONS OF PHA

The PHAs are biocompatible, non-toxic, biodegradable thermoplastics and can be produced from renewable resources. They have a great degree of polymerization, are highly crystalline, optically active, peizoelectric and insoluble in water. These features make them highly competitive with polypropylene. Owing to their novel features, PHAs have a wide range of applications. Initially, PHAs were used in packaging films mainly in bags, containers and paper coatings. PHAs possess applications as those of conventional commodity plastics include the disposable items, such as razors, utensils, diapers, feminine hygiene products, cosmetic containers— shampoo bottles and cups.

In addition to potential as a plastic material, PHAs can serve as chiral precursors for the chemical synthesis of optically active compounds (Senior and Dawes, 1973; Oeding and Schlegel, 1973). They are also used as osteosynthetic material s in the stimulation of bone growth owing to their piezoelectric properties, in bone plates, surgical sutures and blood vessel replacements. However, the medical and pharmaceutical applications are limited due to the slow biodegradation and high hydraulic stability in sterile tissues (Wang and Bakken, 1998).

The PHAs are considered as a source for the synthesis of chiral compounds and are raw materials for the production of paints. PHA can be easily depolymerised to a rich source of optically active, pure, bi-functional hydroxy acids. Plant derived PHA can be depolymerized and used, directly or following esterification, in the manufacture of bulk chemicals (Brandl et al., 1988).

PHAs can be considered for those advanced applications where they cannot be replaced by petroleum-based polymers. Accordingly, PHAs are suited for any such application that requires biocompatibility and/or biodegradability of the polymer. For medical applications, in particular the homopolymers PHB and PHV have been investigated. These scl-PHAs can be processed by melt processes as they are thermoplasts, or by solution processes due to their solubility in a limited number of organic solvents. Keeping in view the promising research results in recent years, the applicability of PHAs in medical areas is more than plausible in the near future as the need for advanced medical devices for drug delivery, tissue engineering and implants and tissue repairs in their broadest sense.

POLYLACTIDES AND POLYGLYCOLIDES

Some other biodegradable plastics that have gained attention are the PLA and polyglycolides (PGA). PLA and PGA are thermoplastics and biodegradable polyesters, which can be low molecular weight and high molecular weight. Low molecular PLA and PGA are made by direct polymerization of lactide and glycolide while as the high molecular PLA and PGA are made by ring-open polymerization of lactide and glycolide.

The degradation times of PLA and PGA range from a few months to years. Dexon, a polyglycolic acid homopolymer, was the first absorbable suture material developed by the American Cyanamid Corporation. The production of lactic acid-based plastics from starchy food wastes and by products is on the increase (Hocking and Marchessault, 1997).They find their importance in medical application as well. They are used as sutures, ligament replacements and screws in orthopedic repairs. In addition they are used in controlled drug release and for arterial grafts. Production requires two key steps, one converts glucose to lactic acid and the other converts lactic acid to polylactic acid. Large-scale fermentation processes are used to manufacture water-resistant bottles, eating utensils and a few other products from aliphatic polyesters. Triglycerides have become the basis for a new category of robust composites. Infusion of glass fiber, hemp, jute fiber, flax, straw and wood or hay with triglycerides is useful in making long lasting durable materials with applications in agricultural equipment, the automobile industry, building construction, etc.

CONCLUSION

Overall, the literature highlights PHA a very promising polymer for a multiple range of applications. For example, it has better barrier properties and mechanical strength than other more widespread bioplastics such as PLA. Different research studies are continuing regarding the enhancement of the PHA yield which includes genetic modification of the bacteria or the use of waste for their growth.

Further a control of its crystallisation could allow even more flexible grades of PHAs or transparent ones to be obtained. This range of interesting properties makes PHA a suitable candidate in various applications PHA exhibits good barrier properties (Miguel et al., 1997; Chen, 2011), and can be used in the packaging industry as a biodegradable plastic thus contributing to solving environmental pollution problems (Chen, 2011). In medical sciences, the monomer of PHB is a normal metabolic in the human blood as the PHB is compatible with the blood and tissues of mammals. It could be used as a surgical implant in surgery for the healing of wounds and blood vessels. PHAs find their use in pharmacology as well, as PHB can be used as microcapsules in therapy or as materials for cell and tablet packaging. It can also be used for packaging applications for deep drawing articles in the food industry, for example, bottles, fast foods, fishnets, laminated foils, sanitary goods, flowerpots, disposable cups, agricultural foils and fibres in textiles.

However, further improvements are still needed to allow a broader market introduction of PHAs. Furthermore efforts must be undertaken by scientists to reduce the production costs and increase the industrial sustainability and commercialization of PHAs (Bhatt et al., 2011). The use of waste feedstock for the culture of the microorganisms accumulating PHAs is encouraged as a route to lead to their greater economic viability and sustainability

The current advances in metabolic engineering supported by the genome information and bioinformatics have opened a cascade of opportunities to introduce new metabolic pathways. This would help us not only to broaden the utilizable substrate range and produce tailor-made PHA but also enhance the current PHA yields.

The studies should also be aimed to understand the host–plasmid interactions so as to develop stable plasmids, such that the wild-type bacteria are surpassed by recombinant bacteria. Transgenic plants harbouring the microbial PHA biosynthesis genes have been recently developed with the purpose of ultimately reducing the polymer price. However, lot more effort has to be done in this area to increase the production of bioplastics to successfully replace the non-degradable plastics.

FUTURE OUTLOOKS

There are benefits and challenges in any new technology thus subsequently those involved with the industry's commencement must be prepared for these hurdles. For PHA to withstand as a value-added product, it must be produced in a large enough scale to be accepted as a material for targeted markets, be biologically achievable, and have an accurate production scenario, however these scenarios are still mainly theoretical. A proper combination of *in vivo* sites of PHA production, ideal host, and ideal growing location for the host increases the complexity of the situation.

Bacterial cells may pose difficulty due to their resilience in the process of cell lysis preceding PHA extraction. Even enzymatic treatments are complex and expensive, and are not realistic for industrial-scale efficiency requirements at this time (Narayan, 2006). PHA processes are mostly environmentally-dependent due to their occurrence in living organisms. Extraction processes result in a very viscous polymer solution, which can be challenging to transport. Furthermore, solvents necessary for the processes can be dangerous, and they are from non-sustainable sources which contradicts with the overall goal of sustainability of the bioplastic production. Non-natural producers of PHA with the inserted genes required for PHA production may become unstable and deleterious effects may result if PHA levels exceed 8%dwt (Suriyamongkol *et al.*, 2007; Narayan, 2006). To date, PHA production costs are 5 to 10-fold higher than those of petroleum plastics (Suriyamongkol *et al.*, 2007). The prime of all these challenges is the difficulty of public acceptance of another large-scale, non-food GM crop.

However many positive changes would be achieved in shifting to bioplastics. PHA can be obtained from many sources. PHA has no known harmful effects on animals and has a net-neutral effect on carbon cycles while reducing greenhouse gas emissions. PHA can directly substitute petroleum plastics and would enhance the biotechnology industry with negligible disposal costs.

Currently used PHA-producing plant strains require few management practice changes and PHA accumulations have been achieved *in vivo*. About half of the solid waste in landfills is biowaste, and its degradation will increase soil value (Snell & Peoples, 2009). After PHA extraction About 10% dry residual material remains and can be used for energy/fuel sources for the recovery process in the bio-refinery, with excess going into the main power grid. Thus, biorefineries have the potential to reach nearly full sustainability.

REFERENCES

ASTM International. (2003). *Specification for biodegradable plastics used as coatings on paper and other compostable substrates*. doi:10.1520/D6868-03

BASF. (2010). *Introduction to biodegradable plastics*. Retrieved from http://www.bioplastics.basf.com

Bhatt, R., Patel, K., & Trivedi, U. (2011). Biodegradation of poly (3-hydroxyalkanoates). In S. K. Sharma & A. Mudhoo (Eds.), *A handbook of applied bio - polymer technology: Synthesis, degradation and applications* (pp. 311–331). London: The Royal Society of Chemistry Publishing. doi:10.1039/9781849733458-00311

Biodegradable Products Institute. (2012). *ASTM D6400 - Test for Compostability*. Retrieved from http://www.bpiworld.org/Default.aspx?pageId=190422

Boopathy, R. (2000). Factor limiting bioremediation technologies. *Bioresource Technology*, *74*(1), 63–67. doi:10.1016/S0960-8524(99)00144-3

Brandl, H., Gross, R. A., Lenz, R. W., & Fuller, R. C. (1988). Pseudomonas oleovorans as a source of poly(B-hydroxyalkanoates) for potential application as biodegradable polyester. *Applied and Environmental Microbiology*, *54*, 1977–1982. PMID:16347708

Bureau de normalisation du Québec. (2014). *Home page*. Retrieved from http://www.bnq.qc.ca/en/

Butt, N., Beyer, H. L., Bennett, J. R., Biggs, D., Maggini, R., Mills, M., ... Possingham, H. P. (2013). Biodiversity risks from fossil fuel extraction. *Science*, *342*(6157), 425–426. doi:10.1126cience.1237261 PMID:24159031

Canadian Association of Petroleum Producers. (2014). *Glossary*. Retrieved from http://www.capp.ca/library/glossary/Pages/default.aspx#p

Chen, G-Q. (2011). Biofunctionalization of polymers and their applications. *Biofunctionalization of Polymers and their Applications, 125*, 29–45. Doi:10.1007/10_2010_89

Chowdhury, A. A. (1963). Poly-β-hydroxybuttersaure abbauende Bakterien und exo-enzyme. *Archives of Microbiology*, *47*, 167–200. doi:10.1007/BF00422523 PMID:14106079

Dawes, E. A., & Senior, P. J. (1973). The role and regulation of energy reserve polymers in micro-organisms. *Advances in Microbial Physiology*, *10*, 135–266. doi:10.1016/S0065-2911(08)60088-0 PMID:4594739

Flechter, A. (1993). *Plastics from Bacteria and for Bacteria: PHA as Natural, Biodegradable Polyesters*. New York: Springer Verlag.

Forni, D., Wenk, C., & Bee, G. (1999a). Digestive utilization of novel biodegradable plastic in growing pigs. *Annales de Zootechnie, 48*, 163-171. doi:10.1051/animres:19990302

Forni, D., Wenk, C., & Bee, G. (1999b). Novel biodegradable plastics in sheep nutrition 1. Effects of untreated plastics on digestibility and metabolic energy and nitrogen utilization. *Journal of Animal Physiology and Animal Nutrition, 81*(1), 31–40. doi:10.1046/j.1439-0396.1999.811189.x

Hannon, M., Gimpel, J., Tran, M., Rasala, B., & Mayfield, S. (2010). Biofuels from algae: Challenges and potential. *Biofuels, 1*(5), 763–784. doi:10.4155/bfs.10.44 PMID:21833344

Haywood, G. W., Anderson, A. J., Ewing, D. F., & Dawes, E. A. (1990). Accumulation of a polyhydroxyalkanoates containing primarily 3- hydroxydecanoate from simple carbohydrate substrates by Pseudomonas sp. stain. *Applied and Environmental Microbiology, 56*, 3354–3359. PMID:16348341

Hocking, P. J., & Marchessault, R. H. (1997). Article. In G. J. L. Griffin (Ed.), Chemistry and Technology of Biodegradable Polymers (pp. 48–96). Chapman & Hall.

Houmiel, K. L., Slater, S., Broyles, D., Casagrande, L., Colburn, S., Gonzalez, K., ... Gruys, K. J. (1999). Poly(*β*-hydroxybutyrate) production in oilseed leukoplasts of *Brassica napus. Planta, 4*(209), 547–550. doi:10.1007004250050760 PMID:10550638

Huang, J., Pray, C., & Rozelle, S. (2002). Enhancing the crops to feed the poor. *Nature, 418*(6898), 678–685. doi:10.1038/nature01015 PMID:12167874

Huang, R., & Reusch, R. N. (1996). Poly(3-hydroxybutyrate) is associated with specific proteins in the cytoplasm and membranes of *Escherichia coli. The Journal of Biological Chemistry, 271*(36), 22196–22202. doi:10.1074/jbc.271.36.22196 PMID:8703033

Huisman, G. W., Leeuwde, O., Eggink, G., & Witholt, B. (1989). Synthesis of poly-3-hydroxyalkanoates is a common feature of fluorescent pseudomonads. *Applied and Environmental Microbiology, 55*, 1949–1954. PMID:2506811

Johnstone, B. (1990). A throw away answer. *Far Eastern Economic Review, 147*(6), 62–63.

Kunasundari, B., & Sudesh, K. (2011). Isolation and recovery of microbial polyhydroxyalkanoates. *Express Polymer Letters, 5*(7), 620–634. doi:10.3144/expresspolymlett.2011.60

Lee, S. Y., Yim, K. S., Chang, H. N., & Chang, Y. K. (1994). Construction of plasmids, estimation of plasmid stability and use of stable plasmids for the production of poly(3-hydroxybutyric) acid by recombinant Escherichia coli. *Journal of Biotechnology, 32*(2), 203–211. doi:10.1016/0168-1656(94)90183-X PMID:7764567

Lemoigne, M. (1926). Produits de dehydration et de polymerisation de l'acide *β*-oxobutyrique. *Bulletin de la Société de Chimie Biologique, 8*, 770–782.

Madison, L. L., & Huisman, G. W. (1999). Metabolic engineering of poly (3-hydroxyalkanoates): From DNA to plastic. *Microbiology and Molecular Biology Reviews, 63*(1), 21–53. PMID:10066830

McLaughlin, S. B., & Kszos, L. A. (2005). Development of switchgrass (*Panicum virgatum*) as a bioenergy feedstock in the United States. *Biomass and Bioenergy*, *28*(6), 515–535. doi:10.1016/j.biombioe.2004.05.006

Metabolix. (2013a). *Why integrate biopolymers into your conversion process?* Retrieved from http://www.metabolix.com/converters

Metabolix. (2013b). *Crop-based technologies.* Retrieved from http://www.metabolix.com/Products/Crop-based-Technologies

Miguel, O., Fernandez-Berridi, M. J., & Iruin, J. J. (1997). Survey on transport properties of liquids, vapors, and gases in biodegradable poly(3-hydroxybutyrate) (PHB). *Journal of Applied Polymer Science*, *64*, 1849–1859. DOI: <1849 doi:10.1002/(sici)1097-4628(19970531)64:9

Narayan, R. (2006). Biobased and biodegradable polymer materials: Rationale, drivers, and technology exemplars. In K. Khemani & C. Scholz (Eds.), *Degradable polymers and materials: Principles and practice* (pp. 282–306). Washington, DC: American Chemical Society. doi:10.1021/bk-2006-0939.ch018

News, R. X. (2013, March 5). "Chemically inducible expression of biosynthetic pathways" in patent application approval process. *Life Science Weekly*. Retrieved from http://www.highbeam.com/doc/1G1-323547527.html

Noda, I., Marchessault, R. H., & Terada, M. (1999). *Polymer data handbook*. London: Oxford University Press.

Oeding, V., & Schlegel, H. G. (1973). Beta-ketothiolase from Hydrogenomonas eutropha HI6 and its significance in the regulation of polybeta- hydroxybutyrate metabolism. *The Biochemical Journal*, *134*(1), 239–248. doi:10.1042/bj1340239 PMID:4198758

PlasticsEurope. (2013a). *How plastic is made*. Retrieved from http://www.plasticseurope.org/what-is-plastic/how-plastic-is-made.aspx

PlasticsEurope. (2013b). *First estimates suggest around 4% increase in plastics global production from 2010*. Retrieved from http://www.plasticseurope.org/information-centre/press-room-1351/press-releases-2012/first-estimates-suggest-around-4-increase-in-plastics-global-production-from-2010.aspx

Reddy, C. S. K. (1594). Evolution, site-specific mutagenesis and development of a PHB synthase protein model. *Biochimica et Biophysica Acta*, (1), 178–190.

Rehm, B.H., Antonio, R.V., Spiekermann, P., Amara, A.A., & Steinb€uchel, A. (2002). *Molecular characterization of the poly(3- hydroxybutyrate) (PHB) synthase from Ralstonia eutropha: in vitro*. Academic Press.

Senior, P. J., Beech, G. A., Ritchie, G. A. F., & Dawes, E. A. (1972). The role of oxygen limitation in the formation of poly-b-hydroxybutyrate during batch and continuous culture of Azobacter beijerinckii. *The Biochemical Journal*, *128*(5), 1193–1201. doi:10.1042/bj1281193 PMID:4643700

Senior, P. J., & Dawes, E. A. (1973). The regulation of poly-beta-hydroxybutyrate metabolism in Azotobacter beirjerinckii. *The Biochemical Journal*, *134*(1), 225–238. doi:10.1042/bj1340225 PMID:4723225

Shivley, J. M. (2006). Preface. In J. M. Shivley (Ed.), *Inclusions in Prokaryotes*. Berlin: Springer-Verlag. doi:10.1007/3-540-33774-1

Snell, K. D., & Peoples, O. P. (2009). PHA Bioplastic: A valueadded coproduct for biomass biorefineries. *Biofuels, Bioproducts & Biorefining*, *3*(4), 456–467. doi:10.1002/bbb.161

Somleva, M. N., Snell, K. D., Beaulieu, J. J., Peoples, O. P., Garrison, B. R., & Patterson, N. A. (2008). Production of polyhydroxybutyrate in switchgrass, a value-added co-product in an important lignocellulosic biomass crop. *Plant Biotechnology Journal*, *6*(7), 663–678. doi:10.1111/j.1467-7652.2008.00350.x PMID:18498309

Song, S. S., Hein, S., & Steinbuchel, A. (1999). Production of poly(4- hydroxybutyric acid) by fed-batch cultures of recombinant strains of Escherichia coli. *Biotechnology Letters*, *21*(3), 193–197. doi:10.1023/A:1005451810844

Sticklen, M. (2008). Plant genetic engineering for biofuel production: Towards affordable cellulosic ethanol. *Nature Reviews. Genetics*, *9*(6), 433–443. doi:10.1038/nrg2336 PMID:18487988

Sudesh, K., Abe, H., & Doi, Y. (2000). Synthesis, structure and properties of polyhydroxyalkanoates: Biological polyesters. *Progress in Polymer Science*, *25*(10), 1503–1555. doi:10.1016/S0079-6700(00)00035-6

Suriyamongkol, P., Weselake, R., Narine, S., Moloney, M., & Shah, S. (2007). Biotechnological approaches for the production of polyhydroxyalkanoates in microorganisms and plants—A review. *Biotechnology Advances*, *25*(2), 148–175. doi:10.1016/j.biotechadv.2006.11.007 PMID:17222526

Tokiwa, Y., Calabia, B. P., Ugwu, C. U., & Aiba, S. (2009). Biodegradability of plastics. *International Journal of Molecular Sciences*, *10*(9), 3722–3742. doi:10.3390/ijms10093722 PMID:19865515

United States Environmental Protection Agency. (2010). *Waste and cleanup risk assessment*. Retrieved from http://www.epa.gov/oswer/riskassessment/glossary.htm

United States Environmental Protection Agency. (2013). *Types of crude oil*. Retrieved from http://www2.epa.gov/emergency-response/types-crude-oil

U.S. Department of Energy. (2013a). *How fossil fuels were formed*. Retrieved from http://www.fe.doe.gov/education/energylessons/coal/gen_howformed.html

U.S. Department of Energy. (2013b). *Total petroleum consumption (thousand barrels per day)*. Retrieved from http://www.eia.gov/cfapps/ipdbproject/iedindex3.cfm?tid=5&pid=5&aid=2&cid=regions&syid=1980&eyid=2010&unit=TBPD

van Veilen, J. B., & Poirier, Y. (2008). Production of renewable polymers from crop plants. *The Plant Journal*, *54*(4), 684–701. doi:10.1111/j.1365-313X.2008.03431.x PMID:18476872

Wang, J. G., & Bakken, L. R. (1998). Screening of soil bacteria for polybeta- hydroxybutyric acid production and its role in the survival of starvation. *Microbial Ecology*, *35*(1), 94–101. doi:10.1007002489900063 PMID:9459662

Wellisch, M., Jungmeier, G., Karbowski, A., Patel, M.K., & Rogulska, M. (2010). Biorefinery systems – potential contributors to sustainable innovation. *Biofuels, Bioproducts & Biorefining*, *4*(3), 275-286. Doi:10.1002/bbb.217

Williamson, D. H., & Wilkinson, J. F. (1958). The isolation and estimation of the poly-beta-hydroxybutyrate inclusions of Bacillus species. *Journal of General Microbiology*, *19*(1), 198–209. doi:10.1099/00221287-19-1-198 PMID:13575768

Zhang, H., Obias, V., Gonyer, K., & Dennis, D. (1994). Production of polyhydroxyalkanoates in sucrose-utilizing recombinant Escherichia coli and Klebsiella strains. *Applied and Environmental Microbiology*, *60*, 1198–1205. PMID:8017916

Section 3
Plastic Waste Management

Chapter 19
Solid Waste Management and Its Impact on the Environment

Ruchi Srivastava
Jiwaji University, India

ABSTRACT

Solid waste consists of household waste, construction and demolition debris, sanitation residue, and waste from streets. This garbage is generated mainly from residential and commercial complexes. With rising urbanization and change in lifestyle and food habits, the amount of solid waste has been increasing rapidly and its composition changing. Solid waste throws back a light on the culture that produces it and affects the health of the people and the environment surrounding it. Globally, people are discarding growing quantities of waste, and its composition is more complex than ever before, as plastic and electronic consumer products diffuse. Solid wastes are hazards as they adversely affect the living as well as nonliving components of the environment. Advanced and new methods of disposal of solid waste such as pyrolysis, pulverization, incineration, and development of sanitary landfills, etc. are used to solve the problem of managing solid waste. Dumping and burning waste is not acceptable practice from environment and health perspective.

INTRODUCTION

Human activities create waste and these wastes are handled, stored, collected and disposed of, which can pose risks to the environment and to public health (Saxena et al., 2010; Zhu et al., 2008). Economic development, urbanization and improved living standards in cities increase the complexity of generated solid waste (Gidde et al., 2008; Rathi, 2007). In discussing solid waste, generally and traditionally certain categories of wastes are well recognized as they are very common. For example, solid wastes include domestic, commercial, industrial, (due to construction and demolition), agricultural, institutional and miscellaneous. Many times domestic and commercial wastes cannot be differentiated and are considered together as urban wastes (Syed, 2006). Municipal solid waste is generally a combination of household and commercial refuse which is generated from the living community (Rajkumar et al., 2010). The continuous indiscriminate disposal of municipal solid waste is accelerating and is linked to poverty, poor

DOI: 10.4018/978-1-5225-9452-9.ch019

governance, urbanization, population growth, poor standards of living, and low level of environmental awareness and inadequate management of environmental knowledge. Municipal solid waste generally includes degradable (paper, textiles, food waste, straw and yard waste), partially degradable (wood, disposable napkins and sludge) and non-degradable materials (leather, plastics, rubbers, metals, glass, ash from fuel burning like coal, briquettes or woods, dust and electronic waste). Rapid industrialization and population explosion in India has led to the migration of people from villages to cities, which generate thousands of tons of MSW daily. Poor collection and inadequate transportation are responsible for the accumulation of MSW at every nook and corner. The management of municipal solid waste is going through a critical phase, due to unavailability of suitable facilities to treat and dispose of the larger amounts of MSW generated daily in metropolitan cities. Adverse impact on all components of the environment and human health occurs due to scientific disposal of MSW (Rathi, 2006; Ray et al., 2005; Sharholy et al., 2005; Jha et al., 2003). Improper management of solid waste has been reported by several researchers in different cities of developing countries (Mohanty et al., 2014; Das and Bhattacharya, 2013; Noorjahan et al., 2012. Due to improper solid waste management, waste has become one of the pollution sources that has caused diverse environment impacts as well as detrimental towards human health and safety. India is one of the least urbanized countries of the world, yet its urban population is second largest amongst the countries of the world. Metropolitan cities (Delhi, Mumbai, Kolkata and Chennai) account for more than 42% of India's urban population (Ghosh and Kansal, 2014) and been a top producer of MSW in India due to its high occupancy.

Solid waste management is a major challenge in urban areas throughout the world. Without an effective and efficient solid waste management program, the waste generated from various human activities, both industrial and domestic, can result in health hazards and have a negative impact on the environment. Understanding the waste generated, the availability of resources, and the environmental conditions of a particular society are important to developing an appropriate waste management system. Solid waste is defined as material that no longer has any value to its original owner and is discarded. The main constituents of solid waste in urban areas are organic waste (including kitchen waste and garden trimmings), paper, glass, metals, and plastics. Ash, dust, and street sweepings can also form a significant portion of the waste. Solid waste management may be defined as the discipline associated with controlling the generation, storage, collection, transfer and transport, processing, and disposal of solid waste in a manner that is in accordance with the best principles of health, economics, engineering, conservation, aesthetics, and other environmental considerations, and that is also responsive to public attitudes.

Solid waste management systems cover all actions that seek to reduce the negative impacts on health, environment and economy. Developing countries are seriously facing the associated problems in collection, transportation and disposal of communal solid waste. Due to unplanned communities and developments in major cities, environmental and sanitary conditions are becoming very complex [Data collection of national study 1996]. Due to a lack of awareness and low income sources, dwellers are forced to live with unhealthy and unhygienic conditions. An improper solid waste management system may contribute to a worsening environmental degradation of the community. Illegal dumping of communal solid waste is responsible for a number of diseases.

CHARACTERIZATION OF WASTES

Solid waste are characterize on the basis of following parameters [U.S Environmental Protection Agency

- Their sources
- By the types of wastes produced
- By generation rates and composition

Accurate information in these areas is necessary in order to monitor and control existing waste management systems and to make regulatory, financial and institutional decisions.

TYPE OF SOLID WASTE

Depending on their source the solid waste may of different type such as [Moeller, D. W. (2005)]

- Residential waste
- Industrial
- Institutional
- Construction and demolition
- Municipal services

CHARACTERISTICS OF SOLID WASTES

- Corrosive: these are wastes that include acids or bases that are capable of corroding mental containers, e.g. tanks[Moeller, D. W. (2005)]
- Ignitability: this is waste that can create fires under certain condition, e.g. waste oils and solvents
- Reactive: these are unstable in nature; they cause explosions, toxic fumes when heated.
- Toxicity: waste which are harmful or fatal when ingested or absorb.

SOLID WASTE TREATMENT

Current treatment strategies are directed towards reducing the amount of solid waste that needs to be landfilled, as well as recovering and utilizing the materials present in the discarded wastes as a resource to the largest possible extent. Different methods are used for treatment of solid waste and the choice of proper method depends upon refuse characteristics, land area available and disposal cost they are as follows [Moeller, D. W. (2005), Centers for Disease and Control. (2009)].

1. Incineration
2. Compaction
3. Pyrolysis
4. Gasification
5. Composting

1. Incineration

It is a controlled combustion process for burning solid wastes in presence of excess air (oxygen) at high temperature of about 1000°C and above to produce gases and residue containing non-combustible material. One of the most attractive features of the incineration process is that it can be used to reduce the original volume of combustible MSW by 80– 90%.

2. Compaction

The waste is compacted or compressed. It also breaks up large or fragile items of waste. This process is conspicuous in the feed at the back end of many garbage collection vehicles. Deposit refuse at bottom of slope for best compaction and control of blowing litter [U.S. Environment Protection Agency (2009)].

3. Pyrolysis

Pyrolysis is defined as thermal degradation of waste in the absence of air to produce char, pyrolysis oil and syngas, e.g. the conversion of wood to charcoal also it is defined as destructive distillation of waste in the absence of oxygen. External source of heat is employed in this process. Because most organic substances are thermally unstable they can upon heating in an oxygen-free atmosphere be split through a combination of thermal cracking and condensation reactions into gaseous, liquid and solid fraction[U.S. Environment Protection Agency (2009)].

4. Gasification

Gasification is a process in which partial combustion of MSW is carried out in the presence of oxygen, but in lesser amount than that is required for complete combustion, to generate a combustible gas (fuel gas) rich in carbon monoxide and hydrogen e.g. the conversion of coal into town gas. When a gasifier is operated at atmospheric pressure with air as the oxidant, the end products of the gasification process are a low-energy gas typically containing (by volume) 20% CO, 15% H_2, 10% CO_2 and 2% CH_4[U.S. Environment Protection Agency (2009)].

5. Composting

Composting is the most responsible technical solution for many developing countries especially, where the climate is arid and the soil is in serious need of organic supplements. The composting process usually follows 2 basic steps, which may be preceded or followed by pre- or post treatments (crushing, sorting, humidification, mixing with other waste, etc. [U.S. Environment Protection Agency (2009)].

TYPICAL ISSUES IN SOLID WASTE MANAGEMENT

The main disposal methods for municipal solid waste in Asian developing countries are open dumping and sanitary landfill. Overall the environmental condition of the uncontrolled dumpsites is extremely vulnerable, with severe environmental pollution. On open dumping grounds, foul odors and air pollution are dangerously affecting the surroundings. Rodents are spreading pathogens in the surrounding areas, and the workers are highly exposed to disease and hazardous waste. Some cities dispose of their waste in sanitary landfills. The landfills are generally well operated and maintained.

STEPS IN SOLID WASTE MANAGEMENT

Solid waste management (SWM) involves the collection, storage, transportation, processing, treatment, recycling, and final disposal of waste. Systems need to be simple, affordable, sustainable (financially, environmentally, and socially) and should be equitable, providing collection services to all.

Many developed countries have formal door-to-door collection systems. However, in low-income countries, waste generators (e.g., householders), domestic helpers, or private waste collectors carry waste to transfer points. This stage is referred to as "primary collection." A transfer point is an intermediate place at which waste is deposited and stored before being transported to the final disposal site. Local authorities then collect waste from the transfer point and convey it to the final disposal site, and this is referred to as "secondary collection." Finally, waste is disposed of to a variety of standards according to available resources and knowledge. This stage is called final disposal. Recyclable materials may be extracted from the waste stream from the points of generation, transfer, or disposal.

Primary Collection

Primary collection is what helps ensure waste enters the waste management process without ending up on streets or blocking drains. Primary collection may be undertaken by waste generators themselves, domestic helpers, or paid waste collectors.

Often primary collection is undertaken by informal sector entrepreneurs who charge a fee for periodic removal of waste. The vehicles used for primary collection are often small and low-cost, such as wheelbarrows, handcarts, or tricycles carts.

Transfer Points

One of the most visible aspects of SWM is the transfer point, providing an interface between primary and secondary collection. These are often poorly designed, involving double handling of waste (once to unload tricycles, again to reload trucks) and unsanitary conditions where transfer points are not properly cleaned.

Where waste generators carry their own waste, transfer points need to be located within easy walking distance (a good guide is nearly 50 m) to discourage indiscriminate dumping. All transfer points and areas should be cleared daily and cleaned as necessary to prevent odors and keep rats and other disease vectors under control. They should also be designed to ensure minimum double handling. There are a number of approaches for achieving this, including "ramp transfer points," which raise primary collection vehicles up to the loading level of demountable containers. Sometimes, however, space does not allow this. Another innovative solution is to use carts that carry a series of small containers that can be easily and safely lifted and emptied into containers.

Secondary Collection

Secondary collection entails the removal and transportation of waste from transfer points to processing and disposal facilities. This is often one of the most costly elements of SWM systems. Waste characterization study data will play an important part in planning secondary collection as it informs us how much waste requires collection, its weight and volume, where it is located, and so on.

Landfill and Incineration

Disposal is one of the most problematic aspects of SWM in low-income countries. Waste characterization data will prove useful in planning disposal options; the quantities of waste generated will help decide what volume of landfill site is required and, according to trends in waste production, enable to project its lifespan. Waste composition data will also help guide your decisions about suitable options: for example the presence of toxic waste will indicate the need for particular care in disposal, and a high organic/ moisture content could make incineration very difficult.

Key planning issues include these:

- identifying and understanding practices at present, including issues (e.g., corruption) that may impact performance now and in the future;
- for land filling, where could a disposal site be situated, what are the pervading geological conditions, where does the water table lie, and what regulations must be adhered to;
- for incineration, is the waste composition suitable is safe technology affordable and would it be feasible to maintain and operate it to sufficiently high standards?

Fully engineered sanitary landfill is the safest disposal option in terms of human health and the environment, and methane can be recovered for electricity generation. However, engineered landfill sites are usually very expensive to construct and operate so may be a more suitable long-term objective. Incineration, involving high-temperature complete combustion of organic material, can be used to reduce volume, and in some situations, energy can be recovered. Open burning of waste is not incineration and is not recommended because it releases toxic smoke. Controlled incinerators can be developed relatively cheaply, but the high moisture content of waste in many low-income countries can cause problems. Most waste incinerators are costly to develop and operate.

In many cases a carefully managed basic landfill site will be more achievable in the short run, involving the following practices:

- preventing all burning;
- locating the site at least 500 m downwind from housing and water sources on a geologically suitable site;
- daily compacting and covering with soil, to increase stability and discourage vermin;
- basic monitoring of dumping, ideally using a weigh-station if available;
- fencing to prevent waste blowing outside the site;
- basic leachate control.

Leachate is liquid runoff, and it is a particular problem in rainy conditions. It has a high "biological oxygen demand" and can damage ecosystems in water bodies. It may also contain toxins such as heavy metals, which can pollute groundwater sources.

METHODS OF WASTE DISPOSAL

The methods for solid waste disposal fall under two segments.

- Waste management: a throwaway or high-waste approach encouraging waste production
- Pollution prevention: a low-waste approach using waste as resources

Solid waste disposal methods fall directly under SWM, and they include the following:

1. Open dumping, sea dumping.
2. Compaction and baling.
3. Sanitary landfill.
4. Composting.
5. Incineration.
6. Reclamation and recycling.

Associated Negative Environmental Impacts Due to Improper Solid Waste Management

Improper solid waste management system results following negative impacts on the environment:

- Dispersed solid waste from the illegal open dumps often blocks the drains and sewers. Ultimately these blockages are creating flooding and unhygienic conditions in the city.
- Flies breeding are directly linked with open solid waste dumps. During the field investigation it was observed that during summer the flies are increasing their population so rapidly due to these waste dumps and they are very effectual vectors that spread disease in the community.
- Associated to the above problems, blocked drains and wastewater flooding in the city due to blocked drains are greatly supporting the mosquitoes breed and they are spreading the malaria and dengue.
- Proportion of food waste in open dumps and waste drains are providing an attractive shelter for rats. It was also reported that these rats are spreading disease, damaging electrical cables and other materials.
- The open burning of collected solid waste causing air pollution issues.
- Uncollected solid wastes from few locations in the cities are degrading the urban environment and discouraging efforts to keep streets and open spaces clean.
- Discarded polythene bags in collected solid waste from Rawalpindi city are generating an aesthetic nuisance and they may also cause the death of grazing animals which eat them [George et al., 1993].

- Due to a lack of health and safety facilities to the waste collection crew in cities, they are specifically facing occupational hazards, including strains from lifting, injuries from sharp objects and traffic accidents.
- Open dumps on the roadside and heavily sized solid waste storage containers are also creating traffic blockage in the areas.
- The cities government is not providing separate waste collection facilities. As a result, a lot of dangerous items (such as broken glass, razor blades, hypodermic needles and other healthcare wastes, aerosol cans and potentially explosive containers and chemicals from industries) may cause risks of injury or poisoning, particularly to scavengers and school going children [Davis & Cornwell., 2009].
- Open body trucks are being used for the collection of solid waste in cities without covers. This practice is totally unhygienic.
- Heavy solid waste collection vehicles are causing significant damage to the road.
- Different segregated solid waste materials, such as plastic bottles and medical supplies, are not being properly cleaned or sterilized by local scavengers.
- During rainy seasons, produced leachate from the open dumped sites is causing serious pollution to water bodies.
- A high percentage of collected solid waste from different cities is being treated or disposed of in unsatisfactory ways, causing a severe aesthetic nuisance in terms of smell and manifestation.
- Liquids and fumes, escaping from deposits of chemical wastes are creating fatal or other serious effects to the community [Akio. 2002].
- Illegal burning of collected solid waste in cities is creating serious negative impacts on outdoor air quality. Furthermore, it is also causing illness and reducing visibility.

IMPACTS OF SOLID WASTE ON HUMAN HEALTH, ANIMALS AND AQUATIC LIFE

There are potential risks to environment and health from improper handling of solid wastes. Direct health risks concern mainly the workers in this field, who need to be protected, as far as possible, from contact with wastes. There are also specific risks in handling wastes from hospitals and clinics. For the general public, the main risks to health are indirect and arise from the breeding of disease vectors, primarily flies and rats [Royal Commission on Environmental Pollution. 1984].

Uncontrolled hazardous wastes from industries mixing up with municipal wastes create potential risks to human health. Traffic accidents can result from toxic spilled wastes. There is specific danger of concentration of heavy metals in the food chain, a problem that illustrates the relationship between municipal solid wastes and liquid industrial effluents containing heavy metals discharged to a drainage/ sewerage system and /or open dumping sites of municipal solid wastes and the wastes discharged thereby maintains a vicious cycle including these some other types of problem are as follows [Royal Commission on Environmental Pollution.1984].

- Chemical poisoning through chemical inhalation
- Uncollected waste can obstruct the storm water runoff resulting in flood
- Low birth weight

- Cancer
- Congenital malformations
- Neurological disease
- Nausea and vomiting
- Mercury toxicity from eating fish with high levels of mercury
- Plastic found in oceans ingested by birds
- Resulted in high algal population in river and sea.
- Degrades water and soil quality

Serious Environmental Issues in Study Area Due to Open Dumping

Open dumps of municipal solid waste are creating serious negative impacts on environment [Summera et al., 2007]. Following negative impacts are being observed due to open dumping of solid waste:

- **Dust and Filthy Dirt**: Strong wind and storm are spreading dust and filth from the open dumps of solid waste to adjacent areas.
- **Odor:** Nearby areas to the open dump sites is being affected due to odor emitting from these dumps.
- **Rats and Other Vermin**: Open dumps of communal solid waste are providing attractive habitat to rats and other vermin.
- **Toxic Gases:** Toxic gases are continuously exposed to the atmosphere.
- **Leachate:** Percolating rainwater through the open dump contaminating ground water resources.
- **Health and Sanitation:** Open dumps of solid waste are a serious threat to human health and sanitation.

Serious Environmental Issues in Study Area Due to Open Burning

It was observed during the field visit that solid waste collected at the communal bins is burnt. The local dwellers were complaining that burning of dumped solid waste is a common practice and creating drastic air pollution.

IMPACTS OF SOLID WASTE ON ENVIRONMENT

The decomposition of waste into constituent chemicals is a common source of local environmental pollution. This problem is especially acute in developing nations. Very few existing landfills in the world's poorest countries would meet environmental standards accepted in industrialized nations, and with limited budgets there are likely to be few sites rigorously evaluated prior to use in the future. The problem is again compounded by the issues associated with rapid urbanization. A major environmental concern is gas release by decomposing garbage. Methane is a by-product of the anaerobic respiration of bacteria, and these bacteria thrive in landfills with high amounts of moisture. Methane concentrations can reach up to 50% of the composition of landfill gas at maximum anaerobic decomposition (Cointreau-Levine, 1997). A second problem with these gasses is their contribution to the enhanced greenhouse gas effect and climate change. Liquid leachate management varies throughout the landfills of the developing world. Leachate poses a threat to local surface and ground water systems.

The use of dense clay deposits at the bottom of waste pits, coupled with plastic sheeting-type liners to prevent infiltration into the surrounding soil, is generally regarded as the optimum strategy to contain excess liquid. In this way, waste is encouraged to evaporate rather than infiltrate.

PREVENTIVE MEASURES FOR REDUCTION OF ADVERSE IMPACT ON ENVIRONMENT AND HUMAN

Proper solid waste management have to be undertaken to ensure that it does not affect the environment and not cause health hazards to the people living there. At the household-level proper segregation of waste has to be done and it should be ensured that all organic matter is kept aside for composting, which is undoubtedly the best method for the correct disposal of this segment of the waste. In fact, the organic part of the waste that is generated decomposes more easily, attracts insects and causes disease. Organic waste can be composted and then used as a fertilizer. These steps may be taken for prevention of impact

- Generation of waste should be decreased.
- Promoting the production of goods which minimize waste generation after use.
- Material recycling and recovery should be increased.
- Promoting the use of plastic recycling identification codes and labels in order to make sorting and recycling of plastic packaging easier.
- Municipalities increasing their level of service to the public regarding sorting of waste.
- Education of producers, the public and people who work in the waste sector should be
- Increased.
- Promoting the use of less hazardous alternatives to hazardous chemicals during production of goods.
- Legislation in the waste sector should be improved.
- Collection of hazardous waste at collection points shall be safe, secure and performed in an environmentally sound manner.

CONCLUSION

The focus of this chapter was on impact of Solid waste due to non engineering and non scientific disposal. It is found that with increase in the global population and the rising demand for food and other essentials, there has been a rise in the amount of waste being generated daily by each household. Waste that is not properly managed especially excreta and other liquid and solid waste from households and the community, are a serious health hazard and lead to the spread of infectious diseases.

REFERENCES

Akio. (2002). Domestic Solid Waste Management in Pakistan. Japan International Corporation Agency.

Alam, P., & Ahmade, K. (2013). Impact of solid waste on health and the environment. *International Journal of Sustainable Development and Green Economics*, *2*(1), 165–168.

Centers for Disease and Control. (2009). *Solid Waste*. Retrieved July 16,from http://www.cdc.gov/nceh/ehs/NALBOH/NALBOH-4.pdf

Das, S., & Bhattacharyya, B. K. (2013). Municipal solid waste characteristics and management in Kolkata, India. In *The 19th International Conference on Industrial Engineering and Engineering Management* (pp. 1399-1409). Springer.

Davis & Cornwell. (n.d.). *Introduction to Environmental Engineering* (2nd ed.). McGraw Hill.

Ghosh, R., & Kansal, A. (2014). Urban challenges in India and the mission for a sustainable habitat. *Interdisciplina, 2*(2).

Gidde, M. R., Todkar, V. V., & Kokate, K. K. (2008). Municipal Solid Waste Management in Emerging Mega Cities: A case study of Pune City. In *Indo Italian Conference on Green and Clean Environment*. MAEER's MIT College of Engineering.

Khan, S. F., Malik, N. E., & Taseer, M. (2007). Impacts Of Municipal Solid Waste Open Dumps On Environment. In *International Conference, ESDev* (*Vol. 1*). Academic Press.

Mandiberg, S. F., & Faure, M. G. (2009). A graduated punishment approach to environmental crimes: Beyond vindication of administrative authority in the United States and Europe. *Colum. J. Envtl. L.*, *34*, 447.

Mohanty, C. R., Mishra, U., & Beuria, P. R. (2014). Municipal solid waste management in Bhubaneswar, India—a review. *Int. J. Latest Trends Eng. Technol*, *3*(3), 303–312.

Nisar, H., Ejaz, N., Naushad, Z., & Ali, Z. (2008). Impacts of solid waste management in Pakistan: A case study of Rawalpindi city. *WIT Transactions on Ecology and the Environment*, *109*, 685–691. doi:10.2495/WM080701

Noorjahan, A., Dhanakumar, S., Mohanraj, R., & Ravichandran, M. (2012). Status of heavy metals distribution in municipal solid waste in Tiruchirappalli City, India. *International Journal of Applied Biology and Pharmaceutical Technology*, *3*(3), 252–258.

Rajkumar, N., Subramani, T., & Elango, L. (2010). Groundwater contamination due to municipal solid waste disposal-A GIS based study in Erode city. *International Journal of Environmental Sciences, 1*(1), 39.

Rathi, S. (2006). Alternative approaches for better municipal solid waste management in Mumbai, India. *Waste Management (New York, N.Y.)*, *26*(10), 1192–1200. doi:10.1016/j.wasman.2005.09.006 PMID:16288861

Rathi, S. (2007). Optimization model for integrated municipal solid waste management in Mumbai, India. *Environment and Development Economics*, *12*(1), 105–121. doi:10.1017/S1355770X0600341X

Royal Commission on Environmental Pollution. (1984). *10th Report tackling pollution—experience and prospects*. London: HMSO.

Saxena, S., Srivastava, R. K., & Samaddar, A. B. (2010). Sustainable Waste Management Issues in India. *IUP Journal of Soil & Water Sciences, 3*(1).

Syed, S. (2006). Solid and liquid waste management. *Emirates J. Eng. Res*, *11*(2), 19–36.

Tchobanoglous, Theisen, & Vigil. (n.d.). *Integrated Solid Waste Management*. McGraw Hill.

Wilson, R. (1995). Nature and Young Children. *Young Children*, *50*(6), 4–11.

Zhu, D., Asnani, P. U., Zurbrugg, C., Anapolsky, S., & Mani, S. K. (2007). *Improving municipal solid waste management in India: A sourcebook for policymakers and practitioners*. The World Bank. doi:10.1596/978-0-8213-7361-3

Chapter 20
Challenges and Factors in Plastics Reutilization/Recycling: A Review

Vaishali Tomar
https://orcid.org/0000-0001-5209-6831
ABH Natures Products, USA

Ankita Dhillon
Banasthali Vidyapith, India

Dinesh Kumar
https://orcid.org/0000-0001-5488-951X
Central University of Gujarat, India

ABSTRACT

Plastics are used worldwide due to the low price, lightweight, and long-lasting availability. It can be molded into different products. Therefore, the invention of plastics has been increased significantly over the last 50-60 years. Several environmental problems are generating due to plastics used across the world. This kind of observation indicates that plastics are not sustainable. It is accumulating in landfills and natural locales due to the stability of the polymers involved. This chapter discusses the structure and uses of plastics. Plastics recycling is a very challenging duty in waste management. This chapter explores the factors affecting the plastic recycling in detail. This chapter also explores the plastic recycling methods and challenges during plastic recycling and deliberates more briefly how the government sector is working to clean most of the plastic waste from landfills to recycling over the next periods. In the last, this chapter highlights the plastic effects on the environment and how we can use again through recycling.

DOI: 10.4018/978-1-5225-9452-9.ch020

INTRODUCTION

Plastics are organic polymers which are derived from petrochemicals and contain high molecular mass. Generally, we can say that it is a group of materials of high molecular weight chains with a carbon backbone. These materials are defined as a monomer which relates to its repeated units to make a polymer. The class of mouldable polymers which can be deformed irreversibly without breaking is known as plasticity (Achilias, 2006; Watanabe, Yasuaki, Takashi, Hiroshi, Toshiyuki & Katsuhiko, 2009). Plastics are a material which consists of an extensive range of synthetic or semi-synthetic organic compounds that can be easily changed into solid substances.

Plastics are produced from fossil oil and gas. Annually 4% of petrochemical is using in the manufacturing of plastics. The energy which is required to produce plastics comes from the regular consumption of fossil fuel (Onu, Vasile, Ciocilteu, Iojoiu & Darie, 1998; Williams& Williams, 1998). Plastics are reducing the use of fossil fuel. Replacement of heavier conventional material like steel by plastic is an example of the reduction of fossil fuel.

Plastics can easily be molded in other substances, and it makes it more useable by the people. People are using plastics due to the low price, low weight, and durability (Achilias, Roupakias, Megalokonomosa, Lappas & Antonakou, 2007). It is also using to substitute heavy materials with weight reduction which give results for 3-7% improvement in fuel efficiency. There are so many examples where plastics are using like packaging, pipes, cable coated materials, structural materials, and agricultural films. The use of plastic is breaking the record every year (Xie, 2008; Zhao, 1996). The plastic industry has been developed due to the different routes for the development of polymers from petrochemical sources. The estimation of the production of the polymer is almost 260 million metric tons per annum which contain synthetic fibers, thermoplastics, and thermoset plastics. Thermoplastic resins are two third part of this production, and globally it is increasing almost 5% per annum (Westerhout, Waanders, Kuipers,& Swaaij, 1997; Yoshioka, Furukawa, Sato & Okuwaki, 1998). Biodegradable plastics are made of bioplastics; bio-plastics are made up of renewable raw materials. Biodegradable plastics can decompose in the environment naturally by a microorganism (Xiao, Ni, Chi, Jin, Xiao, Zhong & Huang, 2009).The advantage of biodegradable plastics on conventional plastics is the manufacturing process. During the manufacturing process, carbon, methane and other forms of pollute does not release when biodegradable plastics burned or recycled. But most of the plastics are not biodegradable, and their longevity is uncertain in the environment. Most of the polymers will be preserved for centuries (Woo, Ayala& Broadbelt, 2000).On the other side, the degradable plastics may be kept for a significant time, and it depends on different factors like ultraviolet light exposure, oxygen, and temperature, and biodegradable plastics rely on the presence of micro-organism(Achilias, 2007). But the degradation factors vary between landfills, terrestrial and aquatic environments. A plastic item reduces due to the impact of weathering; it breaks down into the minor pieces of plastic wreckage. But polymer cannot degrade in the limit timeframe (Wu, Zhou, Zhao, Deng, Zhang& Wang, 2009; Onwudili, Insura& Williams, 2009). The result of this impact is increasing the accumulation of plastics in landfills and as wreckage in the environment and this factor is giving support to waste-management issues and environmental damage.

Plastic recycling is the only factor to reduce this issue from the environment. Recycling is a waste-management method. It is the process which is used to reprocess the material into useful products. Recycling is part of global efforts to decrease the number of plastics in waste watercourse. Approximately 8 million tons of plastic wastes enter the ocean every year (Ward, Goff, Donner, Kaminsky & O'Connor, 2006; Onwudilia & Williams, 2016). The recycling of plastics is more challenging as compared to the recycling of metal due to low density and low cost. There are different technical sprints to overwhelm during recycling. Plastics during the process of recycling are arranged according to their resin type. The resin identification code (RIC) which is a method of categorization of polymer types is useful in sorting the plastics. The society of the plastics industry developed this method in 1988(Oyedun, Gebreegziabher, Ng, & Hui, 2014).Polyethylene terephthalate (PET) is an example to understand the resin code.

This chapter will explore waste management strategy, plastic recycling, challenges and factor during the recycling process.

UNUSABLE MATERIAL MANAGEMENT

There is a wide range of waste management arrangements for the municipal solid waste stream. It is for material who weighted from landfill to incineration process. As per research analysis of different countries, plastics were using around 500kg per person per year, and now it has been increased around 600 kg per person per year (Van, Serrano, Aguado, García & Rojo, 2001; Panda, Singh & Mishra, 2010). Based on domestic and commercially, the use of plastic is 45 kg per person per year which increases 6-9% weight and volume of the municipal solid waste stream. Waste material is improved when they are diverted in landfills. The lightweight of plastic which we use in packaging is visible, and it is rigid and flexible plastic (Van, Serrano, Aguado, García & Rojo, 2001; Panda, Singh& Mishra, 2010). Its arrangements can decrease the quantity of material which is going into useless material management. The process of recycling helps introduce fewer products in the waste stream (Panepinto, Deborah, Tedesco, Vita, Brizio, Enrico, Genon & Giuseppe, 2015).

During the process of recycling, recovered material changed into new products. In the process of recovering the organic materials, it contains energy recovery. During this process, controlled combustion utilized the calorific value of the material (Panda & Singh, 2011; Vilaplana, Ribes-Greus, & Karlsson, 2006). It doesn't affect the demand for the new product in the process of lesser environmental performance than material recovery. This is also possible in the case of polymer and can be manufactured into a reusable container. It can be reusable after waste stream with the restoration of energy (Uemichi, Makino & Kanazuka, 1989; Park, Oh, Lee, Kim,& Yoo,2000). There are some factors which include in the process of the waste management process like landfill, incineration and energy recovery, reprocessing of plastic wrapping, plastics recycling and original material.

LANDFILL

It is a straightforward approach to unusable material management. In some countries, it becomes a different and familiar process to organize waste material. It is a process where the garbage can easily dump (Ulutan, 1998; Park, Oh, Lee, Kim & Yoo, 2000). Many countries are still following this process to dump the garbage. For well-run landfills process for non-hazardous materials, there are two techniques:

1. Restrain waste to as minor an area as probable
2. Dense debris into decrease volume

This process is very cost-effective. Landfill gas can be renovated into natural gas. It is useful in those countries where the large open areas present. But during the time of the earthquake, these areas shakes, and soil liquefaction process occurs (Park, Seo, Lee, Yu & Hwang, 2012). This is a long-time risk of pollution of soils and groundwater too and increases the number of organic pollutants.

INCINERATION AND ENERGY RECOVERY

Incineration is the process of combustion of organic substances. During this process, waste converts into ash, flue gas and heat. Ash is formed from the inorganic constituents of waste materials. Heat which is generated during the process of incineration can be used for electric power. This process decreases the need for the landfill for waste (Achilias, Roupakias, Megalokonomosa, Lappas, Antonakou, 2007). During this process, hazardous materials like polyvinyl chloride and other halogenated complexes are released into the atmosphere. These complexes are mixed in plastics which release furans and polychlorinated biphenyls etc. into the atmosphere (Ukei, Hirose, Horikawa, Takai, Taka, Azuma & Ueno, 2000; Achilias, Giannoulis, & Papageorgiou, 2009). It is useful for the treatment of waste materials in niche areas. This process requires huge investments in infrastructure. Incineration is helpful in the improvement of energy content in the plastic. Energy recovery can be different significantly, but it depends on whether it is used for electricity or combined heat and power (Achilias, Antonakou, Roupakias, Megalokonomos & Lappas, 2008). Incineration is helpful to recycle the waste which deposited on landfill even decades and centuries later. One of the concerned drawbacks of this process is the release of different toxic heavy metals during this process. It is harmful at very minute levels.

PLASTIC WRAP RECYCLING

The plastic film which includes bags and wrap has become part of our daily life. These sources are using in excess amount because of their large quantity and suitability. After the use of this material, they are found buried in landfills or littered in our paths. Through the recycling process, individuals and businesses can reduce the excessive use of bags and wrap. There are some wrapping methods like shrink wrapping, flow wrapping, cello wrapping and bundle wrapping for plastic packaging. These packaging wrapping can be recycled and are in high demand by manufacturers as a raw material. Many years ago, the reuse of packaging materials in the form of bottles was common. A comprehensive application of container reuse is logistical. Some countries follow the process of taking back the refilling process for the marketing of their products. But in Europe, this scheme does not exist (Achilias, Antonakou, Koutsokosta, & Lappas, 2009). Distribution and collection of materials are remote from the product filling companies. Due to brand and marketing purpose, the full range of containers for the process of taking back refilling is less feasible. Bottles and glass are generally used for niche activity for small business to reduce packaging waste. High-value consumer products like electronic products can be manufactured during the recycling process. This is obvious on an industrial scale with the reuse of containers. In some countries, reusable bags are using instead of plastics bags (Achilias, Tsintzou, Nikolaidis, Bikiaris, & Karayannidis, 2011).

Plastics Recycling

It is known that plastic recycling is the part of the waste-management method and it is useful in reprocessing the material into helpful content. It is a useful method to make plastic reusable again. It is a complicated process, but four processes are involved in recycling like primary, secondary, tertiary, and quaternary recycling.

Primary Recycling is the process to reprocess the mechanically into the same products. It is closed loop recycling. It is helpful to recycle waste into equivalents characteristic products like aluminum cans to aluminum cans (Achilias, Redhwi, Siddiqui, Nikolaidis, Bikiaris,& Karayannidis, 2010). It is referred to as the plant recycling process. It is the low-cost process for recycling the clean, unpolluted single-type waste. In this process, products are used merely again in different frameworks (Achilias, Kanellopoulou, Megalokonomos, Antonakou, & Lappas, 2007; Oku, Tanaka &Hata, 2000). This process is very safe to use because there arefewer chances of transmission of diseases.

In the process of closed-looprecycling, different materials like metals, paper, and inks are using in plastic packaging and increasing the problems. It is the most practical process when constituents can be easily separated from the sources of contaminants (Akpanudoh, Gobin & Manos, 2005; Al-Salem, Lettieri, & Baeyens, 2010;Araujo,Fernandes & Fernandes,2002) and can be stabilized against degradation during the reprocessing. The plastic waste stream for reprocessing would involve a slight range of polymer grade to decrease the strain of exchanging the virgin resin. For example, PET bottles are made from the same grade of PET for both the bottle manufacturing process and reprocessing to polyester fibers. Although, HDPE which is used for blow moulding bottles are less suitable for injection moulding applications (Al-Salem, & Lettieri, 2010; Al-Salem, Lettieri, & Baeyens, 2009). The part of post-consumer plastic waste stream which has been recycled in a closed loop manner is PET bottles. Pre-consumer plastic waste like industrial packaging are recycling than post-consumer packaging to a greater extent, and it is pure with greater accessibility from a minor number of sources of higher volume. Post-consumer waste volume is many times larger than industrial waste. But pre and post-consumer waste need to be collected and recycled (Arandes, Abajo, Lopez-Valerio, Fernandez, Azkoiti, Olazar, & Bilbao, 1997; Arandes, Erena, Azkoiti, Olazar, & Bilbao, 2003).

Secondary Recycling is the process to reprocess the products into the lower property. It is also called the downgrading process. This process is very cost effective and shorter lifetime process. In this process, thermoplastic polymers can be used, re-melted and reprocessed into end products. This process does not involve the alteration of the polymer. It is represented by the physical method and can be formed by cutting, shredding or washing into granulates, flakes for manufacturing. By extrusion, it can be melted to make new products (Ward, Goff, Donner, Kaminsky & O'Connor, 2006; Onwudilia & Williams, 2016). This process is helpful to converts waste plastics into different characteristics materials like the conversion of tiresinto rubber products.

Tertiary Recycling is a process of recycling the plastics as a chemical raw material. This process is called feedstock recycling and biological recycling. During this process, there is structural breakdown into the raw components which gives new products. It involves the production of chemicals and fuels from waste plastics (Achilias, Megalokonomos & Karayannidis, 2006). Some products contain a range of different materials which is necessary to remove before the process of recycling like polymers. During this process, there is a reformulation of new products from the waste polymer which depolymerizes

Figure 1. Chemical recycling of PET

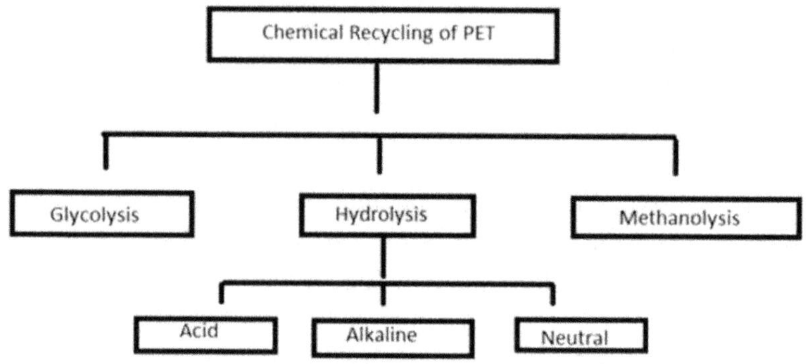

into chemical constituents. The PET recycling process can understand it.(Bajdur, Pajaczkowska, Makarucha, Sulkowska, & Sulkowski, 2002; Aguado, Olazar,San José,Gaisán,& Bilbao, 2002; Aguado, & Serrano, 1999).The recycling of PET has been more winning due to de-polymerization under mild condition. PET broke down into resins through glycolysis and methanolysis process. Figure one shows the diagrammatic representation of chemical recycling of PET. It can be converted back to PET via polymerization reactor (Bockhorn, Hornung, Hornung, & Jakobstroer, 1999).The chemical recycling process has the advantage of recovering the petrochemical constitute of the polymer from manufacturing the other synthetic chemicals (Ballice & Reimert, 2002). It is energy intensive polymerization to carry out plastic manufacture (Nikles & Farahat, 2005).

Quaternary Recycling is a process of energy recovery. During this process energy recovered from the waste plastics. Polymers are the high source of energy recovery (Aguado, Olazar, Gaisan, Prieto, & Bilbao, 2003; Aguayo, Gayubo, Ortega, Olazar, & Bilbao, 1997; Ali &Siddiqui, 2005). These are widely unaccepted to the health risk from toxic air materials like dioxins (in case of heavy metals, chlorine containing polymers, etc.). This is not considered a true recycling process. It includes energy withdrawal by burning and incineration (Passamonti, & Sedran, 2012).

PROCESSING PLASTIC RECYCLING

During the process of recycling, a variety of polymers can be recycled. A single polymer with firm containers is simple to recycle than multi-component materials. It is the process to recover the different types of plastic material into a variety of other products. But some product which is recycled from plastics cannot be reused again (Borgianni, Filippis, Pochetti, & Paolucci, 2002; Cerqueira, Caeiro, Costa & Ramoa Ribeiro, 2008).

Nowadays cross-linked rubber is recycling from the car tires and using to produce the rubber crumb to manufacture the other materials. But in some countries, the landfill of tires and tire waste is banning (Durmus, Koc, Pozan & Kasgoz, 2005; Fernandes, Fernandes & Araujo, 2002). Production of recycled resin from plastics wastes is an important process, and it is not compatible due to the immiscibility at the molecular level and there is the difference at the level of macro scale too (Czernik, Elam, Evans, Meglen, Moens, &Tatsumoto,1998)

PET is polyester which contains the ester functional group can be efficiently cleaved during the different processes like hydrolysis, alcohols, acidolysis, and glycolysis (Elordi, López, Aguado, Olazar & Bilbao, 2007; Elordi, Olazar, Lopez, Amutio, Artetxe, Aguado & Bilbao,2009). PET recycling through microwave reactor has been an effective method to save energy (Elordi, Olazar, Aguado, López, Arabiourrutia & Bilbao, 2007; Faravelli, Bozzano, Colombo, Ranzi & Dente, 2003).

But in case of PVC contaminants, which are present in the PET recycling stream can degrade in the evolution of hydrochloric acid gas at high temperature. And PET in PVC recycles stream is using to produce the solid lumps of undispersed crystalline PET. This process reduces the significance of recycled products (Garcia, Balart, Sanchez & Lopez, 2007; Grause, Predel & Kaminsky, 2006). Table 1 shows the types of plastics with recycled products.

Before recycling of any plastics waste, it goes through different stages. During the process of recycling, it is hard to get the materials with the same color, strength and mechanical properties. There are some factors involved in plastics recycling which are: collection, sorting, cleaning to reduce contamination by polymers(Kim, Kim, Cho, Han & Kim, 2009; Hájeková & Bajus, 2005).

Collection

Collection and disposal of plastic waste is an essential factor during recycling. Roadblocks problems are happening due to the non-degradable nature of plastics (Heyde, & Kremer, 1999; Kim, Kim, Cho, Han& Kim, 2009; La Mantia, 1996; Lee, Cho, Song, Kang, Kim, &Choi, 2003). Curbside, drop-off, buy-back are different ways of collecting the plastics. Curbside recycling is the low-risk process. Materials can be easily obtained in large bins or small open bags (Kruse, Woo & Broadbelt, 2001). It is the good ways which municipal team provides different bags to separate the household's garbage in the colony. It is convenient for community residents (Kim, Lee, Lee, Kim & Choi, 2003).Drop-off recycling is the process where recycling materials are placed at a central collection location. The location for these bags is schools, malls and parks, and so forth (Lee & Song, 2007). For recycled materials, containers are marked to place in them. In this recycling; residents take their garbage to that collection facility. In the

Table 1. Types of plastics, common and recycled products

Types of Plastics	Common Products	Recycled Products
PETE(Polyethylene Terephthalate)	Soda, water, bottles, cups, jars, Trays etc	Clothing, carpet, clamshells, soda etc
HDPE(High-density Polyethylene)	Milk jugs, detergent, shampoo bottles etc	Detergent bottles, flower pot, crates, pipe, decking etc
PVC(Polyvinyl Chloride)	Cleaning supply jugs, pool liners, twine, sheeting, automotive product bottles, sheeting, etc	Pipe, wall siding, binders, carpet backing, flooring, etc
LDPE(Low-Density Polyethylene)	Bread bags, paper towels & tissue overwrap, squeeze bottles, trash bags, six-pack rings etc	Trash bags, plastic lumber, furniture, shipping envelopes, compost bins etc
PP (polypropylene)	Yogurt tubs, cups, juice bottles, straws, hangers, sand & shipping bags, etc	Paint cans, speed bumps, auto parts, food containers, hangers, etc
PS (Polystyrene)	Flatware, hot cups, razors, cd cases etc	Picture frames, crown molding, rulers, flower pots etc
Other	Polycarbonate, nylon, ABS, Acrylic, PLA etc	Electronic housings, auto parts etc

process of refund or buyback, private companies take participation to operate this process. And they pay consumers recycled products which are brought to them (Lee, Noh, Shin, & Seo, 2002; Lee, Yoon, Kim & Park, 2002). In different countries when the container is returned to an authorized center then deposited is fully refunded to the redeemer. Generally, it is started in case of beverage like can or bottle. All these processes help collect plastics bottles from home and other places (Lin& Yen, 2005; Lin& Yen, 2007).

Sorting

Next factor in plastic recycling is sorting. This process occurs through automatic and manually. It is the process where plastic items are separated according to the type of plastics (Liu, Lei, Shitao, Zhiguo & Xiaoping, 2011). It is a problematic process in energy recovery. Manual sorting is useful when the plastic component is available in large quantity. But it is labor demanding process. In automated type techniques, there is one advantage among all wave sorting techniques, but it is not suitable for dark colored plastics. There is a different process which comes under sorting like air sorting, electrostatic sorting, optical sorting, etc. (Bhaskar, Uddin, Murai, Kaneko, Hamano, Kusaba, Muto & Sakata, 2003).

In the process of air sorting, which is based on specific gravity, the lighter particle can be separated from the higher particles (Liu, Zhuo, Shi-Tao, Xiao, Cong-Xia,& Xiao-Ping, 2009). In electrostatic sorting techniques, materials are divided based on electrostatic charge. Clear PET and milk bottles can be separated and identified during the process of separation. Nowadays Fourier-transform near-infrared (FT-NIR) spectroscopy is using to separate the polymer types (Marcilla, Beltran, Hernandez & Navarro, 2004). Optical sorters are also helpful in sorting the colored containers. Other techniques like X-ray detection are also beneficial in the detection of PVC which contains around 60% of chlorine weight (Machado, Rodrigues, Assunc, Soares, Cangani & Cerqueira, 2010).

Cleaning

After the process of sorting, plastics need to be wash properly to remove the impurities like labels, dust, solid pollutants and adhesive. This process increases the quality of the product. During this process, shredder transforms plastics wastes into fractions. These shredders are used to divide the plastics into small parts (Maharana, Negi, & Mohanty, 2007).And prepare them for the recycling process. Washing tanks are useful for this cleaning process. Washing tanks do not contain additives but are filled with cold water for washing. It is helpful to strip out the unwanted materials from the product. An automated washing line is also used to refine the plastic products. It is beneficial to remove the pollution from stuff like PET (Marcilla, Gómez, García, &Olaya, 2002; Mucha, 1976).

Polyolefins can be separated from PVC, PET, etc. through float separation method. Separation of PS from PET is comfortable rather than separation of PVC from PET due to their density overlaps. To remove the low-density film from denser ground plastics, air elutriation is useful to process (Mastral, Berrueco, Gea, & Ceamanos, 2006). There are a lot of methods for separation which are helpful in the separation of plastics. Laser sorting systems are also beneficial to remove the impurities like silicones etc. (Mastral, Esperanza, García,& Juste,2002). This technique uses emission spectra to differentiate the polymers types. Separating the complex mixtures is helpful. This process is using in Europe. During the process of recycling, heat compression is gaining individual demand in different countries (Dawood, & Miura, 2002; De Marco, Caballero, Torres, Laresgoiti, Chomón & Cabrero, 2002; Duangchan, & Samart, 2008; Dawood, & Miura, 2001). This process does not require the matching forms of plastics to be recycled and can be recycled all the plastics in one time. But in the case of monomer process, significant challenges of plastics can be reduced. This process reverses the polymerization reaction to recycle the same type of plastics. It creates new polymer after recycling (Mastellone, Perugini, Ponte &Arena, 2002).

FACTORS BEHIND THE PLASTIC RECYCLING

According to research by Continuous Improvement Fund (CIF), major market trends have shaped the year with the addition of virgin material costs. Major markets are vanishing export markets, swelling transportation costs, and falling supply and demand. CIF is a joint industry-government group who participate in residential recycling programme (Chaupart, Serpe, & Verdu, 1998; Chiu, Chen, & Tsai, 2006). Recycling industries were facing many challenges during the year, but some of the struggles have been outlined as opportunities for investment.

The factors which are included in plastic recycling are:

1. Low energy costs have stimulated an excess amount of new stock in virgin plastics production. According to U.S. expansion projects in Plastics Recycling, there will be histrionic growth in the production of virgin resins in the next three years with lower prices. Polyethylene (PE) followed by polyethylene terephthalate (PET) and polypropylene (PP) will be the biggest impact on the market (Achilias, & Karayannidis, 2004).As per reports, the impact of shale energy has been started in 2018 and move forward past 2020.
2. The restriction in China's import has been shaped the export market in the last few years. According to report, there is effectively elimination to contact to Chinese recycled plastics markets and that so far, it does not seem to be an end date for the restrictions (Beltrame, Bergamasco, Carniti, Castelli, Bertini, & Audisio, 1997). The paper cites which is growing development of Chinese companies are investing in the U.S. for development of material and ship it to China as a pellet (Milne, Behie & Berruti, 1999; Mehta, Biederman, & Shivkumar, 1995). The economics for these types of endeavors are questionable as per the report.
3. Supply and demand are a problem on wider level. Collection volumes have been dropped for PET and high-density polyethylene (HDPE) bottles on the supply side. As per the report, pollution in plastic packages has increased. Meanwhile, dropping in virgin prices and tough-to-find end markets are pulling demand for some low-price recycled plastics. As reports predict that clean film will remain to find use in the bag-to-bag and compound lumber sectors although prices could flip. The highly contaminated film is a different story, mainly in the face of Chinese buyers "withdrawing the market," the report states (Berrueco, Mastral, Esperanza & Ceamanos, 2002). Film rolls generated by Material recovery facilities (MRFs) have difficulty finding markets and those markets will have no price as virgin prices continue to slip as per CIF. CIF has offered a plain opinion on the place of those materials in the stream which sometimes origin bale contamination. It is assuming that the elimination of PVC, PS, PLA, and PETG from plastic packaging stream would significantly improve the economics and quality of PET, PE, and PP, etc. There is no application which currently uses these resins, and it could not be replaced by are cycling-friendly substitute.

It was a year marked by growing transportation costs but in some cases, industry insiders have communicated to Plastics Recycling Update the load costs have been more harmful than the loss of China as an export market (Bockhorn, Donner, Gernsbeck, Hornung, &Hornung,2001; Bodrero, Canivenc & Cansell,1999). As per CIF study, shortage of drivers and compensation are increasing to attract new hires with additional electronic logging device requirements. The plastics recycling sector will be more affected than virgin material producers due to the virgin material sector more frequently relies on the rail as per reports.

CHALLENGES IN THE PLASTIC RECYCLING PROCESS

Recycling of mixed plastics waste is a big challenge in recycling. In the process of recycling, a large portion of the plastics waste can be recycled and increasing the post-consumer collection of packaging. It is helpful to cover a wide range of materials (Marcilla, Gomez, Reyes-Labarta, Giner &Hernandez, 2003). There is a different challenge in a different stage of plastic recycling. It was studied that product who are designing for recycling have strong potential to assist. A regular shopping basket can be recycled from 20 to 50% (Marcilla, Beltran,&Navarro,2007). There are broad running policies which are helpful to promote the use of environmental design principles (Park, 2008).

Recycled resins help increase the process of recycling. Post consumers collection is useful in case of firm packaging, and it is problematic during the stage of collecting and sorting the plastics. Due to the different handling characteristic feature of firm packaging, there is a problem in handling the flexible plastic packaging (Zhang, Hirose, Nishio, Morioka, Azuma, Ueno, Ohkita & Okada, 1995; Achilias, Giannoulis & Papageorgiou, 2009; Olazar, Lopez, Amutio, Elordi, Aguado & Bilbao, 2009). It is a significant challenge in plastic recycling. Low weight to volume ratio of plastic bags makes it less economically valuable. It is less feasible to invest in the collecting and sorting process (Pinto, Franco, Andre, Miranda, Gulyurtlu & Cabrita, 2002). Shrink wrap of pallets and boxes can be recycled into insufficient condition. So, it increases the recycling of films and flexible packaging. This process increases the investment in the sorting process for handling the mixed plastic wastes. For the recycling of mixed plastics, plastics are separated on high levels of purity. This increase the development of polymer recycle stream (Puente & Sedran, 1998).

The efficiency of post-consumer packaging recycling could be noticeably enlarged based on efficient diversity of materials. It is hard to sort the plastics from bottles, jars and PET, etc. and then make the recycled resins with minimum cross-contamination. It is a challenging role in recycling (Ryu, Sharifi& Swithenbank, 2007). In this process, there is a loss of rejected material occurs which increase the significance of resins. Improvement in the area of sorting with recycling the plants gives the possibility for higher recycling volumes. There should be an improvement in maximizing the quantity and quality of resins.

Recycled plastics help produce new products. The production of the virgin polymer decreases the use of oil usages and emissions of greenhouse gases (Sasse & Emig, 1998). If plastics are making the same products after recycling which can easily be produced from wood or other materials, then there will be no requirement of savings the polymers. There will be another way of the benefit for such type of materials usages. It depends on case to case. Chemical recycling technologies assure the principle of materials improvement (Fig.1). But it is costly than mechanical recycling with less favor of the depolymerized process (Scheirs, & Kaminsky, 2006).

The energy which comes from the combustion of waste plastics helps reduce the volume of landfill. It does not decrease the demand for fossil fuels. There are a lot of environmental concerns are associated with this factor (Seo, Lee & Shin, 2003). Due to the low price of petrochemicals in comparison with high process and plant, it is necessary subsidies. The primary target of recycling is to reduce plastic production and save more energy during the recycling process (Serrano, Aguado, Escola, Rodriguez, Morselli & Orsi, 2003). There is a more environmental benefit in mechanical recycling than landfill and incineration.

PUBLIC EFFORTS AND GOVERNMENT SUPPORT FOR RECYCLING

Nowadays people are more aware of sustainable production as well as consumption. It gives support for the recycling process. This awareness is encouraging companies to manufacture recycled products. There is small business have been developing to organize the recyclables at different places. But still, a large portion of the public needs to aware about to understand the value of the environment (Grause, Sugawara, Mizoguchi & Yoshioka,2009).This kind of public need to mindful of the confirmation to recycled content. Recycling of packaging can be a positive characteristic than exaggerated claims for recyclability.

Participation in recycling process comes under the clean environmental support. According to the maximum survey, the population is still participating in kerbside collection (Siddiqui, Achilias, Redhwi, Bikiaris, Katsogiannis, & Karayannidis, 2010).

Governments are providing support for the recycling process. There are a lot of policies started in recycling. For the recovery and recycling of packaging, there is a lot of procedure has been launched. The government provides funds for the reduction of waste activities. The market value has been increased over the last few years (Hayashi, 1998; Kim, Bo-kyung, Youngmin, Myungwan, &Beom-Sik, 2009; Kosmidis, Achilias & Karayannidis, 2001).

To increase the rate of collection of bottles, schemes are effective like container deposited scheme and kerbside collection scheme. In some countries like Australia, the collection rate of recycling bottles are more than in other countries. The number of bottles in the litter was abridged compared to other states (Sifniades, Levy, & Hendrix, 1999).

The feasibility of thermoplastic recycling is affecting due to economic drivers. The recycled polymer compares with a virgin polymer, and the cost of the recycling process is the main factor. An additional issue with this is the quantity and quality supply in comparison to virgin plastic. Lacking in the information on the recycled product increases the discouragement to use recycled material (Singhal, Singhal & Upadhyayula, 2010; Sifniades, Levy, & Hendrix, 1999).

Landfill or incineration is a conventional method for waste disposal. The cost of this process varies among the regions. It depends on geologically and availability of land use (Slapak, Kasteren & Drinkenburg, 1999]. Due to the volcanic effect, landfill process is costly in Japan. Due to the problematic nature of the land, the landfill is hard in Japan. In the Netherlands, it is also expensive due to permeability from the sea. Waste disposal costs are a common economic inducement in the recycling process. Where the population is suitably high, there is more chance to collect the plastic from the household (Suyama, Masafumi, Masamitsu, Hiroyuki, 2010). Collection of bottles varies with locality and sorting the bottles. In rural areas, people deliver their waste for the recycling process. There is a reverse vending machine, which is available in some supermarkets. But in the case of post-consumer waste, it is not active (Smolders & Baeyens, 2004). The cost of virgin oil affects the price of virgin plastic. It is the primary feedstock for plastic production. The plastic recovery is less than virgin plastics. The amount of oil is increasing in the last few years. The quality of recovered plastic is less than virgin plastic. The higher price of oil increases the cost of collection and reprocessing method. It is not technically possible to add recovered plastic to virgin polymer without reducing some quality attributes of the virgin plastics such as color, clarity or mechanical properties. Most uses of recycled resin are to blend the recycled resin with virgin resin or done with polyolefin films for other multi-layer application (Tongamp, Kano, Zhang, & Saito, 2008; Sterling, Walline, & McCoy, 2001; Uemichi, Makino & Kanazuka,1989).

CONCLUSION

In summary, recycling is the process to end the plastics products and make them reusable. It is a good process for economically and environmentally. Nowadays, the recovery of plastics is increasing. It is challenging from a technological factor and social behavior. People are supporting in this recycling process. Government is providing different policies to make life easy for people due to recycling. In some places, people need to encourage more for this recycling process to make the environment clean. People need to use maximum recycle bags to remove waste disposal. Collecting and sorting are the critical factors for recycling which can be easy to support the system.

Recycling of PET bottles gives profit in the emission of greenhouse gas CO_2. Almost 1.6 tonnes of CO_2 during the recycle process provide energy consumption with a reduction in landfill. This emission of CO_2 during the recycling process offers a useful guideline for the policy. A recycling method of virgin PET provides a 30% reduction in emission. In the case of mixed plastics which provide less than 1 tons, CO_2 is a less favorable source of the recycled polymer. Recycling of mixed plastics provides more benefits as compared to landfill and energy recovery (Shin, Yoshioka, & Okuwaki, 1998).

Plastic recycling is one of the major approaches for the end of life of plastic products. It is an approach toward economically as well as environmentally for recycling the plastics. But still, some challenges exist due to technological factor and from social behavior. It is related to collecting the recycle waste and exchange for virgin material. Recycling is an effective way to improve the environment and polymer industry.

ACKNOWLEDGMENT

We gratefully acknowledge support from the Ministry of Science and Technology and Department of Science and Technology, Government of India under the scheme of Establishment of Women Technology Park, for providing the necessary financial support to carry out this study vide letter No, F. No SEED/WTP/063/2014.

REFERENCES

Achilias, D. S. (2006). Chemical recycling of poly (methyl methacrylate). *WSEAS Transactions on Environment and Development*, *2*(2), 85–91.

Achilias, D. S. (2007). Chemical recycling of poly (methyl methacrylate) by pyrolysis. The potential use of the liquid fraction as a raw material for the reproduction of the polymer. *European Polymer Journal*, *43*(6), 2564–2575. doi:10.1016/j.eurpolymj.2007.02.044

Achilias, D. S., Antonakou, E. V., Koutsokosta, E., & Lappas, A. A. (2009). Chemical recycling of polymers from waste electric and electronic equipment. *Journal of Applied Polymer Science*, *114*(1), 212–221. doi:10.1002/app.30533

Achilias, D. S., Antonakou, E. V., Roupakias, C., Megalokonomos, P., & Lappas, A. A. (2008). Recycling techniques of polyolefins from plastic wastes. *Global NEST Journal*, *10*(1), 114–122.

Achilias, D. S., Giannoulis, A., & Papageorgiou, G. Z. (2009). Recycling of polymers from plastic packaging materials using the dissolution/ reprecipitation technique. *Polymer Bulletin*, *63*(3), 449–465. doi:10.100700289-009-0104-5

Achilias, D. S., Kanellopoulou, I., Megalokonomos, P., Antonakou, E., & Lappas, A. (2007). Chemical Recycling of Polystyrene by Pyrolysis: Potential Use of the Liquid Product for the Reproduction of Polymer. *Macromolecular Materials and Engineering*, *292*(8), 923–934. doi:10.1002/mame.200700058

Achilias, D. S., & Karayannidis, G. P. (2004). The chemical recycling of PET in the framework of sustainable development. *Water Air and Soil Pollution Focus*, *4*(4/5), 385–396. doi:10.1023/B:WAFO.0000044812.47185.0f

Achilias, D. S., Megalokonomos, P., & Karayannidis, G. P. (2006). Current trends in chemical recycling of polyolefins. *Journal of Environmental Protection and Ecology*, *7*(2), 407–413.

Achilias, D. S., Redhwi, H. H., Siddiqui, M. N., Nikolaidis, A. K., Bikiaris, D. N., & Karayannidis, G. P. (2010). Glycolytic Depolymerization of PET Waste in a Microwave Reactor. *Journal of Applied Polymer Science*, *118*(5), 3066–3073. doi:10.1002/app.32737

Achilias, D. S., Roupakias, C., Megalokonomosa, P., Lappas, A. A., & Antonakou, E. V. (2007). Chemical recycling of plastic wastes made from polyethylene (LDPE and HDPE) and polypropylene (PP). *Journal of Hazardous Materials*, *149*(3), 536–542. doi:10.1016/j.jhazmat.2007.06.076 PMID:17681427

Achilias, D. S., Tsintzou, G. P., Nikolaidis, A. K., Bikiaris, D. N., & Karayannidis, G. P. (2011). Aminolytic depolymerization of poly (ethylene terephthalate) waste in a microwave reactor. *Polymer International*, *60*(3), 500–506. doi:10.1002/pi.2976

Aguado, J., & Serrano, D. P. (1999). *Feedstock recycling of plastic wastes*. Cambridge, UK: The Royal Society of Chemistry.

Aguado, R., Olazar, M., Gaisan, B., Prieto, R., & Bilbao, J. (2003). Kinetics of polystyrene pyrolysis in a conical spouted bed reactor. *Chemical Engineering Journal*, *92*(1-3), 91–99. doi:10.1016/S1385-8947(02)00119-5

Aguado, R., Olazar, M., San José, M. J., Gaisán, B., & Bilbao, J. (2002). Wax formation in the pyrolysis of polyolefins in a conical sprouted bed reactor. *Energy & Fuels*, *16*(6), 1429–1437. doi:10.1021/ef020043w

Aguayo, A. T., Gayubo, A. G., Ortega, J. M., Olazar, M., & Bilbao, J. (1997). Catalyst deactivation by cooking in the MTG process in fixed and fluidized bed reactors. *Catalysis Today*, *37*(3), 239–248. doi:10.1016/S0920-5861(97)00015-1

Akpanudoh, N. S., Gobin, K., & Manos, G. (2005). Catalytic degradation of plastics waste to liquid fuel over commercial cracking catalyst. *Journal of Molecular Catalysis A Chemical*, *235*(1-2), 67–73. doi:10.1016/j.molcata.2005.03.009

Al-Salem, S. M., & Lettieri, P. (2010). Kinetic study of high-density polyethylene (HDPE) pyrolysis. *Chemical Engineering Research & Design*, *88*(1212A), 1599–1606. doi:10.1016/j.cherd.2010.03.012

Al-Salem, S. M., Lettieri, P., & Baeyens, J. (2009). Recycling and recovery routes of plastic solid waste (PSW): A review. *Waste Management (New York, N.Y.)*, *29*(10), 2625–2643. doi:10.1016/j.wasman.2009.06.004 PMID:19577459

Al-Salem, S. M., Lettieri, P., & Baeyens, J. (2010). The valorization of plastic solid waste (PSW) by primary to quaternary routes: From re-use to energy and chemicals. *Progress in Energy and Combustion Science*, *36*(1), 103–129. doi:10.1016/j.pecs.2009.09.001

Ali, M. F., & Siddiqui, M. N. (2005). Thermal and catalytic decomposition behavior of PVC mixed plastic waste with petroleum residue. *Journal of Analytical and Applied Pyrolysis*, *74*(1-2), 282–289. doi:10.1016/j.jaap.2004.12.010

Arandes, J. M., Abajo, I., Lopez-Valerio, D., Fernández, I., Azkoiti, M. J., Olazar, M., & Bilbao, J. (1997). Transformation of several plastic wastes into fuels by catalytic cracking. *Industrial & Engineering Chemistry Research*, *36*(11), 4523–4529. doi:10.1021/ie970096e

Arandes, J. M., Erena, J., Azkoiti, M. J., Olazar, M., & Bilbao, J. (2003). Thermal recycling of polystyrene and polystyrene-butadiene dissolved in a light cycle oil. *Journal of Analytical and Applied Pyrolysis*, *70*(2), 747–760. doi:10.1016/S0165-2370(03)00056-1

Araujo, A. S., Fernandes, V. J. Jr, & Fernandes, G. J. T. (2002). Thermogravimetric kinetics of polyethylynedegradation over silicoaluminophosphate. *Thermochimica Acta*, *392*, 55–61. doi:10.1016/S0040-6031(02)00072-2

Bajdur, W., Pajaczkowska, J., Makarucha, B., Sulkowska, A., & Sulkowski, W. W. (2002). Effective polyelectrolytes synthesized from expanded polystyrene wastes. *European Polymer Journal*, *38*(2), 299–304. doi:10.1016/S0014-3057(01)00191-4

Ballice, L., & Reimert, R. (2002). Temperature-programmed co-pyrolysis of Turkish lignite with polypropylene. *Journal of Analytical and Applied Pyrolysis*, *65*(2), 207–219. doi:10.1016/S0165-2370(01)00195-4

Beltrame, P. L., Bergamasco, L., Carniti, P., Castelli, A., Bertini, F., & Audisio, G. (1997). Hydrous pyrolysis of polystyrene. *Journal of Analytical and Applied Pyrolysis*, *40*, 451–461. doi:10.1016/S0165-2370(96)00977-1

Berrueco, C., Mastral, F. J., Esperanza, E., & Ceamanos, J. (2002). Production of waxes and tars from the continuous pyrolysis of high-density polyethylene. Influence of operation variables. *Energy & Fuels*, *16*(5), 1148–1153. doi:10.1021/ef020008p

Bhaskar, T., Uddin, M. A., Murai, K., Kaneko, J., Hamano, K., Kusaba, T., ... Sakata, Y. (2003). Comparison of thermal degradation products from real municipal waste plastic and model mixed plastics. *Journal of Analytical and Applied Pyrolysis*, *70*(2), 579–587. doi:10.1016/S0165-2370(03)00027-5

Bockhorn, H., Donner, S., Gernsbeck, M., Hornung, A., & Hornung, U. (2001). Pyrolysis of Polyamide 6 under Catalytic Conditions and its Application to Reutilization of Carpets. *Journal of Analytical and Applied Pyrolysis*, *58*, 79–84. doi:10.1016/S0165-2370(00)00187-X

Bockhorn, H., Hornung, A., Hornung, U., & Jakobstroer, P. (1999). Modeling of isothermal and dynamic pyrolysis of plastics considering nonhomogeneous temperature distribution and detailed degradation mechanism. *Journal of Analytical and Applied Pyrolysis*, *49*(1-2), 53–74. doi:10.1016/S0165-2370(98)00130-2

Bodrero, S., Canivenc, E., & Cansell, F. (1999). Chemical Recycling of Polyamide 6.6 and Polyamide 6 through a Two-Step Ami-/Ammonolysis Process. Presentation at *4th Annual Conference on Recycling of Fibrous Textile and Carpet Waste*, Dalton, GA.

Borgianni, C., Filippis, P.D., Pochetti, F., & Paolucci, M. (2002). *Gasification process of wastes 58 Material Recycling – Trends and Perspectives*. Academic Press.

Cerqueira, H. S., Caeiro, G., Costa, L., & Ramoa Ribeiro, F. (2008). Deactivation of FCC Catalyst. *Journal of Molecular Catalysis. Chem*, *292*, 1–13.

Chaupart, N., Serpe, G., & Verdu, J. (1998). Molecular weight distribution and mass changes during polyamide hydrolysis. *Polymer*, *39*(6-7), 1375–1380. doi:10.1016/S0032-3861(97)00414-X

Chiu, S. J., Chen, S. H., & Tsai, C. T. (2006). Effect of metal chlorides on thermal degradation of (waste) polycarbonate. *Waste Management (New York, N.Y.)*, *26*(3), 252–259. doi:10.1016/j.wasman.2005.03.003 PMID:16387239

Corbin, T., Handermann, A., Kotek, R., Porter, W., Dellinger, J., & Davis, E. (1999). *Reclaiming epsilon-caprolactam from nylon 6 carpet*. U.S. Patent 5,977,193.

Czernik, S., Elam, C., Evans, R., Meglen, R., Moens, L., & Tatsumoto, K. (1998). Catalytic Pyrolysis of Nylon 6 to Recover Caprolactam. *Journal of Analytical and Applied Pyrolysis*, *56*(1), 51–64. doi:10.1016/S0165-2370(98)00068-0

Dawood, A., & Miura, K. (2001). Pyrolysis kinetics of g-irradiated polypropylene. *Polymer Degradation & Stability*, *73*(2), 347–354. doi:10.1016/S0141-3910(01)00096-9

Dawood, A., & Miura, K. (2002). Catalytic pyrolysis of g-irradiated polypropylene (PP) over HY zeolite for enhancing the reactivity and the product selectivity. *Polymer Degradation & Stability*, *76*(1), 45–52. doi:10.1016/S0141-3910(01)00264-6

De Marco, I., Caballero, B., Torres, A., Laresgoiti, M. F., Chomón, M. J., & Cabrero, M. A. (2002). Recycling polymeric wastes by means of pyrolysis. *Journal of Chemical Technology and Biotechnology (Oxford, Oxfordshire)*, *77*(7), 817–824. doi:10.1002/jctb.636

Duangchan, A., & Samart, C. (2008). Tertiary recycling of PVC-containing plastic waste by copyrolysis with cattle manure. *Waste Management (New York, N.Y.)*, *28*(11), 2415–2421. doi:10.1016/j.wasman.2007.12.010 PMID:18314324

Durmus, A., Koc, S. N., Pozan, G. S., & Kasgoz, A. (2005). Thermal-catalytic degradation kinetics of polypropylene over BEA, ZSM-5 and MOR zeolites. *Applied Catalysis B: Environmental*, *61*(3-4), 316–322. doi:10.1016/j.apcatb.2005.06.009

Elordi, G., López, G., Aguado, R., Olazar, M., & Bilbao, J. (2007). Catalytic pyrolysis of high-density polyethylene on a HZSM-5 zeolite catalyst in a conical spouted bed reactor. *International Journal of Chemical Reactor Engineering*, *5*(1), 72. doi:10.2202/1542-6580.1567

Elordi, G., Olazar, M., Aguado, R., López, G., Arabiourrutia, M., & Bilbao, J. (2007). Catalytic pyrolysis of high-density polyethylene in a conical spouted bed reactor. *Journal of Analytical and Applied Pyrolysis*, *79*(1-2), 450–455. doi:10.1016/j.jaap.2006.11.010

Elordi, G., Olazar, M., Lopez, G., Amutio, M., Artetxe, M., Aguado, R., & Bilbao, J. (2009). Catalytic pyrolysis of HDPE in continuous mode over zeolite catalyst spouted bed reactor. *Journal of Analytical and Applied Pyrolysis*, *85*(1-2), 345–351. doi:10.1016/j.jaap.2008.10.015

Faravelli, T., Bozzano, G., Colombo, M., Ranzi, E., & Dente, M. (2003). Kinetic modeling of the thermal degradation of polyethylene and polystyrene mixtures. *Journal of Analytical and Applied Pyrolysis*, *70*(2), 761–777. doi:10.1016/S0165-2370(03)00058-5

Fernandes, G. J. T., Fernandes, V. J. Jr, & Araujo, A. S. (2002). Catalytic degradation of polyethylene over SAPO-37 molecular sieve. *Catalysis Today*, *75*(1-4), 233–238. doi:10.1016/S0920-5861(02)00074-3

Garcia, D., Balart, R., Sanchez, L., & Lopez, J. (2007). Compatibility of recycled PVC/ABS blends effect of previous degradation. *Polymer Engineering and Science*, *47*(6), 789–796. doi:10.1002/pen.20755

Grause, G., Predel, M., & Kaminsky, W. (2006). Monomer recovery from aluminum hydroxide high filled poly (methyl methacrylate) in a fluidized bed reactor. *Journal of Analytical and Applied Pyrolysis*, *75*(2), 236–239. doi:10.1016/j.jaap.2005.06.006

Grause, G., Sugawara, K., Mizoguchi, T., & Yoshioka, T. (2009). Pyrolytic hydrolysis of polycarbonate in the presence of earth-alkali oxides and hydroxides. *Polymer Degradation & Stability*, *94*(7), 1119–1124. doi:10.1016/j.polymdegradstab.2009.03.014

Guisnet, M., Costa, L., & Ribeiro, F. R. (2009). Prevention of zeolite deactivation by cooking. *Journal of Molecular Catalysis A Chemical*, *305*(1-2), 69–83. doi:10.1016/j.molcata.2008.11.012

Hájeková, E., & Bajus, M. (2005). Recycling of low-density polyethylene and polypropylene via copyrolysis of polyalkene oil/waxes with naphtha: Product distribution and coke formation. *Journal of Analytical and Applied Pyrolysis*, *74*(1-2), 270–281. doi:10.1016/j.jaap.2004.11.016

Hayashi, J.-I., Nakahara, T., Kusakabe, K., & Morooka, S. (1998). Pyrolysis of polypropylene in the presence of oxygen. *Fuel Processing Technology*, *55*(3), 265–275. doi:10.1016/S0378-3820(98)00047-2

Heyde, M., & Kremer, S. (1999). LCA Packaging Plastics Waste. LCA Documents. *Material Recycling – Trends and Perspectives, 2*, 60.

Kim, D., Kim, B.-K., Cho, Y., Han, M., & Kim, B. S. (2009). Kinetics of polycarbonate glycolysis in ethylene glycol. *Industrial & Engineering Chemistry Research, 48*(2), 685–691. doi:10.1021/ie8010947

Kim, J. S., Lee, W. Y., Lee, S. B., Kim, S. B., & Choi, M. J. (2003). Degradation of polystyrene waste over base promoted Fe catalysts. *Catalysis Today*, *87*(1-4), 59–68. doi:10.1016/j.cattod.2003.10.004

Kosmidis, V., Achilias, D. S., & Karayannidis, G. P. (2001). Poly (ethylene terephthalate) recycling and recovery of pure terephthalic acid. Kinetics of a phase-transfer catalyzed alkaline hydrolysis. *Macromolecular Materials and Engineering*, *286*(10), 640–647. doi:10.1002/1439-2054(20011001)286:10<640::AID-MAME640>3.0.CO;2-1

Kruse, T. M., Woo, O. S., & Broadbelt, L. J. (2001). Detailed mechanistic modeling of polymer degradation: Application to polystyrene. *Chemical Engineering Science*, *56*, 971–979. doi:10.1016/S0009-2509(00)00312-2

La Mantia, F. P. (1996). *Recycling of PVC and mixed plastic waste*. Toronto: ChemTec Publishing.

Lee, C. G., Cho, Y. J., Song, P. S., Kang, Y., Kim, J. S., & Choi, M. J. (2003). Effects of temperature distribution on the catalytic pyrolysis of polystyrene waste in a swirling fluidizedbed reactor. *Catalysis Today*, *79*, 453–464. doi:10.1016/S0920-5861(03)00060-9

Lee, G.-S., & Song, Y. J. B. (2007). Recycling EAF dust by heat treatment with PVC. *Minerals Engineering*, *20*(8), 739–746. doi:10.1016/j.mineng.2007.03.001

Lee, K. H., Noh, N. S., Shin, D. H., & Seo, Y. (2002). Comparison of plastic types for catalytic degradation of waste plastics into liquid product with spent FCC catalyst. *Polymer Degradation & Stability*, *78*(3), 539–544. doi:10.1016/S0141-3910(02)00227-6

Lee, S. Y., Yoon, J. H., Kim, J. R., & Park, D. W. (2002). Degradation of polystyrene using clinoptilolite catalysts. *Journal of Analytical and Applied Pyrolysis*, *64*(1), 71–83. doi:10.1016/S0165-2370(01)00171-1

Lin, Y.-H., & Yang, M.-H. (2007). Chemical catalysed recycling of waste polymers: Catalytic conversion of polypropylene into fuels and chemicals over spent FCC catalyst in a fluidised-bed reactor. *Polymer Degradation & Stability*, *92*(5), 813–821. doi:10.1016/j.polymdegradstab.2007.01.028

Lin, Y.-H., & Yen, H.-Y. (2005). Fluidised bed pyrolysis of polypropylene over cracking catalysts for producing hydrocarbons. *Polymer Degradation & Stability*, *89*(1), 101–108. doi:10.1016/j.polymdegradstab.2005.01.006

Liu, F.-S., Lei, L., Shitao, Y., Zhiguo, L., & Xiaoping, G. (2011). Methanolysis of polycarbonate catalysed by ionic liquid. *Journal of Hazardous Materials*, *189*(1-2), 249–254. doi:10.1016/j.jhazmat.2011.02.032 PMID:21402441

Liu, F.-S., Zhuo, L., Shi-Tao, Y., Xiao, C., Cong-Xia, X., & Xiao-Ping, G. (2009). Methanolysis and hydrolysis of polycarbonate under moderate conditions. *Journal of Polymers and the Environment*, *17*(3), 208–211. doi:10.100710924-009-0140-0

Machado, H. M. A. M. M. S., Rodrigues, F. G., Assunc, R. M. N., Soares, H. M., Cangani, A. P., & Cerqueira, D. A. (2010). Chemical recycling of poly (vinyl chloride): Application of partially dehydrochlorinated poly (vinyl chloride) for producing a chemically modified polymer. *Journal of Analytical and Applied Pyrolysis*, *115*, 1474–1479.

Maharana, T., Negi, Y. S., & Mohanty, B. (2007). Review Article: Recycling of Polystyrene. *Plastics Technology and Engineering*, *46*(7), 729–736. doi:10.1080/03602550701273963

Marcilla, A., Beltran, M. I., Hernandez, F., & Navarro, R. (2004). HZSM5 and HUSY deactivation during the catalytic pyrolysis of polyethylene. *Applied Catalysis A, General*, *278*(1), 37–43. doi:10.1016/j.apcata.2004.09.023

Marcilla, A., Beltran, M. I., & Navarro, R. (2007). Study of the deactivation process of HZSM5 zeolite during polyethylene pyrolysis. *Applied Catalysis A, General*, *333*(1), 57–66. doi:10.1016/j.apcata.2007.09.004

Marcilla, A., Gómez, A., García, A. N., & Olaya, M. M. (2002). Kinetic study of the catalytic decomposition of the different commercial polyethylenes over an MCM-41 catalyst. *Journal of Analytical and Applied Pyrolysis*, *64*(1), 85–101. doi:10.1016/S0165-2370(01)00174-7

Marcilla, A., Gomez, A., Reyes-Labarta, J. A., Giner, A., & Hernandez, F. (2003). Kinetic study of polypropylene pyrolysis using ZSM-5 and an equilibrium fluid catalytic cracking catalyst. *Journal of Analytical and Applied Pyrolysis*, *68*, 46–48.

Mastellone, M. L., Perugini, F., Ponte, M., & Arena, U. (2002). Fluidized bed pyrolysis of a recycled polyethylene. *Polymer Degradation & Stability*, *76*(3), 479–487. doi:10.1016/S0141-3910(02)00052-6

Mastral, J., Esperanza, E., García, P., & Juste, M. (2002). Pyrolysis of high-density polyethylene in a fluidized bed reactor:influence of the temperature and residence time. *Journal of Analytical and Applied Pyrolysis*, *63*(1), 1–15. doi:10.1016/S0165-2370(01)00137-1

Mastral, J. F., Berrueco, C., Gea, M., & Ceamanos, J. (2006). Catalytic degradation of high-density polyethylene over nanocrystalline HZSM-5 zeolite. *Polymer Degradation & Stability*, *91*(12), 3330–3338. doi:10.1016/j.polymdegradstab.2006.06.009

Mehta, S., Biederman, S., & Shivkumar, S. (1995). Thermal degradation of foamed polystyrene. *Journal of Materials Science*, *30*(11), 2944–2949. doi:10.1007/BF00349667

Milne, B. J., Behie, L. A., & Berruti, F. (1999). Recycling of waste plastics by ultrapyrolysis using an internally circulating fluidized bed reactor. *Journal of Analytical and Applied Pyrolysis*, *51*(1-2), 157–166. doi:10.1016/S0165-2370(99)00014-5

Mucha, M., (1976). Thermogravimetric studies on polymethylenes and polyethylenes. *Journal of Polymer Science*, 25-31.

Nikles, D. E., & Farahat, M. S. (2005). New motivation for the depolymerization products derived from PET waste: A review. *Macromolecular Materials and Engineering*, *290*, 13–30. doi:10.1002/mame.200400186

Oku, A., Tanaka, S., & Hata, S. (2000). Chemical conversion of poly (carbonate) to bis (hydroxyethyl) ether of bisphenol A. An approach to the chemical recycling of plastic wastes as monomers. *Polymer, 41*(18), 6749–6753. doi:10.1016/S0032-3861(00)00014-8

Olazar, M., Lopez, G., Amutio, M., Elordi, G., Aguado, R., & Bilbao, J. (2009). Influence of FCC catalyst steaming on HDPE pyrolysis product distribution. *Journal of Analytical and Applied Pyrolysis, 85*(1-2), 359–365. doi:10.1016/j.jaap.2008.10.016

Onu, P., Vasile, C., Ciocilteu, S., Iojoiu, E., & Darie, H. (1998). Thermal and catalytic decomposition of polyethylene and polypropylene. *Journal of Analytical and Applied Pyrolysis, 49*(1-2), 145–153. doi:10.1016/S0165-2370(98)00109-0

Onwudili, J. A., Insura, N., & Williams, P. T. (2009). Composition of products from the pyrolysis of polyethylene and polystyrene in a closed batch reactor: Effects of temperature and residence time. *Journal of Analytical and Applied Pyrolysis, 86*(2), 293–303. doi:10.1016/j.jaap.2009.07.008

Onwudilia, J. A., & Williams, P. T. (2016). Catalytic supercritical water gasification of plastics with supported RuO2: A potential solution to hydrocarbonwater pollution problem. *Process Safety and Environmental Protection, 102*, 140–149. doi:10.1016/j.psep.2016.02.009

Oyedun, A. O., Gebreegziabher, T., Ng, D. K. S., & Hui, C. W. (2014). Mixed-waste pyrolysis of biomass and plastics waste: A modeling approach to reduce energy usage. *Energy, 75*, 127–135. doi:10.1016/j.energy.2014.05.063

Panda, A. K., & Singh, R. K. (2011). Catalytic performances of kaoline and silica-alumina in the thermal degradation of polypropylene. *Journal of Fuel Chemistry and Technology, 39*(3), 198–202. doi:10.1016/S1872-5813(11)60017-0

Panda, A. K., Singh, R. K., & Mishra, D. K. (2010). Thermolysis of waste plastics to liquid fuel: A suitable method for plastic waste management and manufacture of value-added products - a world prospective. *Renewable & Sustainable Energy Reviews, 14*(1), 233–248. doi:10.1016/j.rser.2009.07.005

Panepinto, D., Tedesco, V., Brizio, E., & Genon, G. (2015). Environmental performances and energy efficiency for MSW gasification treatment. *Waste and Biomass Valorization, 6*(1), 123–135. doi:10.100712649-014-9322-7

Park, H.-J. (2008). Pyrolysis of polypropylene over mesoporous MCM-48 material. *Journal of Physics and Chemistry of Solids, 69*(5-6), 1125–1128. doi:10.1016/j.jpcs.2007.10.083

Park, J. W., Oh, S. C., Lee, H. P., Kim, H. T., & Yoo, K. O. (2000). Kinetic analysis of thermal decomposition of polymer using a dynamic model. *Korean Journal of Chemical Engineering, 17*(5), 489–496. doi:10.1007/BF02707154

Park, S. S., Seo, D. K., Lee, S. H., Yu, T. U., & Hwang, J. (2012). Study on pyrolysis characteristics of refuse plastic fuel using lab-scale tube furnace and thermogravimetric analysis reactor. *Journal of Analytical and Applied Pyrolysis, 97*, 29–38. doi:10.1016/j.jaap.2012.06.009

Passamonti, F. J., & Sedran, U. (2012). Recycling of waste plastics into fuels. LDPE conversion in FCC. *Applied Catalysis B: Environmental, 125*, 499–506. doi:10.1016/j.apcatb.2012.06.020

Pinto, F., Franco, C., Andre, R. N., Miranda, M., Gulyurtlu, I., & Cabrita, I. (2002). Co-gasification study of biomass mixed with plastic wastes. *Fuel*, *3*(81), 291–297. doi:10.1016/S0016-2361(01)00164-8

Puente, D. L. G., & Sedran, U. (1998). Recycling polystyrene into fuels by means of FCC: Performance of various acidic catalysts. *Applied Catalysis B: Environmental*, *19*(3-4), 305–311. doi:10.1016/S0926-3373(98)00084-8

Ryu, C., Sharifi, V. N., & Swithenbank, J. (2007). Waste pyrolysis and generation of storable char. *International Journal of Energy Research*, *31*(2), 177–191. doi:10.1002/er.1241

Sasse, F., & Emig, G. (1998). Chemical recycling of polymer materials. *Chemical Engineering & Technology*, *21*(10), 777–789. doi:10.1002/(SICI)1521-4125(199810)21:10<777::AID-CEAT777>3.0.CO;2-L

Scheirs, J., & Kaminsky, W. (2006). *Feedstock Recycling and Pyrolysis of Waste Plastics. In Converting Waste Plastics into Diesel and Other Fuels*. Wiley – VCH. doi:10.1002/0470021543

Seo, Y.-H., Lee, K.-H., & Shin, D.-H. (2003). Investigation of catalytic degradation of high-density polyethylene by hydrocarbon group type analysis. *Journal of Analytical and Applied Pyrolysis*, *70*(2), 383–398. doi:10.1016/S0165-2370(02)00186-9

Serrano, D. P., Aguado, J., Escola, J. M., Rodriguez, J. M., Morselli, L., & Orsi, R. (2003). Thermal and catalytic cracking of a LDPE-EVA copolymer mixture. *Journal of Analytical and Applied Pyrolysis*, *68–69*, 481–494. doi:10.1016/S0165-2370(03)00037-8

Shin, S.-M., Yoshioka, T., & Okuwaki, A. (1998). Dehydrochlorination behavior of flexible PVC pellets in NaOH solutions at elevated temperature. *Journal of Applied Polymer Science*, *67*(13), 2171–2177. doi:10.1002/(SICI)1097-4628(19980328)67:13<2171::AID-APP7>3.0.CO;2-B

Siddiqui, M. N., Achilias, D. S., Redhwi, H. H., Bikiaris, D. N., Katsogiannis, K.-A. G., & Karayannidis, G. P. (2010). Hydrolytic Depolymerization of PET in a Microwave Reactor. *Macromolecular Materials and Engineering*, *295*(6), 575–584. doi:10.1002/mame.201000050

Sifniades, S., Levy, A., & Hendrix, J. (1999a). *Process for depolymerizing nylon-containing waste to form caprolactam*. U.S. Patent 5,932,724.

Sifniades, S., Levy, A., & Hendrix, J. (1999b). *Process for depolymerizing nylon-containing whole carpet to form caprolactam*. U.S. Patent 5,929,234.

Singhal, R., Singhal, C., & Upadhyayula, S. (2010). Thermal catalytic degradation of polyethylene over silicoaluminophosphate molecular sieves- A thermogravimetric study. *Journal of Analytical and Applied Pyrolysis*, *89*(2), 313–317. doi:10.1016/j.jaap.2010.09.007

Slapak, M. J. P., Kasteren, J. M. N., & Drinkenburg, B. A. A. H. (1999). Hydrothermal recycling of PVC in a bubbling fluidized bed reactor: The influence of bed material and temperature. *Polymers for Advanced Technologies*, *10*(10), 596–602. doi:10.1002/(SICI)1099-1581(199910)10:10<596::AID-PAT913>3.0.CO;2-J

Smolders, K., & Baeyens, J. (2004). Thermal degradation of PMMA in fluidized beds. *Waste Management (New York, N.Y.)*, *24*(8), 849–857. doi:10.1016/j.wasman.2004.06.002 PMID:15381237

Sterling, W. J., Walline, K. S., & McCoy, B. J. (2001). Experimental study of polystyrene thermolysis to moderate conversion. *Polymer Degradation & Stability*, *73*(1), 75–82. doi:10.1016/S0141-3910(01)00069-6

Suyama, K., Masafumi, K., Masamitsu, S., & Hiroyuki, Y. (2010). Chemical recycling of networked polystyrene derivatives using subcritical water in the presence of an aminoalchocol. *Polymer Degradation & Stability*, *95*(9), 1588–1592. doi:10.1016/j.polymdegradstab.2010.05.034

Tongamp, W., Kano, J., Zhang, Q., & Saito, F. (2008). Simultaneous treatment of PVC and oyster-shell wastes by mechanochemical means. *Waste Management (New York, N.Y.)*, *28*(3), 484–488. doi:10.1016/j.wasman.2007.01.022 PMID:17475466

Uemichi, Y., Makino, Y., & Kanazuka, T. (1989). Degradation of polypropylene to aromatic hydrocarbons over Pt- and Fe- containing activated carbon. *Journal of Analytical and Applied Pyrolysis*, *16*(3), 229–238. doi:10.1016/0165-2370(89)80027-0

Ukei, H., Hirose, T., Horikawa, S., Takai, Y., Taka, M., Azuma, N., & Ueno, A. (2000). Catalytic degradation of polystyrene into styrene and design of recyclable polystyrene with dispersed catalysts. *Catalysis Today*, *62*(1), 67–75. doi:10.1016/S0920-5861(00)00409-0

Ulutan, S. (1998). A recycling assessment of PVC bottles by means of heat impact evaluation on its reprocessing. *Journal of Applied Polymer Science*, *69*(5), 865–869. doi:10.1002/(SICI)1097-4628(19980801)69:5<865::AID-APP4>3.0.CO;2-K

Van, G. R., Serrano, D. P., Aguado, J., García, R., & Rojo, C. (2001). Thermal and catalytic Cracking of polyethylene under mild conditions. *Journal of Analytical and Applied Pyrolysis*, *58*, 127–142.

Vilaplana, F., Ribes-Greus, A., & Karlsson, S. (2006). Degradation of recycled high-impact polystyrene: Simulation by reprocessing and thermooxidation. *Polymer Degradation & Stability*, *91*(9), 2163–2170. doi:10.1016/j.polymdegradstab.2006.01.007

Ward, P. G., Goff, M., Donner, M., Kaminsky, W., & O'Connor, K. E. (2006). A two-stepchemo-biotechnological conversion of polystyrene to a biodegradable thermoplastic. *Environmental Science & Technology*, *40*(7), 2433–2437. doi:10.1021/es0517668 PMID:16649270

Watanabe, M., Yasuaki, M., Takashi, M., Hiroshi, I., Toshiyuki, M., & Katsuhiko, H. (2009). Chemical recycling of polycarbonate in high-pressurehigh-temperature steam at 573 K. *Polymer Degradation & Stability*, *94*(12), 2157–2162. doi:10.1016/j.polymdegradstab.2009.09.010

Westerhout, R. W. J., Waanders, J., Kuipers, J. A. M., & Swaaij, W. P. M. (1997). Kinetics of the low-temperature pyrolysis of polyethene, polypropene, and polystyrene modeling, experimental determination, and comparison with literature models and data. *Industrial & Engineering Chemistry Research*, *36*(6), 1955–1964. doi:10.1021/ie960501m

Williams, P.T., & Williams, E.A. (1998). Recycling plastic waste by pyrolysis. *Journal of the Energy Institute*, *71*, 81-93.

Woo, O. S., Ayala, N., & Broadbelt, L. J. (2000). Mechanistic interpretation of base-catalyzed depolymerization of polystyrene. *Catalysis Today*, *55*(1-2), 161–171. doi:10.1016/S0920-5861(99)00235-7

Wu, Y.-H., Zhou, Q., Zhao, T., Deng, M.-L., Zhang, J., & Wang, Y.-Z. (2009). Poly (ethylene glycol) enhanced dehydrochlorination of poly (vinyl chloride). *Journal of Hazardous Materials*, *163*(2-3), 1408–1411. doi:10.1016/j.jhazmat.2008.07.047 PMID:18723284

Xiao, G., Ni, M.-J., Chi, Y., Jin, B.-S., Xiao, R., Zhong, Z.-P., & Huang, Y.-J. (2009). Gasification characteristics of MSW and an ANN prediction model. *Waste Management (New York, N.Y.)*, *29*(1), 240–244. doi:10.1016/j.wasman.2008.02.022 PMID:18420400

Xie, C., Liu, F., Yu, S., Xie, F., Li, L., Zhang, S., & Yang, J. (2008). Catalytic cracking of polypropylene into liquid hydrocarbons over Zr and Mo modified MCM-41 mesoporous molecular sieve. *Catalysis Communications*, *10*(1), 79–82. doi:10.1016/j.catcom.2008.08.001

Yoshioka, T., Furukawa, K., Sato, T., & Okuwaki, A. (1998). Chemical recycling of flexible PVC by oxygen oxidation in NaOH solutions at elevated temperatures. *Journal of Applied Polymer Science*, *70*(1), 129–135. doi:10.1002/(SICI)1097-4628(19981003)70:1<129::AID-APP13>3.0.CO;2-2

Zhang, Z., Hirose, T., Nishio, S., Morioka, Y., Azuma, N., Ueno, A., ... Okada, M. (1995). Chemical recycling of waste polystyrene into styrene over solid acids and bases. *Industrial & Engineering Chemistry Research*, *34*(12), 4514–4519. doi:10.1021/ie00039a044

Zhao, W., Hasegawa, S., Fujita, J., Yoshii, F., Sasaki, T., Makuuchi, K., ... Nishimoto, S. (1996). Effects of zeolites on the pyrolysis polypropylene. *Polymer Degradation & Stability*, *53*(1), 129–135. doi:10.1016/0141-3910(96)00080-8

KEY TERMS AND DEFINITIONS

Challenges: Mixed plastic recycling is a big challenge in plastic recycling. Government and public are doing mixed effort to solve this problem.

Ecological Influences: Recycling constituents requires energy. Recycled plastic products save energy and raw material in comparison to make new products. After dumping the waste in landfills, it will start emitting greenhouse gases when it starts.

Factors: Plastic recycling is a challenging fact for recycling industry. Some of the struggles have been framed as opportunities for investment. Low energy costs are important factor in virgin plastic production.

Plastic Recycling: It is the process in which waste material after reprocessing converts into useful material. It is a global effort to decrease plastic in the waste stream.

Waste Management: It is the process which requires activities and actions to manage the waste from its inception to its final disposal. It includes collection, treatment, monitoring, and regularization of the waste.

Chapter 21
Plastic Pollution and Its Management in the Age of Globalization With Special Reference to India

Summia Rehman
University of Kashmir, India

Bilal Ahmad Parray
Government Degree College Bijbehara, India

ABSTRACT

Globalization as a process has undeniably been involved in an ever-increasing mobility of both men and material. The ever-increasing mobility and free flow of goods, which also include plastic-made commodities, has turned globalization into a severe cause of plastic pollution for developing countries like India. Consequently, in India, consciously or unconsciously, the large-scale consumption of plastic items has potentially opened its gates for plastic pollution. By taking the aspect of free flow of plastic items into consideration, a process perceived as an integral part of globalization, this chapter explores globalization as a prime cause of plastic pollution in India. Further, this chapter locates the need to view globalization and its free flow of plastic commodities critically, so as to manage the menace of plastic pollution in India.

INTRODUCTION

Globalization has over the years become a buzzword. And Globalization as a complex phenomenon has been full of contradictions, complications and multiple meanings. Due to multiple facets, globalization has emerged as one of the most hotly debated issues of the present era. In its face value it promises a utopian world of uniform development and equal opportunities of progress for human societies living across the globe. And on the other hand its practical form and function has proved it far from being what it seems and what it advocates. Under the rubric of economic development it has been able to achieve

DOI: 10.4018/978-1-5225-9452-9.ch021

a neo imperialistic world, much exploitative and devastating, much complex in evolving a greater capitalistic and corporate sector hegemony undermining the role, sovereignty and status of various states and their welfare programmes. The global neo imperialistic order creating claims of homogeneity has inaugurated and extended levels of differentiation and further exploitation of under developed economies. All that and many more evils associated with globalization seem to have turned it into an unceasing form of unchecked corporate anarchy.

Globalization for its multiple implications has been defined differently. For some, it is a cover concept for global capitalism, and rejoinder to imperialism by assigning it a new face, phase and a fundamental structure. Its functioning involves initiatives taken by capitalist countries in collaboration with a microscopic section of underdeveloped economies. Sensing these detrimental features of globalism it has accordingly been condemned as another form of the imposition of the logic of capital and the market on evermore regions of the world and spheres of life. Being perceived differently globalization, for others, acts an evolutionary historical moment seeking nothing but integration and more modernization. Accordingly they would term it a continuation of modernization, a pivotal force of progress, an expression of increased wealth, an era of greater freedom, determination, democracy and happiness.

To the advocates and defenders, globalization is a welcome process, all beneficial and offering fresh economic opportunities. And on political front it enhances political democratization, cooperation, cultural diversity and the opening to an exciting new world. They presume it as an efficient mean to reduce the extent of global inequality for globalization suggests a homogeneous world. However detractors of globalization view it from opposite direction and they presume it as harmful. By treating it as an advanced stage of capitalistic domination and extension of power based on capital, their belief is that, globalization would bring about increased domination and control by the wealthier overdeveloped nations over the poor underdeveloped countries, thus increasing the hegemony of the "haves" over the "have-nots." In addition, globalization critics assert that globalization produces an undermining of democracy, a cultural homogenization, and increased destruction of natural species and the environment. Globalization to them is simply a kind of economic development that takes a serious toll on the environment.

The complexity of globalization is evident from being curial as subject matter of multiple studies and critically involves number of stakeholders with a lot of history and politics. Globalization is viewed as ever increasing phenomena of multiple implications, perceived both positive as well as negative and a result of intentional and unintentional actions and outcome of profit-oriented strategies. Globalization crucially involves many actors varying from social, political, technological and capital. The list includes commercial markets, social relations, flow of trading goods and essential commodities, decisions of capital and capital possessing nations, evolving technologies, ideas, forms of culture, and people across national boundaries via a global networked society (see Castells 1996, 1997,1998; Held et al. 1999). Capitalist domination is buttressed and hence applied by the invisible hands of technology comprised of computerized networks of communication. The rapid development in the means of communication and transportation and technological revolution helps in the free movement of goods, information and peoples across national boundaries to sustain global order of contemporary times. The Internet based technological infrastructure, computerized networks, satellite-communication systems and allied means provides an infrastructure for the global economy and society (see Gilder1989, 2000; Kaku 1997; Best and Kellner 2001). From this perspective, any understanding of globalization requires to comprehend the scientific and technological revolutions offering scope for global restructuring of capital and globalization. The current order of globalization completely relies on scientific infrastructure provided by globally interconnected network of computer and capital.

Theorists of globalization recognize the fundamental importance of scientific and technological revolution assigning space to institutions of capitalism. But at the same time there is a need to avoid the extremes of technological and economic determinism. Jean Baudrillard (1993), believes technologies of information and social reproduction (e.g., simulation) have entered every aspect of society and created a new social environment wherein humanity has left behind reality and modern conceptions, as well as the world of modernity. Due to technological revolution, the human species is evolving into a novel, postindustrial technosociety, culture, and condition in which technology, knowledge, and information are the axial or organizing principles (Bell 1976). Likewise, the ideologues of the information society act as if technology were an autonomous force and either neglect to theorize the co-evolution of capital and technology or use the advancements of technology to legitimate market capitalism (i.e., Gilder 1989, 2000; Gates 1995, 1999; Friedman 1999). From these economist perspectives, globalization is merely a continuation of previous social tendencies-that is, the logic of capital and domination by corporate and commercial interests of the world economy and culture. Defenders of capitalism, by contrast, present globalization as the triumph of free markets, democracy, and individual freedom (Fukuyama 1992; Friedman 1999). The globalization along with economic development has raised many seriousness challenges of environmental deterioration. The economic development, albeit uneven and largely in western countries, had no doubt took place but much at the cost of harmful effects for environment. Globalization has created various forms of pollution including that of plastics as well.

The multiple perspectives of globalization reveal its complexity making it a multifaceted process. It is much deeper and detrimental that it seems at a certain distance. In a balanced perception on it is reasonable to argue that globalization is favourable for the countries that were formerly having colonies and thus a profound capitalistic advancement. Their advancement in the economic and cultural fields with technological and commercial networks sustained their hegemony in the neo-imperialistic era of globalization. And that globalization is a complex phenomenon has been crucial in developing large scale exchanges, both cultural and commercial, that have boosted the overall pattern of global trade. What is however crucial to understand is that the free flow of capital, labour and goods that constitutes the hall marks of globalization have many ramifications for undeveloped economies.

In the process of free flow of goods, globalization proves economically beneficial for the developed countries. Developed countries that had developed industrial sector much before the rudimentary type of industries of underdeveloped countries, exchanged more goods. Like the colonial era industrial production of developed countries increased to flood markets located in the underdeveloped countries. The free flow of goods was substantially a trade in the favour of old capitalistic countries. From undeveloped countries it was labour that floated freely. Certain goods however floated more freely than the others. Plastic goods due to their varied use reached to the underdeveloped countries in huge quantities. The turning of undeveloped countries into markets for foreign goods, especially plastic goods, economic development like notions no doubt developed but it simultaneously created scope for plastic pollution. Globalization while promoting undeveloped world's integration and further exploitation, it necessarily caught them unprepared to tackle efficiently with the menaces of globalization. And one of the menaces of globalization is plastic pollution which underdeveloped countries are facing in contemporary times.

GLOBALIZATION AND UNDEVELOPED WORLD: A CASE OF INDIA

Globalization in Indian context has proved a process with far-reaching consequences. On account of these consequences it has emerged as a much debated theme in academic as well non academic circles. It is widely being asserted that due to globalization technological developments had ushered in an era of greater contacts, of people staying in close touch, togetherness of different cultures, economic prosperity and has opened up vast channels of communication. Though the various pros and cons associated with the process have hugely been debated over and again through different perspectives, the environmental implications of globalization have somehow been marginalized. The multiple perspectives of globalization largely cover its social, political and economical implications. Such perspectives however ignore environmental impact of globalization. Globalization has an ever increasing impact on Environment and plastic pollution is one of them. Plastic pollution is witnessing a tremendous growth due to the increasing mobility of men and materials. A balanced analysis of whole process of globalization makes it obvious that the process needs to be treated as both essential as well inimical in terms of its large scale impacts. Economic development at the cost of environmental degradation and increasing pollution are two essential features of globalization. These two features become more visible from globalization of developing countries like India and its succumbing to plastic pollution.

Both the advocates and opponents of Globalization, despite their overwhelming differences, share a single thread of unanimity by accepting the extensive mobility as an integral aspect of globalization. The Extensive mobility includes exchange of men, materials, knowledge, cultural values and technology. It is however a remarkably free flow of goods that have emerged as a most visible and undisputable feature of Globalization. But in the free flow of goods across different countries and continents, certain goods have travelled more than others, and certain areas have proved more beneficial markets than the rest. On account of revolutionary advancements in the means of communication and transportation globalization has emerged as a process to facilitate in the free flow of goods. Unlike the past, when volume value ratio determines the nature of trade and commerce, the contemporary global era supports trade of articles and commodities of almost every type without being constrained by considerations of distance or bulky goods. While it is true that globalization favors a free flow of men of materials, the over all process of exchange and mobilization is not as simple as it appears. A closer examination of globalization makes it evident that in the process of free flow of goods plastic items have floated more freely. More so, it is largely developing countries that are witnessing a process of proliferation of plastic products and thus succumbing to plastic pollution. India, one of the emerging economies after opening its gates to globalization has witnessed a phenomenal increase in plastic products and consequently witnessing an increasing plastic pollution.

In contemporary times India is considered as one of the major south Asian economies. After gaining independence in 1947, Indian economy flourished in the name of a mixed economy. However by 1990' the mixed economy faced the impact of globalization. At its place, a new economic order termed as liberalization, privatization and globalization (LPG) was introduced which integrated India with the global economy. By getting open for globalization, Indian economic development began to take multiple strides. India's foreign trade developed and industrial sector too witnessed a big leap. One important aspect of India's opening for a global economy was a rapid development in the plastic products. Due to globalization plastic products proliferated more extensively. This proliferation or massive increase took place due to couple of reasons. Due to global and privatization like initiatives private sector developed in India. Number of industries began to receive active assistance from abroad. The increased assistance, in terms of capital, technology and supervision enhanced production of different products including that of plastic products. Secondly, due to globalization Indian markets were flooded with many foreign goods made up of plastic, partially, wholly or having packaging. The ever increasing number of imports brought in massive quantities of plastic due to which India is now reeling under plastic pollution.

PLASTIC INDUSTRY IN INDIA

In India, especially after globalization, the plastic industry has emerged as a fastest growing sector of economy. The main plastic producing industries in India include the Reliance Industries, Indian Oil Corporation Limited, Haldia Petrochemicals, Bharat Petroleum Corporation Limited, and Gas Authority of India Limited. All of them have made considerable development in last few decades. Apart from catering to the domestic needs such industries also export number of plastic products. With an increased growth of 9.5% in the first half of FY 2018, it is estimated that in the current financial year (FY 2018), exports would cross 8 billion USD. With this progressive trend that had set in there is a hope that exports may double in the next 5 years. Besides, the domestic consumption of plastic goods covers now every walk of life in India. Metro cities, capital cities, urban areas and towns' as well rural areas are equally facing the brunt of massive plastic pollution.

With each passing day the consumption of plastic products in India is progressing. At global level the average consumption of plastic is estimated around of 28 kg. In contrast to it, the average per capita consumption of plastic in India is no doubt less than 11 kg, but the picture is by and large an alarming one. Before being open for globalization, the consumption level of plastic items was considerably very low. Prior to LPG, Plastic products due to less production, distribution and consumption were creating relatively less plastic pollution. The ideal form which was hitherto in existence suffered a visible alteration after being associated with globalization. India turned into an active hub of commercial interactions with the rest of the world. In the entire gamut of active commercial interactions India received a phenomenal increase in plastic products. The alarming situation is affirmed by the reports of Ministry of Petroleum and Natural Gas, Government of India which suggests that the annual per capita consumption in India would be 20 kg by 2022. Further, the World Economic Forum suggests that the volume of plastic production and consumption would considerably increase, thus leading to large amounts of plastic waste generation and related GHG emissions by 2050.

The rapid growth of plastic industry is indebted to its wide use in a variety of sectors, such as the automotive, construction, electronics, healthcare, and textiles. The reports of Plast India Foundation suggest a massive growth rate of the industry. It claims that the industry has witnessed a compound annual growth rate (CAGR) of 10%, in volume terms, from 8.33 million metric tonne per annum (MMTPA) in FY 10 to 13.4 MMTPA in FY 15 and is expected to grow at 10.5% from FY 15 to FY 20 to reach 22 MMTPA. The Swadeshi initiatives of India are further going to enhance this sector of economy having huge environmental impacts. The consumption pattern of plastic products is impressive for having covered sectors like packing infrastructure, automobiles, agriculture and other allied sectors.

In comparison to other goods, the free flow of plastic commodities is substantially much higher due to the general increase in plastic production on global level. Plastic products have increased owing to their many advantages over materials made of glass, wood, leather, and metals. Besides, they are versatile, lightweight, flexible, moisture resistant, strong, and relatively inexpensive. Due to all these factors the current global annual production of plastic represents ~40 kg for each of the 7 billion humans on the planet. In the last decades the plastics industry grows at a rate of 3-5% and is driven by growth in end use markets, such as packaging, automotive, infrastructure, transport rails, and telecommunication mainly from emerging economies (China, India, Brazil, South Africa, South Korea, etc.). Polymers and plastic materials in the last decades continuously substitute metals, glass, paper and other traditional materials for a great variety of applications due to their lightweight and strength, the design flexibility they offer for any shape and durability, and especially the low cost. Plastic products have many advantages over older materials they are versatile, lightweight, flexible, moisture resistant, strong, and relatively inexpensive. Those are the attractive qualities that lead people all over the world to increase very fast the consumption of plastic goods. This general increase in global production of plastic products and corresponding pollution is going to impact India hugely through the hands of globalization. On account of globalization the 'Plastics are proving to be much more mobile than other man-made materials such as ceramics, glass, wooden items, metals and paper. It took ceramics, glass, wood and metals thousands of years to achieve anything resembling a global distribution.

Plastic Pollution

The rapid movement of goods that globalization facilitates has turned India into a big market due to its huge population and geographical size. However plastic products and their consumption yielding a number of harmful wastes are making contemporary India a fertile zone for plastic wastes. Like the other parts of the world in India Plastic waste encompasses a wide range of polymeric materials, including, rubbers, elastomers, textiles, fibers, thermosets and thermoplastics, with some 200 plastics families in production including polyethylene (PE), high-density polyethylene (HDPE) and low-density polyethylene (LDPE), polypropylene (PP), polystyrene (PS), polyvinylchloride (PVC) or Vinyl (V), polyethylene terephthalate (PET), Polycarbonate (Other plastic, suitable for food), nylon, polyvinyl alcohol (PVA) and acrylonitrile butadiene styrene (ABS) synthetic rubbers. Plastics can be fabricated from feedstocks derived from petroleum, natural gas, or bio-renewables. Due to wide scale use of plastics the plastic wastes had become difficult to categorize. Scientists are trying to estimate the overall plastic waste in the form of municipal garbage, fishing gears, plastic tools, kitchen utensils, food packaging, pellets, plastic bags and bottles of water and soft drinks.

The increasing plastic pollution has many harmful effects. It affects environment and the various organisms living on earth. Due to plastic pollution the surroundings look ugly, dirty and congested creating number of diseases. The aquatic life is getting disturbed. The Groundwater is becoming toxicated. The Burning of plastic wastes in the open air releases poisonous chemicals which when inhaled by humans and animals affect their health. In India the major components of plastic waste exists in the form of Water and soft drink bottles, food jar, Cables, plumbing pipes, bottles, packaging, Grocery bags, packaging, Bottle caps, medicine bottles, chips packs, Disposal cups, cutlery, packaging foam, Food packaging, electronic goods, and defense gadget and Fishing nets, clothing, ropes.

MANAGEMENT OF PLASTIC POLLUTION

Due to globalization India is facing a challenge of plastic pollution. Both internal productions as well imports have led phenomenal increase in plastic wastes. Being a highly diversified India has no uniform policy to manage. What it posses are certain measures which are far from being able to cope up with the situation.

Role of Municipalities

Spreading in different parts of India, especially urban areas, number of municipal committees and councils are simply accumulating plastic wastes as a part of solid waste management programmes. From number of towns and cities they collect the wastes and collect the same at place with the notion to reduce the size of an affected area. This method of management though quite unscientific is prevalent all across the India. Almost every town and city in India posses a municipality council or town area committee assigned with the job to maintain cleanliness and to put pollutants including plastic wastes away from such areas. In the smaller towns, waste is deposited by the residents at the kerbside/community garbage bins which are picked up by concerned municipalities and transferred to the disposal site. Likewise in larger cities, the house-to-house collection systems exist. However lack processing plants results in crude methods of waste dumping such as land filling of mixed waste.

Open Burning in Air

Large quantities of plastic waste are set on fire in an unorganized manner. In the absence of any proper treatment the plastic wastes are burned openly causing emission of many harmful gasses. There is no scientific data to estimate the extent of open burning but that seems to be one of the widespread waste management mechanisms especially in rural india.in open burning majority of the plastic waste that are being burned include polybags and multilayer pouches used for food packaging, *gutkha*, and so on.

Recycling Methods

Globalization along with other internal developments in India has been a key factor in production of plastic waste. While globalization turned India into a market for foreign goods especially plastics, India's own capability to produce plastic items too has found a phenomenal increase. The overall consumption of plastic products has been further facilitated by the massive urbanization, ever increasing Growth in population, and improving economic conditions. Due all these factors Plastic waste form close to 8% of the generated solid waste in the contemporary country. The per capita waste generation has seen a steady rise from 0.44 kg/day in 2001 to 0.5 kg/day and has been estimated to be growing at a rate of 1.33% per annum. CPCB reports estimate that the collection efficiency was 80.28% in 2014, out of which only 28.4% was treated. The remaining quantities were disposed of in landfills or open dumps. It is estimated that 94% of plastic waste generated is recyclable and belongs to the thermoplastics family, while the rest 6% are non-recyclable thermoset plastics. Recycling which seems to be a suitable way to tackle with large scale plastic wastes is too in operation. But the problem with recycling is to categorize the various wastes at the base level.

Biodegradable Plastic Items

Another method which is being suggested as an effective instrument towards containing the menace of plastic pollution is use of biodegradable paper. But the overall proposal is going to be too much costly and thus much a favorable preference.

Multiple Uses of Plastic Items

In number of places the customers are being motivated to use single plastic items such as polythene bags for multiple uses or to return to the bags in lieu of some concessions.

Legal Enforcements

Use of polythene is being discouraging by means of laws. Number of laws has been made to decreases the extent of plastic wastes. The Solid Waste Management Rules, 2016, defines the material recovery facilities (MRF) as a facility where non-compostable solid waste can be temporarily stored by local bodies or an agency authorized to facilitate segregation, sorting, and recovery of recyclables by the informal sector before waste is delivered or taken up for processing.32 The Solid Waste Management Rules, 2016, mandates ULBs to set-up MRF for processing sorted dry waste.

To Curb the Menace of Globalization

The problematic aspect of plastic waste management in India is failure to understand the nature of globalization. India is producing number of plastic wastes by hosting number of multinational companies. Besides, almost every type of plastic goods is making way into India. Doubts are being expressed that globalization is westernization in deception and people are being turned into consumers for western goods which are plastic goods. If the same trend continued then India's fate is turn into a dustbin for plastic wastes. Whatever plastic items are imported to India are low rate and hard to be recycled. Thus the increasing quantity of plastic wastes and number of other wastes termed as e wastes are increasing rapidly in India. All this needs to curb the global peace of importing plastic wastes to India. Different states have different patterns of sensitiveness to tackle this pollution. And to manage it solid waste policy, discouraging consumption, multiple uses and jute bag like initiatives are being taken.

At present what is however missing is to prevent the global intrusion of plastic items. Due to globalization number of foreign companies is in trade links with India. They are importing to India plastic in terms in various forms. It is expected that being aware of plastic pollution they are giving some form of shape to the plastic in the form of plastic products and selling the same to India. Such items include a huge list of plastic that is either non-renewable of costing much at time of recycling. The endless imported plastic items are regularly enhancing volume of plastic products leading plastic pollution.

CONCLUSION

Globalization has facilitated in the process of economic development of India. Number of industries has developed due to globalization and number of products is being produced to cater to the demands of India. Globalization has relatively been an effective catalyst in the enhancement of plastic products in India. The ever increasing use of plastic products has enlarged plastic pollution. And the increasing plastic pollution thus requires an effective and well coordinated management to protect India from turning into a dustbin for the global plastic wastes. The free flow of plastic items, especially those difficult to recycle have found more attractive market in India. The middle class families in India in their daily use have begun to use electronic gadgets and other products made up of plastic. The plastic used in such products is difficult to recycle. It seems even the foreign countries are importing such items under a planned scheme to do away with the increasing plastic pollution in their respective countries. And consequently all account of excessive importing of plastic products has turned globalization as a plastic pollution menace for India.

REFERENCES

Albrow, M. (1996). *The Global Age*. Cambridge, UK: Polity Press.

Appadurai, A. (1996). *Modernity at Large*. Minneapolis, MN: University of Minnesota Press.

Aronowitz, S., & Giroux, H. (1985). *Education Under Siege*. New York: Bergin and Garvey.

Aronson, R. (1983). *The Dialectics of Disaster*. London, IL: Verso.

Arrighi, G. 1994. The Long Twentieth Centurv. London, UK: Verso.

Axford, B. (1995). *The Global System*. Cambridge, UK: Polity Press.

Axtmann, R. (Ed.). (1998). *Globalization in European Context*. London, UK: Cassells.

Baudrillard, J. (1993). *Symbolic Exchange and Death*. London, UK: Sage.

Bell, D. (1976). *The Coming of Post-Industrial Society*. New York: Basic Books. doi:10.1080/00131727609336501

Best & Kellner. (1991). *Postmodern Theory: Critical Interrogations*. London, UK: Macmillan and Guilford.

Bird, J., Curtis, B., Putnam, T., & Tickner, L. (Eds.). (1993). Mapping the Futures: Local Cultures, Global Change. London, UK: Routledge.

Boggs, C. (2000). *The End of Politics*. New York: Guilford Press.

Borgmann, A. (1994). *Across the Postmodern Divide*. Chicago, IL: University of Chicago Press.

Bowles, S., & Gintis, H. (1986). *On Democracy*. New York: Basic Books.

Brecher, J., & Costello, T. (1994). *Global Village or Global Pillage: Economic Reconstruction from theBottom Up*. Boston, MA: South End Press.

Brecher, J., Costello, T., & Smith, B. (2000). *Globalization from Below*. Boston, MA: South EndPress.

Bronner, S. E., & Kellner, D. (Eds.). (1989). *Critical Theory and Society: A Reader*. New York: Routledge.

Burbach, R. (2001). *Globalization and Postmodern Politics: From Zapatistas to High-Tech Robber Barons*. London, UK: Pluto Press.

Castells, M. (1996). The Information Age: Economy, Society, and Culture.: Vol. 1. *The Rise of the NetworkSociety*. Oxford, UK: Blackwell.

Cohen, J., & Rogers, J. (1983). *On Democracy*. New York: Penguin.

Cvetkovich, A., & Kellner, D. (1997). *Articulating the Global and the Local: Globalization and CulturalStudies*. Boulder, CO: Westview Press.

Cyberatlas. (n.d.). Retrieved from http://cyberatlas.interet.com/big-picture/demographics

Drew, J. (1998). *Global Communications in the Post-Industrial Age: A Study of the Communications Strategies of U.S. Labor Organizations* (Ph.D. dissertation). University of Texas.

Eisenstein, Z. (1998). *Global Obscenities: Patriarchy, Capitalism, and the Lure of Cyberfantasy*. New York: New York University Press.

Ellul, J. (1964). *The Technological Society*. New York: Knopf.

Featherstone, M. (Ed.). (1990). *Global Culture: Nationalism, Globalization, and Modernity*. London, UK: Sage.

Featherstone, M., Lash, S., & Robertson, R. (Eds.). (1995). *Global Modernities*. London, UK: Sage.

Foran, J. (Ed.). (Forthcoming). *The Future of Revolutions: Rethinking Radical Change in the Age of Globalization*. London, UK: Zed Books.

Fredericks, H. (1994). North American NGO Networking Against NAFTA: The Use of Computer Communicationsin Cross-Border Coalition Building. *XVII International Congress of the Latin American Studies Association*, 1-24.

Friedman, T. (1999). *The Lexus and the Olive Tree*. New York: Farrar Straus Giroux.

Fukuyama, F. (1992). *The End of History and the Last Man*. New York: Free Press.

Gilder, G. (1989). *Microcosm*. New York: Simon and Schuster.

Gilroy, P. (1993). *The Black Atlantic: Modernity and Double Consciousness*. Cambridge, MA: Harvard UniversityPress.

Gottdiener, M. (1995). *Postmodern Semiotics*. Oxford, UK: Blackwell.

Grewal, I., & Kaplan, C. (Eds.). (1994). *Scattered Hegemonies: Postmodernity and Transnational FeministPractices*. Minneapolis, MN: University of Minnesota Press.

Hardt, M., & Negri, A. (2000). *Empire*. Cambridge, MA: Harvard University Press.

Harvey, D. (1989). *The Condition of Postmodernity*. Cambridge, MA: Blackwell.University Press.

Held, McGrew, Goldblatt, & Perraton. (1999). *Global Transformations*. Cambridge.

Hirst & Thompson. (1996). *Globalization in Question*. Cambridge, UK: Polity Press.

Huntington, S. (1996). *The Clash of Civilizations and the Remaking of World Order*. New York: Simon and Schuster.

Jameson, F. (1991). *Postmodernism, or the Cultural Logic of Late Capitalism*. Durham, NC: Duke UniversityPress.

Kaku, M. (1997). *Visions: How Science Will Revolutionize the 21st Century*. New York: Anchor Books.

Kelly, K. (1994). *Out of Control: The New Biology of Machines, Social Systems, and the Economic World*. New York: Addison Wesley.

King, A. D. (Ed.). (1991). *Culture, Globalization, and the World-System: Contemporary Conditions for theRepresentation ofIdentity*. Binghamton, NY: SUNY Art Department. doi:10.1007/978-1-349-11902-8

Laclau, E., & Mouffe, C. (1985). *Hegemony and Socialist Strategy: Toward a Radical DemocraticPolitics*. London, UK: Verso.

Lash, S. (1990). *Sociology of Postmodernism*. London: Routledge.

Lash, S., & Urry, J. (1994). *Economies of Signs and Space*. London, UK: Sage.

Latouche, S. (1996). *The Westernizationof the World*. Cambridge, UK: Polity Press.

Lechner, F. J., & Boli, J. (2000). *The Globalization Reader*. Malden, MA: Blackwell.

Luke, A., & Luke, C. (2000). A Situated Perspective on Cultural Globalization. In Globalization and Education. London, UK: Routledge.

Mander, J., & Goldsmith, E. (1996). *The Case Against the Global Economy*. San Francisco, CA: SierraClub Books.

Marx, K., & Engels, F. (1978). *The Marx-Engels Reader* (2nd ed.). New York: W. W. Norton.

McChesney, R. (1995). *Telecommunications, Mass Media, and Democracy: The Battle for the Control of U.S. Broadcasting, 1928-1935*. New York: Oxford University Press.

Moody, K. (1988). *An Injury to One*. London, UK: Verso.

Polyani, K. (1957). *The Great Transformation*. Boston, MA: Beacon Press. (Original work published 1944)

Ritzer, G. (1996). *The McDonaldization of Society*. Thousand Oaks, CA: Pine Forge Press.

Robertson, R. (1991). *Globalization*. London, UK: Sage.

Robins & Webster. (1999). *Times of the Techno culture*. London, UK: Routledge.

Shenk, D. (1997). *Data Smog: Surviving the Information Glut*. New York: HarperCollins.

Sklair, L. (2001). *The Transnational Capitalist Class*. Cambridge, UK: Blackwell.

Slouka, M. (1995). *War of the Worlds*. New York: Harper and Row.

Soja, E. (1989). *Postmodern Geographies*. London, UK: Verso.

Steger, M. (2002). *Globalism: The New Market Ideology*. Lanham, MD: Rowman and Littlefield.

Stiglitz, J. E. (2002). *Globalization and Its Discontents*. New York: Norton.

Stoll, C. (1995). *Silicon Snake Oil: Second Thoughts on the Information Highway*. New York: Doubleday.

Virilio, P. (1998). The Virilio Reader. Malden, MA: Blackwell Publishers.

Waterman, P. (1992). *Internationallabour Communication by Computer: The Fifth International?* Working.

Waters, M. (1995). *Globalization*. London, UK: Routledge.

Watson, J. L. (Ed.). (1997). *Golden Arches East: McDonald's in East Asia*. Palo Alto, CA: Stanford University Press.

Webster, F. (1995). Theories of the Information Society. London, UK: Routledge. doi:10.4324/9780203991367

Chapter 22
Biodegradation of Plastic
An Innovative Solution to Safe the Human Health and Environment

Shalini Singh
University of Lucknow, India

Pushkar Singh Rawat
University of Lucknow, India

ABSTRACT

The use of plastics is increasing gradually, and its degradation is becoming a great threat for society. This chapter raises a question in front of us: Ultimately, how can we balance our needs and safety? Therefore, a term biodegradation is frequently used to explain the ability of microorganism to degrade the organic substance. The chapter would deliver the importance of biodegradation of plastic products, which is a rapidly growing field and offers a new dimension solution with novel properties in waste management areas. Microorganisms like bacteria, fungi, and actinomycetes have developed a special strategy in order to use such materials as energy and carbon source. Biodegradation is the most economic, eco-friendly, and acceptable method. But the detailed characterization of efficient plastic-degrading microbes and microbial enzymes still needs to be carried out. The chapter would also provide a better understanding related to the biodegradation of plastic products that enhances the horizon of knowledge.

INTRODUCTION

Plastic is a synthetic polymer and it made up of carbon, hydrogen, oxygen, chloride, silicon, and nitrogen. The utility of plastics are increasing day by day to complete our basic needs. The uses of plastics are extensively increases because of their unique property like stability and durability which make it differ from other polymers. But due to the lack of safe disposal and efficient degradation methods of these synthetic polymers, they are gradually accumulated in the environment and posing an ecological threat to vegetation and animals (Bhardwaj et al., 2012). In this chapter we tried to explain the hazardous impacts of plastic and its biodegradation mechanism. Apart from this the chapter also deals with

DOI: 10.4018/978-1-5225-9452-9.ch022

other eco-friendly techniques i.e. Bioplastic which is greatly employed in a new era. A large amount of plastic waste is being generated rapidly worldwide. Out of many countries the India, China and UK contribute 16 million tons, 4.5 million tons and 1 million tons of plastic waste, respectively (Kumar et al., 20011).Many reports stated that India produces nearby 10 thousand tons of plastic waste (Puri et al., 2013). The yearly production of plastic was estimated as 57 million tons in Europe in 2012. Plastic waste recycling has not been focused mainly therefore it create such unsuccessful outcomes; of the over 1 trillion plastic bags dumped per annum in the US, only 5% are recycled. Apparently, waste management (bioremediation) is one of the ways to reduce the adverse effects and can serve as a potential tool in plastic waste decomposition (Shah et al., 2008 b; Ojo et al., 2007 & Ali et al., 2014).Plastic waste is the origin of eight complex problems in the aquatic environment: (1) plastic debris pollutes, (2) plastic entangles marine life, (3) consumption of plastic items by marine fauna, (4) petroleum-based plastic polymers biodegradation is time-consuming, (5) broken plastic and its pellets interrupt the food web, (6) interfere the sediment populations, (7) oceanic litter destroying the primary habitat of new emerging life and (8) marine plastic litter also causes a major damage to vessels. A report on 1970s study stated that out of 247 plankton samples in the Atlantic Ocean, 62% of the samples were found as a plastic material. With such kind of challenges, scientists started their ongoing research to explore whether plastics could be designed to become susceptible to microbial attack, making them degradable in microbial lively surroundings. On the other way researcher also start to search the new application of bioremediation. Biodegradation is nature's technique of recycling wastes, or breaking down organic substance into nutrients that can be used and reused by other organisms. In the microbiological words, "biodegradation" refers to the decaying of all organic materials are carried out by an enormous variety of life forms comprising mainly bacteria, fungi, and other organisms. This proves as one of the crucial, natural, biologically mediated processes that convert the hazardous toxic chemicals into non-toxic or less toxic substances. Microorganisms are involved in the degradation and deterioration of both synthetic and natural polymers. The polymers are not directly consumed by microorganisms whereas most of the biochemical processes takes place. Increasing demand of biological degradation of organic compounds may be considered as an economical and efficient tool for remediating hazardous waste-contaminated surroundings. Whereas some environments may be too severely contaminated for initial in situ treatment to be effective, most contaminated media will use some form of biological degradation in the final treatment phase. The sorting out of wide variety of discarded plastic materials is another typical time consuming process. Another element which also develops a serious issue is related to the combustion of plastic waste. Incineration of plastic polymers causes the release of various poisonous compounds such as hydrogen cyanide into the environment. Moreover the additives like pigments, coatings, fillers etc. present in the plastic restrict the use of recycled material. In such a circumstance, biodegradable plastics offer the best solution to the environmental hazard posed by the conventional plastics. As an alternative to synthetic plastics, biodegradable polymers are a newly emerging field. Various mechanistic roles are played by the microbes according to the polymer type's help us to resolve the problem. This chapter also focuses on mechanism of action of various microorganisms that create an idea to research out other facts associated to this and open a new door for microbial application.

SOURCE OF PLASTIC

Plastic is derived from many sources such as crude oil, coal and natural gas. During the refining process of crude oil, petrol, paraffin, lubricating oils and high petroleum gases are produced as bi-products. These gases are broken down into single unit form known as monomers. Monomers are chemical substances consisting of a single molecule. A process called polymerization occurs when thousands of monomers are linked together and result the formation of complex polymers. Most of the polymers are formed due to the combination of the element carbon with one or more other elements such as oxygen, hydrogen, chlorine, fluorine and nitrogen in various compositions.

TYPES OF POLYMERS

Polymers are differentiated according to their chemical nature, structural arrangement and physical properties etc.

Natural Polymers

Biopolymers and dry material of plants found in nature are the abundant source of natural polymers (Leschine et al., 1995). The plant cell wall constitution differs in the composition of the lignocellulosic biomass (cellulose, hemicellulose and lignin), which provides strength to the plants (Premraj et al., 2005). Lignocelluloses play a critical role in developing plant biomass, in which carbohydrate polymer (cellulose, hemicellulose) and an aromatic polymer (lignin) are the major building blocks of the natural polymer (Perez et al., 2002).

Synthetic Polymers

Plastics are manmade compounds that consist of a long chain of polymeric molecules and unusual bonds, with excessive molecular mass and halogen substitutions. Currently the manufacturing process of plastic involves different inorganic and organic materials, including carbon, hydrogen, chloride, oxygen, nitrogen, coal and natural gases (Shah et al., 2008 a). Low-density polyethylene (LDPE), high-density polyethylene (HDPE), polyvinyl chloride, polystyrene and polypropylene with 23, 17.3, 10.7, 12.3 and 18.5%, respectively, and the remaining 9.7% of other types of polymer are contributing as the most widely used polymers of the plastic waste (Puri et al., 2013). The polymer production in 2012 was estimated as polyethylene 30% (LLDPE and LDPE 18%, HDPE 12%), polypropylene 19%, polyvinyl chloride 11%, polystyrene 7%, polyethylene terephthalate 7% and polyurethanes 7% worldwide (Nerland et al., 2014).

On the basis of plastic's thermal properties, it can be dividing in two groups: thermoplastics and thermosetting polymers.

Thermoplastics

Thermoplastics are wide range of polymers that cannot change their chemical composition easily when heated. Therefore the process of heating, shaping, reheating and reforming can be recurring multiple times. Thermoplastics have linear chain molecule which make it differ from thermosetting plastics.

Different types of polymers such as Polyethylene (PE), polypropylene (PP), polystyrene (PS), polyvinyl chloride (PVC) and polytetrafluoroethylene (PTFE) are included in this group. These polymers are also known as common plastics, range from 20,000 to 500,000 AMU in molecular weight and have different numbers of repeating units derived from a simple monomer unit (Gnanavel et al., 2014).

Thermosetting Plastics

Thermosetting polymers comprise various types of plastics. Due to the heavily cross-linked molecules of thermosetting, these plastics are not recyclable (Gnanavel et al., 2012). Thermoplastics are very stable even at high temperatures they can maintain its rigidity and become non-flexible. Some examples of thermosetting include phenol-formaldehyde, polyester resin, urea, polyurethanes, etc.

DEGRADATION MECHANISM OF PLASTIC

Plastic degradation employed by variety of mechanisms such as mechano-chemical, thermal, catalytic, ozone-induced, photoxidation and biodegradation (Figure 1). All the process of plastic deterioration takes an extremely long time which could engage many years (Pramila et al., 2011). Mechano-chemical is the degradation of polymers by mechanical actions such as mixing and high temperature extrusion is a long established technology in the rubber and plastics industry (Kolbert et al., 1996). Thermo degradation means the degradation of polymer by heat energy. It usually obtained oxygen from the atmosphere so this process is also known as thermo-oxidative degradation. The first stage of degradation involves the breaking in the bonds of macromolecules at specific sites. Thermal degradation usually comprises alterations to molecular weight of polymer. The degradation that takes place in the presence of light is termed as "photodegradation." It is initiated first by the absorption of light energy by the appropriate group present in the polymer molecule. Scission of the polymer molecule at an appropriate position of the chain leading to the conversion to smaller fragments is just because of light absorption. Subsequently, photodegradable polymers require either an in-built photo responsive group in the chain or an additive one (Kyrikou et al., 2007). Photodegradation of polymer comprises UV degradation and oxidation. During UV degradation, the UV light is used to degrade the end product. During the oxidation process, heat is used to break down the plastic waste. Many synthetic polymers have shown the resistant against chemical and physical degradation. While the thermal and physical methods of degradation aid in reducing the molecular weight of the plastic and allow it to compatible for biodegradation. But apart from this biodegradation have many applications over other mechanism. Biodegradation is a cheap, non-hazardous and eco-friendly process. That's why a new era mainly focuses on the application of biodegradation and its impact on the society.

BIODEGRADATION

Biological degradation is usually a biochemical phenomenon that refers to the degradation of organic substances by living organisms particularly microbes. It has been considered as a natural process in the microbial world to take up carbon and energy source for their growth and play a key role in the recycling of materials in the natural ecosystem (Strong, 2006). Microorganisms can play a dynamic role

Table 1. Commonly Used Synthetic Plastics and Its Applications

Name of plastic	Symbol	Application
Polypropylene Terephthalate	01 PET	Soft drink, water and dressing bottles, peanut butter, and jam bars
High-density Polyethylene	2 HDPE	Milk, juice and water bottles, trash and retail bags
Polyvinyl Chloride	3 PVC	Juice bottles, cling films, raincoats, visors, shoe soles, garden hoses, and electricity pipes
Low-density Polyethylene	4 LDPE	Frozen food bags, squeezable bottles, flexible container lids
Polypropylene	5 PP	Bottle caps, drinking straws, medicine bottles, car batteries, disposable syringes
Polystyrene	6 PS	Packing materials, laboratory ware, disposable cups, plates, trays, and cutlery
Others (often polycarbonate)	07 O	Beverage bottles, baby milk bottles, electronic casing

in biodegradation, as reported 90 genera of bacteria, fungi and actinomycetes having the capability to degrade plastic (Mahdiyah et al., 2013). Generally, the biodegradation of plastic is a very slow process, and some microorganisms can't degrade certain type of plastics (Singh et al., 2014). The research on degradability of plastics initiated in the early 1980s and numerous papers provide information on the microbial biodegradation of a variety of plastics such as polyhydroxybutyrate (PHB), polycaprolactone

Figure 1. Various Degradation Methods of Plastic Waste

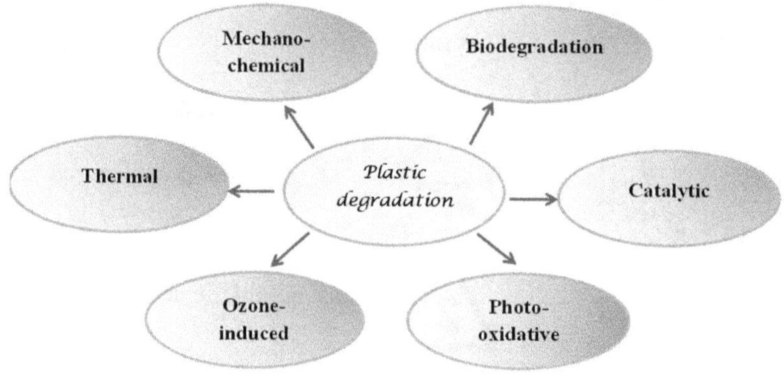

(PCL), polyesters, polylactic acid (PLA), polyurethane PUR, nylon, polyvinyl alcohol (PVA), and polyethylene (PE) (Shimao et al., 2001). Living organisms are involved in the breakdown of plastic material, and consequently the recycled form reverses back to the environment. The term "aging" is used for the change in properties in reference to the polymers. It is utilized as polymer recycling, which reduces the outcome of pollution load (Chandra et al., 1997; Bhardwaj et al., 2012). Anaerobic microbial degradation releases greenhouse gas (methane) in landfills, which increases global warming. Aerobic conditions are essential for fungal degradation while bacterial degradation proceeds in both aerobic as well as anaerobic conditions (Chandra et al., 1998). Plastic can be reduced in an eco-friendly manner with the help of soil microbes and suitable water accessibility. Microorganisms usually involved two types of mechanisms for the biodegradation process.

1. 1. **Aerobic Biodegradation:** This process is well-known as aerobic respiration, aerobic biodegradation play pivotal role in decreasing the natural contaminants at many hazardous waste sites. Aerobic microbes utilize oxygen as an electron acceptor, and break down complex compound into simplest form. Carbon dioxide (CO_2) and water (H_2O) are the by-products of this process (Priyanka et al., 2011).

C plastic + $O_2 \rightarrow CO_2 + H_2O$ + C residual +Biomass

2. 2. **Anaerobic Biodegradation:** Anaerobic biodegradation involves the breakdown of organic contaminants by microorganisms in the absence of oxygen. Various anaerobic microbes use carbon dioxide, nitrate, iron, sulphate and manganese and as their electron acceptors, to break down organic chemicals into smaller compounds.

C plastic $\rightarrow CH_4 + CO_2 + H_2O$ + C residual +Biomass

Polymer molecules are long and insoluble in water so microorganisms are not able to transport the polymers directly into the cells through its outer cell membrane, where most of the biochemical process takes place. In order to use such materials as energy and carbon source, microbes developed a strategy in which they excrete extracellular enzymes that depolymerize the polymers outside the cells and change into simplest form (Gu, 2003; Dvo et al., 2017; Bombelli et al., 2017).The biological degradation of polymeric substances is a complex process involving several subsequent steps induced by the action of various enzymes. The most important type of enzymatic polymer cleavage reaction is hydrolysis (Schink et al., 1992). The bonds such as glycosidic, ester, and peptide linkages are subjected to hydrolysis through nucleophilic attack on the carbonyl carbon atom. Biodegradation mechanism pathways in anaerobic and aerobic conditions are given in Figure 2.

MICROORGANISM INVOLVED IN BIODEGRADATION

Bacteria and fungi are extensively distributed group of microorganisms that play a major role in the treatmentof polymeric compounds in the natural environment(Upreti & Srivastava, 2003).*Micrococcus, Streptomyces*, *Pseudomonas*, *Corynebacterium*, *Arthrobacter*, and *Rhodococcus* are the prominent microbial agents being used for bioremediation (Bhatnagar & Kumari, 2013; Kathiresan, 2003; Dussud & Ghiglione, 2014; Shah et al., 2008a; Kale et al., 2015a, b; Grover et al., 2015; Restrepo-Flórez et al., 2014; Bhardwaj et al., 2012).Some strains that are capable of degrading the PE are *Brevibacillus* spp., *Bacillus* spp., where the proteases synthesize by the bacteriais responsible for degradation(Sivan, 2011). Papain and urease are the other two proteolytic enzymes involve in the degradation of medical polyester PU. Free amine and hydroxyl groups are produced due to the hydrolysis of urethane and urea linkages

Figure 2. Aerobic and Anaerobic Biodegradation Pathways

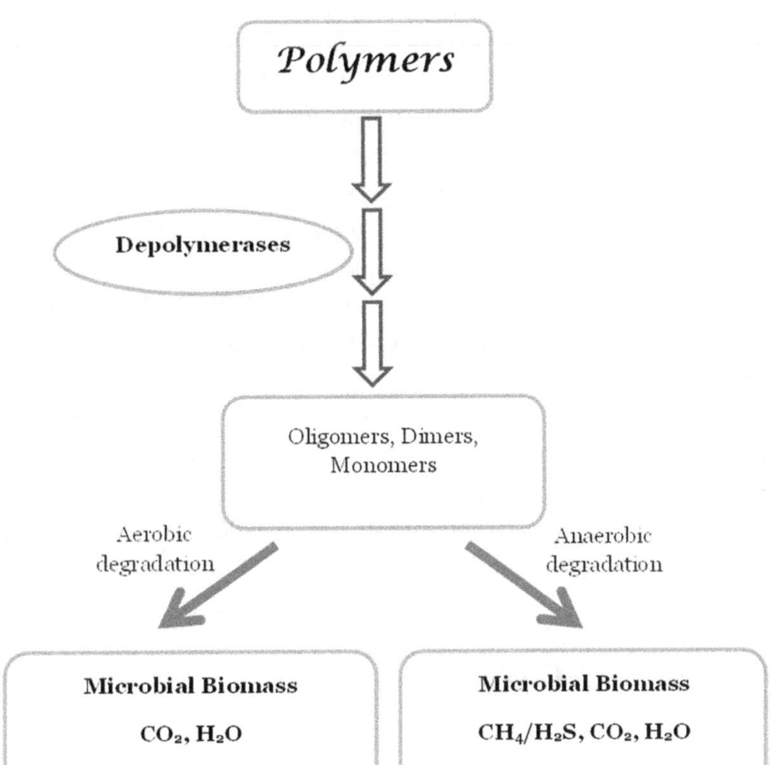

in polymers by papain enzyme (Phua et al., 1987). A newly discovered bacterium, *Ideonella sakaiensis* 201-F6, reported in 2016, by Yoshida et al. having the unusual ability to utilize PET as its major carbon and energy source for growth. Three different kinds of plastic bags HL, VHL, and VN1 with different chemical nature were degraded by a novel thermophilic bacterial strain in shaking liquid medium at 55°C after 30 d isolated from composting agricultural residual in Vietnam. The new strain of bacteria was classified in the *Bacillus* genus according to its morphological property and sequence of partial 16S rRNA coding gene and named as *Bacillus* sp. BCBT21. This strain could produce extracellular hydrolase enzymes including lipase, CMCase, xylanase, chitinase, and protease with different level of activity in the same media (Dang et al., 2018) Manganese peroxidase enzyme, partially purified from the strain of *Phanerochaete chrysosporium* (Lignin-degrading fungi) also help in the degradation of high-molecular weight PE under nitrogen and carbon limited conditions (Shimao, 2001).

Microbial enzymes induce the rate of biodegradation of plastics very effectively without causing any harm to the environment. Researchers are currently investigating ways to augment contained sites with nonnative microbes including genetically engineered microorganisms especially suited to degrading the contaminants of concern at particular site (Kerr et al., 1994). Microbial transformation of organic contaminants normally occurs because the organisms can use the contaminants for their own growth and reproduction. Organic contaminants serve two purposes for the organisms: they provide a source of carbon, which is one of the basic building blocks of new cell constituents, and they provide electrons, which the organisms can extract to obtain energy (Chapelle, 1993). Apart from the bacteria, fungi and actinomycetes were also actively participating in the deterioration of polymers. Some fungi like *Aspergillus niger* and *Aspergillus flavus* produce enzymes that more easily digest aliphatic polyesters derived from 6–12-carbon di-acid monomers than those produced from other monomers (Raaman et al., 2012; Chandra et al., 1997). Fungi were also reported to have cellulase activity, including *Phanerochaete chrysosporium* and *Trichoderma reesei.* Anaerobic biodegradation of cellulose is very complex as compared to aerobic degradation. Leschine et al. (1995), Souza et al. (2013) & Kameshwar et al. (2016) studied CBM1 (carbohydrate- binding module) containing proteins from fungi and Oomycetes (*Phytophthora parasitica*). More interestingly several species of actinomycetes were also participating in the biodegradation of plastic materials like *Streptomyces badius, Streptomyces setonii, Streptomyces viridosporus, Actinetobacter calcoaceticus, Pseudonocardia, Actinoplanes* etc. Especially thermophilic actinomycetes were mainly employed in polyethylene succinate degradation and *Microbispora* were also competent to degrade polyethylene succinate film in 6 days at 50 °C (Duddu et al., 2015; Seretoudi et al., 2002; Hoang et al., 2007). Tseng et al. (2007) reported that 31 isolates belonging to the genus *Saccharomonospora, Streptomyces, Microbispora, Thermoactinomyces* and *Actinomadura* have actively involved in polymer degradation. *Streptomyces* sp. is a thermophilic microorganism isolated from soil having the capability of poly (D-3-hydroxybutyrate) degradation at 50 °C; *Streptomyces* sp. also exhibited a capacity for polyethylene succinate degradation (Calabia & Tokiwa, 2004). All this known evidences summarizes the importance of microbial enzymes during degradation of plastics. Microbial enzymes play a key role during transformation of complex plastic polymers into simplest one.

MECHANISM OF BIODEGRADATION

Biodegradation of polymers involves mainly three broad steps:

Table 2. List of Microorganisms Involved in Biodegradation

Type of Plastic Used	Microorganisms	References
Bacteria		
Polyurethane	*Corynebacterium and Pseudomonas sp.*	Kay et al.,(1991)
LDPE	*Bacillus cereus C1* *Cellulosimicrobium,* *Lysinibacillus*	Suresh et al.,(2011) Muhonja et al., (2018)
Polyurethane	*Pseudomonas cepacia, Pseudomonas sp., and Arthrobacter globiformis*	El-Sayed et al., (1996)
LDPE	*Rhodococcus ruber C208*	Chandra & Rustgi, (1997)
Polyurethane	*Bacillus sp.*	Howard& Blake, (1999)
Degradable plastic	*Pseudomonas sp., Bacillus subtilis, staphylococcus aureus, Streptococcus lactis,Proteus vulgaris, and Micrococcus luteus*	Priyanka & Archana, (2011)
PVC powder	*Pseudomonas aeruginosa*	Peciulyte, (2002)
Degradable polyethylene	*Rhodococcus rhodocorrous ATCC 29672 and Nocardia steroids GK 911*	Bonhomme et al.,(2003)
Polyethylene bags and plastic cups	*Streptococcus sp., Staphylococcus sp.,Micrococcus sp., Moraxella sp., and Pseudomonas sp.*	Kathiresan, (2003)
LDPE	*Pseudomonas stutzeri*	Sharma & Sharma (2004)
LDPE	*Brevibacillus borstelensis707*	Hadad et al.,(2005)
Polyethylene carry bags	*Bacillius cereus, Pseudomonas sp.*	Aswale & Ade, (2008)
Polyethylene carry bags and cups	*Bacillus sp., Staphylococcus sp., Streptococcus sp., Diplococcus sp.,Micrococcus sp., Pseudomonas sp., and Moraxella sp.*	Reddy, (2008)
Degradable polyethylene	*Bacillus mycoides*	Seneviratne et al., (2006)
LDPE	*Rhodococcus ruber C208*	Sivan et al.,(2006)
HDPE and LDPE	*Bacillus sp., Micrococcus p., Listeria sp., and Vibrio sp.*	Kumar et al.,(2007)
Isotactic polypropylene	*Pseudomonas chlororaphis, Pseudomonas stutzeri, and Vibrio sp.*	Cacciari et al.,(1993)
HDPE, LDPE, and LLDPE	*Rhodococcus rhodochorus ATCC 29672*	Fontanella et al.,(2009)
Polyethylene carry bags	*Serratia marcescens*	Aswale & Ade, (2009)
LDPE	*Pseudomonas aeruginosa PAO1 (ATCC 15729), Pseudomonas aeruginosa (ATCC 15692), Pseudomonas putida (KT2440 ATCC 47054), and Pseudomonas syringae (DC3000 ATCC 10862)*	Kyaw et al.,(2012)
HDPE	*Arthrobacter sp. and Pseudomonas sp.*	Balasubramanian et al., (2010)
LDPE powder	*Pseudomonas sp., Staphylococcus sp., andBacillus sp.*	Usha et al.,(2011)
Natural and syntheticpolyethylene	*Pseudomonas sp. (P1, P2, and P3)*	Nanda et al.,(2010)
LDPE	*Staphylococcus epidermis*	Chatterjee et al.,(2010)
LDPE and LLDPE	*Baciilus cereus, Bacillus megaterium, Bacillussubtilis, and Brevibacillus borstelensis*	Abrusci et al., (2011)
Polyethylene carry bags	*Serratia marcescens 724, Bacillus cereus,Pseudomonas aeruginosa, Streptococcusaureus (B-324), and Micrococcus lylae (B-429)*	Aswale, (2010)
Polyethylene bags	*Pseudomonas aeruginosa, Pseudomonas putida, and Bacillus subtilis*	Nwachukwu et al.,(2010)
Fungi		
PVC powder	*Aureobasidium pullulans, Geotrichum candidum, Alternaria alternaria, Cladosporium sp.,Aspergillus sp., Penicillium sp., and Ulocladium atrum*	Peciulyte, (2002)

continued on the following page

Table 2. Continued

Type of Plastic Used	Microorganisms	References
LDPE powder	*Aspergillus nidulans and Aspergillus flavus*	Usha et al., (2011)
PVC	*Poliporusversicolor, Pleurotus sajor caju,Phanerochaete chrysosporium, ME 446, Pleurotus ostreatus, Pleurotus sapidus, Pleurotus eryngii,Pleurotus florida*	Kirbas et al., (1999)
High densitypolyethylene (HDPE)	*Aspergillus niger, Aspergillus oryzae, andAspergillus flavus*	Konduri et al., (2010)
LDPE powder	*Aspergillus versicolor and Aspergillus sp.*	Pramila & Ramesh, (2011)
Degradable plastic	*Phanerochaete chrysosporium*	Lee et al., (1991)
Polyethylene carry bags	*Phanerochaete chrysosporium, Pleurotus ostretus,Aspergillus niger, and Aspergillus glaucus*	Aswale, (2010)
Polyurethane	*Chaetomium globosum and Aspergillus terreus*	Boubendir, (1993)
LDPE	*Aspergillus oryzae*	Konduri et al., (2011)
Degradable polyethylene	*Penicillium frequentans*	Seneviratne et al., (2006)
Disposable plastic films	*Aspergillus flavus and Mucor rouxii NRRL 1835*	El-Shafei et al., (1998)
Degradable polyethylene	*Cladosporium cladosporides*	Bonhomme et al., (2003)
Plasticized PVC	*Aureobasidium pullulans, Rhodotorula aurantiaca, and Kluyveromyces spp.*	Webb et al., (2000)
Degradable plastic	*Aspergillus niger, Aspergillus nidulans, Aspergillus flavus, Aspergillus glaucus, and Penicillium sp.*	Priyanka & Archana(2011)
Polyurethane	*Curvularia senegalensis, Fusarium solani,Aureobasidium pullulans, and Cladosporium sp.*	Crabbe et al., (1994)
Polyethylene bags andplastic cups	*Aspergillus niger and Aspergillus glaucus*	Kathiresan, (2003)
HDPE	*Aspergillus terreus MF12*	Balasubramaniyanet al., (2014)
Plasticized PVC	*Aspergillus versicolor, Aspergillus niger, Aspergillusflavus, Chrysonilia setophila, and Penicillium sp.*	Sachin and Mishra, (2013)
PVC films	*Phanerochaete chrysosporium PV1, Lentinus tigrinus PV2, Aspergillus niger PV3, and Aspergillus sydowii PV4*	Ali et al., (2014)
Polyethylene carry bagsand cups	*Aspergillus niger, Aspergillus ornatus, Aspergillus nidulans, Aspergillus cremeus, Aspergillus flavus,Aspergillus candidus, and Aspergillus glaucus*	Reddy, (2008)
LDPE	*Aspergillus sp.*	Raaman et al., (2012)
Low density polyethylene (LDPE) powder	*Penicillium pinophilium and Aspergillus niger*	Volke-Sepulveda et al., (2002)
Polyethylene bags	*Aspergillus niger*	Nwachukwu et al., (2010)
HDPE	*Phanerochaete chrysosporium ME-446 andTrametes versicolor (IFO 7043, IFO 15413)*	Iiyoshi et al., (1998)
LDPE	*Aspergillus niger, Penicillium funiculosum,Chaetomium globosum, Gliocladium virens, and Pullularia pullulans*	Gilan et al., (2004)
Polyethylene carry bags	*Aspergillus niger*	Aswale & Ade, (2011)
LDPE	*Fusarium sp. AF4*	Shah et al., (2009)
Polyethylene	*Penicillium simplicissmum*	Yamada et al., (2001)
Actinomycetes		
LDPE powder	*Streptomyces KU8, Streptomyces KU5,Streptomyces KU1, and Streptomyces KU6*	Usha et al., (2011)
Starch polyethylene–prooxidant degradable polyethylene	*Streptomyces setonii 75Vi2 and Streptomyces viridosporus T7A*	Pometto et al., (1992)

continued on the following page

Table 2. Continued

Type of Plastic Used	Microorganisms	References
Polyurethane	*Actinetobacter gerneri P7*	Howard et al., (2012)
Polyurethane	*Actinetobacter calcoaceticus*	Halim et al., (1996)
Polyethylene	*Streptomyces sp.*	Mendez et al., (2007)
Polyethylene	*Streptomyces sp., Pseudonocardia, Actinoplanes, Sporichthya*	Sathya et al., (2012)
Disposable plastic films)	*Streptomyces spp. (8 strains)*	El-Shafei et al., (1998)
Starch polyethylene–prooxidant degradable polyethylene	*Streptomyces badius 252*	Lee et al., (1991)

1. Microbial attachment to the surface of the polymer.
2. Microorganisms have the ability to use the polymer as a carbon source for its growth.
3. Finally involve the degradation mechanism of the polymer.

Microorganisms are capable to attach on the surface of polymers, as long as the latter is hydrophilic. Primarily the organism is attached to the surface; it uses the polymer as its carbon source and grows well. First degradation stage involve the secretion of extracellular enzymes by the organism cause the main chain to cleave, leading to the formation of low-molecular weight fragments, like oligomers, dimers or monomers. These low molecular weight compounds are further used by the microbes to drive the energy as described earlier. Small oligomers may also diffuse into the organism and get assimilated in its internal environment.

Other Important Steps of Plastic Degradation by Microorganisms

Different terminologies are used to describe the steps which occur in the plastic biodegradation process (Lucas et al., 2008)

- **Bio-deterioration** defines the action of microbial communities and other decomposer organisms that involve in the physical and chemical deterioration and result a superficial degradation that modifies the mechanical, physical and chemical properties of the plastic.
- **Bio-fragmentation** refers to the catalytic actions that cleave polymeric plastics into oligomers, dimers or monomers by ecto-enzymes or free-radicals secreted by microorganisms.
- **Assimilation** characterizes to the integration of molecules transported in the cytoplasm in the microbial metabolism.
- **Mineralisation** refers to the complete degradation of molecules that resulted in the excretion of completely oxidized metabolites (CO_2, N_2, CH_4, H_2O).

The bio-deterioration seems to be triggered by the formation of a microbial biofilm growing on the surface and inside the plastic. The development of the biofilm is dependent on the composition and the structure of the plastic, but it can also affected by the environmental conditions (Lugauskas et al., 2003). Plastic polymers such as PE and PS are hydrophobic in nature therefore; to form a stable biofilm on these polymers, hydrophobic bacterial surface have also required. For example, the biofilm of *Rhodococcus ruber C208*formed on polyethylene showed high viability and even after 60 days of incubation adhered to the polyethylene without any supplementation of external carbon. The structural components, hugely participate and are important for biofilm formation. The relieve form biofilms of flagellated motile bacteria compared to non-motile bacteria and other structural components such as curli and mannose sensitive type I, IV pili (TfP) encoding genes also play an important role in cell-cell or cell-surface attachments. Type IV pili play a significant role in bacterial motility on the surface and are important for quorum sensing. A functional gene OmpR is reported that promotes the biofilm formation (Prakash et al., 2003; O'Toole et al., 2000; Bogino et al., 2013). Biofilm formation is a highly synchronized event in which many factors are controlled well. Alginate-producing gene *alg*C was reported to enhance the biofilm formation potential by fourfold and is positively regulated by the sigma factor (Kokare et al., 2009),

The microbial biofilm provokes serious physical and chemical deterioration:

- **Physical Deterioration**: Extracellular polymeric substances (EPS) secreted from the microbes is associated to the formation of the microbial biofilm which reinforce the cohesion of the biofilm and adhesion to the plastic surface. The EPS enters the pores and give a way to microorganisms to grow inside, thus increasing the pore size and provoking cracks that weakened the physical properties of the plastic (Bonhomme et al., 2003).
- **Chemical Deterioration**: Highly diverse microbial communities can developed on plastic polymers (Zettler et al. 2013) and result the formation of a biofilm which may release acid compounds such as nitrous acid (e.g. *Nitrosomonas* spp.), nitric acid (e.g. *Nitrobacter* spp.) or sulphuric acid (e.g. *Thiobacillus*spp.) by chemolithotrophic bacteria. Organic acids such as oxalic, citric, fumaric, gluconic, glutaric, glyoxalic, oxalic and oxaloacetic acids may also be released by chemo-organotrophic communities. The pH inside the pores is modified due to acid secretion and performs a progressive degradation that may changes the microstructure of the plastic matrix.

ROLE OF ENZYMES IN BIODEGRADATION

The use of microorganisms for bioremediation is affected with many rate-limiting factors. Costly and time-consuming methods may be necessary to produce microbial cultures. Several factors include physical and chemical treatments, toxins, action of predators and high concentration of pollutants may damage or metabolically inactive the microbial cells. Enzymes exist in every living cell and hence in all microbes. Relative amounts of the various enzymes produced by the microorganisms vary with species and even between strains of the same species. Enzymes are very specific about action on its substrates, so the different enzymes help in the degradation of various types of polymers (Underkofler, 1958). Laccase can help in the oxidation of the hydrocarbon backbone of PE. Gel permeation chromatography (GPC) determine whether cell-free laccase incubated with PE helps in the reduction of average molecular weight and average molecular number of PE by 20% and 15%, respectively(Sivan, 2011). Lignin biodegrading fungi mainly contain laccases that catalyze the oxidation of aromatic compounds. Laccase activity is also known to act on non-aromatic substrates (Mayer & Staples, 2002). Lignin and manganese-dependent peroxidases (LiP and MnP, respectively) and laccases are the three main enzymes of ligninolytic system (Hofrichter et al., 2001).Another one of such example is Xylanases which exist in two forms: endo 1,4 β-xylanase and xylan 1,4 β-xylosidase. Some strains that are capable of degrading the PE are *Brevibacillus* spp., *Bacillus* spp., where proteases are responsible for degradation (Sivan, 2011). *P. chrysosporium*is a white-rot fungus known to produce hemicelluloses that degrade endo-xylanases, acetyl xylan esterases and mannosidases. Heat-stable endo-xylanases are drived from thermophilic fungi, e.g., *Thermoascus aurantiacus*and *Talaromyces emersonii*, while *Butyrivibrio fibrisolvens* (ruminal bacterium) and *Bacillus sterothermophilus* possess β-xylosidase. *Bacillus* spp. produces two types ofalkaline xylanases, i.e., xylanase N and xylanase A, withan active pH range of 5, 7 and 11, respectively(Perez et al., 2002;Jeffrie, 1994; Kameshwar & Qin, 2016). Some helper enzymes like xylan esterases, α-1 arabinofuranosidases and α-4 O-methyl glucuronosidases are required for complete degradation(Perez et al., 2002).Some research work reported that a PETase (PET-digesting enzyme) isolated from Ideonella sakaiensis 201-F6,has the ability to depolymerize aromatic polyester (Austin et al., 2018).

FACTORS AFFECTING THE BIODEGRADATION

Biodegradation is directed by various factors that include polymer characteristics, type of organism, and nature of pretreatment. The characteristics of polymer such as its mobility, crystallinity, molecular weight, type of functional groups, and substituent present in its structure, and plasticizers or additives added to the polymer entire things play a key role in its degradation (Artham et al., 2008; Gu et al., 2000). Biodegradability of polymers is influenced by two main factors such as exposure conditions and characteristic features of polymers. Exposure condition included the abiotic and biotic factors whereas polymer characteristics include flexibility, crystallinity, morphology, functional groups, cross-linking, molecular weight, copolymers, blend, tacticity and additives. Biotic factor refer to the nature of extracellular enzymes, hydrophobicity and biosurfactants while abiotic factors such as temperature, pH, UV radiation and moisture can affect the hydrolysis reaction rates during degradation. The increased temperature and moisture leads to increase in hydrolysis reaction rates and microbial activity (Henton et al., 2005). In high-moisture environmental conditions, there is an increase in hydrolysis reaction, which produces more chain scission and leads to an increase in the available sites for microorganisms to attack the polymer chains, causing faster degradation. Among biotic factors, extracellular enzymes produced by different microorganisms may have active sites with different shapes and hence more able to biodegrade certain polymers. Some factors are mentioned below which affect the degradation mechanism in a common way.

- The presence of functional groups result to increase in hydrophobicity (hydrophilic degradation is faster than hydrophobic).
- The molecular weight and density of the polymer is another important factor (lower degrades faster than higher).
- The morphology of TM: amount of crystalline and amorphous regions (amorphous degrades faster than crystalline).
- Structural complexity such as linearity or the presence of branching in the polymer.
- Presence of easily breakable bonds such as ester or amide bonds. Chain coupling (ester > ether > amide >urethane).
- Molecular composition (blend).
- The nature and physical form of the polymer (e.g., films, pellets, powder or fibers).
- Hardness (Tg) (soft polymers degrade faster than hard ones) (Swift, 1993; Kawai, 1995; Mohan et al., 2010).

Biodegradability Tests

See Table 3.

FORMULA USE TO DETERMINE THE BIODEGRADATION RATE OF THE PLASTIC BAGS

A simple and quick method used to measure the biodegradation of plastic bags was determined by the weight loss of plastic bags after incubation. The weight loss of plastic bags was calculated and based on their weight change according to ASTM D6003-96 (1996) by the formula:

$$\text{WL }(\%) = \frac{mi - mr}{mi} \times 100$$

where WL is the weight loss of samples (%), mi is the initial sample weight (g), and mr is the retention weight of samples after testing (g).

STANDARDS FOR POLYMER DEGRADATION

A well-informed literature on biodegradable products is organized by the US government, in assistance of the Biodegradable Products Institute (BPI). BPI is an organization that deals with academia, industry and government bodies that encourage recycling of polymeric materials (biodegradable) Figure 3. Production of the biodegradable polymer involves the addition of starch and plant fiber extract. BPI provides matter to the ASTM (American Society for Testing and Materials) for assembling ASTM standards (ASTM D6400, D6866). These are the principle databases of degradation which is used to supervise industry. The logo for the compostable product was introduced by the USCC (US Composting Council) and BPI (Kolybaba et al., 2003). Recycling rate and biodegradable products will be increase in future which is also one of the appreciable facts of BPI.

Figure 3. Symbol representing biodegradable grade compostable polymers

Table 3. The analytical tools used to monitor the biodegradation process

S.I.	Test parameters	Description	References
1.	Visual observations	The assessment of visible changes in plastics can be performed in almost all tests. Degradation rate can be check out to see the effects on polymers include the roughening of the surface, formation of holes or cracks, de-fragmentation and changes in colour or formation of biofilms on the surface. These changes point out the first indication of any microbial attack. To obtain information about the degradation mechanism, more sophisticated observations can be made using either scanning by using SEM, transmission optical microscopy or atomic force microscopy (AFM).	(Ikada, 1999)
2.	Alteration in physical properties	Transformation in the physical properties of a polymer such as density, Molecular weight distribution (using GPC), contact angle, viscosity, melting temperature (Tm), glass transition temperature (Tg) with TGA and DSC and changes in the crystalline and amorphous regions by using X-ray diffraction, SAXS and WAXS. Biodegradability is also evaluated by weight loss, tensile strength loss, changes in present elongation and change of polymer molar mass.	(Witt et al., 2001; Sowmya et al., 2014; Erlandsson et al., 1997)
3.	Alteration in chemical properties	Alterations in the chemical properties of the polymer in synthetic media, including the formation or disappearance of functional groups as determined by FTIR, can be measured. The molecular weight and molecular weight distribution of the degraded products or intermediates are observed by techniques such as TLC, NMR and GCMS.	(Arutchelvi et al., 2008)
4.	Quantitative analysis of O_2 and CO_2	Evolution of CO_2 and consumption of O_2: Under aerobic conditions, microbes use oxygen to oxidize carbon, and form carbon dioxide as a major metabolic end product. As a result, the consumption of oxygen (respirometry test) or the formation of carbon dioxide (strum test) is the most often used method to measure biodegradation in laboratory tests, as it gives direct information on the bio-conversion of the carbon backbone of the polymer to metabolic end product.	(Hoffmann et al., 1997)
5.	Analysis of CO_2 and methane	Anaerobic microorganisms predominantly produce a mixture of CO_2 and methane, called biogas, as an extracellular product of their metabolic reactions. This can be tested by using Gas Chromatography, or manually by titrating with barium hydroxide.	(Gartiser et al., 1998;Reischwitz et al., 1997)
6.	Radiolabeling	Radiolabeling is used particularly for investigating slowly degradable materials in a matrix containing carbon sources other than the plastics.	(Albertsson, 1978)
7.	Biological test	A very simple semi-quantitative method is the 'clear-zone' test. This is an agar plate test in which the polymer is dispersed as very fine particles within the synthetic medium agar, which results in the agar having an opaque appearance. After inoculation with microorganisms, the formation of a clear halo around the colony indicates that the organisms are at least able to depolymerize the polymer, which is the first step of biodegradation. This method is usually applied to screen organisms that can degrade a certain polymer. Measurements of clear-zone formation in agar plates and the metabolic activity of the cells in the culture and in the biofilm can be done by ATP assays, protein analysis and FAD analysis.	(Arutchelvi et al., 2008; Nishida et al., 1993; Abou-Zeid et al., 2001)

APPLICATION AND IMPORTANCE OF BIODEGRADATION

Up to the present time, most of the knowledge on the microbial ability to degrade synthetic plastics is based on few bacteria able to grow on culture media, that represent only $<0.1\%$ of the total bacteria. It shows that majority of natural diversity of microorganisms is not fully exploited. By improving -omics technologies (genomic, transcriptomic, proteomic, metabolomics), it is now possible to discover new non-culturable microorganisms involved in plastic colonization and degradation. These technologies provide an opportunity to explore the new properties of microorganisms that arise from the interaction of genes, proteins, other macromolecules, small molecules, and the environment. Among all the biological agents, microbial enzymes are one of the most powerful tools for the biodegradation of plastics. Meanwhile it is cheapest, efficient technology and eco-friendly treatments capable of reducing and even eliminating plastics. There is a huge demand in exploring these microbes which can grow in different conditions and, under specific stress conditions, may be directed to grow and use the plastic polymers as carbon and energy source.

BIOPLASTIC

Bioplastics are plastics derived from renewable biomass sources, such as vegetable fats and oils, corn starch, straw, woodchips, food waste, etc. Bioplastic can be made from agricultural by-products and also from used plastic bottles and other containers using microorganisms. Whereas common plastics, such as fossil-fuel plastics (also called petrobased polymers) are derived from petroleum or natural gas. Production of such plastics tends to require more fossil fuels and to produce more greenhouse gases than the production of biobased polymers (bioplastics). This led to increase the demand of bioplastics obtained from the growth of microorganisms or from plants, which are genetically engineered to build such polymers, are likely to replace currently used plastics at least in some of the fields. Bioplastic material biodegrades rapidly under composting conditions and does not leave toxic residue. The most important are poly (3-hydroxybutyrate) and poly (3-hydroxybutyrate-co-3-hydroxyvalerate).

CONCLUSION

Microorganisms have the capability to degrade inorganic and organic materials, and this is one of the reasons which create an interest to study about the plastic polymers degrading microbes. A term biodegradation arose in past era to describe remediation mechanisms that open a new door to remove out the plastic pollutants in ecofriendly manner. Several plastic-degrading methods existed however; degradation by using microbes is the cheapest, eco-friendly and more acceptable method. Biodegradation is generally considered as consisting of both enzyme-catalyzed hydrolysis and non-enzymatic hydrolysis. More specifically, microorganisms are preferably suited to the task of contaminant destruction because they possess enzymes that allow them to use environmental contaminants as food. *P. aeruginosa*, *P. stutzeri*, *S. badius*, *S. setonii*, *R. ruber*, *C. acidovorans*, *C. thermocellum* and *B. fibrisolvens* are the dominant bacterial species associated with polymer degradation. Whereas many fungi like *Aspergillus niger*, *Aspergillus flavus* and *Streptomyces* are effectively involved in polythene degradation. *Fusarium lini* is involved in synthesizing dehydratase, which is responsible for polyvinyl alcohol degradation with CO_2 and H_2Oformation. *P. cinnabarinus* is also known as white rot fungus and is involved in PVA biodegradation in the presence of Fenton's reagent. The above discussion elucidates the existence of polymer-degrading microorganisms and their application over the other remediation processes. Biodegradable plastics released an approach for novel considerations of waste management strategies, since these materials are designed to degrade under environmental conditions or in municipal and industrial biological waste treatment facilities. Therefore, further studies on the screening of effective microbial strains are necessary to minimize polymer risks for the environment. Meanwhile, new age research should be focused in the field of genomics and proteomics, which could accelerate the degradation process.

Abbreviations

LDPE: low-density polyethylene;
HDPE: high-density polyethylene;
PVA: polyvinylalcohol;
PUR: polyurethane;
PCL: polycaprolactone;
PLA: polylactic acid;
PHB: polyhydroxybutyrate;
PHAs: polyhydroxyalkanoates;
EPS: extracellular polymeric substance;
ISO: International standards Organization;
ASTM: American Society for Testing and Materials;
PE: polyethylene,
PP: polypropylene,
PS: polystyrene,
PVC: polyvinyl chloride,
PTFE: polytetrafluoroethylene,
GPC: Gel permeation chromatography and
AFM: atomic force microscopy

REFERENCES

Abou-Zeid, D. M., Müller, R. J., & Deckwer, W. D. (2001). Degradation of natural and synthetic polyesters under anaerobic conditions. *Journal of Biotechnology*, *86*(2), 113–126. doi:10.1016/S0168-1656(00)00406-5 PMID:11245900

Abrusci, C., Pablos, J. L., Corrales, T., Lopez-Marin, J., Marin, I., & Catalina, F. (2011). Biodegradation of photo-degraded mulching films based on polyethylenes and stearates of calcium and iron as prooxidant additives. *International Biodeterioration & Biodegradation*, *65*(3), 451–459. doi:10.1016/j.ibiod.2010.10.012

Albertsson, A. C. (1978). Biodegradation of synthetic polymers. II. A limited microbial conversion of 14 C in polyethylene to 14 CO_2 by some soil fungi. *Journal of Applied Polymer Science*, *22*(12), 3419–3433. doi:10.1002/app.1978.070221207

Ali, M. I., Ahmed, S., Robson, G., Javed, I., Ali, N., Atiq, N., & Hameed, A. (2014). Isolation and molecular characterization of polyvinyl chloride (PVC) plastic degrading fungal isolates. *Journal of Basic Microbiology*, *54*(1), 18–27. doi:10.1002/jobm.201200496 PMID:23686796

Artham, T., & Doble, M. (2008). Biodegradation of aliphatic and aromatic polycarbonates. *Macromolecular Bioscience*, *8*(1), 14–24. doi:10.1002/mabi.200700106 PMID:17849431

Arutchelvi, J., Sudhakar, M., Arkatkar, A., Doble, M., Bhandari, S., & Uppara, P. V. (2008). Biodegradation of Polyethylene and Polypropylene. *Indian Journal of Biotechnology*, *7*, 9–22.

ASTM D6003-96. (1996). *Standard Test Method for Determining Weight Loss from Plastic Materials Exposed to Simulated Municipal Solid-Waste (MSW) Aerobic Compost Environment*. West Conshohocken, PA: ASTM International.

Aswale, P. (2010). *Studies on bio-degradation of polythene* (PhD thesis). Dr. Babasaheb Ambedkar Marathwada University, Aurangabad, India.

Aswale, P., & Ade, A. (2008). Assessment of the biodegradation of polythene. *Bioinfolet*, *5*, 239.

Aswale, P., & Ade, A. (2009). Effect of pH on biodegradation of polythene by *Serretia marscence*. *The Ecotech*, *1*, 152–153.

Aswale, P., & Ade, A. (2011). Polythene degradation potential of Aspergillus niger. In I. U. Sayed (Ed.), Scholary Articles in Botany. Pune: Academic Press.

Austin, H. P., Allen, M. D., Donohoe, B. S., Rorrer, N. A., & Kearns, F. L. (2018). *Characterization and engineering of a plastic-degrading aromatic polyesterase* (A. T. Bell, Ed.). Berkeley, CA: University of California. doi:10.1073/pnas.1718804115

Balasubramanian, V., Natarajan, K., Hemambika, B., Ramesh, N., Sumathi, C. S., Kottaimuthu, R., & Kannan, V. R. (2010). High-density polyethylene (HDPE) degrading potential bacteria from marine ecosystem of Gulf of Mannar, India. *Letters in Applied Microbiology*, *51*, 205–211. PMID:20586938

Balasubramanian, V., Natarajan, K., Kannan, R. V., & Perumal, P. (2014). Enhancement of *in vitro* high density polyethylene (HDPE) degradation by physical, chemical and biological treatments. *Environmental Science and Pollution Research International*, *21*(21), 12,549–12,562. doi:10.100711356-014-3191-2 PMID:24946709

Bhardwaj, H., Gupta, R., & Tiwari, A. (2012). Microbial Population Associated with Plastic Degradation. *Open Access Scientific Reports*, *5*, 1–4.

Bhatnagar, S., & Kumari, R. (2013). Bioremediation: A sustainable tool for environmental management a review. *Annual Review and Research in Biology*, *3*(4), 974–993.

Bogino, P. C., Oliva, M. D. L. M., Sorroche, F. G., & Giordano, W. (2013). The role of bacterial biofilms and surface components in plant-bacterial associations. *International Journal of Molecular Sciences*, *14*(8), 15838–15859. doi:10.3390/ijms140815838 PMID:23903045

Bombelli, P., Howe, C. J., & Bertocchini, F. (2017). Polyethylene bio-degradation by caterpillars of the wax moth Galleria mellonella. *Current Biology*, *27*(8), R292–R293. doi:10.1016/j.cub.2017.02.060 PMID:28441558

Bonhommea, S., Cuerb, A., Delort, A. M., Lemairea, J., Sancelmeb, M., & Scott, G. (2003). Environmental biodegradation of polyethylene. *Polymer Degradation & Stability*, *81*(3), 441–452. doi:10.1016/S0141-3910(03)00129-0

Boubendir, A. (1993). Purification and biochemical evaluation of polyurethane degrading enzymes of fungal origin. *Dissertation Abstract International, 53*, 4632.

Cacciari, I., Quatrini, P., Zirletta, G., Mincione, E., Vinciguerra, V., Lupatelli, P., & Sermanni, G. G. (1993). Isotactic polypropylene biodegradation by a microbial community: Physicochemical characterization of metabolites produced. *Applied and Environmental Microbiology*, *59*(11), 3695–3700. PMID:8285678

Calabia, B. P., & Tokiwa, Y. (2004). Microbial degradation of poly (D-3-hydroxybutyrate) by a new thermophilic *Streptomyces* isolate. *Biotechnology Letters*, *26*(1), 15–19. doi:10.1023/B:BILE.0000009453.81444.51 PMID:15005145

Chandra, R., & Rustgi, R. (1997). Biodegradation of maleated linear low-density polyethylene and starch blends. *Polymer Degradation & Stability*, *56*(2), 185–202. doi:10.1016/S0141-3910(96)00212-1

Chandra, R., & Rustgi, R. (1998). Biodegradable polymers. *Progress in Polymer Science*, *23*(7), 1273–1335. doi:10.1016/S0079-6700(97)00039-7

Chapelle, F. (1993). *Ground-Water Microbiology & Geochemistry*. New York: John Wiley & Sons, Inc.

Chatterjee, S., Roy, B., Roy, D., & Banerjee, R. (2010). Enzyme-mediated biodegradation of heat treated commercial polyethylene by *Staphylococcal* species. *Polymer Degradation & Stability*, *95*(2), 195–200. doi:10.1016/j.polymdegradstab.2009.11.025

Crabbe, J. R., Campbell, J. R., Thompson, L., Walz, S. L., & Schultz, W. W. (1994). Biodegradation of colloidal ester-based polyurethane by soil fungi. *International Biodeterioration & Biodegradation*, *33*(2), 103–113. doi:10.1016/0964-8305(94)90030-2

Dang, T. C. H., Nguyen, D. T., Thai, H., Nguyen, T. C., Tran, T. T. H., Le, V. H., … Nguyen, T. G. (2018). Plastic degradation by thermophilic *Bacillus* sp. BCBT21 isolated from composting agricultural residual in Vietnam. *Advances in Natural Sciences: Nanoscience and Nanotechnology*, *9*(1).

Duddu, M. K., Tripura, K. L., Guntuku, G., & Divya, D. S. (2015). Biodegradation of low density polyethylene (LDPE) by a new biosurfactant-producing thermophilic *Streptomyces coelicoflavus* NBRC 15399T. *African Journal of Biotechnology*, *14*(4), 327–340. doi:10.5897/AJB2014.14224

Dussud, C., & Ghiglione, J. F. (2014). Bacterial degradation of synthetic plastics. In *CIESM Workshop Monogr* (No. 46). Academic Press.

Dvorák, P., Nikel, P. I., Damborský, J., & de Lorenzo, V. (2017). Bioremediation 3.0: Engineering pollutant-removing bacteria in the times of systemic biology. *Biotechnology Advances*, *35*, 845–866.

El-Sayed, A. H. M. M., Mahmoud, W. M., Davis, E. M., & Coughlin, R. W. (1996). Biodegradation of polyurethane coatings by hydrocarbon- degrading bacteria. *International Biodeterioration & Biodegradation*, *37*(1-2), 69–79. doi:10.1016/0964-8305(95)00091-7

El-Shafei, H. A., El-Nasser, N. H. A., Kansoh, A. L., & Ali, A. M. (1998). Biodegradation of disposable polyethylene by fungi and *Streptomyces* species. *Polymer Degradation & Stability*, *62*(2), 361–365. doi:10.1016/S0141-3910(98)00019-6

Erlandsson, B., Karlson, S., & Albertsson, A. C. (1997). The mode of action of corn starch and a pro oxidant system in LDPE: Influence of thermo-oxidation and UV-irradiation on the molecular weight changes. *Polymer Degradation & Stability*, *55*(2), 237–245. doi:10.1016/S0141-3910(96)00139-5

Fontanella, S., Bonhomme, S., Koutny, M., Husarova, L., Brusson, J. M., Courdavault, J. P., ... Delort, A.-M. (2009). Comparison of the biodegradability of various polyethylene films containing pro-oxidant Additives. *Polymer Degradation & Stability*, *95*(6), 1011–1021. doi:10.1016/j.polymdegradstab.2010.03.009

Gartiser, S., Wallrabenstein, M., & Stiene, G. (1998). Assessment of several test methods for the determination of the anaerobic biodegradability of polymers. *Journal of Environmental Polymer Degradation*, *6*(3), 159–173. doi:10.1023/A:1021869530253

Gilan, I., Hadar, Y., & Sivan, A. (2004). Colonization, biofilm formation and biodegradation of polyethylene by a strain of *Rhodococcus ruber. Applied Microbiology and Biotechnology*, *65*, 97–104. PMID:15221232

Gnanavel, G., Valli, V. M. J., & Thirumarimurugan, M. (2012). A review of biodegradation of plastics waste. *International Journal of Pharmaceutical and Chemical Sciences*, *1*, 670–673.

Gnanavel, G., Valli, V. M. J., Thirumarimurugan, M., & Kannadasan, T. (2014). Degradation of polyethylene in the natural environment. *International Journal of Research in Engineering & Technology*, *2*, 1–6.

Grover, A., Gupta, A., Chandra, S., Kumari, A., & Khurana, S. P. (2015). Polythene and environment. International. *Journal of Environmental Sciences (China)*, *5*(6), 1091–1105.

Gu, J. D. (2003). Microbiological deterioration and degradation of synthetic polymeric materials: Recent research advances. *International Biodeterioration & Biodegradation*, *52*(2), 69–91. doi:10.1016/S0964-8305(02)00177-4

Gu, J. D., Ford, T. E., Mitton, D. B., & Mitchell, R. (2000). Microbial degradation and deterioration of polymeric materials. In The Uhlig Corrosion Handbook (2nd ed.). Wiley.

Hadad, D., Geresh, S., & Sivan, A. (2005). Biodegradation of polyethylene by the thermophilic bacterium *Brevibacillus borstelensis. Journal of Applied Microbiology*, *98*(5), 1093–1100. doi:10.1111/j.1365-2672.2005.02553.x PMID:15836478

Halim El-Sayed, A. H. M. M., Mahmoud, W. M., Davis, E. M., & Coughlin, R. W. (1996). Biodegradation of polyurethane coatings byhydrocarbon-degrading bacteria. *International Biodeterioration & Biodegradation*, *37*(1-2), 69–79. doi:10.1016/0964-8305(95)00091-7

Henton, D. E., Gruber, P., Lunt, J., & Randall, J. (2005). Polylactic acid technology. In A. K. Mohanty, M. Misra, & L. T. Drzal (Eds.), *Natural Fibers, Biopolymers, and Biocomposites* (p. 527). Boca Raton, FL: CRC Press. doi:10.1201/9780203508206.ch16

Hoang, K. C., Tseng, M., & Shu, W. J. (2007). Degradation of polyethylene succinate (PES) by a new thermophilic Microbispora strain. *Biodegradation*, *18*(3), 333–342. doi:10.100710532-006-9067-5 PMID:17109189

Hoffmann, J., Řezníčèková, I., Vaňòková, S., & Kupec, J. (1997). Manometric determination of biological degradability of substances poorly soluble in aqueous environments. *International Biodeterioration & Biodegradation*, *39*(4), 327–332. doi:10.1016/S0964-8305(97)00033-4

Hofrichter, M., Lundell, T., & Hatakka, A. (2001). Conversion of milled pine wood by manganese peroxidase from *Phlebia radiata. Applied and Environmental Microbiology*, *67*(10), 4588–4593. doi:10.1128/AEM.67.10.4588-4593.2001 PMID:11571160

Howard, G. T. (2012). Polyurethane biodegradation. *Microbiol Degrade Xenobiot,* 371–394.

Howard, G. T., & Blake, R. C. (1999). Growth of Pseudomonas fuorescens on a polyester-polyurethane and the purification and characterization of a polyurethanase-protease enzyme. *International Biodeterioration & Biodegradation*, *42*(4), 213–220. doi:10.1016/S0964-8305(98)00051-1

Iiyoshi, Y., Tsutsumi, Y., & Nishida, T. (1998). Polyethylene degradation by lignin-degrading fungi and manganese peroxidase. *Journal of Wood Science*, *44*(3), 222–229. doi:10.1007/BF00521967

Ikada, E. (1999). Electron microscope observation of biodegradation of polymers. *Journal of Environmental Polymer Degradation*, *7*(4), 197–201. doi:10.1023/A:1022882732403

Jeffrie, T. W. (1994). Biodegradation of lignin and hemicelluloses. *Biochemistry of Microbial Degradation,* 233–277.

Kale, S. K., Deshmukh, A. G., Dudhare, M. S., & Patil, V. B. (2015). Microbial degradation of plastic: A review. *Journal of Biochemical Technology*, *6*(2), 952–961.

Kameshwar, A. K. S., & Qin, W. (2016). Recent developments in using advanced sequencing technologies for the genomic studies of lignin and cellulose degrading microorganisms. *International Journal of Biological Sciences*, *12*(2), 156–171. doi:10.7150/ijbs.13537 PMID:26884714

Kathiresan, K. (2003). Polythene and plastics-degrading microbes from the mangrove soil. *Revista de Biología Tropical*, *51*(3), 629–634. PMID:15162769

Kawai, F. (1995). Breakdown of plastics and polymers by microorganisms. *Advances in Biochemical Engineering/Biotechnology*, *52*, 151–194. doi:10.1007/BFb0102319 PMID:7484358

Kay, M. J., Morton, L. H. G., & Prince, E. L. (1991). Bacterial degradation of polyester polyurethane. *International Biodeterioration Bulletin*, *27*(2), 205–222. doi:10.1016/0265-3036(91)90012-G

Kerr, R. S. (1994). *Handbook of Bioremediation*. Boca Raton, FL: CRC Press, Inc. Lewis Publishers.

Kirbas, Z., Keskin, N., & Guner, A. (1999). Biodegradation of polyvinylchloride (PVC) by white rot fungi. *Bulletin of Environmental Contamination and Toxicology*, *63*(3), 335–342. doi:10.1007001289900985 PMID:10475911

Kokare, C. R., Chakraborty, S., Khopade, A. N., & Mahadik, K. R. (2009). Biofilm: Importance and applications. *Indian Journal of Biotechnology*, *8*(2), 159–168.

Kolbert, A. C., Didier, J. G., & Xu, L. (1996). Mechanochemical Degradation of Ethylene–Propylene Copolymers: Characterization of Olefin Chain Ends. *Macromolecules*, *29*(27), 8591–8598. doi:10.1021/ma961099q

Kolybaba, M., Tabil, L. G., Panigrahi, S., Crerar, W. J., Powell, T., & Wang, B. (2003). Biodegradable polymers: past, present, and future. The Society for Engineering in Agricultural Food and Biological System, 1–15.

Konduri, M. K. R., Anupam, K. S., Vivek, J. S., Kumar, R. D. B., & Narasu, M. L. (2010). Synergistic effect of chemical and photo treatment on the rate of biodegradation of high density polyethylene by indigenous fungal isolates. *International Journal of Biotechnology and Biochemistry*, *6*, 157–174.

Konduri, M. K. R., Koteswarareddy, G., Kumar, D. B. R., Reddy, B. V., & Narasu, M. L. (2011). Effect of prooxidants on biodegradation of polyethylene (LDPE) by indigenous fungal isolate, *Aspergillus oryzae*. *Journal of Applied Polymer Science*, *120*(6), 3536–3545. doi:10.1002/app.33517

Kumar, A. A., Karthick, K., & Arumugam, K. P. (2011). Biodegradable polymers and its applications. *International Journal of Bioscience, Biochemistry, Bioinformatics*, *1*(3), 173–176. doi:10.7763/IJBBB.2011.V1.32

Kumar, S., Hatha, A. A. M., & Christi, K. S. (2007). Diversity and effectiveness of tropical mangrove soil microflora on the degradation of polythene carry bags. *Revista de Biología Tropical*, *55*(3-4), 777–786. doi:10.15517/rbt.v55i3-4.5954 PMID:19086383

Kyaw, B. M., Champakalakshmi, R., Sakharkar, M. K., Lim, C. S., & Sakharkar, K. R. (2012). Biodegradation of low density polythene (LDPE) by *Pseudomonas* species. *Indian Journal of Microbiology*, *52*(3), 411–419. doi:10.100712088-012-0250-6 PMID:23997333

Kyrikou, J., & Briassoulis, D. (2007). Biodegradation of agricultural plastic films: A critical review. *Journal of Polymers and the Environment*, *15*(2), 125–150. doi:10.100710924-007-0053-8

Lee, B., Pometto, A. L., Fratzke, A., & Bailey, T. B. (1991). Biodegradation of degradable plastic polyethylene by *Phanerochaete* and *Streptomyces* species. *Applied and Environmental Microbiology*, *57*, 678–685. PMID:16348434

Leschine, S. B. (1995). Cellulose degradation in anaerobic environments. *Annual Review of Microbiology*, *49*(1), 399–426. doi:10.1146/annurev.mi.49.100195.002151 PMID:8561466

Lucas, N., Bienaime, C., Belloy, C., Queneudec, M., Silvestre, F., & Nava-Saucedo, J. E. (2008). Review Polymer biodegradation: Mechanisms and estimation techniques. *Chemosphere*, *73*(4), 429–442. doi:10.1016/j.chemosphere.2008.06.064 PMID:18723204

Lugauskas, A., Levinskaitë, L., & Peciulyte, D. (2003). Micromycetes as deterioration agents of polymeric materials. *International Biodeterioration & Biodegradation*, *52*(4). doi:10.1016/S0964-8305(03)00110-0

Mahdiyah, D., & Mukti, B. H. (2013). Isolation of Polyethylene Plastic degrading-Bacteria. *Biosciences International*, *2*, 29–32.

Mayer, A. M., & Staples, R. C. (2002). Laccase new functions for an old enzyme. *Phytochemistry*, *60*(6), 561–565. doi:10.1016/S0031-9422(02)00171-1 PMID:12126701

Mendez, C. R., Vergaray, G., Vilma, R., Karina, B., & Cardenas, J. (2007). Isolation and characterization of polyethylene-biodegrading mycromycetes. *Revista Peruana de Biología*, *13*(3), 203–205.

Mohan, S. K., & Srivastava, T. (2010). Microbial deterioration and degradation of polymeric materials. *Journal of Biochemical Technology*, *2*, 210–215.

Muhonja, C. N., Makonde, H., Magoma, G., & Imbuga, M. (2018). Biodegradability of polyethylene by bacteria and fungi from Dandora dumpsite Nairobi-Kenya. *PLoS One*, *13*(7), e0198446. doi:10.1371/journal.pone.0198446 PMID:29979708

Nanda, S., Sahu, S. S., Abraham, J. (2010). Studies on the biodegradation of natural and synthetic polyethylene by Pseudomonas sp. *Journal of Applied Sciences & Environmental Management,* (2), 57-60.

Nerland, I. L., Halsband, C., Allan, I., & Thomas, K. V. (2014). *Microplastics in marine environments: occurrence, distribution and effects (Re.no.6754-2014).* Oslo: Norwegian Institute for Water Research.

Nishida, H., & Tokiwa, Y. (1993). Distribution of poly (β-hydroxybutyrate) and poly (ε-caprolactone) aerobic degrading microorganisms in different environments. *Journal of Environmental Polymer Degradation*, *1*(3), 227–233. doi:10.1007/BF01458031

Nwachkwu, S., Obidi, O., & Odocha, C. (2010). Occurrence and recalcitrance of polyethylene bag waste in nigerian soils. *African Journal of Biotechnology*, *9*(37), 6096–6104.

O'Toole, G., Kaplan, H. B., & Kolter, R. (2000). Biofilm formation as microbial development. *Annual Review of Microbiology*, *54*(1), 49–79. doi:10.1146/annurev.micro.54.1.49 PMID:11018124

Ojo, O. A. (2007). Molecular strategies of microbial adaptation to xenobiotics in natural environment. *Biotechnology and Molecular Biology Review*, *2*(1), 1–13.

Peciulyte, D. (2002). Microbial colonization and biodeterioration of plasticized polyvinyl chloride plastics. *Ekologija (Lietuvos Mokslu Akademija)*, *4*, 7–15.

Perez, J., Dorada, J. M., & Rubia, T. D. L. (2002). Biodegradation and biological treatments of cellulose, hemicelluloses and lignin: An overview. *International Microbiology*, *5*(2), 53–63. doi:10.100710123-002-0062-3 PMID:12180781

Phua, S. K., Castillo, E., Anderson, J. M., & Hiltner, A. (1987). Biodegradation of polyurethane *in vitro*. \. *Journal of Biomedical Materials Research*, *21*(2), 231–246. doi:10.1002/jbm.820210207 PMID:3818683

Pometto, A. L., Lee, B., & Johnson, K. E. (1992). Production of an extracellular polyethylene- degrading enzyme(s) by *Streptomyces* species. *Applied and Environmental Microbiology*, *58*(2), 731–733. PMID:1610196

Prakash, B., Veeregowda, B. M., & Krishnappa, G. (2003). Biofilms: A survival strategy of bacteria. *Current Science*, *85*(9), 1299–1307.

Pramila, R., & Ramesh, K. V. (2011). Biodegradation of low density polyethylene (LDPE) by fungi isolated from municipal landfill area. *Journal of Microbiology and Biotechnology Research*, *1*, 131–136.

Premraj, R., & Doble, M. (2005). Biodegradation of polymer. *Indian Journal of Biotechnology*, *4*, 186–193.

Priyanka, N., & Archana, T. (2011). Biodegradability of Polythene and Plastic By The Help of Microorganism: A Way for Brighter Future. *Journal of Environmental & Analytical Toxicology*, 1.

Puri, N., Kumar, B., & Tyagi, H. (2013). Utilization of recycled wastes as ingredients in concrete mix. *International Journal of Innovative Technology and Exploring Engineering*, *2*(2), 74–78.

Raaman, N., Rajitha, N., Jayshree, A., & Jegadeesh, R. (2012). Biodegradation of plastic by Aspergillus spp. isolated from polythene polluted sites around Chennai. *Journal of Academia and Industrial Research*, *1*, 313–316.

Reddy, R. M. (2008). Impact of soil composting using municipal solid waste on biodegradation of plastics. *Indian Journal of Biotechnology*, *7*, 235–239.

Reischwitz, A., Stoppok, E., & Buchholz, K. (1997). Anaerobic degradation of poly-3-hydroxybutyrate and poly-3-hydroxybutyrate-co-3-hydroxyvalerate. *Biodegradation*, *8*(5), 313–319. doi:10.1023/A:1008203525476 PMID:15765610

Restrepo-Flórez, J. M., Bassi, A., & Thompson, M. R. (2014). Microbial degradation and deterioration of polyethylene-a review. *International Biodeterioration & Biodegradation*, *88*, 83–90. doi:10.1016/j.ibiod.2013.12.014

Sachin, S. S., & Mishra, R. L. (2013). Screening and identification of soil fungi with potential of plastic degrading ability. *Indian Journal of Applied Research*, *3*(11), 34–36.

Sathya, R., Ushadevi, T., & Panneerselvam, A. (2012). Plastic degrading actinomycetes isolated from mangrove sediments. *International Journal of Current Research, 4*(10), 1–3.

Schink, B., Janssen, P. H., & Frings, J. (1992). Microbial degradation of natural and of new synthetic polymers. *FEMS Microbiology Reviews*, *103*(2/4), 311–316. doi:10.1111/j.1574-6968.1992.tb05852.x PMID:1476775

Seneviratne, G., Tennakoon, N. S., Weerasekara, M. L. M. A. W., & Nandasena, K. A. (2006). Polyethylene biodegradation by a developed *Penicillium–Bacillus* biofilm. *Current Science*, *90*, 20–22.

Seretoudi, G., Bikiaris, D., & Panayiotou, C. (2002). Synthesis, characterization and biodegradability of poly (ethylene succinate)/poly (ε-caprolactone) block copolymers. *Polymers*, *43*(20), 5405–5415. doi:10.1016/S0032-3861(02)00433-0

Shah, A. A., Hasan, F., Akhter, J., Hameed, A., & Ahmed, S. (2009). Isolation of *Fusarium* sp. AF4 from sewage sludge, with the ability to adhere the surface of polyethylene. *African Journal of Microbiological Research*, *3*, 658–663.

Shah, A. A., Hasan, F., Akhter, J. I., Hameed, A., & Ahmed, S. (2008a). Degradation of polyurethane by novel bacterial consortium isolated from soil. *Annals of Microbiology*, *58*(3), 381–386. doi:10.1007/BF03175532

Shah, A. A., Hasan, F., Hameed, A., & Ahmed, S. (2008b). Biological degradation of plastics: A comprehensive review. *Biotechnology Advances*, *26*(3), 246–265. doi:10.1016/j.biotechadv.2007.12.005 PMID:18337047

Sharma, A., & Sharma, A. (2004). Degradation assessment of low density polythene (LDPE) and polythene (PP) by an indigenous isolate of *Pseudomonas stutzeri. Journal of Scientific and Industrial Research (New Delhi, India)*, *63*, 293–296.

Shimao, M. (2001). Biodegradation of plastics. *Current Opinion in Biotechnology*, *12*(3), 242–247. doi:10.1016/S0958-1669(00)00206-8 PMID:11404101

Singh, J., & Gupta, K. (2014). Screening and Identification of Low density Polyethylene (LDPE) Degrading Soil Fungi Isolated from Polythene Polluted Sites around Gwalior city (MP). *International Journal of Current Microbiology and Applied Sciences*, *3*, 443–448.

Sivan, A. (2011). New perspectives in plastic biodegradation. *Current Opinion in Biotechnology*, *22*(3), 422–426. doi:10.1016/j.copbio.2011.01.013 PMID:21356588

Sivan, A., Szanto, M., & Pavlov, V. (2006). Biofilm development of the polyethylenedegrading bacterium *Rhodococcus ruber. Applied Microbiology and Biotechnology*, *72*(2), 346–352. doi:10.100700253-005-0259-4 PMID:16534612

Souza, W. R. D. (2013). *Microbial degradation of lignocellulosic biomass*. West Palm Beach, FL: InTech.

Sowmya, H., Ramalingappa, M. K., & Thippeswamy, B. (2014). Biodegradation of Polyethylene by Bacillus cereus. *Advances in Polymer Science and Technology. International Journal (Toronto, Ont.)*, *4*, 28–32.

Strong, A. B. (2006). *Plastics: materials and processing* (3rd ed.). Upper Saddle River, NJ: Pearson Prentice Hall.

Suresh, B., Maruthamuthu, S., Palanisamy, N., Ragunathan, R., Pandiyaraj, K. N., & Muralidharan, V. S. (2011). Investigation on biodegradability of polyethylene by *Bacillus cereus* strain Ma-Su isolated from compost soil. *International Research Journal of Microbiology*, *2*, 292–302.

Swift, G. (1993). Directions for environmentally biodegradable polymer research. *Accounts of Chemical Research*, *26*(3), 105–110. doi:10.1021/ar00027a005

Tseng, M., Hoang, K. C., Yang, M. K., Yang, S. F., & Chu, W. S. (2007). Polyester-degrading thermophilic actinomycetes isolated from different environment in Taiwan. *Biodegradation*, *18*(5), 579–583. doi:10.100710532-006-9089-z PMID:17653512

Underkofler, L. A. (1958). Production of microbial enzymes and their applications. *Applied Microbiology*, *6*, 212–221. PMID:13534309

Upreti, M. C., & Srivastava, R. B. (2003). A potential Aspergillus species for biodegradation of polymeric materials. *Current Science*, *84*(11), 1399–1402.

Usha, R., Sangeetha, T., & Palaniswamy, M. (2011). Screening of Polyethylene degrading microorganisms from garbage soil. *Libyan Agricultural Research Center Journal International*, *2*, 200–204.

Volke-Sepulveda, T., Saucedo-Castaneda, G., Gutierrez-Rojas, M., Manzur, A., & Favela-Torres, E. (2002). Thermally treated low density polyethylene biodegradation by *Penicillium pinophilum* and *Aspergillus niger. Journal of Applied Polymer Science*, *83*(2), 305–314. doi:10.1002/app.2245

Webb, J. S., Nixon, M., Eastwood, I. M., Greenhalgh, M., Robson, G. D., & Handley, P. S. (2000). Fungal colonization and biodeterioration of plasticized polyvinyl chloride. *Applied and Environmental Microbiology*, *66*(8), 3194–3200. doi:10.1128/AEM.66.8.3194-3200.2000 PMID:10919769

Witt, U., Einig, T., Yamamoto, M., Kleeberg, I., Deckwer, W. D., & Müller, R. J. (2001). Biodegradation of aliphatic–aromatic copolyesters: Evaluation of the final biodegradability and ecotoxicological impact of degradation intermediates. *Chemosphere, 44*(2), 289–299. doi:10.1016/S0045-6535(00)00162-4 PMID:11444312

Yamada-Onodera, K., Mukumoto, H., Katsuyaya, Y., Saiganji, A., & Tani, Y. (2001). Degradation of polyethylene by a fungus *Penicillium simplicissimum* YK. *Polymer Degradation & Stability, 72*(2), 323–327. doi:10.1016/S0141-3910(01)00027-1

Yoshida, S., Hiraga, K., Takehana, T., Taniguchi, I., Yamaji, H., Maeda, Y., ... Oda, K. (2016). A bacterium that degrades and assimilates polyethylene terephthalate. *Science, 351*(6278), 1196–1199. doi:10.1126cience.aad6359 PMID:26965627

Zettler, E. R., Mincer, T. J., & Amaral-Zettler, L. A. (2013). Life in the "plastisphere": Microbial communities on plastic marine debris. *Environmental Science & Technology, 47*(13), 7137–7146. doi:10.1021/es401288x PMID:23745679

ADDITIONAL READING

Baud, I., Johan, P., & Furedy, C. (2016). Solid Waste Management and Recycling; Actors, Partnerships and Policies in Hyderabad, India and Nairobi, Kenya. The Geo Journal Library, 76.

Feng, H., Zhao, Y., Pelletier, M., Dan, Y., & Zhao, Y. (2009). Synthesis of photo and pH-responsive composite nanoparticles using a two-step controlled radical polymerization method. *Polymer, 50*(15), 3470–3477. doi:10.1016/j.polymer.2009.06.017

Gamerith, C., Vastano, M., Ghorbanpour, S. M., Zitzenbacher, S., Ribitsch, D., Zumstein, M. T., ... Guebitz, G. M. (2017). Enzymatic degradation of aromatic and aliphatic polyesters by P. pastoris expressed cutinase 1 from Thermobifida cellulosilytica. *Frontiers in Microbiology, 8*, 938. doi:10.3389/fmicb.2017.00938 PMID:28596765

Horn, S. J., Sørlie, M., Vårum, K. M., Väljamäe, P., & Eijsink, V. G. H. (2012). In H. J. Gilbert (Ed.), *Measuring processivity. Methods in Enzymology* (Vol. 510, pp. 69–95). San Diego: Academic.

Jendrossek, D. (2001). Microbial degradation of polyesters. In *Biopolyesters* (pp. 293–325). Springer. doi:10.1007/3-540-40021-4_10

Khanam, P. N., & Mariam, A. A. (2015). Processing and characterization of polyethylene-based composites *Advanced Manufacturing. Polymer & Composites Science, 1*, 63–79.

Lederberg, J. (2000). *Encyclopedia of microbiology D-K.* New York: Academic Press.

Wu, H., Wen, B., Zhou, H., Zhou, J., Yu, Z., Cui, L., ... Cao, F. (2015). Synthesis and degradability of copolyesters of 2, 5-furandicarboxylic acid, lactic acid, and ethylene glycol. *Polymer Degradation & Stability, 121*, 100–104. doi:10.1016/j.polymdegradstab.2015.08.009

KEY TERMS AND DEFINITIONS

Biodegradation: Biodegradation is the process by which organic substances are decomposed by micro-organisms (mainly aerobic bacteria) into simpler substances such as carbon dioxide, water and ammonia.

Biofragmentation: A polymer is the lytic process in which bonds within a polymer are cleaved, generating oligomers and monomers in its place.

Bioplastic: Bioplastic is a substance made from organic biomass sources, unlike conventional plastics which are made from petroleum.

Depolymerase: Any enzyme that catalyzes a depolymerization reaction.

Deterioration: A symptom of reduced quality or strength impairment.

Mineralization: In biology, mineralization refers to a process where an inorganic substance precipitates in an organic matrix. This may be due to normal biological processes that take place during the life of an organism such as the formation of bones, eggshells, teeth, coral, and other exoskeletons.

Photo-Oxidation: The degradation of a polymer surface in the presence of oxygen or ozone. The effect is facilitated by radiant energy such as UV or artificial light.

Proteomics: Branch of biotechnology concerned with applying the techniques of molecular biology, biochemistry, and genetics to analyzing the structure, function, and interactions of the proteins produced by the genes of a particular cell, tissue, or organism, with organizing the information in databases, and with applications of the data.

Chapter 23
Framework Proposition Strategy for Collection of Returned Products in Reverse Logistics Environment

Hendrik Lamsali
Universiti Utara Malaysia, Malaysia

ABSTRACT

The importance of reverse logistics and product recovery is evident in various industries as well as in current UNESCO sustainable development goals. This includes plastics and recycling with the former "contributed" significantly towards environmental issues and the latter being one of the primary solutions. The motivations of its implementation are generally divided into legal, economic, and socio-environmental factors. One of the crucial components of plastics recycling and a reverse logistics system is product return channels. The success of other components especially the recovery operations depends on the effectiveness of the return channels. Although numerous investigations on product return channels have been carried out, research on some critical aspects remains wanting. This study presents a review that highlights this deficiency, depicts relevant research development on product return channels, decision-making issues, and direction for future research. At the end of the study, the authors propose a new closed-loop logistics network and future research framework propositions.

INTRODUCTION

Minimizing environmental pollution and industrial waste has become one of the main concerns in many countries. Developed countries such as Japan, United States and the European Union (EU) have already enacted legislation on these issues. It is also acknowledgeable that other related problems such as scarcity of natural resources in certain industries, limited landfill capacities, and the negative effect of discarded products has undesirably amplified over the years. For some companies, engagement in environmental preservation and management of industrial waste is no longer an option. According to

DOI: 10.4018/978-1-5225-9452-9.ch023

Sasikumar, Kannan and Haq (2010), many companies are now engaged in product recovery business due to increasing government pressure, environmental deterioration, economic pressure, resource reduction and social responsibilities. Hence, various governments have started pressuring companies to take responsibility over their products beyond its lifecycle. Sohail and Sohal (2003) stated that legislation aimed at environment-benign production forces manufacturers to take back their products from end-users after they discard them. This is where reverse logistics and reverse supply chain management started.

Logistics network design that encompasses decisions such as determining the numbers, locations, quantity of the flow and capacities of the facilities is one of the most important strategic decisions in the reverse supply chain management (Pishvaee, Kianfar and Karimi, 2010). This network design becomes even more important with the legal implementation of the extended producer responsibility (Alumur, Nickel, Saldanha-da-Gama and Verter, 2012). The extended producer responsibility states that manufacturers are responsible for free taking back and recovery of their end-of-life products and must bear all or a significant part of the collection and treatment costs (Mansour and Zarei, 2008). At the same time, the amount of collected returned products should at least satisfy the required minimum collection rate. It is also noted that collection of used products potentially accounts for a significant part of the total costs of any closed-loop supply chain (Dekker, Fleischmann, Inderfurth, and Van Wassenhove, 2004).

Government regulations concerning product take-back such as a specific minimum level of product returns (minimum percentage of products that firms need to take back) play a major role in the promotion of product recovery. This regulation has been widely practiced in many EU nations and other developed countries such as the United States and Japan. With the enforcement of environmental laws, firms are obliged to come up with suitable ways to manage their discarded products. Other than the requirement to comply with product take-back regulations, there is also the need for firms to devise effective and efficient ways to do so. And this is where the economic factor comes into play. An increasing number of firms are beginning to appreciate the fact that reverse logistics and product recovery management can lead the way towards the realization of business objectives such as profit maximization, cost minimization, resource utilization and production efficiency. Major firms such as Canon, Xerox, Hewlett-Packard, Agfa, Kodak, Daimler-Chrysler, BMW, and Visteon are practicing product recovery management to enhance their profitability and cost competitiveness (while complying with environmental regulations),factors that could lead to better competitive positioning in the market. This brings us to the third driver – consumer pressure. The consumers of today are increasingly environmentally conscious. Termed 'the green consumers' they can be expected to frown on products and firms that are not environmentally friendly. Their influence is gaining in strength, and with the current level of business competition, firms are understandably concerned about their image. Thus, it is not surprising that many firms have implemented environmental campaigns with product recovery themes such as shopping bag recycling (Tesco, Aldi, Carrefour, etc.) and free take back of used products such as personal computers, washing machines and mobile phones. Some firms even go a step further by offering refund payments in a bid to encourage more returns.

In the meantime, the emergence of reverse logistics as the most significant recovery approach in environmental management within the broad supply chain context has long been recognized. The role of reverse logistics in the environmentally-conscious society of today is clearly vital. Implementation of an effective reverse logistics system involving management of product return flows is seen as one of the primary ways of enhancing the competitiveness and profitability of firms (as explained in the previous paragraphs). In other words, the current application of this system in many industries is not only for the purpose of complying with environmental laws but also as a profitable and sustainable business strategy

(Du and Evans, 2007). Briefly, according to Srivastava and Srivastava (2006), environmental issues, sustainable development and legal regulations have resulted in organizations becoming increasingly responsive to reverse logistics and specifically, product recovery management. Persistent problems related to declining landfill capacities and the negative impact of product disposal on the environment have also coerced more nations into employing environmentally friendly measures such as the implementation of a product take-back policy and extending the scope of producer responsibility. The factors mentioned above have significantly encouraged the management of firms to seriously consider the management of product returns which includes product take back and recovery. These are the focal points of this study which comprises two sections. The first section involves a discussion on the selection of product recovery options and the maximum benefits firms can gain from them, while in the second section an investigation is conducted on the ways firms can optimise their profits through the assignment of a location-allocation strategy for product returns.

In a nutshell, this study aims to review relevant studies on product return channels and highlights latest development as well as deficiencies that may lead to potential research propositions in the future. The motivations to embark on this study is to investigate on the "frontline" collection methods of returned products. Latest studies on plastics recycling is also carried out. This paper is organized as follows: First, overview of product return channels and how it is embedded in reverse logistics decision making sequences is highlighted. Next section presents overview of latest studies on plastic recycling then followed by section on product return channels and the collection methods. The issue of collection effectiveness and decisions making in product return channels are then discussed. Then, relevant research development and managerial implications are presented. Potential area for further investigations is then concludes the study.

PLASTICS RECYCLING

Plastics are being manufactured globally at a rate exceeding 335 million tonnes annually and 8.3 billion tonnes have been made since 1960's, with 4.9 billion tonnes accumulating in landfills or in the natural environment (Kosior, Mitchell and Crescenzi, 2018). Electronic waste (e-waste) is the fastest growing waste on the planet, with an annual growth rate of 3–4% and it is estimated that e-waste generation will reach 52.2 million tonnes per annum by 2021 for which only 15% of e-waste is recycled (Sahajwalla and Gaikwad, 2018). Globally plastic waste has been steadily increasing and recycling itself has received much attention because many companies are using it as a strategic tool to serve their customers and to generate good revenue (Satapathy, 2017). Pre-sorting of plastics before recycling is costly and time-intensive, recycling requires large amounts of energy and often leads to low-quality polymers, and current technologies cannot be applied to many polymeric materials (Garcia and Robertson, 2017). In order to increase the plastic recycling returns and reduce the operational cost, managers need to cluster the customers based on the facility location and offer attractive incentives (Sherrif, Subramaniam, Rahman and Jayaram, 2017). Amin, Wu and Karaphillis (2018) investigated plastic pallets recovery methods using three options namely remanufacturing, reusing and recycling. According to Tran and Luc (2018), the highest internal barrier for plastics recycling initiative is limited forecasting and planning for the reverse logistics, and that the perception of poor quality recovered materials is among the external barriers. In the mean time, Hahladakis, Purnell, Iacovidou, Velis and Atseyinku (2018) reported that three main collection schemes are currently implemented in England in which are (i) kerbside collection (KS), (ii) household waste recycling centres (HWRCs), and (iii) bring sites/banks (BSs). The results of their study indicated that: (a) the contribution of KS collection scheme in recovering packaging plastics is higher than HWRCs and BBs, with respective percentages by weight (wt%) 90%, 9% and 1%; (b) alternate weekly collection (AWC) of plastic recyclables in wheeled bins, when collected commingled, demonstrated higher yield in KS collection; (c) only a small percentage (16%) of the total amount of post-consumer plastics collected in the examined period was finally sent to re-processors; (c) nearly a third of Local Authorities (LAs) reported insufficient or poor data; and (d) the most abundant fractions of plastics that finally reached the re-processors were mixed plastic bottles and mixed plastics. Although studies on plastics recycling has been abundant, more research avenues are still continuously being explored and investigated from various perspectives using different approaches. The end goals are absolute; maximization of plastics recovery and collection, as well as minimization of its usage.

PRODUCT RETURN CHANNELS AND THE COLLECTION METHODS

Product return channels can be defined as avenues or facilities for customers to return used or unwanted products back to the producers, collectors, remanufacturers or recyclers. It is part of the broader network design that may encompass both forward and reverse logistics decisions. Producers or remanufacturers are responsible for designing effective network design (collection channels) that may also include other non-logistical factors such as monetary incentives or marketing campaign. Most of the previous research highlighted that product return channels can be divided into either centralized or decentralized return channels (Savaskan and van Wassenhove, 2006). These return channels are actually representing the type of decision making and degree of control practiced by the manufacturers. In the meantime, there are various ways of collecting used or unwanted products back from the consumers. Big companies such as Dell Computer and Hewlett-Packard offers return incentives to their customers in the form of free door-to-door pick up and mail return respectively. Other manufacturers use their retailers or distributors (intermediaries). There are also independent recyclers or remanufacturers that engage directly with customers to collect returned products either using their on-site drop-off facilities or door-to-door pick up services. Apart from that, there are government agencies or local authorities such as the city council offering similar services. In United Kingdom, large hypermarkets such as Tesco and Asda also provide on-site drop-off facilities (recycling centres) in return for loyalty points. It is one of the most important components in reverse logistics and is now viewed as another important avenue for profit making endeavour. Hence, designing the network design and measuring effectiveness of the return channels are also equally critical for the reverse logistics success.

COLLECTION EFFECTIVENESS OF PRODUCT RETURN CHANNELS

Collection effectiveness depends on the consumers' willingness to return used products at the time of disposal (Wojanowski, Verter and Boyaci, 2007). It has been identified that two important factors which influence customers' willingness to return their products are accessibility and incentives. Min and Ko (2009) pointed out that customers' convenience when returning their products should be maximized as it will eventually encourage more future returns. There are three collection methods that are normally used by manufacturers namely mail delivery return, pick up collection and customer drop off. Installing a drop-off facility near residential or commercial areas encourages customers to return their products (easy access). This collection method requires the manufacturer to bear the cost of building or renting as well as operating the drop-off facilities in certain selected area. Nonetheless, the important decision is to decide how many drop-off facilities are needed and its locations. These type of return channels are actually depicting the decision making approach in reverse logistics network. Figure 1 illustrates the collection methods in product return channels. According to Wagner (2012), convenience factors play important roles in the collection effort of solid waste. He identified five key convenience factors to increase collection rate: (1) knowledge requirement, (2) proximity to collection site, (3) opportunity to drop-off materials, (4) the draw of the collection site, and (5) ease of the process. The researcher also developed a performance matrix based on the abovementioned five convenience factors to help solid waste managers make decisions. The study highlighted that the convenience factors also refer to the availability and ease of the collection process for the customers. In other word, minimizing customer's time, effort and travelling cost may positively influence product return rates.

Hence, in practice the facilities need to be located within close proximity to the customers. Some manufacturers use intermediaries such as retailers acting as collection centres to collect returned products from the customers. Previous studies usually group customers based on geographical zones and each zone is served by one particular drop-off facility (Wojanowski et al., 2007; Aras and Aksen, 2008; Aras, Aksen and Tanugur, 2008). In the meantime, incentives play a significant role in influencing customers' willingness to return their products. According to Aras et al., (2008), some manufacturers have been able to influence the quantity of returns by using buy-back campaigns and offering financial incentives to product holders. Apart from an increment in terms of product return quantities, the amount of incentives offered by the manufacturers influences the quality level of the returned products (Aras and Aksen, 2008). Comparatively to Wojanoswki et al., (2007), these two studies examine how the amount of incentives offered to the customers affects manufacturers' profit and collection strategies.

THE COLLECTION CHANNELS AND DECISIONS MAKING ISSUES

Karakayali, Hulya and Akcali (2007) examined decentralized collection and processing end-of-life (EOL) products with aims of developing models to determine optimal acquisition and selling price of the EOL products as well as its remanufactured parts. They also address problems of how to identify when and why OEM would prefer a remanufacturer/collector-driven channel (outsource the processing or collection of returned products). In their model, three channel settings were considered: centralized

Figure 1. Collection methods in product return channels

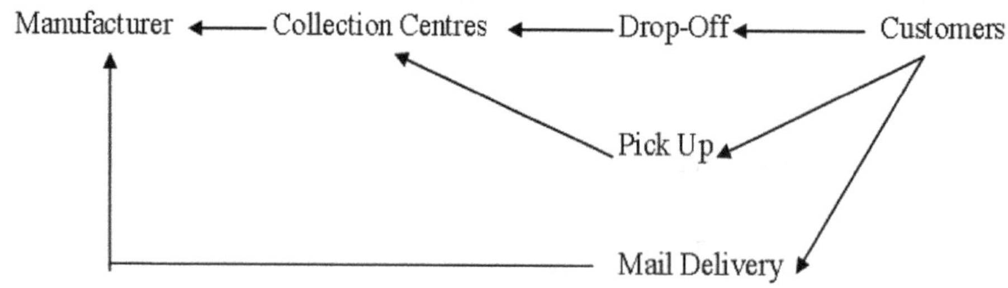

channel, remanufacturer-driven channel and collector driven channel. Findings show that collector-driven channel can increase collection rates and is capable of attaining the same collection rate as the centralized channel due to the pricing behaviour. In the meantime, effective product return network is also very critical to product recovery planning and cost minimization. Many researchers have investigated the effectiveness of a product return network. Nonetheless, Qin and Ji (2010) stated that these investigations have largely been in deterministic environment. They then propose a logistics network configuration with product recovery in fuzzy environment. Based on different decision-making criteria, fuzzy programming approach is employed to formulate three programming models: the expected value model, chance constrained programming and dependent - chance programming. Their work offers an approach for designing practical product recovery network under uncertain environment (using fuzzy programming). In a different study, Savaskan and Wassenhove (2006) discuss about how to understand when a manufacturer would choose to collect returned products directly from consumers or indirectly via the retailers and why. The decision process involves four types of collection channels/models: (1) decentralized direct collection, (2) decentralized indirect collection, (3) centralized direct collection, and (4) centralized indirect collection. The models involve a manufacturer, two retailers and the central planner. In decentralized direct model, the manufacturer sets the wholesale price of the product and the collection effort while the retailers are free to decide the selling price (while considering competition from the other retailer). Figure 2 shows return channel structures as Savaskan and Wassenhove (2006) differentiates each channel into five categories.

In decentralized indirect model, the retailers are responsible for the collection of returned products (in return of a fixed per unit buy-back payment). The applications of decentralized models are illustrated by Wei, Zhao and Sun (2012) in which they highlighted the roles of retailers and third-party collectors in helping manufacturer to gather returned products. In the centralized models, the difference lies upon the role of the central planner who makes the decisions over pricing and collection effort (retailers have no power to decide the selling price or the collection effort). In decentralized models, findings show that retailers prefer direct collection by the manufacturer (to avoid making investment in collection of returned products) while indirect collection benefits the manufacturer in terms of saving the investment costs in collection effort and increase in sales volume (unless retailers' products are considered to be direct substitutes). As for the centralized models, prices have become important determinant; if the retailers have less impact on the prices, then the manufacturer benefits from a direct collection system, and vice versa. Shulman, Coughlan and Savaskan (2010) identified three reverse channels which are (1) vertically integrated system, (2) retailer assuming returns responsibility, and (3) manufacturer assuming returns responsibility. The first is a centralized return channel while the remaining two represent decentralized return structures. The study addresses the relationships between manufacturers and retailers, and how decisions by each party affect each other. The result favours centralized reverse structure in which the manufacturer has greater control over the flow of returned products from customers.

RESEARCH DEVELOPMENT ON PRODUCT RETURN CHANNELS

Most of the studies on product return channels remained focus on network design. In the broadest sense, this involves location and routing problems. Studies by Alumur et al., (2012), Das and Chowdury (2012), Nikbaksh, Eskandarpour and Zegordi (2013), Sherrif, Gunasekaran and Nachiappan (2012), Rogers, Melamed and Lembke (2012), Lieckens and Vandaele (2012), Kannan, Diabat, Alrefai, Govindan and

Figure 2. Product return channel structures

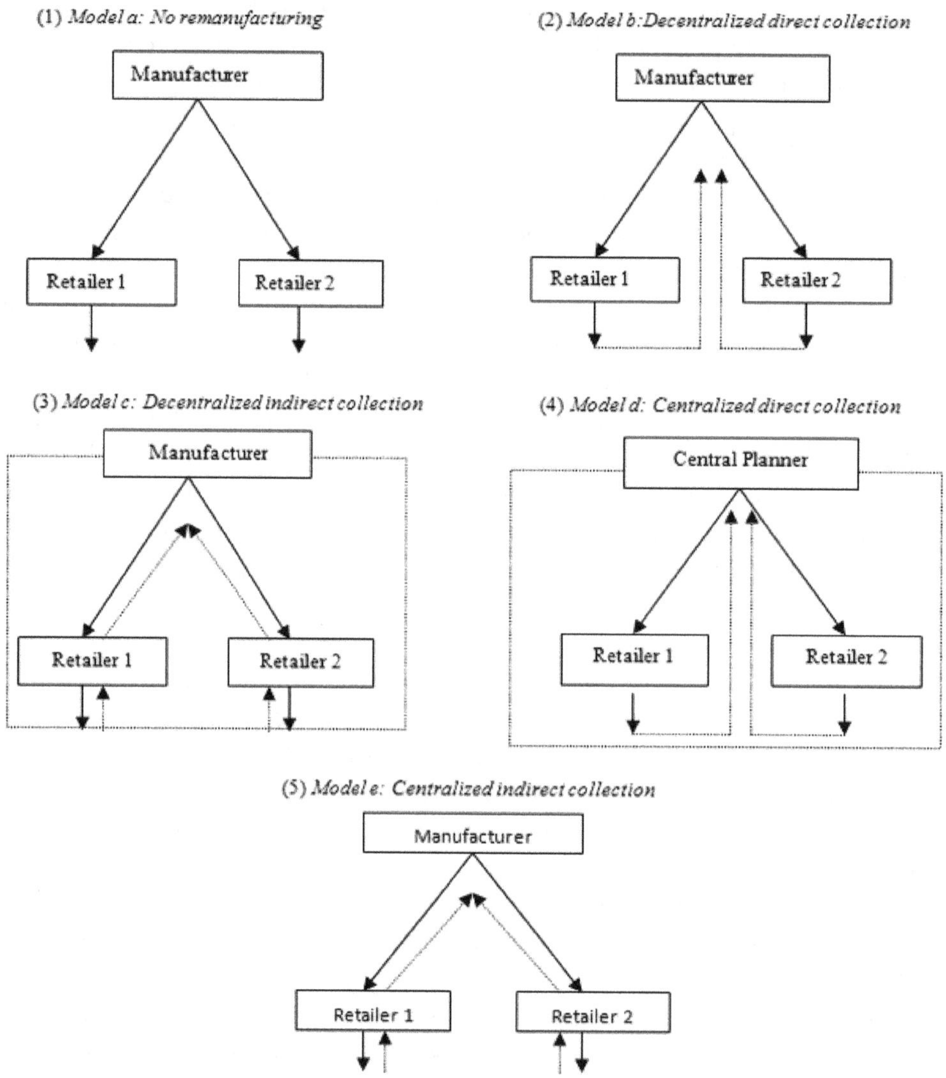

Source: Savaskan and van Wassenhove (2006)

Yong (2012), and John and Sridharan (2013) illustrates discussions on product return channels from the perspective of a network design problem. In the meantime, study by Wei et al., (2012) addresses problem of collecting returned products using game theory and fuzzy theory. Their research represents some similarity with this study in the sense that the main decision is about selecting collection modes and its consequences. They defined collection modes into three categories: (1) manufacturer's direct collection, (2) retailers' collection, and (3) third party collection. Under the (2) and (3) modes, collection rates and retail prices (buyback prices) are determined by retailers and the third party collectors. It resembles a decentralize collection channel. However, the model doesn't specify the exact method of collecting the used products from customers.

Touati-Moungla and Jost (2012) reviewed vehicle routing and scheduling literatures in environmentally-conscious transportation problems. They highlighted that for pick-up delivery routing problem, most studies use insertion-based algorithm (multi-objective) or genetic algorithm (single objective). The research also mentioned about the growing concerns of environmental issues such as public health, global warming and economic safety. Wolfer, Sander and Gogoll (2012) stated that pressing global challenges such as climate change and resources depletion demonstrates the need for structural change in our economic approach towards sustainable development. It appears that most of the location models rely on finite solutions and mixed- integer linear programming which allows for discrete mathematical optimization. Most location- allocation problems also rely on mixed-integer and linear programming model in which number of warehouses, capacities and locations were determined. Jayant, Gupta and Garg (2012) stated that the number of customers supporting environmental protection by delivering their used products to collection points is increasing. In order to minimize the total reverse logistics cost and high utilization rates of collection points, selecting appropriate locations for collection points is critical issues in reverse logistics. In the meantime, study on collection and recycling policies of electronic scraps among countries around the world has been conducted by Oliveira, Bernardes and Gerbase (2012). In their study, they compare policies and collection frameworks of selected European, US, Asian and South American countries. Some countries such as Switzerland and Germany have better comprehensive collection policies and regulations than other countries.

MANAGERIAL IMPLICATIONS

Previous research on product return channels focused more on other 'general' return networks such as centralized and decentralized, and direct or indirect return networks (Savaskan and Wassenhove, 2006; Karakayali et al., 2007; Shulman et al., 2010; Abdessalem, Hadj-Alouane and Riopel, 2012; Bai and Sarkis, 2013; De Brito and Dekker, 2004; Fleischmann, Beullens, Bloemhof-Ruwaard and Wassenhove, 2001; Fleischmann, Bloemhof-Ruwaard, Dekker, van der Laan, van Nunen and Wassenhove, 1997; Fleischmann, Krikke, Dekker and Flapper, 2000; Jayaraman, Guide and Srivastava, 1999; Jayaraman, Patterson and Rolland, 2003; Li and Tee, 2012; Nikolaidis, 2012).

Only several researchers studied the 'groundwork' collection methods albeit focusing on different scope and approach (Sasikumar et al., 2010; Wojanowski et al., 2007; Min and Ko, 2008; Aras and Aksen, 2008; Aras et al., 2008; Wei et al., 2012). Studies on the three collection methods namely drop-off, pick-up and mail return delivery remains insufficient. From the industry point of view, many firms prefer to outsource its reverse logistics function, let alone product collection activity. This scenario is understandable since not many firms able to facilitate three collection methods simultaneously. Costs to offer these facilities such as collection centre's handling and setup costs (drop-off), and related transportation costs (pick-up) are relatively high. Hence, many firms prefer outsourcing some, if not all, of the collection jobs to the third party collectors (Karakayali et al., 2007; Kannan et al., 2012; Oliveira et al., 2012). In some cases, the firm prefers intermediaries such as retailers to collect returned products for them (Savaskan and Wassenhove, 2006; Shulman et al., 2010). These retailers offer drop-off facilities at their premises to the consumers to return their products. However, as more countries around the globe implement the extended producer responsibility legally (Mansour and Zarei, 2008; Sarkis, Helm and Hervani, 2010; Srivastava, 2007; Srivastava and Srivastava, 2006), more firms realize that product recovery is no longer a burden, but an opportunity to make profit from a new avenue. Now, some firms prefer to have direct control over the collection of returned products to better manage and improve the collection rates. Subsequently, having the luxury to offer these three collection methods is a good option for as long as it is feasible. Nevertheless, from the practical point of view, the lack of empirical studies on the three collection methods may affect the abovementioned effort.

POTENTIAL RESEARCH PROPOSITIONS

In product return channel, most previous optimization models treated product return as location problem. Hence, it is more towards managing transportation of returns or finding the best routing strategy rather than looking for optimal assignment. So far, only a handful of study addressed collection problem comprehensively incorporating more than one method (pick-up or drop-off). Literature survey on mail return method is also very limited, if not non-existence (Alumur et al., 2012; Wojanowski et al., 2007; Aras and Aksen, 2008; Aras et al., 2008; Kannan et al., 2012; John and Sridharan, 2013; Akdogan and Coskun, 2012; Baenas, Hojas de Castro, Battistelle and Junior, 2011; Du and Evans, 2007; Ilgin and Gupta, 2010; Krikke, 2011; Ozkir and Basligil, 2012; Parlikad and McFarlane, 2009). Based on the above analysis, follows are some potential research areas in product return channels that can be studied further:

1. Feasibility study on the application of mail return method and its effectiveness.
2. The optimizations of mail return as an alternatives to other collection methods in reverse logistics problem.
3. Developing optimum incentives schemes for mail, drop-off and pick-up collection methods that can benefit firms in terms of collection rates, costs and profit.
4. The applications of different incentives schemes for mail, drop-off and pick-up collection methods under centralized and decentralized decisions making policy. This may include incentives scheme for the return of recyclable plastics.
5. The effectiveness of mail, drop-off and pick-up under direct and indirect collection methods, as well as centralized versus decentralized decisions policy.
6. The effect of quality categorization of returned products in each collection methods. This may also be applicable to plastics.
7. Further studies on plastics reprocessing initiatives and collection strategy.

In the meantime, we propose a new closed-loop logistic framework encompassing both forward and reverse movement of products (Figure 3). In conventional closed - loop logistics network, the reverse movement of products started with collection of returned products. So far, the collection activities have been depicted by a more general product collection avenue such as centralized and decentralized collection or direct and indirect methods. There is a loophole prior to products being send to the recovery facilities. Supposedly, it is not only about decision making policy (*centralized vs decentralized*) or the general return strategy (*direct vs indirect*). Hence, the new framework includes the initial collection methods in which the collection activities are actually happening involving the three methods. The product return channel that is highlighted at the end of the forward flow marks the beginning of the reverse network system. Again it is worth noting that the collection methods of drop-off, pick-up and the mail return has presented significant avenue for future research. Apart from it being the missing link in the previous

Figure 3. New research framework for closed-loop logistics environment

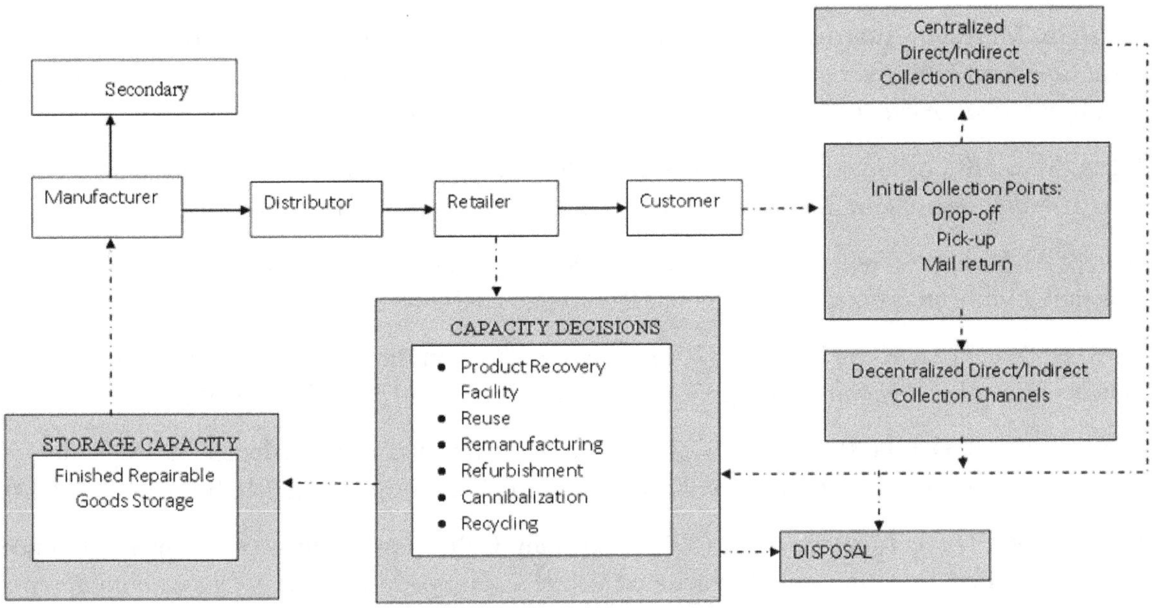

conventional closed-loop logistics network, the importance of these three methods is also undeniably crucial in determining the success of the whole reverse logistics operations.

CONCLUSION

Product recovery management in a closed-loop logistics network encompasses various activities such as collection channels, production (reprocessing, disassembly, separation and inventory management), capacity planning, procurement, warehouse distribution, and recovery networks (such as routings, and location-allocation decisions). This study reviews literature on reverse logistics network in which particular attention is given to the collection activities of returned products (product return channels). The criticality of product recovery management within the reverse logistics context is substantially significant with numerous studies being conducted to address various issues. In product return channels, most research addressed collection of returned products from a broader spectrum; whether collection should be (1) centralized or decentralized, and whether it should be handled (2) directly or indirectly (Savaskan and Wassenhove, 2006; Karakayali et al., 2007). The role and impact of the initial collection points where the first contact between consumers and the return facilities occurs are hardly acknowledged. Relevant studies by Wojanowski et al., (2007), Aras and Aksen (2008), and Aras et al., (2008) acknowledging the optimization of product return' initial collection strategy should be further analysed. At the end of this study, we propose several research areas for further investigation as well as a new framework for a closed-loop logistics network that includes the initial collection methods.

REFERENCES

Abdessalem, M., Hadj–Alouane, A. B., & Riopel, D. (2012). Decision modelling of reverse logistics systems: Selection of recovery operations for end–of–life products. *International Journal of Logistics Systems and Management, 13*(2), 139–161. doi:10.1504/IJLSM.2012.048933

Akdoğan, M. Ş., & Coşkun, A. (2012). Drivers of Reverse Logistics Activities: An Empirical Investigation. *Procedia: Social and Behavioral Sciences, 58*, 1640–1649. doi:10.1016/j.sbspro.2012.09.1130

Alumur, S. A., Nickel, S., Saldanha-da-Gama, F., & Verter, V. (2012). Multi-period reverse logistics network design. *European Journal of Operational Research, 220*(1), 67–78. doi:10.1016/j.ejor.2011.12.045

Amin, S. H., Wu, H., & Karaphillis, G. (2018). A perspective on the reverse logistics of plastic pallets in Canada. *Journal of Remanufacturing, 8*(3), 153–174. doi:10.100713243-018-0051-0

Aras, N., & Aksen, D. (2008). Locating Collection Centers for Distance-and-Incentive-Dependent Returns. *International Journal of Production Economics, 111*(2), 316–333. doi:10.1016/j.ijpe.2007.01.015

Aras, N., Aksen, D., & Tanugur, A. G. (2008). Locating Collection Centers for Incentive-Dependent Returns under a Pick Up Policy with Capacitated Vehicles. *European Journal of Operational Research, 191*(3), 1223–1240. doi:10.1016/j.ejor.2007.08.002

Baenas, J. M., Hojas De Castro, R., Battistelle, R. A. G., & Junior, J. A. G. (2011). A Study of Reverse Logistics Flow Management in Vehicle Battery Industries in the Midwest of the State of Sao Paulo. *Journal of Cleaner Production, 19*(2-3), 168–172. doi:10.1016/j.jclepro.2010.08.018

Bai, C., & Sarkis, J. (2013). Flexibility in Reverse Logistics: A Framework and Evaluation Approach. *Journal of Cleaner Production, 47*, 306–318. doi:10.1016/j.jclepro.2013.01.005

Das, K., & Chowdhury, A. H. (2012). Designing a reverse logistics network for optimal collection, recovery and quality-based product-mix planning. *International Journal of Production Economics, 135*(1), 209–221. doi:10.1016/j.ijpe.2011.07.010

De Brito, M. P., & Dekker, R. (2004). A Framework for Reverse Logistics. In R. Dekker, K. Inderfurth, L. van Wassenhove, & M. Fleischmann (Eds.), *Reverse Logistics. Quantitative Models for Closed- Loop Supply Chains*. Berlin, Germany: Springer-Verlag. doi:10.1007/978-3-540-24803-3_1

Dekker, R., Fleischmann, M., Inderfurth, K., & Van Wassenhove, L. N. (2004). *Reverse Logistics Network Design: Quantitative Models for Closed-Loop Supply Chains*. Berlin: Springer. doi:10.1007/978-3-540-24803-3

Du, F., & Evans, G. W. (2007). A Bi-Objective Reverse Logistics Network Analysis for Post-Sale Service. *Computers & Operations Research.*

Fleischmann, M., Beullens, P., Bloemhof-Ruwaard, J. M., & Van Wassenhove, L. N. (2001). The Impact of Product Recovery on Logistics Network Design. *Production and Operations Management, 10*(2), 156–173. doi:10.1111/j.1937-5956.2001.tb00076.x

Fleischmann, M., Bloemhof-Ruwaard, J. M., Dekker, R., van der Laan, E., van Nunen, J., & Van Wassenhove, L. N. (1997). Quantitative Models for Reverse Logistics: A Review. *European Journal of Operational Research, 103*(1), 1–17. doi:10.1016/S0377-2217(97)00230-0

Fleischmann, M., Krikke, H. R., Dekker, R., & Flapper, S. D. P. (2000). A Characterisation of Logistics Networks for Product Recovery. *Omega, 28*(6), 653–666. doi:10.1016/S0305-0483(00)00022-0

Garcia, J. M., & Robertson, M. L. (2017). The future of plastics recycling. *Science, 358*(6365), 870–872. doi:10.1126cience.aaq0324 PMID:29146798

Hahladakis, J. N., Purnell, P., Iacovidou, E., Velis, C. A., & Atseyinku, M. (2018). Post-consumer plastic packaging waste in England: Assessing the yield of multiple collection-recycling schemes. *Waste Management (New York, N.Y.), 75*, 149–159. doi:10.1016/j.wasman.2018.02.009 PMID:29439928

Ilgin, M. A., & Gupta, S. M. (2010). Environmentally Conscious Manufacturing and Product Recovery (ECMPRO): A Review of the State of the Art. *Journal of Environmental Management, 91*(3), 563–591. doi:10.1016/j.jenvman.2009.09.037 PMID:19853369

Jayant, A., Gupta, P., and Garg, S. K. (2012). Perspectives in Reverse Supply Chain Management (R-SCM): A State of the Art Literature Review. *JJMIE, 6*(1).

Jayaraman, V., Guide, V. D. R. Jr, & Srivastava, R. (1999). Closed-Loop Logistics Model for Remanufacturing. *The Journal of the Operational Research Society, 50*(5), 497–508. doi:10.1057/palgrave.jors.2600716

Jayaraman, V., Patterson, R. A., & Rolland, E. (2003). The Design of Reverse Distribution Networks: Models and Solution Procedures. *European Journal of Operational Research, 150*(1), 128–149. doi:10.1016/S0377-2217(02)00497-6

John, S. T., & Sridharan, R. (2013). Modelling and analysis of network design for a closed–loop supply chain. *International Journal of Logistics Systems and Management, 14*(3), 329–352. doi:10.1504/IJLSM.2013.052064

Kannan, D., Diabat, A., Alrefaei, M., Govindan, K., & Yong, G. (2012). A carbon footprint based reverse logistics network design model. *Resources, Conservation and Recycling, 67*, 75–79. doi:10.1016/j.resconrec.2012.03.005

Karakayali, I., Hulya, E.-F., & Akcali, E. (2007). An Analysis of Decentralized Collection and Processing Of End-Of-Life Products. *Journal of Operations Management, 25*(6), 1161–1183. doi:10.1016/j.jom.2007.01.017

Kosior, E., Mitchell, J., & Crescenzi, I. (2018). Plastics Recycling. *Plastics and the Environment, 47*, 156–176. doi:10.1039/9781788013314-00156

Krikke, H. (2011). Impact of closed-loop network configurations on carbon footprints: A case study in copiers. *Resources, Conservation and Recycling, 55*(12), 1196–1205. doi:10.1016/j.resconrec.2011.07.001

Li, R. C., & Tee, T. J. C. (2012). A Reverse Logistics Model For Recovery Options Of E-waste Considering the Integration of the Formal and Informal Waste Sectors. *Procedia: Social and Behavioral Sciences, 40*, 788–816. doi:10.1016/j.sbspro.2012.03.266

Lieckens, K., & Vandaele, N. (2012). Multi-level reverse logistics network design under uncertainty. *International Journal of Production Research*, *50*(1), 23–40. doi:10.1080/00207543.2011.571442

Mansour, A., & Zarei, M. (2008). A Multi-Period Reverse Logistics Optimization Model for End-Of-Life Vehicles Recovery Based on EU Directive. *International Journal of Computer Integrated Manufacturing*, *21*(7), 764–777. doi:10.1080/09511920701685325

Min, H., & Ko, H.-J. (2008). The Dynamic Design of a Reverse Logistics Network from the Perspective of Third-Party Logistics Service Providers. *International Journal of Production Economics*, *113*(1), 176–192. doi:10.1016/j.ijpe.2007.01.017

Nikbakhsh, E., Eskandarpour, M., & Zegordi, S. H. (2013). Designing a Robust Post-Sales Reverse Logistics Network. *Electrical Engineering and Intelligent Systems*, 313-325.

Nikolaidis, Y. (2012). Reverse Logistics and Quality Management Issues: State-of-the-Art. *Quality Management in Reverse Logistics: A Broad Look on Quality Issues and Their Interaction With Closed-Loop Supply Chains*, 1.

Oliveira, C. R. D., Bernardes, A. M., & Gerbase, A. E. (2012). Collection and recycling of electronic scrap: A worldwide overview and comparison with the Brazilian situation. *Waste Management*.

Özkır, V., & Başlıgil, H. (2012). Multi-objective optimization of closed-loop supply chains in uncertain environment. *Journal of Cleaner Production*.

Parlikad, A. K., & McFarlane, D. (2009). Strategies for product recovery decisions. *International Journal of Product Lifecycle Management*, *4*(1), 186–206. doi:10.1504/IJPLM.2009.031673

Pishvaee, M. S., Kianfar, K., & Karimi, B. (2010). Reverse Logistics Network Design Using Simulated Annealing. *International Journal of Advanced Manufacturing Technology*, *47*(1-4), 269–281. doi:10.100700170-009-2194-5

Qin, Z., & Ji, X. (2010). Logistics Network Design for Product Recovery in Fuzzy Environment. *European Journal of Operational Research*, *202*(2), 479–490. doi:10.1016/j.ejor.2009.05.036

Rogers, D. S., Melamed, B., & Lembke, R. S. (2012). Modeling and Analysis of Reverse Logistics. *Journal of Business Logistics*, *33*(2), 107–117. doi:10.1111/j.0000-0000.2012.01043.x

Sahajwalla, V., & Gaikwad, V. (2018). The present and future of e-waste plastics recycling. *Current Opinion in Green and Sustainable Chemistry*, *13*, 102–107. doi:10.1016/j.cogsc.2018.06.006

Sarkis, J., Helm, M. M., & Hervani, A. A. (2010). Reverse Logistics and Social Sustainability. *Corporate Social Responsibility and Environmental Management*, *17*(6), 337–354. doi:10.1002/csr.220

Sasikumar, P., Kannan, G., & Haq, A. N. (2010). A Multi-Echelon Reverse Logistics Network Design for Product Recovery - Case of Truck Tire Remanufacturing. *International Journal of Advanced Manufacturing Technology*, *49*(9-12), 1223–1234. doi:10.100700170-009-2470-4

Satapathy, S. (2017). An analysis of barriers for plastic recycling in the Indian plastic industry. *Benchmarking: An International Journal*, *24*(2), 415–430. doi:10.1108/BIJ-11-2014-0103

Savaskan, R. C., & van Wassenhove, L. N. (2006). Reverse Channel Design: The Case of Competing Retailers. *Management Science*, *52*(1), 1–14. doi:10.1287/mnsc.1050.0454

Sheriff, K. M., Gunasekaran, A., & Nachiappan, S. (2012). Reverse logistics network design: A review on strategic perspective. *International Journal of Logistics Systems and Management*, *12*(2), 171–194. doi:10.1504/IJLSM.2012.047220

Sheriff, K. M., Subramanian, N., Rahman, S., & Jayaram, J. (2017). Integrated optimization model and methodology for plastics recycling: Indian empirical evidence. *Journal of Cleaner Production*, *153*, 707–717. doi:10.1016/j.jclepro.2016.07.137

Shulman, J. D., Coughlan, A. T., & Savaskan, R. C. (2010). Optimal Reverse Channel Structure for Consumer Product Returns. *Marketing Science*, *29*(6), 1071–1085. doi:10.1287/mksc.1100.0578

Sohail, M. S., & Sohal, A. S. (2003). The Use of Third Party Logistics Services: A Malaysian Perspective. *Technovation*, *23*(5), 401–408. doi:10.1016/S0166-4972(02)00003-2

Srivastava, S. K. (2007). Green Supply-Chain Management: A State-Of-The-Art Literature Review. *International Journal of Management Reviews*, *9*(1), 53–80. doi:10.1111/j.1468-2370.2007.00202.x

Srivastava, S. K., & Srivastava, R. K. (2006). Managing Product Returns for Reverse Logistics. *International Journal of Physical Distribution & Logistics Management*, *36*(7), 524–546. doi:10.1108/09600030610684962

Touati-Moungla, N., & Jost, V. (2012). Combinatorial optimization for electric vehicles management. *Journal of Energy and Power Engineering*, *6*(5), 738–743.

Tran, T. T. H., & Luc, T. T. H. (2018). Reverse Logistics in Plastic Supply Chain: The Current Practice in Vietnam. In Nachhaltige Impulse für Produktion und Logistikmanagement (pp. 219-233). Springer Gabler.

Wagner, T. P. (2012). Examining the concept of convenient collection: An application to extended producer responsibility and product stewardship frameworks. *Waste Management (New York, N.Y.)*, *33*(3), 499–507. doi:10.1016/j.wasman.2012.06.015 PMID:22818910

Wei, J., Zhao, J., & Sun, X. (2012). Reverse channel decisions for a fuzzy closed-loop supply chain. *Applied Mathematical Modelling*.

Wojanowski, R., Verter, V., & Boyaci, T. (2007). Retail-Collection Network Design under Deposit-Refund. *Computers & Operations Research*, *34*(2), 324–345. doi:10.1016/j.cor.2005.03.003

Wolfer, S., Sander, H., & Gogoll, F. (2012). *Reverse Logistics for Waste Electrical and Electronic Equipment (WEEE) in China*. Academic Press.

Compilation of References

Ab Jalil, N., Basri, H., Basri, N. A., & Abushammala, M. F. (2015). The Potential of Biodrying as Pretreatment for municipal solid waste in Malaysia. *Journal of Advanced Review on Scientific Research*, *7*, 5–13.

Abayomi, O. A., Range, P., Al-Ghouti, M. A., Obbard, J. P., Almeer, S. H., & Ben-Hamadou, R. (2017). Microplastics in coastal environments of the Arabian Gulf. *Marine Pollution Bulletin*, *124*(1), 181–188. doi:10.1016/j.marpolbul.2017.07.011 PMID:28739102

Abbasi, M. N., & Sheikh, N. A. (2016). Attitudes and Motivations towards Plastics Recycling: A Multi-tier Supply Chain Approach. *Pakistan Journal of Social Sciences*, *36*(2), 705-722. Retrieved from https://www.bzu.edu.pk/PJSS/Vol36No22016/PJSS-Vol36-No2-10.pdf

Abdessalem, M., Hadj–Alouane, A. B., & Riopel, D. (2012). Decision modelling of reverse logistics systems: Selection of recovery operations for end–of–life products. *International Journal of Logistics Systems and Management*, *13*(2), 139–161. doi:10.1504/IJLSM.2012.048933

Abou-Zeid, D. M., Müller, R. J., & Deckwer, W. D. (2001). Degradation of natural and synthetic polyesters under anaerobic conditions. *Journal of Biotechnology*, *86*(2), 113–126. doi:10.1016/S0168-1656(00)00406-5 PMID:11245900

Abrusci, C., Pablos, J. L., Corrales, T., Lopez-Marín, J., Marín, L., & Catalina, F. (2011). Biodegradation of photo-degraded mulching films based on polyethylene and stearates of calcium and iron as pro-oxidant additives. *International Biodeterioration & Biodegradation*, *65*(3), 451–459. doi:10.1016/j.ibiod.2010.10.012

Abu-Hilal, A., & Al-Najjar, T. (2009). Marine litter in coral reef areas along the Jordan Gulf of Aqaba, Red Sea. *Journal of Environmental Management*, *90*(2), 1043–1049. doi:10.1016/j.jenvman.2008.03.014 PMID:18490098

ACC. (2016). *Biomonitoring data.* Retrieved from https://phthalates.americanchemistry.com/

ACG. (2006). *Allen Consulting Group.* ACG.

Achilias, D. S. (2006). Chemical recycling of poly (methyl methacrylate). *WSEAS Transactions on Environment and Development*, *2*(2), 85–91.

Achilias, D. S. (2007). Chemical recycling of poly (methyl methacrylate) by pyrolysis. The potential use of the liquid fraction as a raw material for the reproduction of the polymer. *European Polymer Journal*, *43*(6), 2564–2575. doi:10.1016/j.eurpolymj.2007.02.044

Achilias, D. S., Antonakou, E. V., Koutsokosta, E., & Lappas, A. A. (2009). Chemical recycling of polymers from waste electric and electronic equipment. *Journal of Applied Polymer Science*, *114*(1), 212–221. doi:10.1002/app.30533

Achilias, D. S., Antonakou, E. V., Roupakias, C., Megalokonomos, P., & Lappas, A. A. (2008). Recycling techniques of polyolefins from plastic wastes. *Global NEST Journal*, *10*(1), 114–122.

Achilias, D. S., Giannoulis, A., & Papageorgiou, G. Z. (2009). Recycling of polymers from plastic packaging materials using the dissolution/ reprecipitation technique. *Polymer Bulletin*, *63*(3), 449–465. doi:10.100700289-009-0104-5

Achilias, D. S., Kanellopoulou, I., Megalokonomos, P., Antonakou, E., & Lappas, A. (2007). Chemical Recycling of Polystyrene by Pyrolysis: Potential Use of the Liquid Product for the Reproduction of Polymer. *Macromolecular Materials and Engineering*, *292*(8), 923–934. doi:10.1002/mame.200700058

Achilias, D. S., & Karayannidis, G. P. (2004). The chemical recycling of PET in the framework of sustainable development. *Water Air and Soil Pollution Focus*, *4*(4/5), 385–396. doi:10.1023/B:WAFO.0000044812.47185.0f

Achilias, D. S., Megalokonomos, P., & Karayannidis, G. P. (2006). Current trends in chemical recycling of polyolefins. *Journal of Environmental Protection and Ecology*, *7*(2), 407–413.

Achilias, D. S., Redhwi, H. H., Siddiqui, M. N., Nikolaidis, A. K., Bikiaris, D. N., & Karayannidis, G. P. (2010). Glycolytic Depolymerization of PET Waste in a Microwave Reactor. *Journal of Applied Polymer Science*, *118*(5), 3066–3073. doi:10.1002/app.32737

Achilias, D. S., Roupakias, C., Megalokonomos, P., Lappas, A. A., & Antonakou, E. V. (2007). Chemical recycling of plastic wastes made from polyethylene (LDPE and HDPE) and polypropylene (PP). *Journal of Hazardous Materials*, *149*(3), 536–542. doi:10.1016/j.jhazmat.2007.06.076 PMID:17681427

Achilias, D. S., Tsintzou, G. P., Nikolaidis, A. K., Bikiaris, D. N., & Karayannidis, G. P. (2011). Aminolytic depolymerization of poly (ethylene terephthalate) waste in a microwave reactor. *Polymer International*, *60*(3), 500–506. doi:10.1002/pi.2976

Adamcova & Vaverkova. (2014). Biodegradable and non-biodegradable Plastic. *Polish J. of Environmental Studies*, *23*(50), 1465-1474.

Adamsson, A., Salonen, V., Paranko, J., & Toppari, J. (2009). Effects of maternal exposure to di-isononylphthalate (DINP) and 1, 1-dichloro-2, 2-bis (p-chlorophenyl) ethylene (p,p′ -DDE)on steroidogenesis is the fetal rat testis and adrenal gland. *Reproductive Toxicology (Elmsford, N.Y.)*, *28*(1), 66–74. doi:10.1016/j.reprotox.2009.03.002 PMID:19490997

Adibi, J. J., Perera, F. P., Jedrychowski, W., Camann, D. E., Barr, D., Jacek, R., & Whyatt, R. M. (2003). Prenatal exposures to phthalates among women in New York City and Krakow, Poland. *Environmental Health Perspectives*, *111*(14), 1719–1722. doi:10.1289/ehp.6235 PMID:14594621

Adibi, J. J., Whyatt, R. M., Hauser, R., Bhat, H. K., Davis, B. J., Calafat, A. M., ... Williams, P. L. (2010). Transcriptional biomarkers of steroidogenesis and trophoblast differentiation in the placenta in relation to prenatal phthalate exposure. *Environmental Health Perspectives*, *118*(2), 291–296. doi:10.1289/ehp.0900788 PMID:20123604

Adibi, J. J., Whyatt, R. M., Williams, P. L., Calafat, A. M., Camann, D., Herrick, R., ... Hauser, R. (2008). Characterization of phthalate exposure among pregnant women assessed by repeat air and urine samples. *Environmental Health Perspectives*, *116*(4), 467–473. doi:10.1289/ehp.10749 PMID:18414628

Aekplakorn, W., Chailurkit, L. O., & Ongphiphadhanakul, B. (2015). Relationship of serum Bisphenol A with diabetes in the Thai population, National Health Examination Survey IV, 2009. *Journal of Diabetes*, *7*(2), 240–249. doi:10.1111/1753-0407.12159 PMID:24720399

Aguado, J., & Serrano, D. P. (1999). *Feedstock recycling of plastic wastes*. Cambridge, UK: The Royal Society of Chemistry.

Aguado, R., Olazar, M., Gaisan, B., Prieto, R., & Bilbao, J. (2003). Kinetics of polystyrene pyrolysis in a conical spouted bed reactor. *Chemical Engineering Journal*, *92*(1-3), 91–99. doi:10.1016/S1385-8947(02)00119-5

Aguado, R., Olazar, M., San José, M. J., Gaisán, B., & Bilbao, J. (2002). Wax formation in the pyrolysis of polyolefins in a conical sprouted bed reactor. *Energy & Fuels*, *16*(6), 1429–1437. doi:10.1021/ef020043w

Aguayo, A. T., Gayubo, A. G., Ortega, J. M., Olazar, M., & Bilbao, J. (1997). Catalyst deactivation by cooking in the MTG process in fixed and fluidized bed reactors. *Catalysis Today*, *37*(3), 239–248. doi:10.1016/S0920-5861(97)00015-1

Ahamad Fausi Ismail, A. B. (2008). The effect of processing conditions on a polyacrylonitrile fiber produced using a solvent-free free coagulation process. *J of Material Science and Engineering A*, *485*(1-2), 251–257. doi:10.1016/j.msea.2007.08.060

Ahmad, S. (2018). *World Environmental Day 2018: Let's beat plastic pollution.* Retrieved from www.waterlogic.com

Ahmadkhaniha, R., Mansouri, M., Yunesian, M., Omidfar, K., Jeddi, M., Larijani, B., ... Rastkari, N. (2014). Association of urinary Bisphenol A concentration with type-2 diabetes mellitus. *Journal of Environmental Health Science & Engineering*, *12*(1), 64. doi:10.1186/2052-336X-12-64 PMID:24625016

Ahsan, N. (1999). Solid waste management plan for Indian megacities. *Indian Journal of Environmental Protection*, *19*, 90–95.

Akdoğan, M. Ş., & Coşkun, A. (2012). Drivers of Reverse Logistics Activities: An Empirical Investigation. *Procedia: Social and Behavioral Sciences*, *58*, 1640–1649. doi:10.1016/j.sbspro.2012.09.1130

Akingbemi, B. T., Ge, R., Klinefelter, G. R., Zirkin, B. R., & Hardy, M. P. (2004). Phthalate-induced Leydig cell hyperplasia is associated with multiple endocrine disturbances. *Proceedings of the National Academy of Sciences of the United States of America*, *101*(3), 775–780. doi:10.1073/pnas.0305977101 PMID:14715905

Akingbemi, B. T., Youker, R. T., Sottas, C. M., Ge, R., Katz, E., Klinefelter, G. R., ... Hardy, M. P. (2001). Modulation of rat Leydig cell steroidogenic function by di (2-ethylhexyl) phthalate. *Biology of Reproduction*, *65*(4), 1252–1259. doi:10.1095/biolreprod65.4.1252 PMID:11566751

Akio. (2002). Domestic Solid Waste Management in Pakistan. Japan International Corporation Agency.

Akpanudoh, N. S., Gobin, K., & Manos, G. (2005). Catalytic degradation of plastics waste to liquid fuel over commercial cracking catalyst. *Journal of Molecular Catalysis A Chemical*, *235*(1-2), 67–73. doi:10.1016/j.molcata.2005.03.009

Alam, R. (2010, July 02). *Environment and the 18th Amendment*. Retrieved from The Express Tribune: https://tribune.com.pk/story/25273/environment-and-the-18th-amendment/

Alam, P., & Ahmade, K. (2013). Impact of solid waste on health and the environment. *International Journal of Sustainable Development and Green Economics*, *2*(1), 165–168.

Albertsson, A. C. (1978). Biodegradation of synthetic polymers. II. A limited microbial conversion of 14 C in polyethylene to 14 CO_2 by some soil fungi. *Journal of Applied Polymer Science*, *22*(12), 3419–3433. doi:10.1002/app.1978.070221207

Albro, P. W., & Lavenhar, S. R. (1989). Metabolism of di(2-ethylhexyl)phthalate. *Drug Metabolism Reviews*, *21*(1), 13–34. doi:10.3109/03602538909029953 PMID:2696633

Albro, P. W., & Moore, B. (1974). Identification of the metabolites of simple phthalate diesters in rat urine. *Journal of Chromatography. A*, *94*, 209–218. doi:10.1016/S0021-9673(01)92368-4 PMID:4844611

Albro, P. W., & Thomas, R. O. (1973). Enzymatic hydrolysis of di-(2-ethylhexyl) phthalate by lipases. *BiochimicaetBiophysica Acta (BBA)- Lipids and Lipid Metabolism*, *306*(3), 380–390. doi:10.1016/0005-2760(73)90176-8

Albrow, M. (1996). *The Global Age*. Cambridge, UK: Polity Press.

Alessa, K. (2016). *Environmental impacts of plastic bags: it can be a danger to animal's life*. Academic Press.

Ali, M. (2017, June 22). *Manufacture, use of non-biodegradable plastic products banned*. Retrieved from https://www.dawn.com/news/1341056

Ali, M., Wang, W., & Chaudhry, N. (2015). Management of wastes from hospitals: A case study of Pakistan. *Waste Management and Research, 34*(1), 87-90.

Ali, M., Wang, W., Chaudhry, N., & Geng, Y. (2017). Hospital waste management in developing countries: A mini review. *Waste Management and Research, 35*(6), 581-592.

Ali, M. F., & Siddiqui, M. N. (2005). Thermal and catalytic decomposition behavior of PVC mixed plastic waste with petroleum residue. *Journal of Analytical and Applied Pyrolysis, 74*(1-2), 282–289. doi:10.1016/j.jaap.2004.12.010

Ali, M. I., Ahmed, S., Robson, G., Javed, I., Ali, N., Atiq, N., & Hameed, A. (2014). Isolation and molecular characterization of polyvinyl chloride (PVC) plastic degrading fungal isolates. *Journal of Basic Microbiology, 54*(1), 18–27. doi:10.1002/jobm.201200496 PMID:23686796

Aljabre, S. H. (2002). Hospital generated waste: A plan for its proper management. *Journal of Family & Community Medicine, 9*(2), 61–65. PMID:23008674

Al-Khatib, I. A., Al-Qaroot, Y. S., & Ali-Shtayeh, M. S. (2009). Management of healthcare waste in circumstances of limited resources: A case study in the hospitals of Nablus city, Palestine. *Waste Management & Research, 27*(4), 305–312. doi:10.1177/0734242X08094124 PMID:19423582

Allsopp, M., Costner, P., & Johnston, P. (2001). Incineration and human health. *Environmental Science and Pollution Research International, 8*(2), 141–145. doi:10.1007/BF02987308 PMID:11400640

Alonso-Magdalena, P., Ropero, A., Rosiano, S., Garcia-Arevalo, M., Ripolli, C., Fuentes, E., ... Nadal, A. (2012). Bisphenol-A acts as a potent estrogen via non-classical estrogentriggered pathways. *Molecular and Cellular Endocrinology, 355*(2), 201–207. doi:10.1016/j.mce.2011.12.012 PMID:22227557

Al-Salem, S. M., & Lettieri, P. (2010). Kinetic study of high-density polyethylene (HDPE) pyrolysis. *Chemical Engineering Research & Design, 88*(1212A), 1599–1606. doi:10.1016/j.cherd.2010.03.012

Al-Salem, S. M., Lettieri, P., & Baeyens, J. (2009). Recycling and recovery routes of plastic solid waste (PSW): A review. *Waste Management (New York, N.Y.), 29*(10), 2625–2643. doi:10.1016/j.wasman.2009.06.004 PMID:19577459

Al-Salem, S. M., Lettieri, P., & Baeyens, J. (2010). The valorization of plastic solid waste (PSW) by primary to quaternary routes: From re-use to energy and chemicals. *Progress in Energy and Combustion Science, 36*(1), 103–129. doi:10.1016/j.pecs.2009.09.001

Alshawafi, A., Analla, M., Alwashali, E., Aheichti, M., & Aksissou, M. (2018). Impacts of Marine Waste, Ingestion of Microplastic in the Fish, Impact on Fishing Yield, M'diq, Morocco. *International Journal of Marine Biology and Research,* 2475-4706.

Altuwair, I. B. (2017). *Environmental Performance Evaluation of Polycarbonates Production Processes. J. of Industrial Engineering & Management, 6*(3), 2–11.

Alumur, S. A., Nickel, S., Saldanha-da-Gama, F., & Verter, V. (2012). Multi-period reverse logistics network design. *European Journal of Operational Research, 220*(1), 67–78. doi:10.1016/j.ejor.2011.12.045

Alzaga, R., Peña, A., & Bayona, J. M. (2003). Determination of phthalic monoesters in aqueous and urine samples by solid-phase microextraction–diazomethane on-fibrederivatization–gas chromatography–mass spectrometry. *Journal of Separation Science*, *26*(1-2), 87–96. doi:10.1002/jssc.200390020

Alzahrani, M. A., Alshanshouri, M. A., & Fakhri, Z. I. (1998). *Guide of healthcare waste management*. Riyadh, Saudi Arabia: Ministry of Health.

American Diabetes Association (ADA). (2011). Diagnosis and classification of diabetes mellitus. *Diabetes Care*, *34*(1), S62–S69. PMID:21193628

Amin, S. H., Wu, H., & Karaphillis, G. (2018). A perspective on the reverse logistics of plastic pallets in Canada. *Journal of Remanufacturing*, *8*(3), 153–174. doi:10.100713243-018-0051-0

Ananth, A. P., Prashanthini, V., & Visvanathan, C. (2010). Healthcare waste management in Asia. *Waste Management (New York, N.Y.)*, *30*(1), 154–161. doi:10.1016/j.wasman.2009.07.018 PMID:19726174

Anastas, P. T., Bickart, P. H., & Kirchhoff, M. M. (2000). Designing safer polymers New York. New York, NY: John Wiley and Sons, Wiley-Interscience.

Anderson, J., Curmen, R., & Miripori, J. (1999). Alternatives to Current Blood Bag Plastic and Plasticizer Materials. *US Department of Health and Human Services Workshop on Plasticizers*.

Anderson, J. C., Park, B. J., & Palace, V. P. (2016). Microplastics in aquatic environments: Implications for Canadian ecosystems. *Environmental Pollution*, *218*, 269–280. doi:10.1016/j.envpol.2016.06.074 PMID:27431693

Andrady, AL & Neal MA (2009). Applications and societal benefitsof plastics. *Phil. Trans. R. Soc. B, 364*, 1977–1984. doi:10.1098/rstb.2008.0304

Andrady, A. (2003). An environmental primer. In A. Andrady (Ed.), *Plastics and theenvironment* (pp. 3–76). Hoboken, NJ: Wiley Interscience. doi:10.1002/0471721557

Andrady, A. L. (2011). Microplastics in the marine environment. *Marine Pollution Bulletin*, *62*(8), 1596–1605. doi:10.1016/j.marpolbul.2011.05.030 PMID:21742351

Andrady, A. L. (2015). Persistence of plastic litter in the oceans. In *Marine anthropogenic litter* (pp. 57–72). Cham: Springer. doi:10.1007/978-3-319-16510-3_3

Anilkumar, A., Sukamaran, D., & Vincent, S. G. T. (2015). Effect of municipal solid waste leachate on groundwater quality of Thiruvananthapuram District, Kerala, India. *Applied Ecology and Environmental Sciences*, *3*, 151–157.

Ansari, Y., Chavan, F. I., & Husain, M. (2017). Effect of plastic grocery bags on environment and its reuse. *International Journal of Advance Research, Ideas and Innovations in Technology*, *3*, 3.

Antonelis, K., Huppert, D., Velasquez, D., & June, J. (2011). Dungeness crab mortality due to lost traps and a cost–benefit analysis of trap removal in Washington State waters of the Salish Sea. *North American Journal of Fisheries Management*, *31*(5), 880–893. doi:10.1080/02755947.2011.590113

Aparacana, S. (2017). Approaches to formalization of the informal waste sector into municipal solid waste management systems in low- and middle-income countries: Review of barriers and success factors. *Waste Management (New York, N.Y.)*, *61*, 593–607. doi:10.1016/j.wasman.2016.12.028 PMID:28038906

APME. (2006). *An Analysis of Plastics Production, Demand and Recovery in Europe*. APME.

Appadurai, A. (1996). *Modernity at Large*. Minneapolis, MN: University of Minnesota Press.

Arambula, S. E., Belcher, S. M., Planchart, A., Turner, S. D., & Patisaul, H. B. (2016). Impact of low dose oral exposure to bisphenol A (BPA) on the neonatal rat hypothalamic and hippocampal transcriptome: A CLAIRTY-BPA Consortium study. Endocrinology, 157(10), 3856–3872. doi:10.1210/en.2016-1339 PubMed doi:10.1210/en.2016-1339 PMID:27571134

Arambula, S. E., Jima, D., & Patisaul, H. B. (2018). Prenatal bisphenol A (BPA) exposure alters the transcriptome of the neonate rat amygdala in a sex-specific manner: A CLARITYBPA consortium study. Neurotoxicology, 65, 207–220. doi:10.1016/j.neuro.2017.10.005 PubMed doi:10.1016/j.neuro.2017.10.005 PMID:29097150

Arandes, J. M., Abajo, I., Lopez-Valerio, D., Fernández, I., Azkoiti, M. J., Olazar, M., & Bilbao, J. (1997). Transformation of several plastic wastes into fuels by catalytic cracking. *Industrial & Engineering Chemistry Research*, *36*(11), 4523–4529. doi:10.1021/ie970096e

Arandes, J. M., Erena, J., Azkoiti, M. J., Olazar, M., & Bilbao, J. (2003). Thermal recycling of polystyrene and polystyrene-butadiene dissolved in a light cycle oil. *Journal of Analytical and Applied Pyrolysis*, *70*(2), 747–760. doi:10.1016/S0165-2370(03)00056-1

Aras, N., & Aksen, D. (2008). Locating Collection Centers for Distance-and-Incentive-Dependent Returns. *International Journal of Production Economics*, *111*(2), 316–333. doi:10.1016/j.ijpe.2007.01.015

Aras, N., Aksen, D., & Tanugur, A. G. (2008). Locating Collection Centers for Incentive-Dependent Returns under a Pick Up Policy with Capacitated Vehicles. *European Journal of Operational Research*, *191*(3), 1223–1240. doi:10.1016/j.ejor.2007.08.002

Araujo, A. S., Fernandes, V. J. Jr, & Fernandes, G. J. T. (2002). Thermogravimetric kinetics of polyethelynedegradation over silicoaluminophosphate. *Thermochimica Acta*, *392*, 55–61. doi:10.1016/S0040-6031(02)00072-2

Arbuckle, T. E., Marro, L., Davis, K., Fisher, M., Ayotte, P., Bélanger, P., . . . Fraser, W. D. (2015). Exposure to free and conjugated forms of bisphenol A and triclosan among pregnant women in the MIREC Cohort. Environmental Health Perspectives, 123(4), 277–284. doi:10.1289/ehp.1408187 PubMed doi:10.1289/ehp.1408187 PMID:25494523

Ardies, C. M., & Dees, C. (1998). Xenoestrogens significantly enhance risk for breast cancer duringgrowth and adolescence. *Medical Hypotheses*, *50*(6), 457–464. doi:10.1016/S0306-9877(98)90262-6 PMID:9710315

Arenholt-Bindslev, D., Breinholt, V., Preiss, A., & Schmalz, G. (1999). Time-related bisphenol-A content and estrogenic activity in saliva samples collected in relation to placement of fissure sealants. *Clinical Oral Investigations*, *3*(3), 120–125. doi:10.1007007840050089 PMID:10803122

Arnkil, R. A., Jarvensivu, A., Korski, P., Piirainen, T., Järvensivu, A., Koski, P., & Piirainen, T. (2010). *Exploring Quadruple Helix: Outlining user-oriented innovation models.* Tampere: The CLIQ. Retrieved from http://tampub.uta.fi/bitstream/handle/10024/65758/978-951-44-8209-0.pdf?sequenc%0Ahttp://www.arnkildialogues.com/files/testataan.kotisivukone.com/julkaisut/exploring_quadruple_helix-2010-1.pdf

Aronowitz, S., & Giroux, H. (1985). *Education Under Siege*. New York: Bergin and Garvey.

Aronson, R. (1983). *The Dialectics of Disaster*. London, IL: Verso.

Arrighi, G. 1994. The Long Twentieth Centurv. London, UK: Verso.

Artham, T., & Doble, M. (2008). Biodegradation of aliphatic and aromatic polycarbonates. *Macromolecular Bioscience*, *8*(1), 14–24. doi:10.1002/mabi.200700106 PMID:17849431

Arutchelvi, J., Sudhakar, M., Arkatkar, A., Doble, M., Bhandari, S., & Uppara, P. V. (2008). Biodegradation of Polyethylene and Polypropylene. *Indian Journal of Biotechnology*, *7*, 9–22.

Ashwood, P., Thompson, R. P., & Powell, J. J. (2007). Fine particles that adsorb lipopolysaccharide via bridging calcium cations may mimic bacterial pathogenicity towards cells. *Experimental Biology and Medicine (Maywood, N.J.), 232*, 107–117. PMID:17202591

Associated Press in Jakarta. (2018). *Indonesia: dead whale had 1,000 pieces of plastic in stomach.* Retrieved November 27, 2018, from The Guardian website: https://www.theguardian.com/environment/2018/nov/20/indonesia-dead-whale-had-1000-pieces-of-plastic-in-stomach

ASTM D6003-96. (1996). *Standard Test Method for Determining Weight Loss from Plastic Materials Exposed to Simulated Municipal Solid-Waste (MSW) Aerobic Compost Environment.* West Conshohocken, PA: ASTM International.

ASTM International. (2003). *Specification for biodegradable plastics used as coatings on paper and other compostable substrates.* doi:10.1520/D6868-03

Aswale, P. (2010). *Studies on bio-degradation of polythene* (PhD thesis). Dr. Babasaheb Ambedkar Marathwada University, Aurangabad, India.

Aswale, P., & Ade, A. (2011). Polythene degradation potential of Aspergillus niger. In I. U. Sayed (Ed.), Scholary Articles in Botany. Pune: Academic Press.

Aswale, P., & Ade, A. (2008). Assessment of the biodegradation of polythene. *Bioinfolet, 5*, 239.

Aswale, P., & Ade, A. (2009). Effect of pH on biodegradation of polythene by *Serretia marscence. The Ecotech, 1*, 152–153.

ATSDR. (1995) Agency for Toxic Substances and Disease Registry. Atlanta, GA: Division of Toxicology.

ATSDR. (1995). Toxicological profile for diethylphthalate, U.S. Department of Health and Human Services, Public Health Service, Agency for Toxic Substances and Disease Registry.

ATSDR. (1997). Toxicological profile for di-n-octylphthalate. U.S. Department of Health and Human Services, Public HealthS ervice, Agency for Toxic Substances and Disease Registry.

ATSDR. (2001). Agency for Toxic Substances and Disease Registry. Atlanta, GA: Division of Toxicology.

ATSDR. (2001). Toxicological profile for di-n-butyl phthalate. Agency for Toxic Substances and Disease Registry, Public Health Service Atlanta, Department of Health and Human Services.

ATSDR. (2002) Agency for Toxic Substances and Disease Registry. Atlanta, GA: Division of Toxicology.

ATSDR. (2002). *Toxicological profile for di(2-ethylhexyl)phthalate (DEHP).* Atlanta, GA: Agency for Toxic Substances and Disease Registry.

ATSDR. (2002). Toxicological profile for di(2-ethylhexyl)phthalate (DEHP). U.S. Department of Health and Human Services, Public Health Service, Agency for Toxic Substances and Disease Registry.

Attina, T. M., & Trasande, L. (2015). Association of exposure to di-2-ethylhexylphthalate replacements with Increased insulin resistance in adolescents from NHANES 2009–2012. *The Journal of Clinical Endocrinology and Metabolism, 100*(7), 2640–2650. doi:10.1210/jc.2015-1686 PMID:25993640

Austin, H. P., Allen, M. D., Donohoe, B. S., Rorrer, N. A., & Kearns, F. L. (2018). *Characterization and engineering of a plastic-degrading aromatic polyesterase* (A. T. Bell, Ed.). Berkeley, CA: University of California. doi:10.1073/pnas.1718804115

Autian, J. (1973). Toxicity and health threats of phthalate esters: Review of the literature. Environmental Health Perspectives, 4, 3–26. doi:10.1289/ehp.73043 PubMed doi:10.1289/ehp.73043 PMID:4578674

Avelar, N. V., Ribeiro, B. C., Rezende, A. A. P., Silva, C. M., Carneiro, A. D. C. O., & Martins, M. A. (2018). Thermal drying of industrial sludge using forced aeration. *Environmental Technology*, 1–11. doi:10.1080/09593330.2018.1470679 PMID:29701122

Axford, B. (1995). *The Global System*. Cambridge, UK: Polity Press.

Axtmann, R. (Ed.). (1998). *Globalization in European Context*. London, UK: Cassells.

Ayala-García, B., López-Santibáñez Guevara, M., Marcos-Camacho, L. I., Fuentes-Farías, A. L., Meléndez-Herrera, E., & Gutiérrez-Ospina, G. (2013). Speciation, phenotypic variation andplasticity: What can endocrine disruptors tell us? *International Journal of Endocrinology*. PMID:23762055

Azzarello, M. Y., & Van Vleet, E. S. (1987). Marine birds and plastic pollution. *Marine Ecology Progress Series*, *37*, 295–303. doi:10.3354/meps037295

Baccarelli, A., Wright, R. O., Bollati, V., Tarantini, L., Litonjua, A. A., Suh, H. H., ... Schwartz, J. (2009). Rapid DNA methylation changes after exposure to traffic particles. *American Journal of Respiratory and Critical Care Medicine*, *179*(7), 572–578. doi:10.1164/rccm.200807-1097OC PMID:19136372

Baenas, J. M., Hojas De Castro, R., Battistelle, R. A. G., & Junior, J. A. G. (2011). A Study of Reverse Logistics Flow Management in Vehicle Battery Industries in the Midwest of the State of Sao Paulo. *Journal of Cleaner Production*, *19*(2-3), 168–172. doi:10.1016/j.jclepro.2010.08.018

Bae, S., Kim, J. H., Lim, Y. H., Park, H. Y., & Hong, Y. C. (2012). Associations of Bisphenol A exposure with heart rate variability and blood pressure. *Hypertension*, *60*(3), 786–793. doi:10.1161/HYPERTENSIONAHA.112.197715 PMID:22851732

Baghotia, K. S. (2009). Biomedical waste management-Delhi experience. *Indian Soc Hosp Waste Management*, *7-8*(1), 29–34.

Bai, C., & Sarkis, J. (2013). Flexibility in Reverse Logistics: A Framework and Evaluation Approach. *Journal of Cleaner Production*, *47*, 306–318. doi:10.1016/j.jclepro.2013.01.005

Bailin, P.D., Byrne, M., Lewis, S., & Liroff, R. (2008). Public awareness drives market for safer alternatives:bisphenol A market analysis report. *Investor Environmental Health Network,* 1-37.

Bajdur, W., Pajaczkowska, J., Makarucha, B., Sulkowska, A., & Sulkowski, W. W. (2002). Effective polyelectrolytes synthesized from expanded polystyrene wastes. *European Polymer Journal*, *38*(2), 299–304. doi:10.1016/S0014-3057(01)00191-4

Bakir, A., Rowland, S. J., & Thompson, R. C. (2014). Transport of persistent organic pollutants by microplastics in estuarine conditions. *Estuarine, Coastal and Shelf Science*, *140*, 14–21. doi:10.1016/j.ecss.2014.01.004

Balakrishnan, A., & Flora, R. M. N. (2017). The Environmental Impact of Plastics and Recycling of Plastic Waste. *International Journal of Engineering Research and Reviews* (Online) *5*(3), (14-20).

Balasubramaniam, M., & Phillott, A. D. (2016, January). Preliminary Observations of Microplastics from Beaches in the Indian Ocean. *Indian Ocean Turtle Newsletter,* (23), 13-16. Retrieved from https://www.iotn.org/wp-content/uploads/2017/05/IOTN-23.pdf#page=15

Balasubramanian, V., Natarajan, K., Hemambika, B., Ramesh, N., Sumathi, C. S., Kottaimuthu, R., & Kannan, V. R. (2010). High-density polyethylene (HDPE) degrading potential bacteria from marine ecosystem of Gulf of Mannar, India. *Letters in Applied Microbiology*, *51*, 205–211. PMID:20586938

Balasubramanian, V., Natarajan, K., Hemambika, B., Ramesh, N., Sumathi, C. S., Kottaimuthu, R., & Kannan, V. R. (2010). High-density polyethylene (HDPE)-degrading potential bacteria from marine ecosystem of Gulf of Mannar, India. *Letters in Applied Microbiology*, *51*, 205–211. PMID:20586938

Balasubramanian, V., Natarajan, K., Kannan, R. V., & Perumal, P. (2014). Enhancement of *in vitro* high density polyethylene (HDPE) degradation by physical, chemical and biological treatments. *Environmental Science and Pollution Research International*, *21*(21), 12,549–12,562. doi:10.100711356-014-3191-2 PMID:24946709

Ballesteros-Gomez, A., Rubio, S., & Perez-Bendito, D. (2009). Analytical methods for the determination of Bisphenol A in food. *Journal of Chromatography. A*, *1216*(3), 449–469. doi:10.1016/j.chroma.2008.06.037 PMID:18635192

Ballice, L., & Reimert, R. (2002). Temperature-programmed co-pyrolysis of Turkish lignite with polypropylene. *Journal of Analytical and Applied Pyrolysis*, *65*(2), 207–219. doi:10.1016/S0165-2370(01)00195-4

Baloch, F. (2018, November 6). *Karachi to become the world's third most populated city by 2030*. Retrieved from Samaa News: https://www.samaa.tv/news/2018/11/karachi-to-become-the-worlds-third-most-populated-city-by-2030/

Bamai, Y. A., Shibata, E., Saito, I., Araki, A., Kanazawa, A., Morimoto, K., ... Chikara, H. (2014). Exposure to house dust phthalates in relation to asthma and allergies in both children and adults. *The Science of the Total Environment*, *485*, 153–163. doi:10.1016/j.scitotenv.2014.03.059 PMID:24704966

Banerjee, T., Srivastava, R. K., & Hung, Y. T. (2012). Plastics waste management in India: an integrated solidwaste management approach. Handbook of Environmental and Waste Management, 2.

Barker, D. J., Eriksson, J. G., Forsen, T., & Osmond, C. (2002). Fetal origins of adult disease: Strength of effects and biological basis. *International Journal of Epidemiology*, *31*(6), 1235–1239. doi:10.1093/ije/31.6.1235 PMID:12540728

Barlow, N. J., & Foster, P. M. (2003). Pathogenesis of male reproductive tract lesions from gestation through adulthood following in utero exposure to di (n-butyl) phthalate. *Toxicologic Pathology*, *31*(4), 397–410. PMID:12851105

Barlow, S. E. (2007). Expert committee recommendations regarding the prevention, assessment, and treatment of child and adolescent overweight and obesity: Summary report. *Pediatrics*, *120*(Supplement 4), S164–S192. doi:10.1542/peds.2007-2329C PMID:18055651

Barnes, D. K. A. (2002). Biodiversity—invasions by marine life on plastic debris. *Nature, 416*, 808–809. doi:10.1038/416808a

Barnes, D. K. A. (2005). Remote islands reveal rapid rise of southern hemisphere sea debris. *Scientific World Journal, 5*, 915–921.

Barnes, D. K. A., Galgani, F., Thompson, R. C., & Barlaz, M. (2009). Accumulation and fragmentation of plastic debris in global environments. *Philosophical Transactions of the Royal Society of London. Series B, Biological Sciences*, *364*(1526), 1985–1998. doi:10.1098/rstb.2008.0205 PMID:19528051

Barr, D. B., Silva, M. J., Kato, K., Reidy, J. A., Malek, N. A., Hurtz, D., ... Calafat, A. M. (2003). Assessing human exposure to phthalates using monoesters and their oxidized metabolites as biomarkers. *Environmental Health Perspectives*, *111*(9), 1148–1151. doi:10.1289/ehp.6074 PMID:12842765

Barreiros, J. P., & Guerreiro, O. (2014). Notes on a plastic debris collar on a juvenile Pagellus acarne (Perciformes : Sparidae) from Terceira Island, Azores, NE Atlantic. *Bothalia Journal*, *44*(4), 42–45.

Barreiros, J. P., & Raykov, V. S. (2014). Lethal lesions and amputation caused by plastic debris and fishing gear on the loggerhead turtle Caretta caretta (Linnaeus, 1758). Three case reports from Terceira Island, Azores (NE Atlantic). *Marine Pollution Bulletin*, *86*(1–2), 518–522. doi:10.1016/j.marpolbul.2014.07.020 PMID:25066455

Barroso, M. (2011). Commission Directive 2011/8/EU of 28 January 2011 Amending Directive2002/72/EC as Regards the Restriction of Use of Bisphenol A in Plastic Infant Feeding Bottles (Text with EEA relevance).

BASF. (2010). *Introduction to biodegradable plastics*. Retrieved from http://www.bioplastics.basf.com

Batholomew, P., Cycyota, M., Petrilli, L., Rosauer, D., Scharf, M., & Giovanetto, S. (1994). Recycling post-consumer hospital wastes. In *87th Annual Meeting and Exhibition, Air & Waste Manage. Assoc.* (Paper No. 94-FA-154.02)

Batool, S. A., & Chaudhry, M. N. (2008). The impact of municipal solid waste treatment methods on greenhouse gas emissions in Lahore, Pakistan. *Waste Management (New York, N.Y.)*, *29*(1), 63–69. doi:10.1016/j.wasman.2008.01.013 PMID:18387288

Batool, S. A., Chaudhry, N., & Majeed, K. (2008). Economic potential of recycling business in Lahore, Pakistan. *Waste Management (New York, N.Y.)*, *28*(2), 294–298. doi:10.1016/j.wasman.2006.12.007 PMID:17475469

Baudrillard, J. (1993). *Symbolic Exchange and Death*. London, UK: Sage.

Bauer, S. M., Roy, A., Emo, J., Chapman, T. J., Georas, S. N., & Lawrence, B. P. (2012). The effects of maternal exposure to bisphenol A on allergic lung inflammation into adulthood. Toxicological Sciences, 130(1), 82–93. doi:10.1093/toxsci/kfs227 PubMed doi:10.1093/toxsci/kfs227 PMID:22821851

Beck, C. A., & Barros, N. B. (1991). The impact of debris on the Florida manatee. *Marine Pollution Bulletin*, *22*(10), 508–510. doi:10.1016/0025-326X(91)90406-I

Becker, K., Goen, T., Seiwert, M., Conrad, A., Pick-Fuss, H., Muller, J., & … . (2009). Gere's IV: Phthalate metabolites and Bisphenol A in urine of German children. *International Journal of Hygiene and Environmental Health*, *212*(6), 685–692. doi:10.1016/j.ijheh.2009.08.002 PMID:19729343

Begum, Z. (2010). *Plastics and environment. Dissemination Paper for the Ministryof Environment and Forest*. Government of India.

Bekö, G., Weschler, C. J., Langer, S., Callesen, M., Toftum, J., & Clausen, G. (2013). Children's phthalate intakes and resultant cumulative exposures estimated from urine compared with estimates from dust ingestion, inhalation and dermal absorption in their homes and day care centers. *PLoS One*, *8*(4), e62442. doi:10.1371/journal.pone.0062442 PMID:23626820

Bellas, J., Martínez-Armental, J., Martínez-Cámara, A., Besada, V., & Martínez-Gómez, C. (2016). Ingestion of microplastics by demersal fish from the Spanish Atlantic and Mediterranean coasts. *Marine Pollution Bulletin*, *109*(1), 55–60. doi:10.1016/j.marpolbul.2016.06.026 PMID:27289284

Bell, D. (1976). *The Coming of Post-Industrial Society*. New York: Basic Books. doi:10.1080/00131727609336501

Beltrame, P. L., Bergamasco, L., Carniti, P., Castelli, A., Bertini, F., & Audisio, G. (1997). Hydrous pyrolysis of polystyrene. *Journal of Analytical and Applied Pyrolysis*, *40*, 451–461. doi:10.1016/S0165-2370(96)00977-1

Benjamin, S., Pradeep, S., Josh, M. S., Kumar, S., & Masai, E. (2015). A monograph on the remediation of hazardous phthalates. *Journal of Hazardous Materials*, *298*(15), 58–72. doi:10.1016/j.jhazmat.2015.05.004 PMID:26004054

Benjamin, S., Prakasan, P., Sreedharan, S., Wright, A. D. G., & Spener, F. (2015). Pros and cons of CLA consumption: An insight from clinical evidences. *Nutrition & Metabolism*, *12*(1), 1. doi:10.1186/1743-7075-12-4 PMID:25972911

Ben-Jonathan, N., Hugo, E. R., & Brandebourg, T. D. (2009). Effects of Bisphenol A on adipokine release from human adipose tissue: Implications for the metabolic syndrome. *Molecular and Cellular Endocrinology*, *304*(1-2), 49–54. doi:10.1016/j.mce.2009.02.022 PMID:19433247

Bergmann, M., & Klages, M. (2012). Increase of litter at the Arctic deep-sea observatory HAUSGARTEN. *Marine Pollution Bulletin*, *64*(12), 2734–2741. doi:10.1016/j.marpolbul.2012.09.018 PMID:23083926

Bergmann, M., Sandhop, N., Schewe, I., & D'Hert, D. (2016). Observations of floating anthropogenic litter in the Barents Sea and Fram Strait, Arctic. *Polar Biology*, *39*(3), 553–560. doi:10.100700300-015-1795-8

Berman, T., Hochner-Celnikier, D., Calafat, A. M., Needham, L. L., Amitai, Y., Wormser, U., & Richter, E. (2009). Phthalate exposure among pregnant women in Jerusalem, Israel: Results of a pilotstudy. *Environment International*, *35*(2), 353–357. doi:10.1016/j.envint.2008.08.010 PMID:18824263

Bern, H. (1992). The fragile fetus. In T. Colborn, & C. Clement (Eds.), Chemically-Induced Alterations in Sexual and Functioal Development: The Wildlife/Human Connection. Princeton, NJ: Princeton Scientific Publishing Co.

Berrueco, C., Mastral, F. J., Esperanza, E., & Ceamanos, J. (2002). Production of waxes and tars from the continuous pyrolysis of high-density polyethylene. Influence of operation variables. *Energy & Fuels*, *16*(5), 1148–1153. doi:10.1021/ef020008p

Bertelsen, R. J., Carlsen, K. C. L., Calafat, A. M., Hoppin, J. A., Håland, G., Mowinckel, P., ... Løvik, M. (2013). Urinary biomarkers for phthalates associated with asthma in Norwegianchildren. *Environmental Health Perspectives (Online)*, *121*(2), 251–256. doi:10.1289/ehp.1205256 PMID:23164678

Besseling, E., Wegner, A., Foekema, E. M., Van Den Heuvel-Greve, M. J., & Koelmans, A. A. (2012). Effects of microplastic on fitness and PCB bioaccumulation by the lugworm Arenicola marina (L.). *Environmental Science & Technology*, *47*(1), 593–600. doi:10.1021/es302763x PMID:23181424

Best & Kellner. (1991). *Postmodern Theory: Critical Interrogations*. London, UK: Macmillan and Guilford.

Betts, K. (2008). Why small plastic particles may pose a big problem in the oceans. *Environmental Science & Technology*, *42*(24), 8996. doi:10.1021/es802970v PMID:19174862

Bezboruah, A. N., & Bhargava, D. S. (2003). Vermicomposting of municipal solid waste from a campus. *Indian Journal of Environmental Protection*, *23*, 1120–1136.

Bhardwaj, H., Gupta, R., & Tiwari, A. (2012). Microbial Population Associated with Plastic Degradation. *Open Access Scientific Reports*, *5*, 1–4.

Bhaskar, D. (2019). *88 square kilometer land will be needed only for garbage management*. Academic Press.

Bhaskar, T., Uddin, M. A., Murai, K., Kaneko, J., Hamano, K., Kusaba, T., ... Sakata, Y. (2003). Comparison of thermal degradation products from real municipal waste plastic and model mixed plastics. *Journal of Analytical and Applied Pyrolysis*, *70*(2), 579–587. doi:10.1016/S0165-2370(03)00027-5

Bhatnagar, S., & Kumari, R. (2013). Bioremediation: A sustainable tool for environmental management a review. *Annual Review and Research in Biology*, *3*(4), 974–993.

Bhatt, R., Patel, K., & Trivedi, U. (2011). Biodegradation of poly (3-hydroxyalkanoates). In S. K. Sharma & A. Mudhoo (Eds.), *A handbook of applied bio - polymer technology: Synthesis, degradation and applications* (pp. 311–331). London: The Royal Society of Chemistry Publishing. doi:10.1039/9781849733458-00311

Bhide, A. D., & Shekdar, A. V. (1998). Solid waste management in Indian urban centers. *International Solid Waste Association Times*, *1*, 26–28.

Biedermann, S., Tschudin, P., & Grob, K. (2010). Transfer of Bisphenol A from thermal printer paper to the skin. *Analytical and Bioanalytical Chemistry*, *398*(1), 571–576. doi:10.100700216-010-3936-9 PMID:20623271

Biello & David. (2011). Are Biodegradeable Plastics Doing More Harm Than Good? *Scientific American*.

Biodegradable Products Institute. (2012). *ASTM D6400 - Test for Compostability*. Retrieved from http://www.bpiworld.org/Default.aspx?pageId=190422

Birchard, K. (2002). Out of sight, out of mind...the medical waste problem. *Lancet*, *359*(9300), 56. doi:10.1016/S0140-6736(02)07256-2 PMID:11809202

Bird, J., Curtis, B., Putnam, T., & Tickner, L. (Eds.). (1993). Mapping the Futures: Local Cultures, Global Change. London, UK: Routledge.

Biswas, P., & Wu, C. Y. (2005). Nanoparticles and the environment. *Journal of the Air & Waste Management Association*, *55*(6), 708–746. doi:10.1080/10473289.2005.10464656 PMID:16022411

Bjorndal, K. A., Bolten, A. B., & Lagueux, C. J. (1994). Ingestion of marine debris by juvenile sea turtles in coastal Florida habitats. *Marine Pollution Bulletin*, *28*(3), 154–158. doi:10.1016/0025-326X(94)90391-3

Black, M., Karki, J., Lee, A. C., Makai, P., Barai, Y. R., Kritsotakis, E. I., ... Heckmann, A. F. (2019). The health risks of informal waste workers in the Kathmandu Valley: A cross-sectional survey. *Public Health*, *166*, 10–18. doi:10.1016/j.puhe.2018.09.026 PMID:30419409

Blettler, M. C., Abrial, E., Khan, F. R., Sivri, N., & Espinola, L. A. (2018). Freshwater plastic pollution: Recognizing research biases and identifying knowledge gaps. *Water Research*, *143*, 416–424. doi:10.1016/j.watres.2018.06.015 PMID:29986250

Bloom, M. S., Kim, D., VomSaal, F. S., Taylor, J. A., Cheng, G., Lamb, J. D., & Fujimoto, V. Y. (2011a). Bisphenol A exposure reduces the estradiol response to gonadotropin stimulation during *in vitro* fertilization. *Fertility and Sterility*, *96*(3), 672–7.e2. doi:10.1016/j.fertnstert.2011.06.063 PMID:21813122

Bloom, M. S., VomSaal, F. S., Kim, D., Taylor, J. A., Lamb, J. D., & Fujimoto, V. Y. (2011b). Serum unconjugated bisphenol A concentrations in men may influence embryo quality indicators during in vitrofertilization. *Environmental Toxicology and Pharmacology*, *32*(2), 319–323. doi:10.1016/j.etap.2011.06.003 PMID:21843814

Blount, B. C., Milgram, K. E., Silva, M. J., Malek, N. A., Reidy, J. A., Needham, L. L., & Brock, J. W. (2000). Quantitative detection of eight phthalate metabolites in human urine using HPLC– APCI-MS/MS. *Analytical Chemistry*, *72*(17), 4127–4134. doi:10.1021/ac000422r PMID:10994974

Blount, B. C., Silva, M. J., Caudill, S. P., Needham, L. L., Pirkle, J. L., Sampson, E. J., ... Brock, J. W. (2000). Levels of seven urinary phthalate metabolites in a human reference population. *Environmental Health Perspectives*, *108*(10), 979–982. doi:10.1289/ehp.00108979 PMID:11049818

Boas, M., Frederiksen, H., Feldt-Rasmussen, U., Skakkebæk, N. E., Hegedus, L., Hilsted, L., ... Main, K. M. (2010). Childhood exposure to phthalates: Associations with thyroid function, insulinlike growth factor I and growth. *Environmental Health Perspectives*, *118*(10), 1458–1464. doi:10.1289/ehp.0901331 PMID:20621847

Bockhorn, H., Donner, S., Gernsbeck, M., Hornung, A., & Hornung, U. (2001). Pyrolysis of Polyamide 6 under Catalytic Conditions and its Application to Reutilization of Carpets. *Journal of Analytical and Applied Pyrolysis*, *58*, 79–84. doi:10.1016/S0165-2370(00)00187-X

Bockhorn, H., Hornung, A., Hornung, U., & Jakobstroer, P. (1999). Modeling of isothermal and dynamic pyrolysis of plastics considering nonhomogeneous temperature distribution and detailed degradation mechanism. *Journal of Analytical and Applied Pyrolysis*, *49*(1-2), 53–74. doi:10.1016/S0165-2370(98)00130-2

Bodrero, S., Canivenc, E., & Cansell, F. (1999). Chemical Recycling of Polyamide 6.6 and Polyamide 6 through a Two-Step Ami-/Ammonolysis Process. Presentation at *4th Annual Conference on Recycling of Fibrous Textile and Carpet Waste*, Dalton, GA.

Boerger, C. M., Lattin, G. L., Moore, S. L., & Moore, C. J. (2010). Plastic ingestion by planktivorous fishes in the North Pacific Central Gyre. *Marine Pollution Bulletin*, *60*(12), 2275–2278. doi:10.1016/j.marpolbul.2010.08.007 PMID:21067782

Boetzkes, A. (2016). Plastic, Oil Culture, and the Ethics of Waste. In C. Mauch (Ed.), *Out of Sight, Out of Mind: The Politics and Culture of Waste* (pp. 51–58). Berlin, Germany: Federal Ministry of Education and Research, Germany. Retrieved from http://www.environmentandsociety.org/sites/default/files/2016_i1.pdf

Boggs, C. (2000). *The End of Politics*. New York: Guilford Press.

Bogino, P. C., Oliva, M. D. L. M., Sorroche, F. G., & Giordano, W. (2013). The role of bacterial biofilms and surface components in plant-bacterial associations. *International Journal of Molecular Sciences*, *14*(8), 15838–15859. doi:10.3390/ijms140815838 PMID:23903045

Boh, S. (2018). *Singapore-Indonesia deep-sea expedition team discovers over a dozen species new to science*. Retrieved May 29, 2018, from The Straits Times website: https://www.straitstimes.com/singapore/singapore-indonesia-deep-sea-expedition-team-discover-over-a-dozen-species-new-to-science

Bombelli, P., Howe, C. J., & Bertocchini, F. (2017). Polyethylene bio-degradation by caterpillars of the wax moth Galleria mellonella. *Current Biology*, *27*(8), R292–R293. doi:10.1016/j.cub.2017.02.060 PMID:28441558

Bonds, R. S., & Midoro-Horiuti, T. (2013). Estrogen effects in allergy and asthma. Current Opinion in Allergy and Clinical Immunology, 13(1), 92–99. doi:10.1097/ACI.0b013e32835a6dd6 PubMed doi:10.1097/ACI.0b013e32835a6dd6 PMID:23090385

Bonefeld-Jorgensen, E. C., Long, M., Hofmeister, M. V., & Vinggaard, A. M. (2007). Endocrine-disrupting potential of bisphenol A, bisphenol A dimethacrylate, 4-n-nonylphenol, and 4-n-octylphenol in vitro: New data and a brief review. Environmental Health Perspectives, 115(Suppl 1), 69–76. doi:10.1289/ehp.9368 PubMed doi:10.1289/ehp.9368 PMID:18174953

Bonhomme, S., Cuer, A., Delort, A. M., Lemaire, J., Sancelme, M., & Scott, G. (2003). Environmental biodegradation of polyethylene. *Polymer Degradation & Stability*, *81*(3), 441–452. doi:10.1016/S0141-3910(03)00129-0

Bønnelykke, K., Raaschou-Nielsen, O., Tjønneland, A., Ulrik, C. S., Bisgaard, H., & Andersen, Z. J. (2015). Postmenopausal hormone therapy and asthma-related hospital admission. The Journal of Allergy and Clinical Immunology, 135(3), 813–816.e5. doi:10.1016/j.jaci.2014.11.019 PubMed doi:10.1016/j.jaci.2014.11.019 PMID:25579482

Boopathy, R. (2000). Factor limiting bioremediation technologies. *Bioresource Technology*, *74*(1), 63–67. doi:10.1016/S0960-8524(99)00144-3

Booth, C. H., Christianson, A. D., Lawrence, J. M., Pham, L. D., Lashley, J. C., & Drymiotis, F. R. (2007). Ytterbium divalency and lattice disorder in near-zero thermal expansion YbGaGe. *Physical Review B: Condensed Matter and Materials Physics*, *75*(1), 401–407. doi:10.1103/PhysRevB.75.012301

Borch, J., Axelstad, M., Vinggaard, A. M., & Dalgaard, M. (2006). Diisobutyl phthalate has comparable anti-androgenic effects to di-n-butyl phthalate in fetal rat testis. *Toxicology Letters*, *163*(3), 183–190. doi:10.1016/j.toxlet.2005.10.020 PMID:16458459

Borch, J., Dalgaard, M., & Ladefoged, O. (2005). Early testicular effects in rats perinatally exposed to DEHP in combination with DEHA—Apoptosis assessment and immunohistochemical studies. *Reproductive Toxicology (Elmsford, N.Y.), 19*(4), 517–525. doi:10.1016/j.reprotox.2004.11.004 PMID:15749266

Borgianni, C., Filippis, P.D., Pochetti, F., & Paolucci, M. (2002). *Gasification process of wastes 58 Material Recycling – Trends and Perspectives*. Academic Press.

Borgmann, A. (1994). *Across the Postmodern Divide*. Chicago, IL: University of Chicago Press.

Bornehag, C. G., Carlstedt, F., Jönsson, B. A., Lindh, C. H., Jensen, T. K., Bodin, A., ... Swan, S. H. (2015). Prenatal phthalate exposures and anogenital distance in Swedish boys. *Environmental Health Perspectives, 123*(1), 101–107. doi:10.1289/ehp.1408163 PMID:25353625

Bornehag, C. G., Lundgren, B., Weschler, C. J., Sigsgaard, T., Hagerhed-Engman, L., & Sundell, J. (2005). Phthalates in indoor dust and their association with building characteristics. *Environmental Health Perspectives, 113*(10), 1399–1404. doi:10.1289/ehp.7809 PMID:16203254

Bornehag, C. G., & Nanberg, E. (2010). Phthalate exposure and asthma in children. *International Journal of Andrology, 33*, 333–345.

Bornehag, C. G., Sundell, J., Weschler, C. J., Sigsgaard, T., Lundgren, B., Hasselgren, M., & Hägerhed-Engman, L. (2004). The association between asthma and allergic symptoms in children and phthalates in house dust: A nested case–control study. *Environmental Health Perspectives, 112*(14), 1393–1397. doi:10.1289/ehp.7187 PMID:15471731

Bošnir, J., Puntarić, D., Galić, A., Škes, I., Dijanić, T., Klarić, M., ... Šmit, Z. (2007). Migration of phthalates from plastic containers into soft drinks and mineral water. *Food Technology and Biotechnology, 45*, 91–95.

Boubendir, A. (1993). Purification and biochemical evaluation of polyurethane degrading enzymes of fungal origin. *Dissertation Abstract International, 53*, 4632.

Bouwmeester, H., Hollman, P. C. H., & Peters, R. J. B. (2015). Potential Health Impact of Environmentally Released Micro- and Nanoplastics in the Human Food Production Chain: Experiences from Nanotoxicology. *Environmental Science & Technology, 49*(15), 8932–8947. doi:10.1021/acs.est.5b01090 PMID:26130306

Bowles, S., & Gintis, H. (1986). *On Democracy*. New York: Basic Books.

BPF. (2016). *A History of Plastics*. Retrieved from British Plastic Federation website: http://www.bpf.co.uk/plastipedia/plastics_history/default.aspx

Bradley, E. L., Burden, R. A., Bentayeb, K., Driffield, M., Harmer, N., Mortimer, D. N., & Castle, L. (2013). Exposure to phthalic acid, phthalate diesters and phthalate monoesters from foodstuffs: UK total diet study results. *Food Additives & Contaminants: Part A, 30*(4), 735–742. doi:10.1080/19440049.2013.781684 PMID:23641808

Brandão, M. L., Braga, K. M., & Luque, J. L. (2011). Marine debris ingestion by Magellanic penguins, *Spheniscus magellanicus* (Aves: Sphenisciformes), from the Brazilian coastal zone. *Marine Pollution Bulletin, 62*(10), 2246–2249. doi:10.1016/j.marpolbul.2011.07.016 PMID:21864861

Brandl, H., Gross, R. A., Lenz, R. W., & Fuller, R. C. (1988). Pseudomonas oleovorans as a source of poly(B-hydroxyalkanoates) for potential application as biodegradable polyester. *Applied and Environmental Microbiology, 54*, 1977–1982. PMID:16347708

Braun, J. M., Kalkbrenner, A. E., Calafat, A. M., Baneft, J. T., Pornkunwilai, S., Ye, X., Silva, M. J., … Lanphear, B. P. (2011). Variability and predictors of urinary Bisphenol A concentrations during pregnancy. *Environmental and Health Perspective, 119*(1), 131-137.

Braun, J. M., Kalkbrenner, A. E., Calafat, A. M., Yolton, K., Ye, X., Dietrich, K. N., & Lanphear, B. P. (2011). Impact ofearly-life bisphenol A exposure on behavior and executive function in children. *Pediatrics*, *128*(5), 873–882. doi:10.1542/peds.2011-1335 PMID:22025598

Braun, J. M., Sathyanarayana, S., & Hauser, R. (2013). Phthalate exposure and children's health. *Current Opinion in Pediatrics*, *25*(2), 247–254. doi:10.1097/MOP.0b013e32835e1eb6 PMID:23429708

Braunrath, R., Podlipna, D., Padlesak, S., & Cichna-Markl, M. (2005). Determination of Bisphenol A in canned foods by immunoaffinity chromatography, HPLC, and fluorescence detection. *Journal of Agricultural and Food Chemistry*, *53*(23), 8911–8917. doi:10.1021/jf051525j PMID:16277382

Brecher, J., & Costello, T. (1994). *Global Village or Global Pillage: Economic Reconstruction from theBottom Up*. Boston, MA: South End Press.

Brecher, J., Costello, T., & Smith, B. (2000). *Globalization from Below*. Boston, MA: South EndPress.

Brinton, W. F. Jr. (2005). Characterization of man-made foreign matter and its presence in multiple size fractions from mixed waste composting. *Compost Science & Utilization*, *13*(4), 274–280. doi:10.1080/1065657X.2005.10702251

Bronner, S. E., & Kellner, D. (Eds.). (1989). *Critical Theory and Society: A Reader*. New York: Routledge.

Browne, M. A., Crump, P., Niven, S. J., Teuten, E., Tonkin, A., Galloway, T., & Thompson, R. (2011). Accumulation of microplastic on shorelines woldwide: Sources and sinks. *Environmental Science & Technology*, *45*(21), 9175–9179. doi:10.1021/es201811s PMID:21894925

Browne, M. A., Dissanayake, A., Galloway, T. S., Lowe, D. M., & Thompson, R. C. (2008). Ingested microscopic plastic translocates to the circulatory system of the mussel, *Mytilus edulis* (L.). *Environmental Science & Technology*, *42*(13), 5026–5031. doi:10.1021/es800249a PMID:18678044

Brunner, P. H., & Rechberger, H. (2015). Waste to energy – key element for sustainable waste management. *Waste Management*, 373–12.

Brunner, P. H., & Ernst, W. R. (1986). Alternative methods for the analysis of municipal solid waste. *Waste Management & Research*, *4*(1), 147–160. doi:10.1177/0734242X8600400116

Bruson. (1942). Acrylonitrile -Butadiene –Styrene. *Journal of the American Chemical Society*, *64*(10), 2457–2461.

Buckley, J. P., Palmieri, R. T., Matuszewski, J. M., Herring, A. H., Baird, D. D., Hartmann, K. E., & Hoppin, J. A. (2012). Consumer product exposures associated with urinary phthalate levels in pregnant women. Journal of Exposure Science & Environmental Epidemiology, 22(5), 468–475. doi:10.1038/jes.2012.33 PubMed doi:10.1038/jes.2012.33 PMID:22760436

Burbach, R. (2001). *Globalization and Postmodern Politics: From Zapatistas to High-Tech Robber Barons*. London, UK: Pluto Press.

Bureau de normalisation du Québec. (2014). *Home page*. Retrieved from http://www.bnq.qc.ca/en/

Burnley, S. J. (2007). The use of chemical composition data in waste management planning –a case study. *Waste Management (New York, N.Y.)*, *27*(3), 327–336. doi:10.1016/j.wasman.2005.12.020 PMID:16647255

Buser, M. C., Murray, H. E., & Scinicariello, F. (2014). Age and sex differences in childhood and adulthood obesity association with phthalates: Analyses of NHANES 2007–2010. *International Journal of Hygiene and Environmental Health*, *217*(6), 687–694. doi:10.1016/j.ijheh.2014.02.005 PMID:24657244

Bushnik, T, Haines, D., Levallois, P., Levesque, J., van Oostdam, J., & Viau, C. (2010). Lead and Bisphenol A concentrations in the Canadian population. *Health Reproduction,* 217-218.

Butt, N., Beyer, H. L., Bennett, J. R., Biggs, D., Maggini, R., Mills, M., ... Possingham, H. P. (2013). Biodiversity risks from fossil fuel extraction. *Science*, *342*(6157), 425–426. doi:10.1126cience.1237261 PMID:24159031

Cabaton, N. J., Wadia, P. R., Rubin, B. S., Zalko, D., Schaeberle, C. M., Askenase, M. H., ... Soto, A. M. (2011). Perinatal exposure to environmentally relevant levels of Bisphenol A decreases fertility and fecundity in CD-1 mice. *Environmental Health Perspectives*, *119*(4), 547–552. doi:10.1289/ehp.1002559 PMID:21126938

Cacciari, I., Quatrini, P., Zirletta, G., Mincione, E., Vinciguerra, V., Lupatelli, P., & Sermanni, G. G. (1993). Isotactic polypropylene biodegradation by a microbial community: Physicochemical characterization of metabolites produced. *Applied and Environmental Microbiology*, *59*(11), 3695–3700. PMID:8285678

Cadogan, D., Papez, M., Poppe, A. C., Pugh, D. M., & Scheubel, J. (1994). Assessment of the release, occurrence and possible effects of plasticizers in the environment. *Progress in Rubber and Plastics Technology*, *10*(1), 1–19.

Calabia, B. P., & Tokiwa, Y. (2004). Microbial degradation of poly (D-3-hydroxybutyrate) by a new thermophilic *Streptomyces* isolate. *Biotechnology Letters*, *26*(1), 15–19. doi:10.1023/B:BILE.0000009453.81444.51 PMID:15005145

Calafat, A. M., Kuklenyik, Z., Reidy, J. A., Caudill, S. P., Ekong, J., & Needham, L. L. (2005). Urinary concentrations of bisphenol A and 4-nonylphenol in a human reference population. *Environmental Health Perspectives*, *113*(4), 391–395. doi:10.1289/ehp.7534 PMID:15811827

Calafat, A. M., & McKee, R. H. (2006). Integrating biomonitoring exposure data into the risk assessment process: Phthalates [diethyl phthalate and di (2-ethylhexyl) phthalate] as a case study. *Environmental Health Perspectives*, *114*(11), 1783–1789. doi:10.1289/ehp.9059 PMID:17107868

Calafat, A. M., Slakman, A. R., Silva, M. J., Herbert, A. R., & Needham, L. L. (2004). Automated solid phase extraction and quantitative analysis of human milk for 13 phthalate metabolites. *Journal of Chromatography. B, Analytical Technologies in the Biomedical and Life Sciences*, *805*(1), 49–56. doi:10.1016/j.jchromb.2004.02.006 PMID:15113539

Calafat, A. M., Weuve, J., Ye, X., Jia, L. T., Hu, H., Ringer, S., ... Hauser, R. (2009). Exposure to Bisphenol A and other phenols in neonatal intensive care unit premature infants. *Environmental Health Perspectives*, *117*(4), 639–644. doi:10.1289/ehp.0800265 PMID:19440505

Calafat, A. M., Ye, X., Wong, L. Y., Reidy, J. A., & Needham, L. L. (2008). Exposure of the U.S. population to Bisphenol A and 4-tertiary-octylphenol: 2003–2004. *Environmental Health Perspectives*, *116*(1), 39–44. doi:10.1289/ehp.10753 PMID:18197297

Caldwell, J. C. (2012). DEHP: Genotoxicity and potential carcinogenic mechanisms—a review. *Mutation Research/Reviews in Mutation Research*, *751*(2), 82–157. doi:10.1016/j.mrrev.2012.03.001 PMID:22484601

Callegari, C., Everett, S., Ross, M., & Brasel, J. A. (1987). Anogenital ratio: Measure of fetal virilization in premature and full-term newborn infants. *The Journal of Pediatrics*, *111*(2), 240–243. doi:10.1016/S0022-3476(87)80075-6 PMID:3612396

Campioli, E., Martinez-Arguelles, D. B., & Papadopoulos, V. (2014). In utero exposure to the endocrine disruptor di-(2-ethylhexyl) phthalate promotes local adipose and systemic inflammation in adult male offspring. *Nutrition & Diabetes*, *4*(5), e115. doi:10.1038/nutd.2014.13 PMID:24799162

Canadian Association of Petroleum Producers. (2014). *Glossary*. Retrieved from http://www.capp.ca/library/glossary/Pages/default.aspx#p

Cao, X. L. (2008). Determination of phthalates and adipate in bottled water by headspace solid-phase microextraction and gas chromatography/mass spectrometry. *Journal of Chromatography. A*, *1178*(1-2), 231–238. doi:10.1016/j.chroma.2007.11.095 PMID:18082753

Cao, X. L. (2010). Phthalate esters in foods: Sources, occurrence, and analytical methods. *Comprehensive Reviews in Food Science and Food Safety*, *9*(1), 21–43. doi:10.1111/j.1541-4337.2009.00093.x

Cao, X. L., & Corriveau, J. (2008). Migration of Bisphenol A from polycarbonate baby and water bottles into water under severe conditions. *Journal of Agricultural and Food Chemistry*, *56*(15), 6378–6381. doi:10.1021/jf800870b PMID:18636679

Cao, X. L., Corriveau, J., & Popovic, S. (2009). Levels of Bisphenol A in canned soft drink products in Canadian markets. *Journal of Agricultural and Food Chemistry*, *57*(4), 1307–1311. doi:10.1021/jf803213g PMID:19170636

Cao, X. L., Corriveau, J., & Popovic, S. (2010). Bisphenol A in canned food products from canadian markets. *Journal of Food Protection*, *73*(6), 1085–1089. doi:10.4315/0362-028X-73.6.1085 PMID:20537264

Cao, X. L., Corriveau, J., Popovic, S., Clement, G., Beraldin, F., & Dufresne, G. (2009). Bisphenol A in baby food products in glass jars with metal lids from Canadian markets. *Journal of Agricultural and Food Chemistry*, *57*(12), 5345–5351. doi:10.1021/jf9006888 PMID:19459630

Carayannis, E. G., Barth, T. D., & Campbell, D. F. (2012). The Quintuple Helix innovation model: global warming as a challenge and driver for innovation. *Journal of Innovation and Entrepreneurship*. doi:10.1186/2192-5372-1-2

Carayannis, E. G., & Campbell, D. F. J. (2011). Open Innovation Diplomacy and a 21st Century Fractal Research, Education and Innovation (FREIE) Ecosystem: Building on the Quadruple and Quintuple Helix Innovation Concepts and the "Mode 3" Knowledge Production System. *Journal of the Knowledge Economy*, *2*(3), 327–372. doi:10.100713132-011-0058-3

Carbery, M., O'Connor, W., & Palanisami, T. (2018). Trophic transfer of microplastics and mixed contaminants in the marine food web and implications for human health. *Environment International*, *115*, 400–409. doi:10.1016/j.envint.2018.03.007 PMID:29653694

Carey, M. J. (2011). Intergenerational transfer of plastic debris by Short-tailed Shearwaters (Ardenna tenuirostris). *Emu-Austral Ornithology*, *111*(3), 229–234. doi:10.1071/MU10085

Carisse, H., Thomas, M., & Sumi, M. (2018). *Combating plastic and air pollution on earth day*. Vital Strategies Environmental Health Division.

Carlsson, K. (1986). Heavy metals from "energy from waste" plants– comparison of gas cleaning systems. *Waste Management & Research*, *4*(1), 15–20. doi:10.1177/0734242X8600400103

Carlstedt, F., Jönsson, B., & Bornehag, C. (2013). PVC flooring is related to human uptake of phthalates in infants. Indoor Air, 23(1), 32–39. doi:10.1111/j.1600-0668.2012.00788.x PubMed doi:10.1111/j.1600-0668.2012.00788.x PMID:22563949

Carpenter, E. J., & Smith, K. L. (1972). Plastics on the Sargasso Sea surface. *Science*, *175*(4027), 1240–1241. doi:10.1126cience.175.4027.1240 PMID:5061243

Carr, S. A., Liu, J., & Tesoro, A. G. (2016). Transport and fate of microplastic particles in wastewater treatment plants. *Water Research*, *91*, 174–182. doi:10.1016/j.watres.2016.01.002 PMID:26795302

Carwile, J.L., & Michels, K.B. (2011). Urinary bisphenol A and obesity: NHANES 2003-2006. *Environmental Research*, *111*(6), 825-30. doi: : 21676388. doi:10.1016/j.envres.2011.05.014PMID

Carwile, J. L., & Michels, K. B. (2011). Urinary Bisphenol A and obesity: NHANES 2003–2006. *Environmental Research, 111*(6), 825–830. doi:10.1016/j.envres.2011.05.014 PMID:21676388

Casals-Casas, C., & Desvergne, B. (2011). Endocrine disruptors: From endocrine to metabolic disruption. *Annual Review of Physiology, 73*(1), 135–162. doi:10.1146/annurev-physiol-012110-142200 PMID:21054169

Casas, M., Valvi, D., Luque, N., Ballesteros-Gomez, A., Carsin, A. E., Fernandez, M. F., ... Vrijheid, M. (2013). Dietary and sociodemographic determinants of Bisphenol A urine concentrations in pregnant women and children. *Environment International, 56*, 10–18. doi:10.1016/j.envint.2013.02.014 PMID:23542682

Castaño-Vinyals, G., Carrasco, E., Lorente, J. A., Sabaté, Y., Cirac-Claveras, J., Pollán, M., & Kogevinas, M. (2012). Anogenital distance and the risk of prostate cancer. *BJU International, 110*(11b), E707–E710. doi:10.1111/j.1464-410X.2012.11516.x PMID:22984847

Castells, M. (1996). The Information Age: Economy, Society, and Culture.: Vol. 1. *The Rise of the NetworkSociety*. Oxford, UK: Blackwell.

Cavalieri, E. L., & Rogan, E. G. (2010). Is Bisphenol A a weak carcinogen like the natural estrogens and diethylstilbestrol? *IUBMB Life, 62*(10), 746–751. doi:10.1002/iub.376 PMID:20945454

CDC. (2003). Second national report on human exposure to environmental chemicals. Atlanta, GA: National Center for Environmental Health, Division of Laboratory Sciences.

CDC. (2003). Second national report on human exposure to environmental chemicals. US Department of Health and Human Services, Centers for Disease Control and Prevention, National Center for Environmental Health, Division of Laboratory Sciences.

CDC. (2005). Third national report on human exposure to environmental chemicals. Atlanta, GA: National Center for Environmental Health, Division of Laboratory Sciences.

CDC. (2005). Third national report on human exposure to environmental chemicals. US Department of Health and Human Services, Centers for Disease Control and Prevention, National Center for Environmental Health, Division of Laboratory Sciences.

Cedervall, T., Hansson, L. A., Lard, M., Frohm, B., & Linse, S. (2012). Food chain transport of nanoparticles affects behaviour and fat metabolism in fish. *PLoS One, 7*(2), e32254. doi:10.1371/journal.pone.0032254 PMID:22384193

Center for the Evaluation of Risks to Human Reproduction (CERHR). (2000). *NTP-CERHR Expert Panel Report on Di(2-ethyl- hexyl) Phthalate*. Alexandria, VA: Science International, Inc.

Centers for Disease and Control. (2009). *Solid Waste*. Retrieved July 16,from http://www.cdc.gov/nceh/ehs/NALBOH/NALBOH-4.pdf

Centers for Disease Control and Prevention. (2018). Fourth Report on Human Exposure to Environmental Chemicals, Updated Tables. Atlanta, GA: U.S. Department of Health and Human Services, Centers for Disease Control and Prevention. Retrieved from

Central Pollution Control Board (CPCB). (2013). *Overview of Plastic Waste Management*. Author.

Central Pollution Control Board (CPCB). (2017). *Consolidated guidelines for segregation, collection and disposal of plastic waste*. Author.

Central Pollution Control Board. (2013). *Overview of Plastic Waste Management, India*. Author.

Central Pollution Control Board. (2015). Assessment & Characterisation of Plastic Waste Generation in 60 Major Cities, India. Author.

Central Pollution Control Board. (2017). India, Life cycle assessment study of plastics packaging products. Author.

Cerqueira, H. S., Caeiro, G., Costa, L., & Ramoa Ribeiro, F. (2008). Deactivation of FCC Catalyst. *Journal of Molecular Catalysis. Chem*, *292*, 1–13.

Cha, C. Y., & Carlisle, C. T. (2001). Microwave process for volatile organic compound abatement. *Journal of the Air & Waste Management Association*, *51*(12), 1628–1641. doi:10.1080/10473289.2001.10464389 PMID:15666467

Chae, Y., Kim, D., Kim, S. W., & An, Y. J. (2018). Trophic transfer and individual impact of nano-sized polystyrene in a four-species freshwater food chain. *Scientific Reports*, *8*(1), 284. doi:10.103841598-017-18849-y PMID:29321604

Chakrabarty, P., Srivastava, V. K., & Chakrabarti, S. N. (1995). Solid waste disposal and the environment–a review. *Indian Journal of Environmental Protection*, *15*, 39–43.

Chandra, R., & Rustgi, H. (1998). Biodegradable polymers. *Progress in Polymer Science*, *23*(7), 1273–1335. doi:10.1016/S0079-6700(97)00039-7

Chandra, R., & Rustgi, R. (1997). Biodegradation of maleated linear low-density polyethylene and starch blends. *Polymer Degradation & Stability*, *56*(2), 185–202. doi:10.1016/S0141-3910(96)00212-1

Chang, B. V., Yang, C. M., Cheng, C. H., & Yuan, S. Y. (2004). Biodegradation of phthalate esters by two bacteria strains. *Chemosphere*, *55*(4), 533–538. doi:10.1016/j.chemosphere.2003.11.057 PMID:15006506

Chang, J. W., Lee, C. C., Pan, W. H., Chou, W. C., Huang, H. B., Chiang, H. C., & Huang, P. C. (2017). Estimated daily intake and cumulative risk assessment of phthalates in the general Taiwanese after the 2011 DEHP food scandal. *Scientific Reports*, *7*(1), 45009. doi:10.1038rep45009 PMID:28327585

Chanprateep, S. (2010). Current trends in biodegradable polyhydroxylakanoates. *Journal of Bioscience and Bioengineering*, *110*(6), 621–632. doi:10.1016/j.jbiosc.2010.07.014 PMID:20719562

Chao, W. L., Lin, C. M., Shiung, I. I., & Kuo, Y. L. (2006). Degradation of di-butyl-phthalate by soil bacteria. *Chemosphere*, *63*(8), 1377–1383. doi:10.1016/j.chemosphere.2005.09.021 PMID:16289698

Chapelle, F. (1993). *Ground-Water Microbiology & Geochemistry*. New York: John Wiley & Sons, Inc.

Chatonnet, P., Boutou, S., & Plana, A. (2014). Contamination of wines andspirits by phthalates: Types of contaminants present, contamination sources and means of prevention. *Food Addit. Contam. Part A*, *31*(9), 1605–1615. doi:10.1080/19440049.2014.941947 PMID:25099435

Chatterjee, S., Roy, B., Roy, D., & Banerjee, R. (2010). Enzyme-mediated biodegradation of heat treated commercial polyethylene by Staphylococcal species. *Polymer Degradation Stability, 95,* 195-200.

Chatterjee, S., Roy, B., Roy, D., & Banerjee, R. (2010). Enzyme-mediated biodegradation of heat treated commercial polyethylene by *Staphylococcal* species. *Polymer Degradation & Stability*, *95*(2), 195–200. doi:10.1016/j.polymdegradstab.2009.11.025

Chaturvedi, B. (2002). *The source of this information is a press release of NoPlastics in the Environment (Nope) Imports Versus Surplus: A Glut of Plasticsin India Today*. Chintan Environmental Organization.

Chaupart, N., Serpe, G., & Verdu, J. (1998). Molecular weight distribution and mass changes during polyamide hydrolysis. *Polymer*, *39*(6-7), 1375–1380. doi:10.1016/S0032-3861(97)00414-X

Chen, G-Q. (2011). Biofunctionalization of polymers and their applications. *Biofunctionalization of Polymers and their Applications, 125*, 29–45. Doi:10.1007/10_2010_89

Chen, C. M. (2008). Overview of obesity in Mainland China. *Obesity Reviews, 9*(1), 14–21. doi:10.1111/j.1467-789X.2007.00433.x PMID:18307694

Chen, F. P., & Chien, M. H. (2014). Lower concentrations of phthalates induce proliferation in humanbreast cancer cells. *Climacteric, 17*(4), 377–384. doi:10.3109/13697137.2013.865720 PMID:24228746

Cheng, Y. W., Sung, F. C., Yang, Y., Lo, Y. H., Chung, Y. T., & Li, K.-C. (2009). Medical waste production at hospitals and associated factors. *Waste Management (New York, N.Y.), 29*(1), 440–444. doi:10.1016/j.wasman.2008.01.014 PMID:18359619

Chen, K.-S., & Hsu, R.-F. (2007). Evaluation of environmental effects on mechanical properties and characterization of creep behaviour of PMMA. *Zhongguo Gongcheng Xuekan, 30*(2), 267–274. doi:10.1080/02533839.2007.9671253

Chen, Y.-C. (2018). Effects of urbanization on municipal solid waste composition. *Waste Management (New York, N.Y.), 79*, 828–836. doi:10.1016/j.wasman.2018.04.017 PMID:30078496

Chiappone, M., Dienes, H., Swanson, D. W., & Miller, S. L. (2005). Impacts of lost fishing gear on coral reef sessile invertebrates in the Florida Keys National Marine Sanctuary. *Biological Conservation, 121*(2), 221–230. doi:10.1016/j.biocon.2004.04.023

Chiu, S. J., Chen, S. H., & Tsai, C. T. (2006). Effect of metal chlorides on thermal degradation of (waste) polycarbonate. *Waste Management (New York, N.Y.), 26*(3), 252–259. doi:10.1016/j.wasman.2005.03.003 PMID:16387239

Choi, J., Eom, J., Kim, J., Lee, S., & Kim, Y. (2014). Association between some endocrine-disruptingchemicals and childhood obesity in biological samples of young girls: A cross-sectional study. *Environmental Toxicology and Pharmacology, 38*(1), 51–57. doi:10.1016/j.etap.2014.04.004 PMID:24908636

Chowdhury, A. A. (1963). Poly-β-hydroxybuttersaure abbauende Bakterien und exo-enzyme. *Archives of Microbiology, 47*, 167–200. doi:10.1007/BF00422523 PMID:14106079

Citizens Environmental Coalition (CEC). (1993). Managing Medical Waste, CEC Fact Sheet #6. Albany, NY: CEC.

Cladiere, M., Gasperi, J., Lorgeoux, C., Bonhomme, C., Rocher, V., & Tassin, B. (2013). Alkylphenolic compounds and bisphenol A contamination within heavily urbanized area: Case study of Paris. *Environmental Science and Pollution Research International, 20*(5), 2973–2983. doi:10.100711356-012-1220-6 PMID:23054786

Claereboudt, M. R. (2004). Shore litter along sandy beaches of the Gulf of Oman. *Marine Pollution Bulletin, 49*(9–10), 770–777. doi:10.1016/j.marpolbul.2004.06.004 PMID:15530520

Claessens, M., De Meester, S., Van Landuyt, L., De Clerck, K., & Janssen, C. R. (2011). Occurrence and distribution of microplastics in marine sediments along the Belgian coast. *Marine Pollution Bulletin, 62*(10), 2199–2204. doi:10.1016/j.marpolbul.2011.06.030 PMID:21802098

Clapp, J., & Swantoon, L. (2009). Environmental Policies. Centre for International Governance Innovation.

Clayton, J. A., & Collins, F. S. (2014). NIH to balance sex in cell and animal studies. Nature, 509(7500), 282–283. doi:10.1038/509282a PubMed doi:10.1038/509282a PMID:24834516

Cliff, G., Dudley, S. F., Ryan, P. G., & Singleton, N. (2002). Large sharks and plastic debris in KwaZulu-Natal, South Africa. *Marine & Freshwater Research, 53*(2), 575–581. doi:10.1071/MF01146

Cobellis, L. (2003). High plasma concentrations of di-(2-ethylhexyl)-phthalate in women with endometriosis. *Human Reproduction (Oxford, England)*, *18*(7), 1512–1515. doi:10.1093/humrep/deg254 PMID:12832380

Cocci, P., Mosconi, G., Arukwe, A., Mozzicafreddo, M., Angeletti, M., Aretusi, G., & Palermo, F. A. (2015). Effects of diisodecyl phthalate on PPAR: RXR-dependent gene expression pathways inSea Bream hepatocytes. *Chemical Research in Toxicology*, *28*(5), 935–947. doi:10.1021/tx500529x PMID:25825955

Colacino, J. A., Harris, T. R., & Schecter, A. (2010). Dietary intake is associated with phthalate body burden in a nationally representative sample. *Environmental Health Perspectives*, *118*(7), 998–1003. doi:10.1289/ehp.0901712 PMID:20392686

Colborn, T., vom Saal, F. S., & Soto, A. M. (1993). Developmental effects of endocrine-disrupting chemicals in wildlife and humans. Environmental Health Perspectives, 101(5), 378–384. doi:10.1289/ehp.93101378 PubMed doi:10.1289/ehp.93101378 PMID:8080506

Colin, A., Bach, C., Rosin, Ch., Munoz, J.-F., & Dauchy, X. (2013). Is drinking water a major route of human exposure toalkylphenol and bisphenol contaminants in France? *Archives of Environmental Contamination and Toxicology*, *66*(1), 86–99. doi:10.100700244-013-9942-0 PMID:23921451

Colmenero, A. I., Barría, C., Broglio, E., & García-Barcelona, S. (2017). Plastic debris straps on threatened blue shark Prionace glauca. *Marine Pollution Bulletin*, *115*(1-2), 436–438. doi:10.1016/j.marpolbul.2017.01.011 PMID:28089553

Colomer-Mendoza, F. J., Robles-Martinez, F., Herrera-Prats, L., Gallardo-Izquierdo, A., & Bovea, M. D. (2012). Bio-drying as a biological process to diminish moisture in gardening and harvest wastes. *Environment, Development and Sustainability*, *14*(6), 1013–1026. doi:10.100710668-012-9369-1

Colón, I., Caro, D., Bourdony, C. J., & Rosario, O. (2000). Identification of phthalate esters in the serum of young Puerto Rican girls with premature breast development. *Environmental Health Perspectives*, *108*(9), 895. PMID:11017896

Comanita, E.-D., Hlihor, R. M., Ghinea, C., & Gavrilescu, M. (2016). Occurrence of plastic waste in the environment: Ecological and health risks. *Environmental Engineering and Management Journal*, *15*(3), 675–685. doi:10.30638/eemj.2016.073

Commission Staff Working Document on the Implementation of the Community Strategy for Endocrine Disrupters. (2007). *A Range of Substances Suspected of Interfering with the Hormone Systems of Humans and Wildlife; CEC*. Brussels: Commission of the European Communities.

Coors, A., Jones, P., Giesy, J., & Ratte, H. (2003). Removal of estrogenic activity from municipal waste landfill leachate assessed with a bioassay based on reporter gene expression. *Environmental Science & Technology*, *37*(15), 3430–3434. doi:10.1021/es0300158 PMID:12966991

Corbin, T., Handermann, A., Kotek, R., Porter, W., Dellinger, J., & Davis, E. (1999). *Reclaiming epsilon-caprolactam from nylon 6 carpet*. U.S. Patent 5,977,193.

Cordova, M. R., Hadi, T. A., & Prayudha, B. (2018). Occurrence and abundance of microplastics in coral reef sediment : A case study in Sekotong, Lombok-Indonesia. *Advances in Environmental Sciences Bioflux*, *10*(1), 23–29. doi:10.5281/zenodo.1297719

Cordova, M. R., & Wahyudi, A. J. (2016). Microplastic in the Deep-Sea Sediment of Southwestern Sumatran Waters. *Marine Research in Indonesia*, *41*(1), 27. doi:10.14203/mri.v41i1.99

Cozar, A., Echevarria, F., Gonzalez-Gordillo, J. I., Irigoien, X., Ubeda, B., Hernandez-Leon, S., ... Duarte, C. M. (2014). Plastic debris in the open ocean. *Proceedings of the National Academy of Sciences*, *111*(28), 10239–10244. 10.1073/pnas.1314705111

Crabbe, J. R., Campbell, J. R., Thompson, L., Walz, S. L., & Schultz, W. W. (1994). Biodegradation of colloidal ester-based polyurethane by soil fungi. *International Biodeterioration & Biodegradation*, *33*(2), 103–113. doi:10.1016/0964-8305(94)90030-2

Crain, D. A., Eriksen, M., Iguchi, T., Jobling, S., Laufer, H., LeBlanc, G. A., & Guillette, L. J. Jr. (2007). An ecological assessment of bisphenol-A: Evidence from comparative biology. *Reproductive Toxicology (Elmsford, N.Y.)*, *24*(2), 225–239. doi:10.1016/j.reprotox.2007.05.008 PMID:17604601

Crawford, C. B., & Quinn, B. (2017). The contemporary history of plastics. In Microplastic Pollutants (pp. 19–37). Academic Press. doi:10.1016/B978-0-12-809406-8.00002-5

Csan'ady, G., Oberste-Frielinghaus, H., Semder, B., Baur, C., Schneider, K., & Filser, J. (2002). Distribution and unspecific protein binding of the xenoestrogens Bisphenol A and daidzein. *Archives of Toxicology*, *76*(5-6), 299–305. doi:10.100700204-002-0339-5 PMID:12107647

Cucchiella, F., D'Adamo, I., Koh, S. C., & Rosa, P. (2015). Recycling of WEEEs: An economic assessment of present and future e-waste streams. *Renewable & Sustainable Energy Reviews*, *51*, 263–272. doi:10.1016/j.rser.2015.06.010

Cunha, S., Cunha, C., Ferreira, A., & Fernandes, J. (2012). Determination of bisphenol A and bisphenol B in canned seafood combining QuEChERS extraction with dispersive liquid-liquid microextraction followed by gaschromatography-mass spectrometry. *Analytical and Bioanalytical Chemistry*, *404*(8), 2453–2463. doi:10.100700216-012-6389-5 PMID:22995997

Cunha, S., & Fernandes, J. (2013). Assessement of bisphenol A and bisphenol B in canned vegetables and fruits by gaschromatography-mass spectrometry after QuEChERS and dispersive liquid-liquid microextraction. *Food Control*, *33*(2), 549–555. doi:10.1016/j.foodcont.2013.03.028

Cvetkovich, A., & Kellner, D. (1997). *Articulating the Global and the Local: Globalization and CulturalStudies*. Boulder, CO: Westview Press.

Cyberatlas. (n.d.). Retrieved from http://cyberatlas.interet.com/big-picture/demographics

Czernik, S., Elam, C., Evans, R., Meglen, R., Moens, L., & Tatsumoto, K. (1998). Catalytic Pyrolysis of Nylon 6 to Recover Caprolactam. *Journal of Analytical and Applied Pyrolysis*, *56*(1), 51–64. doi:10.1016/S0165-2370(98)00068-0

da Costa, J. P., Santos, P. S., Duarte, A. C., & Rocha-Santos, T. (2016). (Nano) plastics in the environment–sources, fates and effects. *The Science of the Total Environment*, *566*, 15–26. doi:10.1016/j.scitotenv.2016.05.041 PMID:27213666

Damstra, T., Barlow, S., Bergman, A., Kavlock, R., & Van Der Kraak, G. (Eds.). (2004). *Global assessment of the state of the science of endocrine disruptors*. International Programme on Chemical Safety. Retrieved from http://ehp.niehs.nih.gov/who/

Dang, T. C. H., Nguyen, D. T., Thai, H., Nguyen, T. C., Tran, T. T. H., Le, V. H., … Nguyen, T. G. (2018). Plastic degradation by thermophilic *Bacillus* sp. BCBT21 isolated from composting agricultural residual in Vietnam. *Advances in Natural Sciences: Nanoscience and Nanotechnology*, *9*(1).

Dara, P. K., Terfa, A. M., & Deng, B. P. (2018). Beating the plastic pollution: A review. *International Journal of Innovative Research in Science, Engineering and Technology, 7*, 6.

Darbre, P. D., & Charles, A. K. (2010). Environmental oestrogens and breast cancer: Evidence for combined involvement of dietary, household and cosmetic xenoestrogens. *Anticancer Research*, *30*, 815–827. PMID:20393002

Dargnat, C., Teil, M. J., Chevreuil, M., & Blanchard, M. (2009). Phthalate removal throughout wastewater treatment plant: Case study of Marne Aval station (France). *The Science of the Total Environment*, *407*(4), 1235–1244. doi:10.1016/j.scitotenv.2008.10.027 PMID:19036415

Das, S., & Bhattacharyya, B. K. (2013). Municipal solid waste characteristics and management in Kolkata, India. In *The 19th International Conference on Industrial Engineering and Engineering Management* (pp. 1399-1409). Springer.

Das, K., & Chowdhury, A. H. (2012). Designing a reverse logistics network for optimal collection, recovery and quality-based product-mix planning. *International Journal of Production Economics*, *135*(1), 209–221. doi:10.1016/j.ijpe.2011.07.010

Das, M. T., Ghosh, P., & Thakur, I. S. (2014). Intake estimates of phthalate esters for South Delhi population based on exposure media assessment. *Environmental Pollution*, *189*, 118–125. doi:10.1016/j.envpol.2014.02.021 PMID:24657605

Daspatnaik. (2016). Retrieved from http://www.ecoideaz.com/expert-corner/finding-solutions-to-plastic-waste-management-in-india

Datta, P., Mohi, G. K., & Chander, J. (2018). Biomedical waste management in India: Critical appraisal. *Journal of Laboratory Physicians*, *10*(1), 6–14. doi:10.4103/JLP.JLP_89_17 PMID:29403196

Dau, B. K., Gilardi, K. V., Gulland, F. M., Higgins, A., Holcomb, J. B., Leger, J. S., & Ziccardi, M. H. (2009). Fishing gear–related injury in California marine wildlife. *Journal of Wildlife Diseases*, *45*(2), 355–362. doi:10.7589/0090-3558-45.2.355 PMID:19395745

David, R. M., McKee, R. H., Butala, J. H., Barter, R. A., &Kayser, M. (2001). Esters of Aromatic Mono-, Di-, and Tricarboxylic Acids, Aromatic Diacids and Di-, Tri-, OrPolyalcohols. *Patty's Toxicology*.

Davidson, T. M. (2012). Boring crustaceans damage polystyrene floats under docks polluting marine waters with microplastic. *Marine Pollution Bulletin*, *64*(9), 1821–1828. doi:10.1016/j.marpolbul.2012.06.005 PMID:22763283

Davis & Cornwell. (n.d.). *Introduction to Environmental Engineering* (2nd ed.). McGraw Hill.

Davis, A. P., Murphy, C. G., Saraceni-Richards, C. A., Rosenstein, M. C., Wiegers, T. C., & Mattingly, C. J. (2009). Comparative Toxicogenomics Database: A knowledgebase and discovery tool for chemical–gene–disease networks. *Nucleic Acids Research*, *37*(Database), 786–792. doi:10.1093/nar/gkn580 PMID:18782832

Davis, B. J., Maronpot, R. R., & Heindel, J. J. (1994). Di-(2-ethylhexyl) phthalate suppresses estradiol and ovulation in cycling rats. *Toxicology and Applied Pharmacology*, *128*(2), 216–223. doi:10.1006/taap.1994.1200 PMID:7940536

Davis, B. J., Weaver, R., Gaines, L. J., & Heindel, J. J. (1994). Mono-(2-ethylhexyl) phthalate suppresses estradiol production independent of FSH-cAMP stimulation in rat granulosa cells. *Toxicology and Applied Pharmacology*, *128*(2), 224–228. doi:10.1006/taap.1994.1201 PMID:7940537

Dawes, E. A., & Senior, P. J. (1973). The role and regulation of energy reserve polymers in micro-organisms. *Advances in Microbial Physiology*, *10*, 135–266. doi:10.1016/S0065-2911(08)60088-0 PMID:4594739

Dawood, A., & Miura, K. (2001). Pyrolysis kinetics of g-irradiated polypropylene. *Polymer Degradation & Stability*, *73*(2), 347–354. doi:10.1016/S0141-3910(01)00096-9

Dawood, A., & Miura, K. (2002). Catalytic pyrolysis of g-irradiated polypropylene (PP) over HYzeolite for enhancing the reactivity and the product selectivity. *Polymer Degradation & Stability*, *76*(1), 45–52. doi:10.1016/S0141-3910(01)00264-6

De Brito, M. P., & Dekker, R. (2004). A Framework for Reverse Logistics. In R. Dekker, K. Inderfurth, L. van Wassenhove, & M. Fleischmann (Eds.), *Reverse Logistics. Quantitative Models for Closed- Loop Supply Chains*. Berlin, Germany: Springer-Verlag. doi:10.1007/978-3-540-24803-3_1

De Coster, S., & van Larebeke, N. (2012). Endocrine-disrupting chemicals: Associated disorders and mechanisms of action. *Journal of Environmental and Public Health*. PMID:22991565

De Marco, I., Caballero, B., Torres, A., Laresgoiti, M. F., Chomón, M. J., & Cabrero, M. A. (2002). Recycling polymeric wastes by means of pyrolysis. *Journal of Chemical Technology and Biotechnology (Oxford, Oxfordshire)*, *77*(7), 817–824. doi:10.1002/jctb.636

de Sá, L. C., Oliveira, M., Ribeiro, F., Rocha, T. L., & Futter, M. N. (2018). Studies of the effects of microplastics on aquatic organisms: What do we know and where should we focus our efforts in the future? *The Science of the Total Environment*, *645*, 1029–1039. doi:10.1016/j.scitotenv.2018.07.207 PMID:30248828

Debicka, M., Zygadlo, M., & Latosinska, J. (2013). Investigations of bio– drying process of municipal solid waste. *Ecological Chemistry and Engineering A*, *20*, 1–28.

Dekker, R., Fleischmann, M., Inderfurth, K., & Van Wassenhove, L. N. (2004). *Reverse Logistics Network Design: Quantitative Models for Closed-Loop Supply Chains*. Berlin: Springer. doi:10.1007/978-3-540-24803-3

Delfosse, V., Grimaldi, M., Pons, J. L., Boulahtouf, A., le Maire, A., Cavailles, V., ... Balaguer, P. (2012). Structural and mechanistic insights into bisphenols action provide guidelines for risk assessment and discovery of Bisphenol A substitutes. *Proceedings of the National Academy of Sciences of the United States of America*, *109*(37), 14930–14935. doi:10.1073/pnas.1203574109 PMID:22927406

Derraik, J. G. B. (2002). The pollution of the marine environment by plastic debris: Areview. *Marine Pollution Bulletin*, *44*(9), 842–852. doi:10.1016/S0025-326X(02)00220-5 PMID:12405208

Desforges, J. P. W., Galbraith, M., & Ross, P. S. (2015). Ingestion of microplastics by zooplankton in the Northeast Pacific Ocean. *Archives of Environmental Contamination and Toxicology*, *69*(3), 320–330. doi:10.100700244-015-0172-5 PMID:26066061

Desvergne, B., Feige, J. N., & Casals-Casas, C. (2009). PPAR-mediated activity of phthalates: A link to the obesity epidemic? *Molecular and Cellular Endocrinology*, *304*(1-2), 43–48. doi:10.1016/j.mce.2009.02.017 PMID:19433246

Devriese, L. I., van der Meulen, M. D., Maes, T., Bekaert, K., Paul-Pont, I., Frère, L., & Vethaak, A. D. (2015). Microplastic contamination in brown shrimp (*Crangon crangon*, Linnaeus 1758) from coastal waters of the Southern North Sea and Channel area. *Marine Pollution Bulletin*, *98*(1-2), 179–187. doi:10.1016/j.marpolbul.2015.06.051 PMID:26456303

Dianin, A. P. (1891). "О продуктах конденсации кетонов с фенолами" [Condensation of ketones with phenols]. Журнал Русского Физико-Химического Общества. *Journal of the Russian Physical and Chemical Society*, *23*, 488–517.

Díaz-Torres, E. R., Ortega-Ortiz, C. D., Silva-Iñiguez, L., Nene-Preciado, A., & Orozco, E. T. (2017). Floating Marine Debris in waters of the Mexican Central Pacific. *Marine Pollution Bulletin*, *115*(1–2), 225–232. doi:10.1016/j.marpolbul.2016.11.065 PMID:27974156

Dietert, R. R., DeWitt, J. C., Germolec, D. R., & Zelikoff, J. T. (2010). Breaking patterns of environmentally influenced disease for health risk reduction: Immune perspectives. *Environmental Health Perspectives*, *118*(8), 1091–1099. doi:10.1289/ehp.1001971 PMID:20483701

Dirinck, E., Dirtu, A. C., Geens, T., Covaci, A., Van Gaal, L., & Jorens, P. G. (2015). Urinary phthalate metabolites are associated with insulin resistance in obese subjects. *Environmental Research*, *137*, 419–423. doi:10.1016/j.envres.2015.01.010 PMID:25622280

Dirtu, A. C., Geens, T., Dirinck, E., Malarvannan, G., Neels, H., Van Gaal, L., ... Covaci, A. (2013). Phthalate metabolites in obese individuals undergoing weight loss: Urinary levels and estimation of the phthalates daily intake. *Environment International*, *59*, 344–353. doi:10.1016/j.envint.2013.06.023 PMID:23892227

Dirven, H. A. A. M., Van Den Broek, P. H. H., & Jongeneelen, F. J. (1993). Determination of four metabolites of the plasticizer di (2-ethylhexyl) phthalate in human urine samples. *International Archives of Occupational and Environmental Health*, *64*(8), 555–560. doi:10.1007/BF00517700 PMID:8314613

Do, L. A. T., Boonmongkon, P., Paek, S. C., & Guadamuz, T. E. (2017). *'Hu Hong' (bad thing): parental perceptions of teenagers' sexuality in urban Vietnam*. doi:10.118612889-017-4133-y

Dodds, E. C., & Lawson, W. (1936). Synthetic estrogenic agents without the phenantthrene nucleus. *Nature*, *137*(3476), 996. doi:10.1038/137996a0

Dodds, E. C., & Lawson, W. (1938). Molecular structure in relation to oestrogenic activity. Compounds without a phenanthrene nucleus. *Proceedings of the Royal Society*, *125*, 222–232.

Dodiuk, H., & Goodman, S. H. (2013). Handbook of Thermoset Plastics. In Handbook of Thermoset Plastics. doi:10.1016/C2011-0-09694-1

Dodson, R. E., Nishioka, M., Standley, L. J., Perovich, L. J., Brody, J. G., & Rudel, R. A. (2012). Endocrine disruptors and asthma-associated chemicals in consumer products. Environmental Health Perspectives, 120(7), 935–943. doi:10.1289/ehp.1104052 PubMed doi:10.1289/ehp.1104052 PMID:22398195

Doelman, C. J. A., Borm, P. J. A., & Bast, A. (1990). Plasticizers and bronchial hyper reactivity. *Lancet*, *335*(8691), 725. doi:10.1016/0140-6736(90)90839-W PMID:1969080

Dohan, K., & Maximenko, N. (2010). Monitoring Ocean Currents with Satellite Sensors. *Oceanography (Washington, D.C.)*, *23*(4), 94–103. doi:10.5670/oceanog.2010.08

Dolinoy, D. C., Huang, D., & Jirtle, R. L. (2007). Maternal nutrient supplementation counteracts Bisphenol A-induced DNA hypomethylation in early development. *Proceedings of the National Academy of Sciences of the United States of America*, *104*(32), 13056–13061. doi:10.1073/pnas.0703739104 PMID:17670942

Dorger. (2019). Retrieved from https://www.thestreet.com/world/countries-most-plastic-waste-14878534

Doull, J., Cattley, R., Elcombe, C., Lake, B. G., Swenberg, J., Wilkinson, C., ... Van Gemert, M. (1999). A cancer risk assessment of di (2-ethylhexyl) phthalate: Application of the new US EPA Risk Assessment Guidelines. *Regulatory Toxicology and Pharmacology*, *29*(3), 327–357. doi:10.1006/rtph.1999.1296 PMID:10388618

Doyle, T. J., Bowman, J. L., Windell, V. L., McLean, D. J., & Kim, K. H. (2013). Transgenerationaleffects of di-(2-ethylhexyl) phthalate on testicular germ cell associations and spermatogonial stemcells in mice. *Biology of Reproduction*, *88*(5), 112. doi:10.1095/biolreprod.112.106104 PMID:23536373

Drew, J. (1998). *Global Communications in the Post-Industrial Age: A Study of the Communications Strategies of U.S. Labor Organizations* (Ph.D. dissertation). University of Texas.

Dris, R., Gasperi, J., Saad, M., Mirande, C., & Tassin, B. (2016). Synthetic fibers in atmospheric fallout: A source of microplastics in the environment? *Marine Pollution Bulletin*, *104*(1-2), 290–293. doi:10.1016/j.marpolbul.2016.01.006 PMID:26787549

Duangchan, A., & Samart, C. (2008). Tertiary recycling of PVC-containing plastic waste by copyrolysis with cattle manure. *Waste Management (New York, N.Y.)*, *28*(11), 2415–2421. doi:10.1016/j.wasman.2007.12.010 PMID:18314324

Duddu, M. K., Tripura, K. L., Guntuku, G., & Divya, D. S. (2015). Biodegradation of low density polyethylene (LDPE) by a new biosurfactant-producing thermophilic *Streptomyces coelicoflavus* NBRC 15399T. *African Journal of Biotechnology, 14*(4), 327–340. doi:10.5897/AJB2014.14224

Du, F., & Evans, G. W. (2007). A Bi-Objective Reverse Logistics Network Analysis for Post-Sale Service. *Computers & Operations Research.*

Duraisamy, M., & Shrinithivihahshini, N. D. (2017). Need for regulatory policies in India, on the use of bisphenol A in food contact plastic containers. *Current Science, 113*(5), 861-868. Retrieved from https://web.a.ebscohost.com/abstract?direct=true&profile=ehost&scope=site&authtype=crawler&jrnl=00113891&AN=125124518&h=oIMQUSRyn1d%2b6Xbkfq8CFnbQ0hlJEVdR7NYqWIh58E0eHLEL6FDlS1DjZhW3EVKknYFr2yO1apriRXga4GTrSQ%3d%3d&crl=c&resultNs=AdminWebAuth&resultLocal=

Durmaz, E., Özmert, E. N., Erkekoğlu, P., Giray, B., Derman, O., Hıncal, F., & Yurdakök, K. (2010). Plasma phthalate levels in pubertal gynecomastia. *Pediatrics*, *125*(1), e122–e129. doi:10.1542/peds.2009-0724 PMID:20008419

Durmus, A., Koc, S. N., Pozan, G. S., & Kasgoz, A. (2005). Thermal-catalytic degradation kinetics of polypropylene over BEA, ZSM-5 and MOR zeolites. *Applied Catalysis B: Environmental*, *61*(3-4), 316–322. doi:10.1016/j.apcatb.2005.06.009

Dussud, C., & Ghiglione, J. F. (2014). Bacterial degradation of synthetic plastics. In *CIESM Workshop Monogr* (No. 46). Academic Press.

Duty, S. M., Ackerman, R. M., Calafat, A. M., & Hauser, R. (2005). Personal care product use predicts urinary concentrations of some phthalate monoesters. Environmental Health Perspectives, 113(11), 1530–1535. doi:10.1289/ehp.8083 PubMed doi:10.1289/ehp.8083 PMID:16263507

Duty, S. M., Calafat, A. M., Silva, M. J., Brock, J. W., Ryan, L., Chen, Z., ... Hauser, R. (2004). The relationship between environmental exposure to phthalates and computer-aided sperm analysis motion parameters. *Journal of Andrology*, *25*(2), 293–302. doi:10.1002/j.1939-4640.2004.tb02790.x PMID:14760016

Duty, S. M., Calafat, A. M., Silva, M. J., Ryan, L., & Hauser, R. (2005). Phthalate exposure and reproductive hormones in adult men. *Human Reproduction (Oxford, England)*, *20*(3), 604–610. doi:10.1093/humrep/deh656 PMID:15591081

Duty, S. M., Mendonca, K., Hauser, R., Calafat, A. M., Ye, X., Meeker, J. D., ... Ringer, S. (2013). Potential sources of Bisphenol A in the neonatal intensive care unit. *Pediatrics*, *131*(3), 483–489. doi:10.1542/peds.2012-1380 PMID:23420909

Duty, S. M., Silva, M. J., Barr, D. B., Brock, J. W., Ryan, L., Chen, Z., ... Hauser, R. (2003). Phthalate exposure and human semen parameters. *Epidemiology (Cambridge, Mass.)*, *14*(3), 269–277. doi:10.1097/01.EDE.0000059950.11836.16 PMID:12859026

Duty, S. M., Singh, N. P., Silva, M. J., Barr, D. B., Brock, J. W., Ryan, L., ... Hauser, R. (2003). The relationship between environmental exposures to phthalates and DNA damage in human sperm using the neutral comet assay. *Environmental Health Perspectives*, *111*(9), 1164–1169. doi:10.1289/ehp.5756 PMID:12842768

Du, Y. Y., Fang, Y. L., Wang, Y. X., Zeng, Q., Guo, N., Zhao, H., & Li, Y. F. (2016). Follicular fluid and urinary concentrations of phthalate metabolites among infertile women and associations with in vitro fertilization parameters. *Reproductive Toxicology (Elmsford, N.Y.)*, *61*, 142–150. doi:10.1016/j.reprotox.2016.04.005 PMID:27067915

Dvorák, P., Nikel, P. I., Damborský, J., & de Lorenzo, V. (2017). Bioremediation 3.0: Engineering pollutant-removing bacteria in the times of systemic biology. *Biotechnology Advances*, *35*, 845–866.

Eckenfelder, W. W., & O'Connor, D. J. (2013). Biological waste treatment. Elsevier.

EEA. (2010). *The European environment — state and outlook 2010: synthesis*. Copenhagen: European Environment Agency.

Ehrlich, S., Williams, P. L., Missmer, S. A., Flaws, J. A., Ye, X., Calafat, A. M., ... Hauser, R. (2012). Urinary Bisphenol A concentrations and early reproductive health outcomes among women undergoing IVF. *Human Reproduction (Oxford, England), 27*(12), 3583–3592. doi:10.1093/humrep/des328 PMID:23014629

Eigenheer, E., & Zanon, U. (1991). O quefazer com osresiduoshospitaleres. Propostaparaclassificacao, embalagem, coleta e destinacao final. *Arquivos Brasileiros de Medicina, 65*(3), 233–237.

Eisenstein, Z. (1998). *Global Obscenities: Patriarchy, Capitalism, and the Lure of Cyberfantasy*. New York: New York University Press.

Ejaredar, M., Nyanza, E. C., Ten Eycke, K., & Dewey, D. (2015). Phthalate exposure and childrensneurodevelopment: A systematic review. *Environmental Research, 142*, 51–60. doi:10.1016/j.envres.2015.06.014 PMID:26101203

Eleana-Diana, C., & Rosca, M. (2015). Environmental impacts of polyvinyl chloride (PVC) production process. *Health and Bioengineering Conference*.

Elias, H. G. (2005). *Plastics, General Survey*. Ullmann's Encyclopedia of Industrial Chemistry.

Ellul, J. (1964). *The Technological Society*. New York: Knopf.

Elordi, G., López, G., Aguado, R., Olazar, M., & Bilbao, J. (2007). Catalytic pyrolysis of high-density polyethylene on a HZSM-5 zeolite catalyst in a conical spouted bed reactor. *International Journal of Chemical Reactor Engineering, 5*(1), 72. doi:10.2202/1542-6580.1567

Elordi, G., Olazar, M., Aguado, R., López, G., Arabiourrutia, M., & Bilbao, J. (2007). Catalytic pyrolysis of high-density polyethylene in a conical spouted bed reactor. *Journal of Analytical and Applied Pyrolysis, 79*(1-2), 450–455. doi:10.1016/j.jaap.2006.11.010

Elordi, G., Olazar, M., Lopez, G., Amutio, M., Artetxe, M., Aguado, R., & Bilbao, J. (2009). Catalytic pyrolysis of HDPE in continuous mode over zeolite catalyst spouted bed reactor. *Journal of Analytical and Applied Pyrolysis, 85*(1-2), 345–351. doi:10.1016/j.jaap.2008.10.015

El-Sayed, A. H. M. M., Mahmoud, W. M., Davis, E. M., & Coughlin, R. W. (1996). Biodegradation of polyurethane coatings by hydrocarbon- degrading bacteria. *International Biodeterioration & Biodegradation, 37*(1-2), 69–79. doi:10.1016/0964-8305(95)00091-7

El-Shafei, H. A., Abd El-Nasser, N. H., Kansoh, A. L., & Ali, A. M. (1998). Biodegradation of disposable polyethylene by fungi Streptomyces species. *Polymer Degradation & Stability, 62*(2), 361–365. doi:10.1016/S0141-3910(98)00019-6

Ema, M., & Miyawaki, E. (2001). Effects of monobutyl phthalate on reproductive function in pregnant and pseudopregnant rats. *Reproductive Toxicology (Elmsford, N.Y.), 15*(3), 261–267. doi:10.1016/S0890-6238(01)00131-9 PMID:11390170

Engel, S. M., Miodovnik, A., Canfield, R. L., Zhu, C., Silva, M. J., Calafat, A. M., & Wolff, M. S. (2010). Prenatal phthalate exposure is associated with childhood behavior and executive functioning. *Environmental Health Perspectives, 118*(4), 565–571. doi:10.1289/ehp.0901470 PMID:20106747

Engel, S. M., Zhu, C., Berkowitz, G. S., Calafat, A. M., Silva, M. J., Miodovnik, A., & Wolff, M. S. (2009). Prenatal phthalate exposure and performance on the Neonatal Behavioral Assessment Scale in a multiethnic birth cohort. *Neurotoxicology, 30*(4), 522–528. doi:10.1016/j.neuro.2009.04.001 PMID:19375452

Engler, R. E. (2012). The complex interaction between marine debris and toxic chemicals in the ocean. *Environmental Science & Technology, 46*(22), 12302–12315. doi:10.1021/es3027105 PMID:23088563

EPA. (2012). *Phthalates action plan.* Retrieved from https://www.epa.gov/sites/production/files/2015- 09/documents/phthalates_actionplan_revised_2012-03-14.pdf

EPA. (2015). *On phthalates.* Retrieved from https://www.epa.gov/assessing-and-managing-chemicals-undertsca/

EPA. (2015). *Phthalates.* Retrieved from https://www.epa.gov/ace/biomonitoring-phthalates

Eriksen, M., Lebreton, L. C. M., Carson, H. S., Thiel, M., Moore, C. J., Borerro, J. C., ... Reisser, J. (2014). Plastic Pollution in the World's Oceans: More than 5 Trillion Plastic Pieces Weighing over 250,000 Tons Afloat at Sea. *PLoS One*, *9*(12), e111913. doi:10.1371/journal.pone.0111913 PMID:25494041

Erlandsson, B., Karlson, S., & Albertsson, A. C. (1997). The mode of action of corn starch and a pro oxidant system in LDPE: Influence of thermo-oxidation and UV-irradiation on the molecular weight changes. *Polymer Degradation & Stability*, *55*(2), 237–245. doi:10.1016/S0141-3910(96)00139-5

Errico, S., Bianco, M., Mita, L., Migliaccio, M., Rossi, S., Nicolucci, C., ... Diano, N. (2014). Migration of Bisphenol A into canned tomatoes produced in Italy: Dependence on temperature and storage conditions. *Food Chemistry*, *160*, 157–164. doi:10.1016/j.foodchem.2014.03.085 PMID:24799222

Eskenazi, B., Warner, M., Samuels, S., Young, J., & Gerthoux, P. M. (2007). Serum dioxin concentrations and risk of uterine leiomyomain the Seveso Women's Health Study. *American Journal of Epidemiology*, *166*, 79–87. doi:10.1093/aje/kwm048

EU Scientific Committee on Toxicity Ecotoxicity and the Environment (CSTEE). (2017). *Opinion on phthalate migration from soft PVC toys and child-care articles.* Brussels: Author.

European Commission. (2011). *Commission Regulation (EU) No 10/2011 of 14 January 2011 on Plastic materials and articles intended to come into contact with food.* Author.

European Food Safety Authority (EFSA). (2003a). *Opinion of the Scientific Panel on food additives, flavourings, processing aids and materials in contact with food (AFC) related to Butylbenzylphthalate (BBP) for use in food contact materials.* Author.

European Food Safety Authority (EFSA). (2003b). *Opinion of the scientific panel on food additives, flavouring, processing aids and material in contact with food on a request from the Commission related to di-isodecylphthalate (DIDP) for use in food contact materials.* Author.

European Food Safety Authority (EFSA). (2005a). *Opinion of the Scientific Panel on food additives, flavourings, processing aids and material in contact with food (AFC) related to di-Butylphthalate (DBP) for use in food contact materials.* Author.

European Food Safety Authority (EFSA). (2005b). *Opinion of the Scientific Panel on food additives, flavourings, processing aids and materials in contact with food (AFC) related to Bis(2-ethylhexyl)phthalate (DEHP) for use in food contact materials.* Author.

European Food Safety Authority (EFSA). (2005c). *Opinion of the scientific panel on food additives, flavouring, processing aids and material in contact with food on a request from the Commission related to di-isononylphthalate (DINP) for use in food contact materials.* Author.

European Union. (2008). *European Union Risk Assessment Report e Bisphenol A. EINECS No: 201-245-8.* Retrieved from http://esis.jrc.ec.europa.eu/doc/existingchemicals/risk_assessment/REPORT/bisphenolareport325

EuropeP. (2012). *The Plastics Portal.* Retrieved from http://www. plasticseurope.org/

Evans, R. M., Barish, G. D., & Wang, Y. X. (2004). PPARs and the complex journey to obesity. *Nature Medicine*, *10*(4), 355–361. doi:10.1038/nm1025 PMID:15057233

Evans, S. M., Ashwood, P., Warley, A., Berisha, F., Thompson, R. P. H., & Powell, J. J. (2002). The role of dietary microparticles and calcium in apoptosis and interleukin-1β release of intestinal macrophages. *Gastroenterology*, *123*(5), 1543–1553. doi:10.1053/gast.2002.36554 PMID:12404229

Fabjan, E., Hulzebos, E., Mennes, W., & Piersma, A. H. (2006). A category approach for reproductive effects of phthalates. *Critical Reviews in Toxicology*, *36*(9), 695–726. doi:10.1080/10408440600894914 PMID:17050082

Faravelli, T., Bozzano, G., Colombo, M., Ranzi, E., & Dente, M. (2003). Kinetic modeling of the thermal degradation of polyethylene and polystyrene mixtures. *Journal of Analytical and Applied Pyrolysis*, *70*(2), 761–777. doi:10.1016/S0165-2370(03)00058-5

Farrell, P., & Nelson, K. (2013). Trophic level transfer of microplastic: Mytilus edulis (L.) to Carcinus maenas (L.). *Environmental Pollution*, *177*, 1–3. doi:10.1016/j.envpol.2013.01.046 PMID:23434827

FDA. (2001). Food and Drug Administration Total Diet Study; summary of residues found ordered by pesticide market baskets 91-3--99-1. Rockville, MD: Office of Plant and Dairy Foods and Beverages.

FDA. (2012). *Bisphenol A (BPA): Use in Food Contact Application.* Retrieved from http://www.fda.gov/newsevents/publichealthfocus/ucm064437

Featherstone, M. (Ed.). (1990). *Global Culture: Nationalism, Globalization, and Modernity.* London, UK: Sage.

Featherstone, M., Lash, S., & Robertson, R. (Eds.). (1995). *Global Modernities.* London, UK: Sage.

Feldman, D. (2014). Poly (vinyl chloride) Nanocomposites. *J. of Macromolecular Science Part-A*, *51*(8), 659–667. doi:10.1080/10601325.2014.925265

Fendall, L. S., & Sewell, M. A. (2009). Contributing to marine pollution by washing your face: Microplastics in facial cleansers. *Marine Pollution Bulletin*, *58*(8), 1225–1228. doi:10.1016/j.marpolbul.2009.04.025 PMID:19481226

Ferguson, K. K., Loch-Caruso, R., & Meeker, J. D. (2011). Urinary phthalate metabolites in relation to biomarkers of inflammation and oxidative stress: NHANES 1999–2006. *Environmental Research*, *111*(5), 718–726. doi:10.1016/j.envres.2011.02.002 PMID:21349512

Ferguson, M. S., Graham, O. H., Bang, F. B., & Hairston, N. G. (1946). Studies on Schistosomiasis japonica. V. Protection experiments against Schistosomiasis japonica. *American Journal of Epidemiology*, *44*(3), 367–378. doi:10.1093/oxfordjournals.aje.a119103 PMID:20274589

Fernandes, P. (2018). *Beware, plastic could be in everything you eat.* Academic Press.

Fernandes, G. J. T., Fernandes, V. J. Jr, & Araujo, A. S. (2002). Catalytic degradation of polyethylene over SAPO-37 molecular sieve. *Catalysis Today*, *75*(1-4), 233–238. doi:10.1016/S0920-5861(02)00074-3

Fernandez, M. F., Arrebola, J. P., Taoufiki, J., Navalón, A., Ballesteros, O., Pulgar, R., ... Olea, N. (2007). Bisphenol-A and chlorinated derivatives in adipose tissue of women. *Reproductive Toxicology (Elmsford, N.Y.)*, *24*(2), 259–264. doi:10.1016/j.reprotox.2007.06.007 PMID:17689919

Fernandez, S. V., Huang, Y., Snider, K. E., Zhou, Y., Pogash, T. J., & Russo, J. (2012). Expression and DNA methylation changes in human breast epithelial cells after bisphenol A exposure. *International Journal of Oncology*, *41*(1), 369–377. doi:10.3892/ijo.2012.1444 PMID:22576693

Fierens, T., Servaes, K., Van Holderbeke, M., Geerts, L., De Henauw, S., Sioen, I., & Vanermen, G. (2012). Analysis of phthalates in food products and packaging materials sold on the Belgian market. *Food and Chemical Toxicology*, *50*(7), 2575–2583. doi:10.1016/j.fct.2012.04.029 PMID:22554646

Fierens, T., Van Holderbeke, M., Willems, H., De Henauw, S., & Sioen, I. (2012). Transfer of eight phthalates through the milk chain - A case study. *Environment International*, *2013*(51), 1–7. PMID:23138015

Fierens, T., Vanermen, G., Van Holderbeke, M., De Henauw, S., & Sioen, I. (2012). Effect of cooking at home on the levels of eight phthalates in foods. *Food and Chemical Toxicology*, *50*(12), 4428–4435. doi:10.1016/j.fct.2012.09.004 PMID:22985986

Fiori, L., Bassoa, D., Castelloa, D., & Baratierib, M. (2014). Hydrothermal carbonization of biomass: Design of a batch reactor and preliminary experimental results. *Chemical Engineering Transactions*, *37*, 55–60.

Fisher, J. S., Macpherson, S., Marchetti, N., & Sharpe, R. M. (2003). Human 'testicular dysgenesis syndrome': A possible model using in-utero exposure of the rat to dibutyl phthalate. *Human Reproduction (Oxford, England)*, *18*(7), 1383–1394. doi:10.1093/humrep/deg273 PMID:12832361

Flechter, A. (1993). *Plastics from Bacteria and for Bacteria: PHA as Natural, Biodegradable Polyesters*. New York: Springer Verlag.

Fleischmann, M., Beullens, P., Bloemhof-Ruwaard, J. M., & Van Wassenhove, L. N. (2001). The Impact of Product Recovery on Logistics Network Design. *Production and Operations Management*, *10*(2), 156–173. doi:10.1111/j.1937-5956.2001.tb00076.x

Fleischmann, M., Bloemhof-Ruwaard, J. M., Dekker, R., van der Laan, E., van Nunen, J., & Van Wassenhove, L. N. (1997). Quantitative Models for Reverse Logistics: A Review. *European Journal of Operational Research*, *103*(1), 1–17. doi:10.1016/S0377-2217(97)00230-0

Fleischmann, M., Krikke, H. R., Dekker, R., & Flapper, S. D. P. (2000). A Characterisation of Logistics Networks for Product Recovery. *Omega*, *28*(6), 653–666. doi:10.1016/S0305-0483(00)00022-0

Flint, S., Markle, T., Thomson, S., & Wallace, E. (2012). Bisphenol Aexposure effects and policy; a wildlife perspective. *Journal of Environmental Management*, *104*, 19–34. doi:10.1016/j.jenvman.2012.03.021 PMID:22481365

Foin, N., Lee, R. D., Torii, R., Guitierrez-Chico, J. L., Mattesini, A., Nijjer, S., ... Wong, P. (2014). Impact of stent strut design in metallic stents and biodegradable scaffolds. *International Journal of Cardiology*, *177*(3), 800–808. doi:10.1016/j.ijcard.2014.09.143 PMID:25449502

Fontanella, S., Bonhomme, S., Koutny, M., Husarova, L., Brusson, J. M., Courdavault, J. P., ... Delort, A.-M. (2009). Comparison of the biodegradability of various polyethylene films containing pro-oxidant Additives. *Polymer Degradation & Stability*, *95*(6), 1011–1021. doi:10.1016/j.polymdegradstab.2010.03.009

Food and Drug Administration. (2000). Guidance for Industry and Other Stakeholders Toxicological Principles for the Safety Assessment of Food Ingredients. Redbook, 1-5.

Food and Drug Administration. (2007) Guidance for Industry and Other Stakeholders Toxicological Principles for the Safety Assessment of Food Ingredients. Redbook. Retrieved from https://www.fda.gov/Food/GuidanceRegulation/GuidanceDocuments RegulatoryInformation/IngredientsAdditivesGRASPackaging/ ucm2006826.htm

Food, U. S., & Adminstration, D. (2001). *Safety Assessment of Di (2-ethylhexyl) phthalate (DEHP) Released from PVC Medical Devices*. Rockville, MD: Center for Devices and Radiological Health, US Food and Drug Administration.

Foran, J. (Ed.). (Forthcoming). *The Future of Revolutions: Rethinking Radical Change in the Age of Globalization.* London, UK: Zed Books.

Forni, D., Wenk, C., & Bee, G. (1999a). Digestive utilization of novel biodegradable plastic in growing pigs. *Annales de Zootechnie, 48*, 163-171. doi:10.1051/animres:19990302

Forni, D., Wenk, C., & Bee, G. (1999b). Novel biodegradable plastics in sheep nutrition 1. Effects of untreated plastics on digestibility and metabolic energy and nitrogen utilization. *Journal of Animal Physiology and Animal Nutrition, 81*(1), 31–40. doi:10.1046/j.1439-0396.1999.811189.x

Foster, P. M. (2006). Disruption of reproductive development in male rat offspring following in utero exposure to phthalate esters. *International Journal of Andrology, 29*(1), 140–147. doi:10.1111/j.1365-2605.2005.00563.x PMID:16102138

Foster, P. M. D., Mylchreest, E., Gaido, K. W., & Sar, M. (2001). Effects of phthalate esters on the developing reproductive tract of male rats. *APMIS, 109*(S103), S272–S277. doi:10.1111/j.1600-0463.2001.tb05776.x PMID:11392369

Foster, P. M., Thomas, L. V., Cook, M. W., & Gangolli, S. D. (1980). Study of the testicular effects and changes in zinc excretion produced by some n-alkyl phthalates in the rat. *Toxicology and Applied Pharmacology, 54*(3), 392–398. doi:10.1016/0041-008X(80)90165-9 PMID:7394794

Fowler, C. W. (1987). Marine debris and northern fur seals: A case study. *Marine Pollution Bulletin, 18*(6), 326–335. doi:10.1016/S0025-326X(87)80020-6

Fox, C. S., Pencina, M. J., D'Agostino, R. B., Murabito, J. M., Seely, E. W., Pearce, E. N., & Vasan, R. S. (2008). Relations of thyroid function to body weight: Cross-sectional and longitudinal observations in a community-based sample. *Archives of Internal Medicine, 168*, 587–592. doi:10.1001/archinte.168.6.587 PMID:18362250

Fredericks, H. (1994). North American NGO Networking Against NAFTA: The Use of Computer Communicationsin Cross-Border Coalition Building. *XVII International Congress of the Latin American Studies Association*, 1-24.

Frederiksen, H., Aksglaede, L., Sorensen, K., Nielsen, O., Main, K. M., Skakkebaek, N. E., ... Andersson, A.-M. (2013). Bisphenol A and other phenols in urine from Danish children and adolescents analyzed by isotope diluted TurboFlow- LC-MSMS. *International Journal of Hygiene and Environmental Health, 216*(6), 710–720. doi:10.1016/j.ijheh.2013.01.007 PMID:23491025

Frederiksen, H., Nielsen, J. K., Morck, T. A., Hansen, P. W., Jensen, J. F., Nielsen, O., ... Knudsen, L. E. (2013). Urinary excretion of phthalate metabolites, phenols and parabens in rural and urban Danish mother-child pairs. *International Journal of Hygiene and Environmental Health, 216*(6), 772–783. doi:10.1016/j.ijheh.2013.02.006 PMID:23528233

Frederiksen, H., Sørensen, K., Mouritsen, A., Aksglaede, L., Hagen, C. P., Petersen, J. H., ... Juul, A. (2012). High urinary phthalate concentration associated with delayed pubarche in girls. *International Journal of Andrology, 35*(3), 216–226. doi:10.1111/j.1365-2605.2012.01260.x PMID:22428786

Friedman, T. (1999). *The Lexus and the Olive Tree.* New York: Farrar Straus Giroux.

Fromme, H., Gruber, L., Seckin, E., Raab, U., Zimmermann, S., Kiranoglu, M., ... Völkel, W. (2011). Phthalates and their metabolites in breast milk—Results from the Bavarian Monitoring of Breast Milk (BAMBI). *Environment International, 37*(4), 715–722. doi:10.1016/j.envint.2011.02.008 PMID:21406311

Fukuyama, F. (1992). *The End of History and the Last Man.* New York: Free Press.

Fu, P., Kawamura, K., & Barrie, L. A. (2008). Photochemical and other sources of organic compounds in the Canadian high Arctic aerosol pollution during winter– spring. *Environmental Science & Technology, 43*(2), 286–292. doi:10.1021/es803046q PMID:19238953

Galgani, F., Hanke, G., & Maes, T. (2015). Global distribution, composition and abundance of marine litter. In Marine Anthropogenic Litter (pp. 29–56). doi:10.1007/978-3-319-16510-3_2

Galgani, F., Hanke, G., Werner, S., & De Vrees, L. (2013). Marine litter within the European Marine Strategy Framework Directive. *ICES Journal of Marine Science*, *70*(6), 1055–1064. doi:10.1093/icesjms/fst122

Galgani, F., Leaute, J. P., Moguedet, P., Souplet, A., Verin, Y., Carpentier, A., ... Nerisson, P. (2000). Litter on the sea floor along European coasts. *Marine Pollution Bulletin*, *40*(6), 516–527. doi:10.1016/S0025-326X(99)00234-9

Galgani, F., Pham, C. K., Claro, F., & Consoli, P. (2018). Marine animal forests as useful indicators of entanglement by marine litter. *Marine Pollution Bulletin*, *135*, 735–738. doi:10.1016/j.marpolbul.2018.08.004 PMID:30301092

Gallego-Schmid, A., Mendoza, J. M. F., Jeswani, H. K., & Azapagic, A. (2016). Life cycle environmental impacts of vacuum cleaners and the effects of European regulation. *The Science of the Total Environment*, *559*, 192–203. doi:10.1016/j.scitotenv.2016.03.149 PMID:27060658

Galliou, F., Markakis, N., Fountoulakis, M. S., Nikolaidis, N., & Manios, T. (2018). Production of organic fertilizer from olive mill wastewater by combining solar greenhouse drying and composting. *Waste Management (New York, N.Y.)*, *75*, 305–311. doi:10.1016/j.wasman.2018.01.020 PMID:29366800

Gallo, F., Fossi, C., Weber, R., Santillo, D., Sousa, J., Ingram, I., ... Romano, D. (2018). Marine litter plastics and microplastics and their toxic chemicals components: The need for urgent preventive measures. *Environmental Sciences Europe*, *30*(1), 13. doi:10.118612302-018-0139-z PMID:29721401

Galloway, T. S., Baglin, N., Lee, B. P., Kocur, A. L., Shepherd, M. H., Steele, A. M., & Harries, L. W. (2018). An engaged research study to assess the effect of a 'real-world' dietary intervention on urinary bisphenol A (BPA) levels in teenagers. *BMJ Open*, *8*(2), e018742. doi:10.1136/bmjopen-2017-018742 PMID:29431133

Gangolli, S. D. (1982). Testicular effects of phthalate esters. *Environmental Health Perspectives*, *45*, 77–84. doi:10.1289/ehp.824577 PMID:6754364

Gao, D., Li, Z., Wen, Z., & Ren, N. (2014). Occurrence and fate of phthalate esters in full-scale domestic wastewater treatment plants and their impact on receiving waters along the Songhua River in China. *Chemosphere*, *95*, 24–32. doi:10.1016/j.chemosphere.2013.08.009 PMID:24001662

Garcia, D., Balart, R., Sanchez, L., & Lopez, J. (2007). Compatibility of recycled PVC/ABS blends effect of previous degradation. *Polymer Engineering and Science*, *47*(6), 789–796. doi:10.1002/pen.20755

Garcia, J. M., & Robertson, M. L. (2017). The future of plastics recycling. *Science*, *358*(6365), 870–872. doi:10.1126cience.aaq0324 PMID:29146798

Garlotta, D. (2001). A Literature Review of Poly(Lactic Acid). *Journal of Polymers and the Environment*, *9*(2), 63–84. doi:10.1023/A:1020200822435

Gartiser, S., Wallrabenstein, M., & Stiene, G. (1998). Assessment of several test methods for the determination of the anaerobic biodegradability of polymers. *Journal of Environmental Polymer Degradation*, *6*(3), 159–173. doi:10.1023/A:1021869530253

Gascon, M., Casas, M., Morales, E., Valvi, D., Ballesteros-Gómez, A., Luque, N., ... Sunyer, J. (2015). Prenatal exposure to bisphenol A and phthalatesand childhood respiratory tract infections and allergy. *The Journal of Allergy and Clinical Immunology*, *135*(2), 370–378. doi:10.1016/j.jaci.2014.09.030 PMID:25445825

Gasperi, J., Garnaud, S., Rocher, V., & Moilleron, R. (2008). Priority pollutants in wastewater and combined sewer overflow. *The Science of the Total Environment*, *407*(1), 263–272. doi:10.1016/j.scitotenv.2008.08.015 PMID:18814902

Geens, T., Roosens, L., Neels, H., & Covaci, A. (2009). Assessment of human exposure to bisphenol-A, triclosan andtetrabromobisphenol-A through indoor dust intake in Belgium. *Chemosphere*, *76*(6), 755–760. doi:10.1016/j.chemosphere.2009.05.024 PMID:19535125

Gentilcore, D., Porreca, I., Rizzo, F., Ganbaatar, E., Carchia, E., Mallorado, M., ... Ambrosino, C. (2013). Bisphenol Ainterferes with thyroid specific gene expression. *Toxicology*, *304*(8), 21–31. doi:10.1016/j.tox.2012.12.001 PMID:23238275

Ge, R. S., Chen, G. R., Tanrikut, C., & Hardy, M. P. (2007). Phthalate ester toxicity in Leydig cells: Developmental timing and dosage considerations. *Reproductive Toxicology (Elmsford, N.Y.)*, *23*(3), 366–373. doi:10.1016/j.reprotox.2006.12.006 PMID:17258888

GESAMP Joint Group of Experts on the Scientific Aspects of Marine Environmental Protection. (2015). Sources, fate and effects of microplastics in the marine environment: A global assessment. *Reports and Studies GESAMP*, *90*, 96. doi:10.13140/RG.2.1.3803.7925

Gesner, B. D. (1965). Environmental surface effects on ABS resins. *Journal of Applied Polymer Science*, *9*(11), 3701–3706. doi:10.1002/app.1965.070091117

Gewert, B; Plassmann, M. M., & MacLeod, M. (2015). Pathways for degradation of plastic polymers floating in the marine environment. *Environmental Science Processes Impacts, 17*, 1095-1513.

Geyer, R., Jambeck, J. R., & Law, K. L. (2017). Production, use, and fate of all plastics ever made. *Science Advances*, *3*(7), e1700782. doi:10.1126ciadv.1700782 PMID:28776036

Ghisari, M., & Bonefeld-Jorgensen, E. C. (2009). Effects of plasticizers and their mixtures on estrogen receptor and thyroid hormone functions. *Toxicology Letters*, *189*(1), 67–77. doi:10.1016/j.toxlet.2009.05.004 PMID:19463926

Ghosh, R., & Kansal, A. (2014). Urban challenges in India and the mission for a sustainable habitat. *Interdisciplina, 2*(2).

Gidde, M. R., Todkar, V. V., & Kokate, K. K. (2008). Municipal Solid Waste Management in Emerging Mega Cities: A case study of Pune City. In *Indo Italian Conference on Green and Clean Environment*. MAEER's MIT College of Engineering.

Gigault, J., Pedrono, B., Maxit, B., & Ter Halle, A. (2016). Marine plastic litter: The unanalyzed nano-fraction. *Environmental Science. Nano*, *3*(2), 346–350. doi:10.1039/C6EN00008H

Gilan, I., Hadar, Y., & Sivan, A. (2004). Colonization, biofilm formation and biodegradation of polyethylene by a strain of *Rhodococcus ruber. Applied Microbiology and Biotechnology*, *65*, 97–104. PMID:15221232

Gilder, G. (1989). *Microcosm*. New York: Simon and Schuster.

Gill, M. (2014). Bioplastic: A better alternative to plastics. *International Journal of Research in Applied Natural Sciences*, *2*(8), 115–120.

Gilman, E. (2016). Abandoned, lost and discarded gillnets and trammel nets. Methods to estimate ghost fishing mortality, and the status of regional monitoring and management. In E. Gilman, F. Chopin, P. Suuronen, & B. Kuemlangan (Eds.), *FAO Fisheries Technical Paper* (Vol. 600). Retrieved from www.fao.org/3/a-i5051e.pdf

Gilroy, P. (1993). *The Black Atlantic: Modernity and Double Consciousness*. Cambridge, MA: Harvard UniversityPress.

Giordano, P. M., Behel, A. D., Lawrence, J. E., Soileau, J. M., & Bradford, B. N. (1983). Mobility in soil and plant availability of metals derived from incinerated municipal refuse. *Environmental Science & Technology*, *17*(4), 193–198. doi:10.1021/es00110a003 PMID:22304633

Gnanavel, G., Valli, V. M. J., & Thirumarimurugan, M. (2012). A review of biodegradation of plastics waste. *International Journal of Pharmaceutical and Chemical Sciences, 1*, 670–673.

Gnanavel, G., Valli, V. M. J., Thirumarimurugan, M., & Kannadasan, T. (2014). Degradation of polyethylene in the natural environment. *International Journal of Research in Engineering & Technology, 2*, 1–6.

Gokhale, S. (2017). How safe is your hospital - doctor? *Medical Journal, Armed Forces India, 52*(2), 120–123. doi:10.1016/S0377-1237(17)30858-4 PMID:28769360

Goldberg. (1994). The pollution of the marine environment by plastic debris: a review, *Marine Pollution Bulletin, 44,* 842-852.

Goldberg, E. D. (1997). Plasticizing the seafloor: An overview. *Environmental Technology (United Kingdom), 18*(2), 195–201. doi:10.1080/09593331808616527

Goldstein, M. C., Rosenberg, M., & Cheng, L. (2012). Increased oceanic microplastic debris enhances oviposition in an endemic pelagic insect. *Biology Letters, 8*(5), 817–820. doi:10.1098/rsbl.2012.0298 PMID:22573831

Golub, M. S., Wu, K. L., Kaufman, F. L., Li, L. H., Moran-Messen, F., Zeise, L., ... Donald, J. M. (2010). Bisphenol A: Developmental toxicity from early prenatal exposure. *Birth Defects Research. Part B, Developmental and Reproductive Toxicology, 89*(6), 441–466. doi:10.1002/bdrb.20275 PMID:21136531

Goodson, A., Robin, H., Summerfield, W., & Cooper, I. (2004). Migration of Bisphenol A from can coatings – effects of damage, storage conditions and heating. *Food Additives and Contaminants, 21*(10), 1015–1026. doi:10.1080/02652030400011387 PMID:15712526

Goodson, A., Summerfield, W., & Cooper, I. (2002). Survey of Bisphenol A and Bisphenol F in canned foods. *Food Additives and Contaminants, 19*(8), 796–802. doi:10.1080/02652030210146837 PMID:12227943

Gore, A. C., Chappell, V. A., Fenton, S. E., Flaws, J. A., Nadal, A., Prins, G. S., Toppari, J., & Zoeller, R. T. (2015). Executive summary to EDC-2: The Endocrine Society's Second Scientific Statement on endocrine-disrupting chemicals. Endocr. Rev. 36, 593. E1–E150.

Gottdiener, M. (1995). *Postmodern Semiotics*. Oxford, UK: Blackwell.

Gould, J. C., Leonard, L. S., Maness, S. C., Wagner, B. L., Conner, K., Zacharewski, T., ... Gaido, K. W. (1998). Bisphenol A interacts with the estrogen receptor _ in a distinct manner from estradiol. *Molecular and Cellular Endocrinology, 142*(1-2), 203–214. doi:10.1016/S0303-7207(98)00084-7 PMID:9783916

Gourmelon, G. (2015, January 27). *Global Plastic Production Rises, Recycling Lags.* Retrieved from World Watch Institute: http://worldwatch.net/sites/default/files/vital_signs_trend_plastic_full_pdf.pdf

Government of the Punjab. (2004, May 18). *The Punjab Polythene Bag Rules 2004.* Retrieved from Environment Protection Department Punjab: https://epd.punjab.gov.pk/system/files/The_Punjab_Polythene_Bag_Rules_2004.pdf

Graham, P. R. (1973). Phthalate ester plasticizers–why and how they are used. Environmental Health Perspectives, 3, 3–12. PubMed PMID:4712540

Graham, E. R., & Thompson, J. T. (2009). Deposit- and suspension-feeding sea cucumbers (Echinodermata) ingest plastic fragments. *Journal of Experimental Marine Biology and Ecology, 368*(1), 22–29. doi:10.1016/j.jembe.2008.09.007

Graham, M., Mac, W., Intyre, S., & Alldredge, A. L. (1999). Diel variations of marine snow concentration in surface waters and implications for particle flux in the sea. *Deep-sea Research. Part I, Oceanographic Research Papers, 47*(3), 367–395. doi:10.1016/S0967-0637(99)00063-1

Grause, G., Predel, M., & Kaminsky, W. (2006). Monomer recovery from aluminum hydroxide high filled poly (methyl methacrylate) in a fluidized bed reactor. *Journal of Analytical and Applied Pyrolysis*, *75*(2), 236–239. doi:10.1016/j.jaap.2005.06.006

Grause, G., Sugawara, K., Mizoguchi, T., & Yoshioka, T. (2009). Pyrolytic hydrolysis of polycarbonate in the presence of earth-alkali oxides and hydroxides. *Polymer Degradation & Stability*, *94*(7), 1119–1124. doi:10.1016/j.polymdegradstab.2009.03.014

Gray, L. E., Ostby, J., Furr, J., Price, M., Veeramachaneni, D. N., & Parks, L. (2000). Perinatal exposure to the phthalates DEHP, BBP, and DINP, but not DEP, DMP, or DOTP, alters sexual differentiation of the male rat. Toxicological Sciences, 58(2), 350–365. doi:10.1093/toxsci/58.2.350 PubMed doi:10.1093/toxsci/58.2.350 PMID:11099647

Gray, T. J. B., & Beamand, J. A. (1984). Effect of some phthalate esters and other testicular toxins on primary cultures of testicular cells. *Food and Chemical Toxicology*, *22*(2), 123–131. doi:10.1016/0278-6915(84)90092-9 PMID:6538161

Greenberg, R. R., Zoller, W. H., & Gordon, G. E. (1978). Composition and size distributions of particles released in refuse incineration. *Environmental Science & Technology*, *12*(5), 566–573. doi:10.1021/es60141a011

Green, R., Hauser, R., Calafat, A. M., Weuve, J., Schettler, T., Ringer, S., ... Hu, H. (2005). Use of di(2-ethylhexyl) phthalate-containing medical products and urinary levels of mono(2-ethylhexyl) phthalate in neonatal intensive care unit infants. *Environmental Health Perspectives*, *113*(9), 1222–1225. doi:10.1289/ehp.7932 PMID:16140631

Greentravelife. (2016). *Midway Island: An Environmental Tragedy*. Retrieved from Greentravelife.com.

Gregory, M. R. (2009). Environmental implications of plastic debris in marinesettings-entanglement ingestion smothering hangers-on hitch-hiking and alieninvasions. *Philosophical Transactions of the Royal Society of London. Series B, Biological Sciences*, *364*(1526), 2013–2025. doi:10.1098/rstb.2008.0265 PMID:19528053

Grewal, I., & Kaplan, C. (Eds.). (1994). *Scattered Hegemonies: Postmodernity and Transnational FeministPractices*. Minneapolis, MN: University of Minnesota Press.

Groh, K. J., Backhaus, T., Carney-Almorth, B., Geueke, B., Inostroza, P. A., Lennquist, A., ... Muncke, J. (2019). Overview of known plastic packaging-associated chemicals and their hazards. *The Science of the Total Environment*, *651*(Part 2), 3253–3268. doi:10.1016/j.scitotenv.2018.10.015 PMID:30463173

Gross, C., & Colony, J. (1972). An Etiological Study of Phthalate Self-Contamination of Spacecraft and Contamination from Their Earthly Environs. Retrieved from

Grossman, S. R., Dahlem, D., & Huffington Post. (2017). *Heartbreaking photos show what your trash does to animals*. Retrieved from www.huffingtonpost.in

Grover, Gupta, Shivani, Kumari, & Khorana. (2015). Polythene and environment. *International Journal ofEnvironmental Sciences, 5*(6), 1091-1104.

Grover, A., Gupta, A., Chandra, S., & Kumari, A., & Khurana, P. S. M. (2015). Polythene and environment. *International Journal of Environmental Sciences*, *5*, 6.

Grover, A., Gupta, A., Chandra, S., Kumari, A., & Khurana, S. P. (2015). Polythene and environment. International. *Journal of Environmental Sciences (China)*, *5*(6), 1091–1105.

Grumetto, L., Montesano, D., Seccia, S., Albrizio, S., & Barbato, F. (2008). Determination of Bisphenol A and bisphenol B residues in canned peeled tomatoes by reversed-phase liquid chromatography. *Journal of Agricultural and Food Chemistry*, *56*(22), 10633–10637. doi:10.1021/jf802297z PMID:18959420

Grun, F., & Blumberg, B. (2006). Environmental obesogens: Organotins and endocrine disruption via nuclear receptor signaling. *Endocrinology*, *147*(6), S50–S55. doi:10.1210/en.2005-1129 PMID:16690801

Grun, F., & Blumberg, B. (2009). Minireview: The case for obesogens. *Molecular Endocrinology (Baltimore, Md.)*, *23*(8), 1127–1134. doi:10.1210/me.2008-0485 PMID:19372238

Grun, F., & Blurnberg, B. (2009). Endocrine disrupters as obesogens. *Molecular and Cellular Endocrinology*, *304*(1-2), 19–29. doi:10.1016/j.mce.2009.02.018 PMID:19433244

Grun, F., Watanabe, H., Zamanian, Z., Maeda, L., Arima, K., Cubacha, R., ... Blumberg, B. (2006). Endocrine-disrupting organotin compounds are potent inducers of adipogenesis in vertebrates. *Molecular Endocrinology (Baltimore, Md.)*, *20*(9), 2141–2155. doi:10.1210/me.2005-0367 PMID:16613991

Grynkiewicz-Bylina, B. (2011). Dangerous phthalates in children's environment. *Ecological Chemistry and Engineering. S*, *18*(4), 455–463.

Gu, J. D., Ford, T. E., Mitton, D. B., & Mitchell, R. (2000). Microbial degradation and deterioration of polymeric materials. In The Uhlig Corrosion Handbook (2nd ed.). Wiley.

Guisnet, M., Costa, L., & Ribeiro, F. R. (2009). Prevention of zeolite deactivation by cooking. *Journal of Molecular Catalysis A Chemical*, *305*(1-2), 69–83. doi:10.1016/j.molcata.2008.11.012

Gu, J. D. (2003). Microbiological deterioration and degradation of synthetic polymeric materials: Recent research advances. *International Biodeterioration & Biodegradation*, *52*(2), 69–91. doi:10.1016/S0964-8305(02)00177-4

Gundarov, V. P., & Kavalerov, G. I. (2001). Development of standardization and certification of the quality of medical devices. *Meditsinskaia Tekhnika*, (3): 4–8. PMID:11515269

Guo, H., Han, B., Qin, L., Li, B., You, H., Yang, J., . . . Yang, X. (2012). Pulmonary toxicity and adjuvant effect of di-(2-exylhexyl) phthalate in ovalbumin-immunized BALB/c mice. PLoS One, 7(6), e39008. doi:10.1371/journal.pone.0039008 PubMed doi:10.1371/journal.pone.0039008 PMID:22701742

Guo, Y., Zhang, Z., Liu, L., Li, Y., Ren, N., & Kannan, K. (2012). Occurrence and profiles of phthalates in foodstuffs from China and their implications for human exposure. *Journal of Agricultural and Food Chemistry*, *60*(27), 6913–6919. doi:10.1021/jf3021128 PMID:22703192

Guyton, K. Z., Chiu, W. A., Bateson, T. F., Jinot, J., Siegel Scott, C., Brown, R. C., & Caldwell, J. C. (2009). A reexamination of the PPAR-alpha activation mode of action as a basis for assessing human cancer risks of environmental contaminants. *Environmental Health Perspectives*, *117*(11), 1664–1672. doi:10.1289/ehp.0900758 PMID:20049115

Gyawali, S., Rathore, D. S., Shankar, P. R., & Kumar, K. V. (2013). Strategies and challenges for safe injection practice in developing countries. *Journal of Pharmacology & Pharmacotherapeutics*, *4*(1), 8–12. doi:10.4103/0976-500X.107634 PMID:23662018

Hadad, D., Geresh, S., & Sivan, A. (2005). Biodegradation of polyethylene by the thermophilic bacterium *Brevibacillus borstelensis*. *Journal of Applied Microbiology*, *98*(5), 1093–1100. doi:10.1111/j.1365-2672.2005.02553.x PMID:15836478

Hafeez, S., Mahmood, A., Syed, J. H., Li, J., Ali, U., Malik, R. N., & Zhang, G. (2016). Waste dumping sites as a potential source of POPs and associated health risks in perspective of current waste management practices in Lahore city, Pakistan. *The Science of the Total Environment*, *562*, 953–961. doi:10.1016/j.scitotenv.2016.01.120 PMID:27153484

Hahladakis, J. N., & Aljabri, H. M. (2019). Delineating the plastic waste status in the State of Qatar: Potential opportunities, recovery and recycling routes. *The Science of the Total Environment*, *653*, 294–299. doi:10.1016/j.scitotenv.2018.10.390 PMID:30412874

Hahladakis, J. N., Purnell, P., Iacovidou, E., Velis, C. A., & Atseyinku, M. (2018). Post-consumer plastic packaging waste in England: Assessing the yield of multiple collection-recycling schemes. *Waste Management (New York, N.Y.)*, *75*, 149–159. doi:10.1016/j.wasman.2018.02.009 PMID:29439928

Hahladakis, J. N., Velis, C. A., Weber, R., Iacovidou, E., & Purnell, P. (2018). An overview of chemical additives present in plastics: Migration, release, fate and environmental impact during their use, disposal and recycling. *Journal of Hazardous Materials*, *344*, 179–199. doi:10.1016/j.jhazmat.2017.10.014 PMID:29035713

Hájeková, E., & Bajus, M. (2005). Recycling of low-density polyethylene and polypropylene via copyrolysis of polyalkene oil/waxes with naphtha: Product distribution and coke formation. *Journal of Analytical and Applied Pyrolysis*, *74*(1-2), 270–281. doi:10.1016/j.jaap.2004.11.016

Halden, R. U. (2010). Plastics and health risks. *Annual Review of Public Health*, *31*(1), 179–194. doi:10.1146/annurev.publhealth.012809.103714 PMID:20070188

Ha, M., Kwon, H. J., Leem, J. H., Kim, H. C., Lee, K. J., Park, I., ... Lee, B.-E. (2014). Korean Environmental Health Survey in Children and Adolescents (KorEHS-C): Survey design and pilot study results on selected exposure biomarkers. *International Journal of Hygiene and Environmental Health*, *217*(2-3), 260–270. doi:10.1016/j.ijheh.2013.06.001 PMID:23831304

Hameed, K., Riaz, O., Nassar u Minallah, M., & Munawar, H. (2017). Types of Hospital Waste and Waste Generation Rate in Different Hospitals of Faisalabad City, Pakistan. *Journal of Basic & Applied Scienes, 13*, 386-391. Retrieved from http://lifescienceglobal.com/pms/index.php/jbas/article/view/4777/2709

Han, H. (2017). Environmental Injustice in the Production and Disposal of Plastics. *The Undergraduate Sociological Journal of Boston College,* (8), 47-53. Retrieved from https://pdfs.semanticscholar.org/751d/3f07b908ed69303c03797b0f2a4b45fba521.pdf#page=47

Han, Y., Wang, X., Chen, G., Xu, G., Liu, X., Zhu, W., . . . Miao, J. (2014). Di-(2-ethylhexyl) phthalate adjuvantly induces imbalanced humoral immunity in ovalbumin-sensitized BALB/c mice ascribing to T follicular helper cells hyperfunction. Toxicology, 324, 88–97. doi:10.1016/j.tox.2014.07.011 PubMed doi:10.1016/j.tox.2014.07.011 PMID:25093321

Hanaoka, T., Kawamura, N., Hara, K., & Tsugane, S. (2002). Urinary bisphenol A and plasma hormone concentrations in male workers exposed to bisphenol A diglycidyl ether and mixed organic solvents. *Occupational and Environmental Medicine*, *59*(9), 625–628. doi:10.1136/oem.59.9.625 PMID:12205237

Hanna, C. W., Bloom, M. S., Robinson, W. P., Kim, D., Parsons, P. J., vom Saal, F. S., ... Fujimoto, V. Y. (2012). DNA methylation changes in whole blood is associated with exposure to the environmental contaminants, mercury, lead, cadmium and bisphenol A, in women undergoing ovarian stimulation for IVF. *Human Reproduction (Oxford, England)*, *27*(5), 1401–1410. doi:10.1093/humrep/des038 PMID:22381621

Hannas, B. R., Lambright, C. S., Furr, J., Howdeshell, K. L., Wilson, V. S., & Gray, L. E. Jr. (2011). Dose-response assessment of fetal testosterone production and gene expression levels in rat testes following in utero exposure to diethylhexyl phthalate, diisobutyl phthalate, diisoheptyl phthalate, and diisononyl phthalate. *Toxicological Sciences*, *123*(1), 206–216. doi:10.1093/toxsci/kfr146 PMID:21633115

Hannon, M., Gimpel, J., Tran, M., Rasala, B., & Mayfield, S. (2010). Biofuels from algae: Challenges and potential. *Biofuels*, *1*(5), 763–784. doi:10.4155/bfs.10.44 PMID:21833344

Han, S. W., Lee, H., Han, S. Y., Lim, D. S., Jung, K. K., Kwack, S. J., ... Lee, B. M. (2009). An exposure assessment of di-(2-ethylhexyl) phthalate (DEHP) and di-n-butyl phthalate (DBP) in human semen. *Journal of Toxicology and Environmental Health. Part A.*, *72*(21-22), 1463–1469. doi:10.1080/15287390903212972 PMID:20077219

Hansen, J. (1999). Risk for testicular cancer after occupational exposure to plastics. *International Journal of Cancer*, *82*(6), 911–912. doi:10.1002/(SICI)1097-0215(19990909)82:6<911::AID-IJC23>3.0.CO;2-O PMID:10446462

Hao, C., Cheng, X., Xia, H., & Ma, X. (2012). The endocrine disruptor mono-(2-ethylhexyl) phthalate promotes adipocyte differentiation and induces obesity in mice. *Bioscience Reports*, *32*(6), 619–629. doi:10.1042/BSR20120042 PMID:22953781

Hardell, L., Ohlson, C. G., & Fredrikson, M. (1997). Occupational exposure to polyvinyl chloride as a risk factor for testicular cancer evaluated in a case-control study. *International Journal of Cancer*, *73*(6), 828–830. doi:10.1002/(SICI)1097-0215(19971210)73:6<828::AID-IJC10>3.0.CO;2-0 PMID:9399660

Hardt, M., & Negri, A. (2000). *Empire*. Cambridge, MA: Harvard University Press.

Hargreaves, J. C., Adl, M. S., & Warman, P. R. (2008). A review of the use of composted municipal solid waste in agriculture. *Agriculture, Ecosystems & Environment*, *123*(1-3), 1–14. doi:10.1016/j.agee.2007.07.004

Harris, C., Henttu, P., Parker, M. G., & Sumpter, J. P. (1997). The estrogenicexposures are not associated with testicular toxicity.4activity of phthalate esters in vitro. *Environmental Health Perspectives*, *105*, 802–811. doi:10.1289/ehp.97105802 PMID:9347895

Hartline, N. L., Bruce, N. J., Karba, S. N., Ruff, E. O., Sonar, S. U., & Holden, P. A. (2016). Microfiber masses recovered from conventional machine washing of new or aged garments. *Environmental Science & Technology*, *50*(21), 11532–11538. doi:10.1021/acs.est.6b03045 PMID:27689236

Hartmann, L., & Rolim, A. (2002). Post-consumer plastic recycling as a sustainable development tool: a case study. *GPEC 2002: plastics impact on the environment, Conf. Proc.*, 431–438.

Harvey, D. (1989). *The Condition of Postmodernity*. Cambridge, MA: Blackwell.University Press.

Hasselerharm, R. P. E., Falahudin, D., Peeters, E. T., & Koelmans, A. A. (2018). Microplastic effect thresholds for freshwater benthic macroinvertebrates. *Environmental Science & Technology*, *52*(4), 2278–2286. doi:10.1021/acs.est.7b05367 PMID:29337537

Hatch, E. E., Nelson, J. W., Qureshi, M. M., Weinberg, J., Moore, L. L., Singer, M., & Webster, T. F. (2008). Association of urinary phthalate metabolite concentrations with body mass index and waist circumference: A cross-sectional study of NHANES data, 1999–2002. *Environmental Health*, *7*(27), 1–15. PMID:18522739

Hatch, E. E., Nelson, J. W., Stahlhut, R. W., & Webster, T. F. (2010). Association of endocrine disruptorsand obesity: Perspectives from epidemiological studies. *International Journal of Andrology*, *33*(2), 324–332. doi:10.1111/j.1365-2605.2009.01035.x PMID:20113374

Hauser, R. (2008). *Urinary phthalate metabolites and semen quality:a review of a potential biomarker of susceptibility*. Academic Press.

Hauser, R., & Calafat, A. M. (2005). Phthalates and human health. Occupational and Environmental Medicine, 62(11), 806–818. doi:10.1136/oem.2004.017590 PubMed doi:10.1136/oem.2004.017590 PMID:16234408

Hauser, R., Duty, S., Godfrey-Bailey, L., & Calafat, A. M. (2004). Medications as a source of human exposure to phthalates. *Environmental Health Perspectives*, *112*(6), 751–753. doi:10.1289/ehp.6804 PMID:15121520

Hauser, R., Gaskins, A. J., Souter, I., Smith, K. W., Dodge, L. E., Ehrlich, S., ... Williams, P. L. (2015). Urinary phthalate metabolite concentrations and reproductive outcomes among women undergoing in vitro fertilization: Results from the EARTH study. *Environmental Health Perspectives*, *124*(6), 831–839. doi:10.1289/ehp.1509760 PMID:26545148

Hauser, R., Meeker, J. D., Duty, S., Silva, M. J., & Calafat, A. M. (2006). Altered semen quality in relation to urinary concentrations of phthalate monoester and oxidative metabolites. *Epidemiology (Cambridge, Mass.), 17*(6), 682–691. doi:10.1097/01.ede.0000235996.89953.d7 PMID:17003688

Hauser, R., Meeker, J. D., Park, S., Silva, M. J., & Calafat, A. M. (2004b). Temporal variability of urinary phthalate metabolite levels in men of reproductive age. *Environmental Health Perspectives, 112*(17), 1734–0. doi:10.1289/ehp.7212 PMID:15579421

Hauser, R., Meeker, J. D., Singh, N. P., Silva, M. J., Ryan, L., Duty, S., & Calafat, A. M. (2006). DNA damage in human sperm is related to urinary levels of phthalate monoester and oxidative metabolites. *Human Reproduction (Oxford, England), 22*(3), 688–695. doi:10.1093/humrep/del428 PMID:17090632

Hayashi, J.-I., Nakahara, T., Kusakabe, K., & Morooka, S. (1998). Pyrolysis of polypropylene in the presence of oxygen. *Fuel Processing Technology, 55*(3), 265–275. doi:10.1016/S0378-3820(98)00047-2

Hays, S. M., Aylward, L. L., Kirman, C. R., Krishnan, K., & Nong, A. (2011). Biomonitoring equivalents for di-isononyl phthalate (DINP). *Regulatory Toxicology and Pharmacology, 60*(2), 181–188. doi:10.1016/j.yrtph.2011.03.013 PMID:21466828

Haywood, G. W., Anderson, A. J., Ewing, D. F., & Dawes, E. A. (1990). Accumulation of a polyhydroxyalkanoates containing primarily 3- hydroxydecanoate from simple carbohydrate substrates by Pseudomonas sp. stain. *Applied and Environmental Microbiology, 56*, 3354–3359. PMID:16348341

He, M., Inoue, K.-I., Yoshida, S., Tanaka, M., Takano, H., Sun, G., & Ichinose, T. (2013). Effects of airway exposure to di-(2-ethylhexyl) phthalate on allergic rhinitis. Immunopharmacology and Immunotoxicology, 35(3), 390–395. doi:10.3109/08923973.2013.787432 PubMed doi:10.3109/08923973.2013.787432 PMID:23672524

He, Y., Miao, M., Herrinton, L. J., Wu, C., Yuan, W., Zhou, Z., & Li, D. K. (2009). Bisphenol A levels in blood and urine in a Chinese population and the personal factors affecting the levels. *Environmental Research, 109*(5), 629–633.

Heffeman, A. L., Aylward, L. L., Toms, L. M., Eaglesham, G., Hobson, P., Sly, P. D., & ... (2013). Age related trends in urinary excretion of Bisphenol A in Australian children and adults: Evidence from a pooled sample study using samples of convenience. *Journal of Toxicology and Environmental Health, 76*(18), 1039–1055. doi:10.1080/15287394.2013.834856 PMID:24188190

Heindel, J. J., & Vandenberg, L. N. (2015). Developmental origins of health and disease: A paradigm for understanding disease etiology and prevention. Current Opinion in Pediatrics, 27(2), 248–253. doi:10.1097/MOP.0000000000000191 PubMed doi:10.1097/MOP.0000000000000191 PMID:25635586

Heindel, J. J., Newbold, R. R., Bucher, J. R., Camacho, L., Delclos, K. B., Lewis, S. M., . . . Schug, T. T. (2015). NIEHS/FDA CLARITYBPA research program update. Reproductive Toxicology (Elmsford, N.Y.), 58, 33–44. doi:10.1016/j.reprotox.2015.07.075 PubMed doi:10.1016/j.reprotox.2015.07.075 PMID:26232693

Heindel, J. J. (2003). Endocrine disruptors and the obesity epidemic. *Toxicological Sciences, 76*(2), 247–249. doi:10.1093/toxsci/kfg255 PMID:14677558

Heindel, J. J., & vom Saal, F. S. (2009). Role of nutrition and environmental endocrine disrupting chemicals during the perinatal period on the etiology of obesity. *Molecular and Cellular Endocrinology, 304*(1-2), 90–96. doi:10.1016/j.mce.2009.02.025 PMID:19433253

Held, McGrew, Goldblatt, & Perraton. (1999). *Global Transformations*. Cambridge.

Henton, D. E., Gruber, P., Lunt, J., & Randall, J. (2005). Polylactic acid technology. In A. K. Mohanty, M. Misra, & L. T. Drzal (Eds.), *Natural Fibers, Biopolymers, and Biocomposites* (p. 527). Boca Raton, FL: CRC Press. doi:10.1201/9780203508206.ch16

Herr, C., zurNieden, A., Koch, H. M., Schuppe, H. C., Fieber, C., Angerer, J., ... Stilianakis, N. I. (2009). Urinary di (2-ethylhexyl) phthalate (DEHP)—Metabolites and male human markers of reproductive function. *International Journal of Hygiene and Environmental Health*, *212*(6), 648–653. doi:10.1016/j.ijheh.2009.08.001 PMID:19733116

Herzke, D., Anker-Nilssen, T., Nost, T. H., Gotsch, A., Christensen-Dalsgaard, S., Langset, M., ... Koelmans, A. A. (2016). Negligible impact of ingested microplastics on tissue concentrations of persistent organic pollutants in northern fulmars off coastal Norway. *Environmental Science & Technology*, *50*(4), 1924–1933. doi:10.1021/acs.est.5b04663 PMID:26694206

Hester, R. E., & Harrison, R. M. (2011). Marine Pollution and Human Health. Royal Society of Chemistry, 84-85.

Heudorf, U., Mersch-Sundermann, V., & Angerer, J. (2007). Phthalates: Toxicology and exposure. International Journal of Hygiene and Environmental Health, 210(5), 623–634. doi:10.1016/j.ijheh.2007.07.011 PubMed doi:10.1016/j.ijheh.2007.07.011 PMID:17889607

Heyde, M., & Kremer, S. (1999). LCA Packaging Plastics Waste. LCA Documents. *Material Recycling – Trends and Perspectives, 2*, 60.

Higuchi, T. T., Palmer, J. S., Gray, L. E. Jr, & Veeramachaneni, D. R. (2003). Effects of dibutyl phthalate in male rabbits following in utero, adolescent, or postpubertal exposure. *Toxicological Sciences*, *72*(2), 301–313. doi:10.1093/toxsci/kfg036 PMID:12655036

Hine, C. H., Kodama, J. K., Anderson, H. H., Simonson, D. W., & Wellington, J. S. (1958). The toxicology of epoxy resins. Arch. Indust. Heal., 17, 129–144. PubMed PMID:13497307

Hines, E. P., Calafat, A. M., Silva, M. J., Mendola, P., & Fenton, S. E. (2009). Concentrations ofphthalate metabolites in milk, urine, saliva, and serum of lactating North Carolina women. *Environmental Health Perspectives*, *117*(1), 86–92. doi:10.1289/ehp.11610 PMID:19165392

Hirai, H., Takada, H., Ogata, Y., Yamashita, R., Mizukawa, K., Saha, M., ... Ward, M. W. (2011). Organic micropollutants in marine plastics debris from the open ocean and remote and urban beaches. *Marine Pollution Bulletin*, *62*(8), 1683–1692. doi:10.1016/j.marpolbul.2011.06.004 PMID:21719036

Hiroi, H., Tsutsumi, O., Momoeda, M., Takai, Y., Osuga, Y., & Taketani, Y. (1999). Differential interactions of bisphenol A and 17 beta-estradiol with estrogen receptor alpha (ERalpha) and ERbeta. Endocrine Journal, 46(6), 773–778. doi:10.1507/endocrj.46.773 PubMed doi:10.1507/endocrj.46.773 PMID:10724352

Hirst & Thompson. (1996). *Globalization in Question*. Cambridge, UK: Polity Press.

Hisham, A. (2016). Polypropylene as a Promising Plastic: A Review. *American Journal of Political Science*, *6*(1), 1–11.

Hoang, K. C., Tseng, M., & Shu, W. J. (2007). Degradation of polyethylene succinate (PES) by a new thermophilic Microbispora strain. *Biodegradation*, *18*(3), 333–342. doi:10.100710532-006-9067-5 PMID:17109189

Hocking, P. J., & Marchessault, R. H. (1997). Article. In G. J. L. Griffin (Ed.), Chemistry and Technology of Biodegradable Polymers (pp. 48–96). Chapman & Hall.

Hocking. (1991). *Relative merits of polystyrene foam and paper in hot drink cups: Implications for packaging*. Academic Press.

Hoegh-Guldberg, O., Cai, R., Poloczanska, E. S., Brewer, P. G., Sundby, S., Hilmi, K., ... Jung, S. (2015). The ocean. *Climate Change 2014: Impacts, Adaptation and Vulnerability: Part B: Regional Aspects. Working Group II Contribution to the Fifth Assessment Report of the Intergovernmental Panel on Climate Change, 347*(6223), 1655–1734. doi:10.1017/CBO9781107415386.010

Hoekstra, E. J., & Simoneau, C. (2013). Release of Bisphenol A from polycarbonate-a review. *Critical Reviews in Food Science and Nutrition, 53*(4), 386–402. doi:10.1080/10408398.2010.536919 PMID:23320909

Hoffmann, J., Řezníčèková, I., Vaňòková, S., & Kupec, J. (1997). Manometric determination of biological degradability of substances poorly soluble in aqueous environments. *International Biodeterioration & Biodegradation, 39*(4), 327–332. doi:10.1016/S0964-8305(97)00033-4

Hofrichter, M., Lundell, T., & Hatakka, A. (2001). Conversion of milled pine wood by manganese peroxidase from *Phlebia radiata. Applied and Environmental Microbiology, 67*(10), 4588–4593. doi:10.1128/AEM.67.10.4588-4593.2001 PMID:11571160

Högberg, J., Hanberg, A., Berglund, M., Skerfving, S., Remberger, M., Calafat, A. M., ... Håkansson, H. (2008). Phthalate diesters and their metabolites in human breast milk, blood or serum, and urine as biomarkers of exposure in vulnerable populations. *Environmental Health Perspectives, 116*(3), 334–339. doi:10.1289/ehp.10788 PMID:18335100

Holm, A., Solbu, K., Molander, P., Lundanes, E., & Greibrokk, T. (2004). Sensitive biomonitoring of phthalate metabolites in human urine using packed capillary column switching liquid chromatography coupled to electrospray ionization ion-trap mass spectrometry. *Analytical and Bioanalytical Chemistry, 378*(7), 1762–1768. doi:10.100700216-003-2488-7 PMID:14758462

Holmes, L. A., Turner, A., & Thompson, R. C. (2014). Interactions between trace metals and plastic production pellets under estuarine conditions. *Marine Chemistry, 167*, 25–32. doi:10.1016/j.marchem.2014.06.001

Hong, Y. C., Park, E. Y., Park, M. S., Ko, J. A., Oh, S.-Y., Kim, H., ... Ha, E.-H. (2009). Community level exposure to chemicals and oxidative stress in adult population. *Toxicology Letters, 184*(2), 139–144. doi:10.1016/j.toxlet.2008.11.001 PMID:19049859

Hoornweg, D., & Bhada-Tata, P. (2012). What a Waste: a Global Review of Solid Waste Management. *Urban Development Series Knowledge Papers*, 151–198.

Hoornweg, D., & Bhada-Tata, P. (2012). *What a Waste: A Global Review of Solid Waste Management*. Washington, DC: The World Bank. Retrieved from https://openknowledge.worldbank.org/handle/10986/17388

Hopewell, J., Dvorak, R., & Kosior, E. (2009). Plastics recycling: Challenges and opportunities. *Philosophical Transactions of the Royal Society of London. Series B, Biological Sciences, 364*(1526), 2115–2126. doi:10.1098/rstb.2008.0311 PMID:19528059

Hoppin, J. A., Jaramillo, R., London, S. J., Bertelsen, R. J., Salo, P. M., Sandler, D. P., & Zeldin, D. C. (2013). Phthalate exposure and allergy in the US population: Results from NHANES 2005-2006. *Environmental Health Perspectives (Online), 121*(10), 1129–1134. doi:10.1289/ehp.1206211 PMID:23799650

Hoppin, J. A., Ulmer, R., & London, S. J. (2004). Phthalate exposure and pulmonary function. *Environmental Health Perspectives, 112*(5), 571–574. doi:10.1289/ehp.6564 PMID:15064163

Hormann, A. M., vom Saal, F. S., Nagel, S. C., Stahlhut, R. W., Moyer, C. L., Ellersieck, M. R., . . . Taylor, J. A. (2014). Holding thermal receipt paper and eating food after using hand sanitizer results in high serum bioactive and urine total levels of bisphenol A (BPA). PLoS One, 9(10), e110509. doi:10.1371/journal.pone.0110509 PubMed doi:10.1371/journal.pone.0110509 PMID:25337790

Houmiel, K. L., Slater, S., Broyles, D., Casagrande, L., Colburn, S., Gonzalez, K., ... Gruys, K. J. (1999). Poly(β-hydroxybutyrate) production in oilseed leukoplasts of *Brassica napus*. *Planta*, *4*(209), 547–550. doi:10.1007004250050760 PMID:10550638

Howard, G. T. (2012). Polyurethane biodegradation. *Microbiol Degrade Xenobiot,* 371–394.

Howard, G. T., & Blake, R. C. (1999). Growth of Pseudomonas fuorescens on a polyester-polyurethane and the purification and characterization of a polyurethanase-protease enzyme. *International Biodeterioration & Biodegradation*, *42*(4), 213–220. doi:10.1016/S0964-8305(98)00051-1

Hsieh, T. H., Tsai, C. F., Hsu, C. Y., Kuo, P. L., Lee, J. N., Chai, C. Y., ... Tsai, E. M. (2012). Phthalates induce proliferation and invasiveness of estrogen receptor-negative breast cancer through the AhR/HDAC6/c-Myc signaling pathway. *The FASEB Journal*, *26*(2), 778–787. doi:10.1096/fj.11-191742 PMID:22049059

Huang, H. B., Chen, H. Y., Su, P. H., Huang, P. C., Sun, C. W., Wang, C. J., ... Wang, S. L. (2015). Fetal and childhood exposure to phthalate diesters and cognitive function in children up to 12 years of age: Taiwanese maternal and infant cohort study. *PLoS One*, *10*(6), e0131910. doi:10.1371/journal.pone.0131910 PMID:26121592

Huang, J., Pray, C., & Rozelle, S. (2002). Enhancing the crops to feed the poor. *Nature*, *418*(6898), 678–685. doi:10.1038/nature01015 PMID:12167874

Huang, P. C., Kuo, P. L., Chou, Y. Y., Lin, S. J., & Lee, C. C. (2009). Association between prenatal exposure to phthalates and the health of newborns. *Environment International*, *35*(1), 14–20. doi:10.1016/j.envint.2008.05.012 PMID:18640725

Huang, P. C., Kuo, P. L., Guo, Y. L., Liao, P. C., & Lee, C. C. (2007). Associations between urinary phthalate monoesters and thyroid hormones in pregnant women. *Human Reproduction (Oxford, England)*, *22*(10), 2715–2722. doi:10.1093/humrep/dem205 PMID:17704099

Huang, R., & Reusch, R. N. (1996). Poly(3-hydroxybutyrate) is associated with specific proteins in the cytoplasm and membranes of *Escherichia coli*. *The Journal of Biological Chemistry*, *271*(36), 22196–22202. doi:10.1074/jbc.271.36.22196 PMID:8703033

Huang, Y. W., Wong, C. K. C., Zheng, J. S., Bouwman, H., Barra, R., Wahlstrom, B., ... Wong, M. H. (2012). Bisphenol A (BPA) in China: A review of sources, environmental levels, and potential human health impacts. *Environment International*, *42*, 91–99. doi:10.1016/j.envint.2011.04.010 PMID:21596439

Huang, Z., Ding, A., Guo, H., Lu, G., & Huang, X. (2016). Construction of Nontoxic Polymeric UV-Absorber with Great Resistance to UV-Photoaging. *Scientific Reports*, *6*(1), 25508. doi:10.1038rep25508 PMID:27138547

Huber, W. W., Grasl-Kraupp, B., & Schulte-Hermann, R. (1996). Hepatocarcinogenic potential of di (2-ethylhexyl) phthalate in rodents and its implications on human risk. *Critical Reviews in Toxicology*, *26*(4), 365–481. doi:10.3109/10408449609048302 PMID:8817083

Huc, L., Lemarie, A., Gueraud, F., & H'elie's-Toussaint, C. (2012). Low concentrations of Bisphenol A induce lipid accumulation mediated by the production of reactive oxygen, species in the mitochondria of HepG2 cells. *Toxicology In Vitro*, *26*(5), 709–717. doi:10.1016/j.tiv.2012.03.017 PMID:22515966

Hu, G. X., Lian, Q. Q., Ge, R. S., Hardy, D. O., & Li, X. K. (2009). Phthalate-induced testicular dysgenesis syndrome: Leydig cell influence. *Trends in Endocrinology and Metabolism*, *20*(3), 139–145. doi:10.1016/j.tem.2008.12.001 PMID:19278865

Hugo, E. R., Brandebourg, T. D., Woo, J. G., Loftus, J., Alexander, J. W., & Ben-Jonathan, N. (2008). Bisphenol A at environmentally relevant doses inhibits adiponectin release from human adipose tissue explants and adipocytes. *Environmental Health Perspectives*, *116*(12), 1642–1647. doi:10.1289/ehp.11537 PMID:19079714

Huisman, G. W., Leeuwde, O., Eggink, G., & Witholt, B. (1989). Synthesis of poly-3-hydroxyalkanoates is a common feature of fluorescent pseudomonads. *Applied and Environmental Microbiology*, *55*, 1949–1954. PMID:2506811

Hu, L., Su, L., Xue, Y., Mu, J., Zhu, J., Xu, J., & Shi, H. (2016). Uptake, accumulation and elimination of polystyrene microspheres in tadpoles of Xenopustropicalis. *Chemosphere*, *164*, 611–617. doi:10.1016/j.chemosphere.2016.09.002 PMID:27635643

Huntington, S. (1996). *The Clash of Civilizations and the Remaking of World Order*. New York: Simon and Schuster.

Hussain, N., Jaitley, V., & Florence, A. T. (2001). Recent advances in the understanding of uptake of microparticulates across the gastrointestinal lymphatics. *Advanced Drug Delivery Reviews*, *50*(1), 107–142. doi:10.1016/S0169-409X(01)00152-1 PMID:11489336

Hyland, R. G. (1993). Regulatory developments affecting medical waste disposal. In *86th Annual Meeting and Exhibition.* Air & Waste Manage. Assoc. (Paper No. 93-TA-47.03)

Hyland, R. G., Drum, D. A., & Bulley, M. (1994). Disposal medical wastes. In *87th Annual Meeting and Exhibition.* Air & Waste Manage. Assoc. (Paper No. 94-RP-123B.02)

IARC. (2000). *IARC monographs on the evaluation of carcinogenic risks to humans*. Lyon7 Some Industrial Chemicals.

IARC. (2013). Working Group on the Evaluation of Carcinogenic Risks to Humans. Some chemicals present in industrial and consumer products, food and drinking-water. *IARC Monographs on the Evaluation of Carcinogenic Risks to Humans*, *101*, 9–549. PMID:24772663

Iiyoshi, Y., Tsutsumi, Y., & Nishida, T. (1998). Polyethylene degradation by lignin-degrading fungi and manganese peroxidase. *Journal of Wood Science*, *44*(3), 222–229. doi:10.1007/BF00521967

Ikada, E. (1999). Electron microscope observation of biodegradation of polymers. *Journal of Environmental Polymer Degradation*, *7*(4), 197–201. doi:10.1023/A:1022882732403

Ikezuki, Y., Tsutsumi, O., Takai, Y., Kamei, Y., & Taketani, Y. (2002). Determination of bisphenol a concentrations in human biologicalfluids reveals significant early prenatal exposure. *Human Reproduction (Oxford, England)*, *17*(11), 2839–2841. doi:10.1093/humrep/17.11.2839 PMID:12407035

Ilgin, M. A., & Gupta, S. M. (2010). Environmentally Conscious Manufacturing and Product Recovery (ECMPRO): A Review of the State of the Art. *Journal of Environmental Management*, *91*(3), 563–591. doi:10.1016/j.jenvman.2009.09.037 PMID:19853369

Imanishi, S., Manabe, N., Nishizawa, H., Morita, M., Sugimoto, M., Iwahori, M., & Miyamoto, H. (2003). Effects of oral exposure of bisphenol A on mRNA expression of nuclear receptors in murine placentae assessed by DNA microarray. *The Journal of Reproduction and Development*, *49*(5), 329–336. doi:10.1262/jrd.49.329 PMID:14967926

Imhof, H. K., & Laforsch, C. (2016). Hazardous or not–Are adult and juvenile individuals of Potamopyrgusantipodarum affected by non-buoyant microplastic particles? *Environmental Pollution*, *218*, 383–391. doi:10.1016/j.envpol.2016.07.017 PMID:27431695

Imran, M., Haydar, S., Kim, J., Awam, M. R., & Bhatti, A. A. (2017). E-waste flows, resource recovery and improvement of legal framework in Pakistan. *Resources, Conservation and Recycling*, *125*, 131–138. doi:10.1016/j.resconrec.2017.06.015

Inoue, H., Yuki, G., Yokota, H., & Kato, S. (2003). Bisphenol A glucuronidation and absorption in rat intestine. *Drug Metabolism and Disposition: the Biological Fate of Chemicals*, *31*(1), 140–144. doi:10.1124/dmd.31.1.140 PMID:12485963

International Trade Administration. (2018, September 8). *Pakistan - Waste Management*. Retrieved from https://www.export.gov/article?id=Pakistan-Waste-Management

Iqbal, M., Breivik, K., Syed, J. H., Malik, R. N., Li, J., Zhang, G., & Jones, K. C. (2015). Emerging issue of e-waste in Pakistan: A review of status, research needs and data gaps. *Environmental Pollution*, *207*, 308–318. doi:10.1016/j.envpol.2015.09.002 PMID:26433180

Itoh, H., Yoshida, K., & Masunaga, S. (2007). Quantitative identification of unknown exposure pathways of phthalates based on measuring their metabolites in human urine. *Environmental Science & Technology*, *41*(13), 4542–4547. doi:10.1021/es062926y PMID:17695894

Ito, Y., Yamanoshita, O., Asaeda, N., Tagawa, Y., Lee, C. H., Aoyama, T., ... Nakajima, T. (2007). Di (2-ethylhexyl) phthalate induces hepatictumorigenesis through a peroxisome proliferator-activated receptor-α independentPathway. *Journal of Occupational Health*, *49*(3), 172–182. doi:10.1539/joh.49.172 PMID:17575397

IUCN. (2005). *Environmental Law in Pakistan: Governing Natural Resources and the Process and Instituitions that Affect Them.* Karachi: IUCN, Environmental Law Programme. Retrieved from https://portals.iucn.org/library/sites/library/files/documents/ELC-016-1.pdf

Ivar do Sul, J. A., & Costa, M. F. (2014). The present and future of microplastic pollution in the marine environment. *Environmental Pollution*, *185*, 352–364. doi:10.1016/j.envpol.2013.10.036 PMID:24275078

Jaakkola, J. J. K., & Knight, T. L. (2008). The role of exposure to phthalates from polyvinyl chloride products in the development of asthma and allergies: A systematic review and meta-analysis. *Environmental Health Perspectives*, *116*(7), 845–853. doi:10.1289/ehp.10846 PMID:18629304

Jaakkola, J. J., Oie, L., Nafstad, P., Botten, G., Samuelsen, S. O., & Magnus, P. (1999). Interior surface materials in the home and the development of bronchial obstruction in young children in Oslo, Norway. *American Journal of Public Health*, *89*(2), 188–192. doi:10.2105/AJPH.89.2.188 PMID:9949747

Jaakkola, J. J., Parise, H., Kislitsin, V., Lebedeva, N. I., & Spengler, J. D. (2004). Asthma, wheezing, and allergies in Russian schoolchildren in relation to new surface materials in the home. *American Journal of Public Health*, *94*(4), 560–562. doi:10.2105/AJPH.94.4.560 PMID:15054004

Jaakkola, J. J., Verkasalo, P. K., & Jaakkola, N. (2000). Plastic wall materials in the home and respiratory health in young children. *American Journal of Public Health*, *90*(5), 797–799. doi:10.2105/AJPH.90.5.797 PMID:10800434

Jabeen, K., Su, L., Li, J., Yang, D., Tong, C., Mu, J., & Shi, H. (2017). Microplastics and mesoplastics in fish from coastal and fresh waters of China. *Environmental Pollution*, *221*, 141–149. doi:10.1016/j.envpol.2016.11.055 PMID:27939629

Jacobsen, J. K., Massey, L., & Gulland, F. (2010). Fatal ingestion of floating net debris by two sperm whales (*Physeter macrocephalus*). *Marine Pollution Bulletin*, *60*(5), 765–767. doi:10.1016/j.marpolbul.2010.03.008 PMID:20381092

Jaeger, R. J., & Rubin, R. J. (1970). Plasticizers from plastic devices: Extraction, metabolism, and accumulation by biological systems. Science, 170(3956), 460–462. doi:10.1126/science.170.3956.460 PubMed doi:10.1126cience.170.3956.460 PMID:5460077

Jafari-Sales, Shahniani, & Bagherizadeh. (2017). Bioplastics and the Environment, Electronic. *Journal of Biology*, *13*(3), 274–279.

Jalil, A., Mian, N., & Rahman, K. M. (2013). Using plastic bags and its damaging impact on Environment and Agriculture: An alternative proposal. *International Journal of Learning & Development, 17*, 3-4.

Jambeck, J. R., Geyer, R., Wilcox, C., Siegler, T. R., Perryman, M., Andrady, A., . . . Law, K. L. (2015). Plastic waste inputs from land into the ocean. *Science Magazine*. Retrieved from http://wedocs.unep.org/bitstream/handle/20.500.11822/17969/Plastic_waste_inputs_from_land_into_the_ocean.pdf?sequence=1&isAllowed=y

Jambeck, J. R., Geyer, R., Wilcox, C., Siegler, T. R., Perryman, M., Andrady, A., ... Law, K. L. (2015). Plastic waste inputs from land into the ocean. *Science, 347*(6223), 768–771. doi:10.1126cience.1260352 PMID:25678662

Jameson, F. (1991). *Postmodernism, or the Cultural Logic of Late Capitalism*. Durham, NC: Duke UniversityPress.

Jang, S. W., Kim, D. H., Seong, K. T., Chung, Y. H., & Yoon, H. J. (2014). Analysis of floating debris behaviour in the Nakdong River basin of the southern Korean peninsula using satellite location tracking buoys. *Marine Pollution Bulletin, 88*(1–2), 275–283. doi:10.1016/j.marpolbul.2014.08.031 PMID:25261180

Jang, Y. C., Lee, C., Yoon, O. S., & Kim, H. (2006). Medical waste management in Korea. *Journal of Environmental Management, 80*(2), 107–115. doi:10.1016/j.jenvman.2005.08.018 PMID:16338054

Janjua, N. R., Mortensen, G. K., Andersson, A. M., Kongshoj, B., Skakkebæk, N. E., & Wulf, H. C. (2007). Systemic uptake of diethyl phthalate, dibutyl phthalate, and butyl paraben following whole-body topical application and reproductive and thyroid hormone levels in humans. *Environmental Science & Technology, 41*(15), 5564–5570. doi:10.1021/es0628755 PMID:17822133

Javed, N., Majeed, K., Farhan, K., & Nadeem, K. (2016). *Healthcare Waste Treatment and Disposal Lahore*. Lahore: The Urban Unit.

Jayant, A., Gupta, P., and Garg, S. K. (2012). Perspectives in Reverse Supply Chain Management (R-SCM): A State of the Art Literature Review. *JJMIE, 6*(1).

Jayaraman, V., Guide, V. D. R. Jr, & Srivastava, R. (1999). Closed-Loop Logistics Model for Remanufacturing. *The Journal of the Operational Research Society, 50*(5), 497–508. doi:10.1057/palgrave.jors.2600716

Jayaraman, V., Patterson, R. A., & Rolland, E. (2003). The Design of Reverse Distribution Networks: Models and Solution Procedures. *European Journal of Operational Research, 150*(1), 128–149. doi:10.1016/S0377-2217(02)00497-6

Jayasiri, H. B., Purushothaman, C. S., & Vennila, A. (2013). Quantitative analysis of plastic debris on recreational beaches. *Marine Pollution Bulletin, 77*(1), 107–112. doi:10.1016/j.marpolbul.2013.10.024 PMID:24210947

Jeffrie, T. W. (1994). Biodegradation of lignin and hemicelluloses. *Biochemistry of Microbial Degradation*, 233–277.

Jenkins, S., Raghuraman, N., Eltoum, I., Carpenter, M., Russo, J., & Lamartiniere, C. A. (2009). Oral exposure to Bisphenol A increases dimethyl benzanthraceneo-induced mammary cancer in rats. *Environmental Health Perspectives, 117*(6), 910–915. doi:10.1289/ehp.11751 PMID:19590682

Jha, M. K., Sondhi, O. A. K., & Pansare, M. (2003). Solid waste management – a case study. *Indian Journal of Environmental Protection, 23*, 1153–1160.

Jiang, Y., Cole, T., Pan, H., Lin, Z., Ju, M., & ... . (2007). Construction of height and weight percentile references for Shanghai children and adolescents. *Shanghai Journal of Preventive Medicine, 19*, 544–547.

Joardar, S. D. (2000). Urban residential solid waste management in India. *Public Works Management & Policy, 4*(4), 319–330. doi:10.1177/1087724X0044006

Joensen, U. N., Frederiksen, H., Jensen, M. B., Lauritsen, M. P., Olesen, I. A., Lassen, T. H., ... Jørgensen, N. (2012). Phthalate excretion pattern and testicular function: A study of 881 healthy Danish men. *Environmental Health Perspectives*, *120*(10), 1397–1403. doi:10.1289/ehp.1205113 PMID:22832070

John, S. T., & Sridharan, R. (2013). Modelling and analysis of network design for a closed–loop supply chain. *International Journal of Logistics Systems and Management*, *14*(3), 329–352. doi:10.1504/IJLSM.2013.052064

Johns, L. E., Ferguson, K. K., Soldin, O. P., Cantonwine, D. E., Rivera-González, L. O., Del Toro, L. V. A., ... Meeker, J. D. (2015). Urinary phthalate metabolites in relation to maternal serum thyroid and sex hormone levels during pregnancy: A longitudinal analysis. *Reproductive Biology and Endocrinology*, *13*(1), 1. doi:10.1186/1477-7827-13-4 PMID:25596636

Johnstone, B. (1990). A throw away answer. *Far Eastern Economic Review*, *147*(6), 62–63.

Jonsson, B. A. (2005). Urinary phthalate metabolites and biomarkers of reproductive function in young men. *Epidemiology (Cambridge, Mass.)*, *16*, 487–493. doi:10.1097/01.ede.0000164555.19041.01 PMID:15951666

Josh, M. S., Pradeep, S., Adarsh, V. K., Vijayalekshmi Amma, K. S., Sudha Devi, R., Balachandran, S., ... Benjamin, S. (2014a). *In silico* evidences for the binding of phthalates onto human estrogen receptor α, β subtypes and human estrogen-related receptor γ. *Molecular Simulation*, *40*(5), 408–417. doi:10.1080/08927022.2013.814131

Josh, M. S., Pradeep, S., Balachandran, S., Devi, R. S., Amma, K. V., & Benjamin, S. (2012). Temperatureand solvent-dependent migrations of di (2-ethylhexyl) phthalate, the hazardous plasticizer from commercial PVC blood storage bag. *Journal of Polymer Research*, *19*(7), 1–9. doi:10.100710965-012-9915-4

Josh, M. S., Pradeep, S., Balan, A. K., Sreejith, M. N., & Benjamin, S. (2016). Accessing the molecular interactions of phthalates and their primary metabolites with the human pregnane X receptor using in silico profiling. *Journal of Applied Toxicology*, *36*(12), 1599–1604. doi:10.1002/jat.3321 PMID:27071811

Josh, M. S., Pradeep, S., Vijayalekshmi Amma, K. S., Balachandran, S., Abdul-Jaleel, U. C., Mukesh, D., ... Sailas, B. (2014b). Phthalates efficiently bind to human peroxisome proliferator activated receptor and retinoid X receptor α, β, γ subtypes: An *in silico* approach. *Journal of Applied Toxicology*, *34*(7), 754–765. doi:10.1002/jat.2902 PMID:23843199

Josh, M. S., Pradeep, S., Vijayalekshmy Amma, K. S., Sudha Devi, R., Balachandran, S., Sreejith, M. N., & Benjamin, S. (2015). Human ketosteroid receptors interact with hazardous phthalate plasticizers and their metabolites: An *in silico* study. *Journal of Applied Toxicology*, *36*(6), 836–843. doi:10.1002/jat.3221 PMID:26304264

Jovanović, B. (2017). Ingestion of microplastics by fish and its potential consequences from a physical perspective. *Integrated Environmental Assessment and Management*, *13*(3), 510–515. doi:10.1002/ieam.1913 PMID:28440941

Jugan, M. L., Levi, Y., & Blondeau, J. P. (2010). Endocrine disruptors and thyroid hormone physiology. *Biochemical Pharmacology*, *79*(7), 939–947. doi:10.1016/j.bcp.2009.11.006 PMID:19913515

Jurica, K., Brčić Karačonji, I., Lasić, D., Vukić Lušić, D., Anić Jurica, S., & Lušić, D. (2016). Determination of phthalates in plum spirit and their occurrence during plum spirit production. *Acta Alimentaria*, *45*(1), 141–148. doi:10.1556/066.2016.45.1.17

Just, A. C., Miller, R. L., Perzanowski, M. S., Rundle, A. G., Chen, Q., Jung, K. H., . . . Whyatt, R. M. (2015). Vinyl flooring in the home is associated with children's airborne butylbenzyl phthalate and urinary metabolite concentrations. Journal of Exposure Science & Environmental Epidemiology, 25(6), 574–579. doi:10.1038/jes.2015.4 PubMed doi:10.1038/jes.2015.4 PMID:25690585

Kadowaki, T., Yamauchi, T., Kubota, N., Hara, K., Ueki, K., & Tobe, K. (2006). Adiponectin and adiponectin receptors in insulin resistance, diabetes, and the metabolic syndrome. *The Journal of Clinical Investigation*, *116*(7), 1784–1792. doi:10.1172/JCI29126 PMID:16823476

Kaiser, B., Eagan, P. D., & Shaner, H. (2001). Solutions to Health Care Waste: Life-Cycle Thinking and "Green" Purchasing. *Environmental Health Perspectives*, *109*(3), 205–207. doi:10.1289/ehp.01109205 PMID:11333178

Kaku, M. (1997). *Visions: How Science Will Revolutionize the 21st Century*. New York: Anchor Books.

Kale, S. K., Deshmukh, A. G., Dudhare, M. S., & Patil, V. B. (2015). Microbial degradation of plastic: A review. *Journal of Biochemical Technology*, *6*(2), 952–961.

Kameshwar, A. K. S., & Qin, W. (2016). Recent developments in using advanced sequencing technologies for the genomic studies of lignin and cellulose degrading microorganisms. *International Journal of Biological Sciences*, *12*(2), 156–171. doi:10.7150/ijbs.13537 PMID:26884714

Kamrin, M. A. (2009). Phthalate risks, phthalate regulation, and public health: A review. *J. Toxicol. Environ. Health B*, *12*(2), 157–174. doi:10.1080/10937400902729226 PMID:19235623

Kamrin, M. A. (2009). Phthalate risks, phthalate regulation, and public health: A review. *Journal of Toxicology and Environmental Health. Part B*, *12*(2), 157–174.

Kang, J. H., Kito, F., & Katayama, Y. (2006). Human exposure to Bisphenol A. *Toxicology*, *226*(2-3), 79–89. doi:10.1016/j.tox.2006.06.009 PMID:16860916

Kang, J. H., Kito, K., & Kondo, F. (2003). Factors influencing the migration of bisphenol A from cans. *Journal of Food Protection*, *66*(8), 1444–1447. doi:10.4315/0362-028X-66.8.1444 PMID:12929833

Kannan, D., Diabat, A., Alrefaei, M., Govindan, K., & Yong, G. (2012). A carbon footprint based reverse logistics network design model. *Resources, Conservation and Recycling*, *67*, 75–79. doi:10.1016/j.resconrec.2012.03.005

Kanno, Y., Okada, H., Kobayashi, T., Takenaka, T., & Suzuki, H. (2007). Effects of endocrine disrupting substance on estrogen receptor gene transcription in dialysis patients. *Therapeutic Apheresis and Dialysis*, *11*(4), 262–265. doi:10.1111/j.1744-9987.2007.00472.x PMID:17661831

Kansal, A. (2002). Solid waste management strategies for India. *Indian Journal of Environmental Protection*, *22*, 444–448.

Kaposi, K. L., Mos, B., Kelaher, B. P., & Dworjanyn, S. A. (2014). Ingestion of microplastic has limited impact on a marine larva. *Environmental Science & Technology*, *48*(3), 1638–1645. doi:10.1021/es404295e PMID:24341789

Karakayali, I., Hulya, E.-F., & Akcali, E. (2007). An Analysis of Decentralized Collection and Processing Of End-Of-Life Products. *Journal of Operations Management*, *25*(6), 1161–1183. doi:10.1016/j.jom.2007.01.017

Kashiwada, S. (2006). Distribution of nanoparticles in the see-through medaka (Oryzias latipes). *Environmental Health Perspectives*, *114*(11), 1697–1702. doi:10.1289/ehp.9209 PMID:17107855

Kathiresan, K. (2003). Polythene and plastic degrading microbes from mangrove soil. *Revista de Biología Tropical*, *51*, 629–633. PMID:15162769

Kathiresan, K. (2003). Polythene and plastics-degrading microbes from the mangrove soil. *Revista de Biología Tropical*, *51*(3), 629–634. PMID:15162769

Kato, K., Shoda, S., Takahashi, M., Doi, N., Yoshimura, Y., & Nakazawa, H. (2003). Determination of three phthalate metabolites in human urine using on-line solid-phase extraction–liquid chromatography–tandem mass spectrometry. *Journal of Chromatography. B, Analytical Technologies in the Biomedical and Life Sciences*, *788*(2), 407–411. doi:10.1016/S1570-0232(03)00041-2 PMID:12705982

Kato, K., Silva, M. J., Brock, J. W., Reidy, J. A., Malek, N. A., Hodge, C. C., ... Barr, D. B. (2003). Quantitative detection of nine phthalate metabolites in human serum using reversed-phase high-performance liquid chromatography-electrospray ionization-tandem mass spectrometry. *Journal of Analytical Toxicology*, *27*(5), 284–289. doi:10.1093/jat/27.5.284 PMID:12908941

Kato, K., Silva, M. J., Needham, L. L., & Calafat, A. M. (2005). Determination of 16 phthalate metabolites in urine using automated sample preparation and on-line preconcentration/high-performance liquid chromatography/tandem mass spectrometry. *Analytical Chemistry*, *77*(9), 2985–2991. doi:10.1021/ac0481248 PMID:15859620

Kato, K., Silva, M. J., Reidy, J. A., Hurtz, D. III, Malek, N. A., Needham, L. L., ... Calafat, A. M. (2004). Mono(2-Ethyl-5-Hydro- xyhexyl) phthalate and Mono(2-Ethyl-5-Oxohexyl) phtha- late as biomarkers for human exposure assessment to Di(2-Ethylhexyl) phthalate. *Environmental Health Perspectives*, *112*(3), 327–330. doi:10.1289/ehp.6663 PMID:14998748

Kato, K., Yamauchi, T., Higashiyama, K., & Nakazawa, H. (2003). High Throughput Analysis of Di-(2-Ethylhexyl) phthalate Metabolites in Urine for Exposure Assessment. *Journal of Liquid Chromatography & Related Technologies*, *26*(13), 2167–2176. doi:10.1081/JLC-120022401

Kavlock, R., Barr, D., Boekelheide, K., Breslin, W., Breysse, P., Chapin, R., ... Williams, P. (2006). NTP-CERHR Expert Panel update on the reproductive and developmental toxicity of di(2-ethylhexyl) phthalate. *Reproductive Toxicology (Elmsford, N.Y.)*, *22*(3), 291–399. doi:10.1016/j.reprotox.2006.04.007 PMID:17068859

Kawagoshi, Y., Fujita, Y., Kishi, I., & Fukunaga, I. (2003). Estrogenic chemicals and estrogenic activity in leachate from municipal waste landfill determined by yeast two-hybrid assay. *Journal of Environmental Monitoring*, *5*(2), 269–274. doi:10.1039/b210962j PMID:12729267

Kawai, F. (1995). Breakdown of plastics and polymers by microorganisms. *Advances in Biochemical Engineering/Biotechnology*, *52*, 151–194. doi:10.1007/BFb0102319 PMID:7484358

Kay, M. J., Morton, L. H. G., & Prince, E. L. (1991). Bacterial degradation of polyester polyurethane. *International Biodeterioration Bulletin*, *27*(2), 205–222. doi:10.1016/0265-3036(91)90012-G

Kelly, K. (1994). *Out of Control: The New Biology of Machines, Social Systems, and the Economic World.* New York: Addison Wesley.

Keresztes, S., Tatár, E., Czégény, Z., Záray, G., & Mihucz, V. G. (2013). Study on the leaching of phthalates from polyethylene terephthalate bottles into mineral water. *The Science of the Total Environment*, *458-460*, 451–458. doi:10.1016/j.scitotenv.2013.04.056 PMID:23688967

Keri, R. A., Ho, S.-M., Hunt, P., Knudsen, K., Soto, A. M., & Prins, G. S. (2007). An evaluation of evidence for the carcinogenic acivity of Bisphenol A. *Reproductive Toxicology (Elmsford, N.Y.)*, *24*(2), 240–252. doi:10.1016/j.reprotox.2007.06.008 PMID:17706921

Kerr, R. S. (1994). *Handbook of Bioremediation*. Boca Raton, FL: CRC Press, Inc. Lewis Publishers.

Kershaw, D. P. J. (2015). *Biodegradable Plastics & Marine Litter. Misconceptions, concerns and impacts on marine environments.* United Nations Environment Programme (UNEP). Retrieved from http://wedocs.unep.org/handle/20.500.11822/7468

Khajuria, A., & Kumar, A. (2007). Assessment of healthcare waste generated by government hospitals in Agra. *Our Nature*, *5*(1), 25–30. doi:10.3126/on.v5i1.794

Khalil, N., Ebert, J. R., Wang, L., Belcher, S., Lee, M., Czerwinski, S. A., & Kannan, K. (2014). Bisphenol A and cardiometabolic risk factors in obese children. *Science of the Total Environment,* 470-471, 726-732.

Khan, A. (2018). *Pakistan uses 55 billion shopping bags every year.* Retrieved from The Nation: https://nation.com.pk/17-Dec-2018/pakistan-uses-55-billion-shopping-bags-every-year

Khan, S. F., Malik, N. E., & Taseer, M. (2007). Impacts Of Municipal Solid Waste Open Dumps On Environment. In *International Conference, ESDev* (*Vol. 1*). Academic Press.

Khan, Z. A. (2018, March 19). *Hazardous plastic scraps imports continue unabated in Pakistan.* Retrieved from https://www.dawn.com/news/1396102

Khan, A., Nawaz, K., Usama, M., & Ashraf, Z. (2015). Feasibility Study of Municipal Plastic Waste for Power Generation in Lahore City, Pakistan. *Journal of Chemical Engineering & Process Technology*, *229*(6). doi:10.4172/2157-7048.1000229

Khan, F. R., Syberg, K., Shashoua, Y., & Bury, N. R. (2015). Influence of polyethylene microplastic beads on the uptake and localization of silver in zebrafish (*Danio rerio*). *Environmental Pollution*, *206*, 73–79. doi:10.1016/j.envpol.2015.06.009 PMID:26142753

Khan, M., Chaudhry, M. N., Ahmad, S. R., Saif, S., & Mehmood, A. (2018). Challenges to EIA consultants whilst dealing with stakeholders in Punjab, Pakistan. *Environmental Impact Assessment Review*, *73*, 201–209. doi:10.1016/j.eiar.2018.09.001

Khan, R. R. (1994). Environmental management of municipal solid wastes. *Indian Journal of Environmental Protection*, *14*, 26–30.

Khedr, A. (2013). Optimized extraction method for LC-MS determination of bisphenol A, melamine and di(2-ethylhexyl) phthalate in selected soft drinks, syringes, and milk powder. *Journal of Chromatography. B, Analytical Technologies in the Biomedical and Life Sciences*, *930*, 98–103. doi:10.1016/j.jchromb.2013.04.040 PMID:23727873

Kim, K., Park, H., Yang, W., & Lee, J. H. (2011). Urinary concentrations of bisphenol A and triclosan and associations with demographic factors in the Korean population. Environmental Research, 111(8), 1280–1285. doi:10.1016/j.envres.2011.09.003 PubMed doi:10.1016/j.envres.2011.09.003 PMID:21925656

Kimber, I., & Dearman, R. J. (2010). An assessment of the ability of phthalates to influence immune and allergic responses. *Toxicology*, *271*(3), 73–82. doi:10.1016/j.tox.2010.03.020 PMID:20371260

Kim, D., Kim, B.-K., Cho, Y., Han, M., & Kim, B. S. (2009). Kinetics of polycarbonate glycolysis in ethylene glycol. *Industrial & Engineering Chemistry Research*, *48*(2), 685–691. doi:10.1021/ie8010947

Kim, J. S., Lee, W. Y., Lee, S. B., Kim, S. B., & Choi, M. J. (2003). Degradation of polystyrene waste over base promoted Fe catalysts. *Catalysis Today*, *87*(1-4), 59–68. doi:10.1016/j.cattod.2003.10.004

Kim, K., & Park, H. (2013). Association between urinary concentrations of Bisphenol A and type 2 diabetes in Korean adults: A population based cross-sectional study. *International Journal of Hygiene and Environmental Health*, *216*(4), 467–471. doi:10.1016/j.ijheh.2012.07.007 PMID:22921714

Kim, S. H., & Park, M. J. (2014). Phthalate exposure and childhood obesity. *Annals of Pediatric Endocrinology & Metabolism*, *19*(2), 69–75. doi:10.6065/apem.2014.19.2.69 PMID:25077088

Kim, Y. H., Kim, C. S., Park, S., Han, S. Y., Pyo, M. Y., & Yang, M. (2003). Gender differences in the levels of Bisphenol A metabolites in urine. *Biochemical and Biophysical Research Communications*, *312*(2), 441–448. doi:10.1016/j.bbrc.2003.10.135 PMID:14637157

King, A. D. (Ed.). (1991). *Culture, Globalization, and the World-System: Contemporary Conditions for theRepresentation of Identity*. Binghamton, NY: SUNY Art Department. doi:10.1007/978-1-349-11902-8

Kirbas, Z., Keskin, N., & Guner, A. (1999). Biodegradation of polyvinylchloride (PVC) by white rot fungi. *Bulletin of Environmental Contamination and Toxicology*, *63*(3), 335–342. doi:10.1007001289900985 PMID:10475911

Klangsin, P., & Harding, A. (1998). Medical waste treatment and disposal methods used by hospitals in Oregon, Washington and Idaho. *Journal of the Air & Waste Management Association*, *48*(6), 516–526. doi:10.1080/10473289.1998.10463706 PMID:9949738

Klaunig, J. E., Babich, M. A., Baetcke, K. P., Cook, J. C., Corton, J. C., David, R. M., ... Roberts, R. A. (2003). PPARα agonist-induced rodent tumors: Modes of action and human relevance. *Critical Reviews in Toxicology*, *33*(6), 655–780. doi:10.1080/713608372 PMID:14727734

Knudsen, N., Laurberg, P., Rasmussen, L. B., Bulow, I., Perrild, H., Ovesen, L., & Jorgensen, T. (2005). Small differences in thyroid function may be important for body mass index and the occurrence of obesity in the population. *The Journal of Clinical Endocrinology and Metabolism*, *90*(7), 4019–4024. doi:10.1210/jc.2004-2225 PMID:15870128

Koch, H. M., Bolt, H. M., & Angerer, J. (2004). Di(2-ethylhexyl)phthalate (DEHP) metabolites in human urine and serum after a single oral dose of deuterium-labelled DEHP. Archives of Toxicology, 78(3), 123–130. doi:10.1007/s00204-003-0522-3 PubMed doi:10.100700204-003-0522-3 PMID:14576974

Koch, H. M., Bolt, H. M., Preuss, R., & Angerer, J. (2005). New metabolites of di(2-ethylhexyl)phthalate (DEHP) in human urine and serum after single oral doses of deuteriumlabelled DEHP. Archives of Toxicology, 79(7), 367–376. doi:10.1007/s00204-004-0642-4 PubMed doi:10.100700204-004-0642-4 PMID:15700144

Koch, H. M., Lorber, M., Christensen, K. L. Y., Pälmke, C., Koslitz, S., & Brüning, T. (2013). Identifying sources of phthalate exposure with human biomonitoring: Results of a 48h fasting study with urine collection and personal activity patterns. International Journal of Hygiene and Environmental Health, 216(6), 672–681. doi:10.1016/j.ijheh.2012.12.002 PubMed doi:10.1016/j.ijheh.2012.12.002 PMID:23333758

Koch, H. M., & Calafat, A. M. (2009). Human body burdens of chemicals used in plastic manufacture. *Philosophical Transactions of the Royal Society of London. Series B, Biological Sciences*, *364*(1526), 2063–2078. doi:10.1098/rstb.2008.0208 PMID:19528056

Koch, H. M., Drexler, H., & Angerer, J. (2003). An estimation of the daily intake of di (2-ethylhexyl) phthalate (DEHP) and other phthalates in the general population. *International Journal of Hygiene and Environmental Health*, *206*(2), 77–83. doi:10.1078/1438-4639-00205 PMID:12708228

Koch, H. M., Drexler, H., & Angerer, J. (2004). Internal exposure of nursery-school children and their parents and teachers to di (2-ethylhexyl) phthalate (DEHP). *International Journal of Hygiene and Environmental Health*, *207*(1), 15–22. doi:10.1078/1438-4639-00270 PMID:14762970

Koch, H. M., Gonzalez-Reche, L. M., & Angerer, J. (2003). On-line clean-up by multidimensional liquid chromatography–electrospray ionization tandem mass spectrometry for high throughput quantification of primary and secondary phthalate metabolites in human urine. *Journal of Chromatography. B, Analytical Technologies in the Biomedical and Life Sciences*, *784*(1), 169–182. doi:10.1016/S1570-0232(02)00785-7 PMID:12504195

Koch, H. M., Rossbach, B., Drexler, H., & Angerer, J. (2003). Internal exposure of the general population to DEHP and other phthalates—Determination of secondary and primary phthalate monoester metabolites in urine. *Environmental Research*, *93*(2), 177–185. doi:10.1016/S0013-9351(03)00083-5 PMID:12963402

Kokare, C. R., Chakraborty, S., Khopade, A. N., & Mahadik, K. R. (2009). Biofilm: Importance and applications. *Indian Journal of Biotechnology*, *8*(2), 159–168.

Kolarik, B., Naydenov, K., Larsson, M., Bornehag, C.-G., & Sundell, J. (2008). The association between phthalates in dust and allergic diseases among Bulgarian children. Environmental Health Perspectives, 116(1), 98–103. doi:10.1289/ehp.10498 PubMed doi:10.1289/ehp.10498 PMID:18197306

Kolbert, A. C., Didier, J. G., & Xu, L. (1996). Mechanochemical Degradation of Ethylene–Propylene Copolymers: Characterization of Olefin Chain Ends. *Macromolecules*, *29*(27), 8591–8598. doi:10.1021/ma961099q

Kolybaba, M., Tabil, L. G., Panigrahi, S., Crerar, W. J., Powell, T., & Wang, B. (2003). Biodegradable polymers: past, present, and future. The Society for Engineering in Agricultural Food and Biological System, 1–15.

Konduri, M. K. R., Anupam, K. S., Vivek, J. S., Kumar, R. D. B., & Narasu, M. L. (2010). Synergistic effect of chemical and photo treatment on the rate of biodegradation of high density polyethylene by indigenous fungal isolates. *International Journal of Biotechnology and Biochemistry*, *6*, 157–174.

Konduri, M. K. R., Koteswarareddy, G., Kumar, D. B. R., Reddy, B. V., & Narasu, M. L. (2011). Effect of prooxidants on biodegradation of polyethylene (LDPE) by indigenous fungal isolate, *Aspergillus oryzae*. *Journal of Applied Polymer Science*, *120*(6), 3536–3545. doi:10.1002/app.33517

Konieczna, A., Rutkowska, A., & Rachon, D. (2015). Health risk of exposure to Bisphenol A (BPA). Roczniki Panstwowego Zakladu Higieny, 66(1), 5–11. PubMed PMID:25813067

Korai, M. S., Mahar, R. B., & Uqaili, M. A. (2017). The feasibility of municipal solid waste for energy generation and its existing management practices in Pakistan. *Renewable & Sustainable Energy Reviews*, *72*, 338–353. doi:10.1016/j.rser.2017.01.051

Kortenkamp, A., & Faust, M. (2010). Combined exposures to anti-androgenic chemicals: Steps towards cumulative risk assessment. *International Journal of Andrology*, *33*(2), 463–474. doi:10.1111/j.1365-2605.2009.01047.x PMID:20487045

Kosior, E., Mitchell, J., & Crescenzi, I. (2018). Plastics Recycling. *Plastics and the Environment*, *47*, 156–176. doi:10.1039/9781788013314-00156

Kosmidis, V., Achilias, D. S., & Karayannidis, G. P. (2001). Poly (ethylene terephthalate) recycling and recovery of pure terephthalic acid. Kinetics of a phase-transfer catalyzed alkaline hydrolysis. *Macromolecular Materials and Engineering*, *286*(10), 640–647. doi:10.1002/1439-2054(20011001)286:10<640::AID-MAME640>3.0.CO;2-1

Kostigen, T. M., & Magazine, F. D. (2008). The world's largest dump: the great pacific garbage patch. *Discover Magazine*. Retrieved from http://discovermagazine. com/2008/jul/10theworldslargestdump.

Kosti, R. I., & Panagiotakos, D. B. (2006). The epidemic of obesity in children and adolescents in the world. *Central European Journal of Public Health*, *14*(4), 151–159. doi:10.21101/cejph.a3398 PMID:17243492

Kostka, G., Urbanek-Olejnik, K., & Wiadrowska, B. (2010). Di-butyl phthalate—Induced hypomethylation of the c-myc gene in ratliver. *Toxicology and Industrial Health*, *26*(7), 407–416. doi:10.1177/0748233710369124 PMID:20504828

Koushal, V., Sharma, R., Sharma, M., Sharma, R., & Sharma, V. (2014). Plastics: Issues Challenges and Remediation. *Int J Waste Resources*, *4*, 134. doi:10.4172/2252-5211.1000134

Koushal, V., Sharma, R., Sharma, M., Sharma, R., & Sharma, V. (2014). Plastics: Issues Challenges and Remediation. *International Journal of Waste Resources*, *4*(1), 2–6.

Kransler, K. M., Bachman, A. N., & McKee, R. H. (2013). Estimates of daily di-isodecyl phthalate (DIDP) intake calculated from urinary biomonitoring data. *Regulatory Toxicology and Pharmacology*, *65*(1), 29–33. doi:10.1016/j.yrtph.2012.11.004 PMID:23174424

Krewski, D., ... (2010). Toxicity testing in the 21st century: A vision and a strategy. J. Toxicol. Environ. Heal. B. Critical Review, 13, 51–138. PubMed PMID:20574894

Krikke, H. (2011). Impact of closed-loop network configurations on carbon footprints: A case study in copiers. *Resources, Conservation and Recycling*, *55*(12), 1196–1205. doi:10.1016/j.resconrec.2011.07.001

Krishnan, A., Stathis, P., Permuth, S. F., Tokes, L., & Feldman, D. (1993). Bisphenol-A: An estrogenic substance is released from polycarbonate flasks during autoclaving. Endocrinology, 132(6), 2279–2286. doi:10.1210/endo.132.6.8504731 PubMed doi:10.1210/endo.132.6.8504731 PMID:8504731

Kruse, G. H., & Kimker, A. (1993). *Degradable escape mechanisms for pot gear: a summary report to the Alaska Board of Fisheries*. Alaska Department of Fish & Game, Division of Commercial Fisheries.

Kruse, T. M., Woo, O. S., & Broadbelt, L. J. (2001). Detailed mechanistic modeling of polymer degradation: Application to polystyrene. *Chemical Engineering Science*, *56*, 971–979. doi:10.1016/S0009-2509(00)00312-2

Kühn, S., Bravo Rebolledo, E. L., & Van Franeker, J. A. (2015). Deleterious effects of litter on marine life. In Marine Anthropogenic Litter (pp. 75–116). doi:10.1007/978-3-319-16510-3_4

Kuhn, T. S. (1970). The structure of scientific revolutions (2nd ed.). The University of Chicago Press.

Kuiper, G. G., Lemmen, J. G., Carlsson, B., Corton, J. C., Safe, S. H., Van Der Saag, P. T., ... Gustafsson, J. A. (1998). Interaction of estrogenic chemicals and phytoestrogens with estrogen receptor β. *Endocrinology*, *139*(10), 4252–4263. doi:10.1210/endo.139.10.6216 PMID:9751507

Kumar, A. A., Karthick, K., & Arumugam, K. P. (2011). Biodegradable polymers and its applications. *International Journal of Bioscience, Biochemistry, Bioinformatics*, *1*(3), 173–176. doi:10.7763/IJBBB.2011.V1.32

Kumar, A. A., Sivakumar, R., Reddy, Y. S. R., Bhagya Raja, M. V., Nishanth, T., & Revanth, V. (2016). Preliminary study on marine debris pollution along Marina beach, Chennai, India. *Regional Studies in Marine Science*, *5*, 35–40. doi:10.1016/j.rsma.2016.01.002

Kumar, S., Hatha, A. A. M., & Christi, K. S. (2007). Diversity and effectiveness of tropical mangrove soil microflora on the degradation of polythene carry bags. *Revista de Biología Tropical*, *55*(3-4), 777–786. doi:10.15517/rbt.v55i3-4.5954 PMID:19086383

Kunasundari, B., & Sudesh, K. (2011). Isolation and recovery of microbial polyhydroxyalkanoates. *Express Polymer Letters*, *5*(7), 620–634. doi:10.3144/expresspolymlett.2011.60

Kuo, C. H., Hsieh, C.-C., Kuo, H.-F., Huang, M.-Y., Yang, S.-N., Chen, L.-C., . . . Hung, C.-H. (2013). Phthalates suppress type I interferon in human plasmacytoid dendritic cells via epigenetic regulation. Allergy, 68(7), 870–879. doi:10.1111/all.12162 PubMed doi:10.1111/all.12162 PMID:23738920

Kuo, C. C., Moon, K., Thayer, K. A., & Navas-Acien, A. (2013). Environmental chemicals and type 2 diabetes: An updated systematic review of the epidemiologic evidence. *Current Diabetes Reports*, *13*(6), 831–849. doi:10.100711892-013-0432-6 PMID:24114039

Kurata, Y., Kidachi, F., Yokoyama, M., Toyota, N., Tsuchitani, M., & Katoh, M. (1998). Subchronic toxicity of di (2-ethylhexyl) phthalate in common marmosets: Lack of hepatic peroxisome proliferation, testicular atrophy, or pancreatic acinar cell hyperplasia. *Toxicological Sciences*, *42*(1), 49–56. PMID:9538047

Kuruto-Niwa, R., Tateoka, Y., Usuki, Y., & Nozawa, R. (2007). Measurement of bisphenol A concentrations in human colostrum. *Chemosphere*, *66*(6), 1160–1164. doi:10.1016/j.chemosphere.2006.06.073 PMID:16904728

Kyaw, B. M., Champakalakshmi, R., Sakharkar, M. K., Lim, C. S., & Sakharkar, K. R. (2012). Biodegradation of Low Density Polythene (LDPE) by Pseudomonas species. *Indian Journal of Medical Microbiology*, *52*(3), 411–419. doi:10.100712088-012-0250-6 PMID:23997333

Kyrides, L. P. (1933). U.S. Pat. No. 1,923,938.

Kyrikou, J., & Briassoulis, D. (2007). Biodegradation of agricultural plastic films: A critical review. *Journal of Polymers and the Environment*, *15*(2), 125–150. doi:10.100710924-007-0053-8

La Kind, J. S., & Naiman, D. Q. (2011). Daily intake of bisphenol A and potential sources of exposure: 2005-2006 National Health and Nutrition Examination Survey. Journal of Exposure Science & Environmental Epidemiology, 21(3), 272–279. doi:10.1038/jes.2010.9 PubMed doi:10.1038/jes.2010.9 PMID:20237498

La Mantia, F. P. (1996). *Recycling of PVC and mixed plastic waste*. Toronto: ChemTec Publishing.

Laclau, E., & Mouffe, C. (1985). *Hegemony and Socialist Strategy: Toward a Radical DemocraticPolitics*. London, UK: Verso.

Lacy, P., & Rutqvist, J. (2015). *Waste to Wealth: The Circular Economy Advantage*. New York: Palgrave Macmillan. Retrieved from https://books.google.com.pk/books?hl=en&lr=&id=DmKkCgAAQBAJ&oi=fnd&pg=PP1&dq=plastic+pollution+circular+economy+pakistan&ots=7WOHBD1Rc5&sig=sR30Noypse-sYRhuHTQFtA2bk74#v=onepage&q&f=false

Lai, P., & Michelangeli, F. (2012). Bis(2-hydroxy-3-tert-butyl-5-methyl-phenyl)-methane (bisphenol) is a potent and selective inhibitor of the secretory pathway Ca2+ ATPase (SPCA1). *Biochemical and Biophysical Research Communications*, *424*(3), 616–619. doi:10.1016/j.bbrc.2012.07.004 PMID:22796571

Laist, D. W. (1997). Impacts of marine debris: Entanglement of marine life in marine debris including a comprehensive list of species with entanglement and ingestion records. In Marine Debris (pp. 99-139). New York, NY: Springer.

Laist, D. W. (1997). Impacts of Marine Debris: Entanglement of Marine Life in Marine Debris Including a Comprehensive List of Species with Entanglement and Ingestion Records. In J. M. Coe & D. B. Rogers (Eds.), *Marine Debris* (pp. 99–139). Springer Series on Environmental Management. doi:10.1007/978-1-4613-8486-1_10

Lakind, J. S., & Naiman, D. Q. (2008). Bisphenol A (BPA) daily intakesin the United States: Estimates from the 2003–2004 NHANES urinary BPA data. *Journal of Exposure Science & Environmental Epidemiology*, *18*(6), 608–615. doi:10.1038/jes.2008.20 PMID:18414515

Lal, A. K. (1996). Environmental status of Delhi. *Indian Journal of Environmental Protection*, *16*, 1–11.

Lambert, S., Sinclair, C. J., Bradley, E. L., & Boxall, A. B. A. (2013). Effects of environmental conditions on latex degradation in aquatic systems. *The Science of the Total Environment*, *447*, 225–234. doi:10.1016/j.scitotenv.2012.12.067 PMID:23384646

Lambert, S., & Wagner, M. (2016). Characterisation of nanoplastics during the degradation of polystyrene. *Chemosphere*, *145*, 265–268. doi:10.1016/j.chemosphere.2015.11.078 PMID:26688263

Lambrot, R., Muczynski, V., Lécureuil, C., Angenard, G., Coffigny, H., Pairault, C., ... Rouiller-Fabre, V. (2009). Phthalates impair germ cell development inthe human fetal testis in vitro without change in testosterone production. *Environmental Health Perspectives, 117*(1), 32–37. doi:10.1289/ehp.11146 PMID:19165384

Lam, S.-S., Ramanathan, S., Carbery, M., Gray, K., Vanka, K. S., Maurin, C., ... Palanisami, T. (2018). A Comprehensive Analysis of Plastics and Microplastic Legislation Worldwide. *Water, Air, and Soil Pollution*, 229–345. doi:10.100711270-018-4002-z

Lang, I. A., Galloway, T. S., Scarlett, A., Henley, W. E., Depledge, M., Wallace, R. B., & Melzer, D. (2008). Association of urinary bisphenol A concentration with medical disorders and laboratory abnormalities in adults. *Journal of American Medical Association, 300*, 1303–1310. doi:.11.1303 doi:10.1001/jama.300

Lang, I. A., Galloway, T. S., & Scarlett, A. (2008). Association of Urinary Bisphenol A Concentration With Medical Disorders and Laboratory Abnormalities in Adults. *Journal of the American Medical Association, 300*(11), 1303–1310. doi:10.1001/jama.300.11.1303 PMID:18799442

LaRocca, J., Binder, A. M., McElrath, T. F., & Michels, K. B. (2014). The impact of first trimester phthalate and phenol exposure on IGF2/H19 genomic imprinting and birth outcomes. *Environmental Research, 133*, 396–406. doi:10.1016/j.envres.2014.04.032 PMID:24972507

Larsen, S. T., Hansen, J. S., Hansen, E. W., Clausen, P. A., & Nielsen, G. D. (2007). Airway inflammation and adjuvant effect after repeated airborneexposures to di-(2-ethylhexyl) phthalate and ovalbumin in BALB/c mice. *Toxicology, 235*(1), 119–129. doi:10.1016/j.tox.2007.03.010 PMID:17462807

Lash, S. (1990). *Sociology of Postmodernism*. London: Routledge.

Lash, S., & Urry, J. (1994). *Economies of Signs and Space*. London, UK: Sage.

Latini, G., Del Vecchio, A., Massaro, M., Verrotti, A., & De Felice, C. (2006). *In utero exposure to phthalates and fetal development*. Academic Press.

Latini, G., De Felice, C., Presta, G., Del Vecchio, A., Paris, I., Ruggieri, F., & Mazzeo, P. (2003). Exposure to di (2-ethylhexyl) phthalate in humans during pregnancy. *Neonatology, 83*(1), 22–24. doi:10.1159/000067012 PMID:12566679

Latini, G., De Felice, C., Presta, G., Del Vecchio, A., Paris, I., Ruggieri, F., & Mazzeo, P. (2003). In utero exposure to di-(2-ethylhexyl) phthalate and duration of human pregnancy. *Environmental Health Perspectives, 111*(14), 1783–1785. doi:10.1289/ehp.6202 PMID:14594632

Latini, G., Gallo, F., & De Felice, C. (2004). Birth characteristics and hepatoblastoma risk in young children. *Cancer: Interdisciplinary International Journal of the American Cancer Society, 101*(1), 210–210. doi:10.1002/cncr.20357 PMID:15222013

Latini, G., Knipp, G., Mantovani, A., Marcovecchio, M. L., Chiarelli, F., & Soder, O. (2010). Endocrine disruptors and human health. *Mini-Reviews in Medicinal Chemistry, 10*(9), 846–855. doi:10.2174/138955710791608271 PMID:20482499

Latini, G., Verrotti, A., & De Felice, C. (2004). Di-2-ethylhexyl phthalate and endocrine disruption: A review. *Current Drug Targets. Immune, Endocrine and Metabolic Disorders, 4*(1), 37–40. doi:10.2174/1568008043340017 PMID:15032624

Latouche, S. (1996). *The Westernizationof the World*. Cambridge, UK: Polity Press.

Lavers, J. L., Bond, A. L., & Hutton, I. (2014). Plastic ingestion by flesh-footed shearwaters (Puffinus carneipes): Implications for fledgling body condition and the accumulation of plastic-derived chemicals. *Environmental Pollution, 187*, 124–129. doi:10.1016/j.envpol.2013.12.020 PMID:24480381

Law, K. (2017). Plastics in the marine environment. In Environmental Toxicology and Chemistry (Vol. 33). doi:10.1146/annurev-marine-010816-060409

Laws, S. C., Carey, S. A., Ferrell, J. M., Bodman, G. J., & Cooper, R. L. (2000). Estrogenic activity of octylphenol, nonylphenol, Bisphenol A and methoxychlor in rats. *Toxicological Sciences*, *54*(1), 154–167. doi:10.1093/toxsci/54.1.154 PMID:10746942

le Maire, A., Bourguet, W., & Balaguer, P. (2010). A structural view of nuclear hormone receptor: Endocrine disruptor interactions. *Cellular and Molecular Life Sciences*, *67*(8), 1219–1237. doi:10.100700018-009-0249-2 PMID:20063036

Le Moal, J., Sharpe, R. M., Jϕrgensen, N., Levine, H., Jurewicz, J., Mendiola, J., … Toppari, J. (2015). Toward a multi-country monitoring system of reproductive health in the context of endocrine disrupting chemical exposure. *The European Journal of Public Health.*

Leblank, R. (2019). *The Decomposition of Waste in Landfills: A Story of Time and Materials*. Available at: https://www.thebalancesmb.com/how-long-does-it-take-garbage-to-decompose-2878033

Lebreton, L. C. M., & Borrero, J. C. (2013). Modeling the transport and accumulation floating debris generated by the 11 March 2011 Tohoku tsunami. *Marine Pollution Bulletin*, *66*(1-2), 53–58. doi:10.1016/j.marpolbul.2012.11.013 PMID:23219397

Lebreton, L. C. M., Greer, S. D., & Borrero, J. C. (2012). Numerical modelling of floating debris in the world's oceans. *Marine Pollution Bulletin*, *64*(3), 653–661. doi:10.1016/j.marpolbul.2011.10.027 PMID:22264500

Lebreton, L. C. M., Van Der Zwet, J., Damsteeg, J. W., Slat, B., Andrady, A., & Reisser, J. (2017). River plastic emissions to the world's oceans. *Nature Communications*, *8*, 15611. doi:10.1038/ncomms15611 PMID:28589961

Lechner, F. J., & Boli, J. (2000). *The Globalization Reader*. Malden, MA: Blackwell.

Lee, B. K., Ellenbecker, M. J., & Moure-Eraso, R. (2002). Analyses of the recycling potential of medical plastic wastes. *Waste Management, 22*(5), 461–470.

Lee, B. K., Moure-Eraso, R., & Ellenbecker, M. J. (1995). Potential dioxin and furan sources from hospital solid waste streams: a pilot study. *J. Korea Air Pollution Research Assoc.*, *11*(E), 13–21.

Lee, H. C., Yamanouchi, K., & Nishihara, M. (2006). Effects of perinatal exposure to phthalate/Adipateesters on hypothalamic gene expression and sexual behavior in rats. *Journal of Reproduction and Development, 52*(3), 343-352.

Lee, B. K., Ellenbecker, M. J., & Moure-Ersaso, R. (2004). Alternatives for Treatment and Disposal Cost Reduction of Regulated Medical Wastes. *Waste Management (New York, N.Y.)*, *24*(2), 143–151. doi:10.1016/j.wasman.2003.10.008 PMID:14761753

Lee, B., Pometto, A. L., Fratzke, A., & Bailey, T. B. (1991). Biodegradation of degradable plastic polyethylene by phanerochaete and streptomyces species. *Applied and Environmental Microbiology*, *57*, 678–685. PMID:16348434

Lee, B., Pometto, A. L., Fratzke, A., & Bailey, T. B. (1991). Biodegradation of degradable plastic polyethylene by *Phanerochaete* and *Streptomyces* species. *Applied and Environmental Microbiology*, *57*, 678–685. PMID:16348434

Lee, C. G., Cho, Y. J., Song, P. S., Kang, Y., Kim, J. S., & Choi, M. J. (2003). Effects of temperature distribution on the catalytic pyrolysis of polystyrene waste in a swirling fluidizedbed reactor. *Catalysis Today*, *79*, 453–464. doi:10.1016/S0920-5861(03)00060-9

Lee, Ch.-Ch., Jiang, L.-Y., Kuo, Y.-L., Hsieh, Ch., Chen, C. S., & Tien, C.-J. (2013). The potential role of water quality parameters on occurrence of nonylphenol and bisphenol A and identificationof their discharge sources in the river ecosystems. *Chemosphere*, *91*(7), 904–911. doi:10.1016/j.chemosphere.2013.02.006 PMID:23473432

Lee, D. I., Cho, H. S., & Jeong, S. B. (2006). Distribution characteristics of marine litter on the sea bed of the East China Sea and the South Sea of Korea. *Estuarine, Coastal and Shelf Science*, *70*(1–2), 187–194. doi:10.1016/j.ecss.2006.06.003

Lee, G.-S., & Song, Y. J. B. (2007). Recycling EAF dust by heat treatment with PVC. *Minerals Engineering*, *20*(8), 739–746. doi:10.1016/j.mineng.2007.03.001

Lee, H., & Peart, T. (2000). Bisphenol A contamination in Canadian municipal and industrial wastewater and sludge samples. *Water Quality Research Journal of Canada*, *35*(2), 283–298. doi:10.2166/wqrj.2000.018

Lee, K. H., Noh, N. S., Shin, D. H., & Seo, Y. (2002). Comparison of plastic types for catalytic degradation of waste plastics into liquid product with spent FCC catalyst. *Polymer Degradation & Stability*, *78*(3), 539–544. doi:10.1016/S0141-3910(02)00227-6

Lee, K. W., Shim, W. J., Kwon, O. Y., & Kang, J. H. (2013). Size-dependent effects of micro polystyrene particles in the marine copepod *Tigriopus japonicus*. *Environmental Science & Technology*, *47*(19), 11278–11283. doi:10.1021/es401932b PMID:23988225

Lee, S. Y., Yim, K. S., Chang, H. N., & Chang, Y. K. (1994). Construction of plasmids, estimation of plasmid stability and use of stable plasmids for the production of poly(3-hydroxybutyric) acid by recombinant Escherichia coli. *Journal of Biotechnology*, *32*(2), 203–211. doi:10.1016/0168-1656(94)90183-X PMID:7764567

Lee, S. Y., Yoon, J. H., Kim, J. R., & Park, D. W. (2002). Degradation of polystyrene using clinoptilolite catalysts. *Journal of Analytical and Applied Pyrolysis*, *64*(1), 71–83. doi:10.1016/S0165-2370(01)00171-1

Le, H. H., Carlson, E. M., Chua, J. P., & Belcher, S. M. (2008). Bisphenol A is released from polycarbonate drinking bottles and mimics the neurotoxic actions of estrogen in developing cerebellar neurons. *Toxicology Letters*, *176*(2), 149–156. doi:10.1016/j.toxlet.2007.11.001 PMID:18155859

Lemoigne, M. (1926). Produits de dehydration et de polymerisation de l'acide β-oxobutyrique. *Bulletin de la Société de Chimie Biologique*, *8*, 770–782.

Leonardi, A., Cofini, M., Rigante, D., Lucchetti, L., Cipolla, C., Penta, L., & Esposito, S. (2017). The Effect of Bisphenol A on Puberty: A Critical Review of the Medical Literature. *International Journal of Environmental Research and Public Health*, *14*(9), 1044. doi:10.3390/ijerph14091044 PMID:28891963

Leranth, C., Hajszan, T., Szigeti-Buck, K., Bober, J., & MacLusky, N. J. (2008). Bisphenol A prevents the synaptogenic response to estradiol in hippocampus and prefrontal cortex of ovariectomized nonhuman primates. *Proceedings of the National Academy of Sciences of the United States of America*, *105*(37), 14187–14191. doi:10.1073/pnas.0806139105 PMID:18768812

Leranth, C., Szigeti-Buck, K., MacLusky, N. J., & Hajszan, T. (2008). Bisphenol A prevents the synaptogenic response to testosterone in the brain of adult male rats. *Endocrinology*, *149*(3), 988–994. doi:10.1210/en.2007-1053 PMID:18048497

Leschine, S. B. (1995). Cellulose degradation in anaerobic environments. *Annual Review of Microbiology*, *49*(1), 399–426. doi:10.1146/annurev.mi.49.100195.002151 PMID:8561466

Levendis, Y., Atal, A., Carlson, J., & Quintana, M. (2001). PAH and soot emissions from burning components of medical waste: Examination/surgical gloves and cotton pads. *Chemosphere*, *42*(5-7), 775–783. doi:10.1016/S0045-6535(00)00251-4 PMID:11219703

Lewis, H., Gertsakis, J., Grant, T., Morelli, N., & Sweatman, A. (2017). *Design + Envrionment: A Global Guide to Designing Greener Goods*. London: Routledge. Retrieved from https://www.taylorfrancis.com/books/9781351282208

Li, D. K., Zhou, Z., Miao, M., He Y., Wang, J., Ferber, J., ... Yuan, W. (2011). Urine bisphenol-A (BISPHENOL A) level in relation to semen quality. *Fertility and Sterility, 95,* 625–630. doi:10.1016/j.fertnstert.2010.09.026

Li, J., Li, L., Zuo, H., Ke, C., Yan, B., Wen, H., . . . Yang, X. (2014). T-helper type-2 contact hypersensitivity of Balb/c mice aggravated by dibutyl phthalate via long-term dermal exposure. PLoS One, 9(2), e87887. doi:10.1371/journal.pone.0087887 PubMed doi:10.1371/journal.pone.0087887 PMID:24498391

Li, L. X., Chen, L., Meng, X.-Z., Chen, B.-H., Chen, S.-Q., Zhao, Y., . . . Zhang, Y.-H. (2013). Exposure levels of environmental endocrine disruptors in mother-newborn pairs in China and their placental transfer characteristics. PLoS One, 8(5), e62526. doi:10.1371/journal.pone.0062526 PubMed doi:10.1371/journal.pone.0062526 PMID:23667484

Li, N., Mahat, D., & Park, S. (2009). *Reduce Reuse and Replace: A Study on Solutions to Plastic Wastes.* An Interactive Qualifying Project Submitted to the faculty of Worcester Polytechnic Institute.

Li, Q.A., Li, H., Du, G.F., Xu, Z. H. (2010). Electrochemical detection of Bisphenol A mediated by [Ru(bpy)(3)](2+) on an ITO electrode. *Journal of Hazardous Materials, 180,* 703–709. doi:10.. doi:10.1016/j.jhazmat

Liao, Wu, Zhu, & Yi. (n.d.). Synthesis and properties of novel styrene acrylonitrile/polypropylene blends with enhanced toughness. *Chemistry Central Journal.*

Liao, Ch., Liu, F., & Kannan, K. (2012). Bisphenol S, a new bisphenol analogue in paper products and currency bills and its association with bisphenol A residues. *Environmental Science & Technology*, *46*(12), 6515–6522. doi:10.1021/es300876n PMID:22591511

Li, D. K., Zhou, Z., Miao, M., He, Y., Qing, D., Wu, T., ... Yuan, W. (2010a). Relationship between urine bisphenol-A level and declining male sexual function. *Journal of Andrology*, *31*(5), 500–506. doi:10.2164/jandrol.110.010413 PMID:20467048

Li, D., Zhou, Z., Qing, D., He, Y., Wu, T., Miao, M., ... Yuan, W. (2009). Occupational exposure to bisphenol-A (BPA) and the risk of self-reported male sexual dysfunction. *Journal of Human Reproduction*, *25*(2), 519–527. doi:10.1093/humrep/dep381

Lieckens, K., & Vandaele, N. (2012). Multi-level reverse logistics network design under uncertainty. *International Journal of Production Research*, *50*(1), 23–40. doi:10.1080/00207543.2011.571442

Li, H., & Kim, K. H. (2003). Effects of mono-(2-ethylhexyl) phthalate on fetal and neonatal rat testis organ cultures. *Biology of Reproduction*, *69*(6), 1964–1972. doi:10.1095/biolreprod.103.018895 PMID:12904314

Li, J., Yang, D., Li, L., Jabeen, K., & Shi, H. (2015). Microplastics in commercial bivalves from China. *Environmental Pollution*, *207*, 190–195. doi:10.1016/j.envpol.2015.09.018 PMID:26386204

Li, L., Zhang, T., Qin, X. S., Ge, W., Ma, H. G., Sun, L. L., ... Shen, W. (2014). Exposure to diethylhexyl phthalate (DEHP) results in a heritable modification of imprint genes DNA methylation in mouse oocytes. *Molecular Biology Reports*, *41*(3), 1227–1235. doi:10.100711033-013-2967-7 PMID:24390239

Lim, H., & Hoag, S. W. (2013). Plasticizer effects on physical-mechanical properties of solvent cast Soluplus® films. *AAPS PharmSciTech*, *14*(3), 903–910. doi:10.120812249-013-9971-z PMID:23689959

Lind, P. M., Zethelius, B., & Lind, L. (2012). Circulating levels of phthalate metabolites are associated with prevalent diabetes in the elderly. *Diabetes Care, 35*(7), 1519-1524. doi:10.2337/dc11-2396

Lindberg, M., Lindgren, M., & Packendorff, J. (2014). Quadruple Helix as a Way to Bridge the Gender Gap in Entrepreneurship: The Case of an Innovation System Project in the Baltic Sea Region. *Journal of the Knowledge Economy*, *5*(1), 94–113. doi:10.100713132-012-0098-3

Lind, P. M., Roos, V., Ronn, M., Johansson, L., Ahlstrom, H., Kullberg, J., & Lind, L. (2012). Serumconcentrations of phthalate metabolites are related to abdominal fat distribution two years later in elderly women. *Environmental Health*, *11*(21), 10–1186. PMID:22472124

Lin, L. C., Wang, S. L., Chang, Y. C., Huang, P. C., Cheng, J. T., Su, P. H., & Liao, P. C. (2011). Associations between maternal phthalate exposure and cord sex hormones in human infants. *Chemosphere*, *83*(8), 1192–1199. doi:10.1016/j.chemosphere.2010.12.079 PMID:21272909

Lin, S., Ku, H. Y., Su, P. H., Chen, J. W., Huang, P. C., Angerer, J., & Wang, S. L. (2011). Phthalateexposure in pregnant women and their children in central Taiwan. *Chemosphere*, *82*(7), 947–955. doi:10.1016/j.chemosphere.2010.10.073 PMID:21075419

Lin, Y.-H., & Yang, M.-H. (2007). Chemical catalysed recycling of waste polymers: Catalytic conversion of polypropylene into fuels and chemicals over spent FCC catalyst in a fluidised-bed reactor. *Polymer Degradation & Stability*, *92*(5), 813–821. doi:10.1016/j.polymdegradstab.2007.01.028

Lin, Y.-H., & Yen, H.-Y. (2005). Fluidised bed pyrolysis of polypropylene over cracking catalysts for producing hydrocarbons. *Polymer Degradation & Stability*, *89*(1), 101–108. doi:10.1016/j.polymdegradstab.2005.01.006

Lin, Z. P., Ikonomou, M. G., Jing, H., Mackintosh, C., & Gobas, F. A. (2003). Determination of phthalate ester congeners and mixtures by LC/ESI-MS in sediments and biota of an urbanized marine inlet. *Environmental Science & Technology*, *37*(10), 2100–2108. doi:10.1021/es026361r PMID:12785513

Li, R. C., & Tee, T. J. C. (2012). A Reverse Logistics Model For Recovery Options Of E-waste Considering the Integration of the Formal and Informal Waste Sectors. *Procedia: Social and Behavioral Sciences*, *40*, 788–816. doi:10.1016/j.sbspro.2012.03.266

Lithner, D., Larsson, A., & Dave, G. (2011). Environmental and health hazard ranking and assessment of plastic polymers based on chemical composition. *The Science of the Total Environment*, *409*(18), 3309–3324. doi:10.1016/j.scitotenv.2011.04.038 PMID:21663944

Lithner, D., Nordensvan, I., & Dave, G. (2012). Comparative acute toxicity of leachates from plastic products made of polypropylene, polyethylene, PVC, acrylonitrile-butadiene-styrene, and epoxy to Daphnia magna. *Environmental Science and Pollution Research International*, *19*(5), 1763–1772. doi:10.100711356-011-0663-5 PMID:22183785

Liu, F.-S., Lei, L., Shitao, Y., Zhiguo, L., & Xiaoping, G. (2011). Methanolysis of polycarbonate catalysed by ionic liquid. *Journal of Hazardous Materials*, *189*(1-2), 249–254. doi:10.1016/j.jhazmat.2011.02.032 PMID:21402441

Liu, F.-S., Zhuo, L., Shi-Tao, Y., Xiao, C., Cong-Xia, X., & Xiao-Ping, G. (2009). Methanolysis and hydrolysis of polycarbonate under moderate conditions. *Journal of Polymers and the Environment*, *17*(3), 208–211. doi:10.100710924-009-0140-0

Liu, J., Yu, P., Qian, W., Li, Y., Zhao, J., Huan, F., ... Xiao, H. (2013). Perinatal bisphenol A exposure and adult glucose homeostasis: Identifying critical windows of exposure. *PLoS One*, *8*(5), e64143. doi:10.1371/journal.pone.0064143 PMID:23675523

Liu, L., Bao, H., Liu, F., Zhang, J., & Shen, H. (2012). Phthalates exposure of Chinese reproductive age couples and its effect on male semen quality, a primary study. *Environment International*, *42*, 78–83. doi:10.1016/j.envint.2011.04.005 PMID:21524797

Liu, T. K., Wang, M. W., & Chen, P. (2013). Influence of waste management policy on the characteristics of beach litter in Kaohsiung, Taiwan. *Marine Pollution Bulletin*, *72*(1), 99–106. doi:10.1016/j.marpolbul.2013.04.015 PMID:23673204

Liu, Z., Liu, Z., & Li, X. (2006). Status and prospect of the application of municipal solid waste incineration in China. *Applied Thermal Engineering*, *26*(11-12), 1193–1197. doi:10.1016/j.applthermaleng.2005.07.036

Li, W., Zhou, J., & Xu, Y. (2015). Study of the *in vitro* cytotoxicity testing of medical devices. *Biomedical Reports*, *3*(5), 617–620. doi:10.3892/br.2015.481 PMID:26405534

Lobelle, D., & Cunliffe, M. (2011). Early microbial biofilm formation on marine plastic debris. *Marine Pollution Bulletin*, *62*(1), 197–200. doi:10.1016/j.marpolbul.2010.10.013 PMID:21093883

Loganathan, S., & Kannan, K. (2011). Occurrence of bisphenol A in indoor dust from two locations in the Eastern United States and implications for human exposures. *Archives of Environmental Contamination and Toxicology*, *61*(1), 68–73. doi:10.100700244-010-9634-y PMID:21221962

López-Carrillo, L., Hernández-Ramírez, R. U., Calafat, A. M., Torres-Sánchez, L., Galván-Portillo, M., Needham, L. L., & Cebrián, M. E. (2009). Exposure to phthalates and breast cancer risk in northern Mexico. *Environmental Health Perspectives*, *118*(4), 539–544. doi:10.1289/ehp.0901091 PMID:20368132

Lorenz, C., Von Goetz, N., Scheringer, M., Wormuth, M., & Hungerbühler, K. (2011). Potential exposure of German consumers to engineered nanoparticles in cosmetics and personal care products. *Nanotoxicology*, *5*(1), 12–29. doi:10.3109/17435390.2010.484554 PMID:21417685

Lottrup, G., Andersson, A. M., Leffers, H., Mortensen, G. K., Toppari, J., Skakkebaek, N. E., & Main, K. M. (2006). Possible impact of phthalates on infant reproductive health. *International Journal of Andrology*, *29*(1), 172–180. doi:10.1111/j.1365-2605.2005.00642.x PMID:16466537

Louis, G. M. B., Sundaram, R., Sweeney, A. M., Schisterman, E. F., Maisog, J., & Kannan, K. (2014). Urinary bisphenol A, phthalates, and couple fecundity: The Longitudinal Investigation of Fertility and the Environment (LIFE) Study. *Fertility and Sterility*, *101*(5), 1359–1366. doi:10.1016/j.fertnstert.2014.01.022 PMID:24534276

Lovekamp-Swan, T., & Davis, B. J. (2003). Mechanisms of phthalate ester toxicity in the female reproductive system. *Environmental Health Perspectives*, *111*(2), 139–145. doi:10.1289/ehp.5658 PMID:12573895

Lovekamp, T. N., & Davis, B. J. (2001). Mono-(2-ethylhexyl) phthalate suppresses aromatase transcript levels and estradiol production in cultured rat granulosa cells. *Toxicology and Applied Pharmacology*, *172*(3), 217–224. doi:10.1006/taap.2001.9156 PMID:11312650

Lucas, N., Bienaime, C., Belloy, C., Queneudec, M., Silvestre, F., & Nava-Saucedo, J. E. (2008). Review Polymer biodegradation: Mechanisms and estimation techniques. *Chemosphere*, *73*(4), 429–442. doi:10.1016/j.chemosphere.2008.06.064 PMID:18723204

Lugauskas, A., Levinskaitė, L., & Peciulyte, D. (2003). Micromycetes as deterioration agents of polymeric materials. *International Biodeterioration & Biodegradation*, *52*(4). doi:10.1016/S0964-8305(03)00110-0

Luke, A., & Luke, C. (2000). A Situated Perspective on Cultural Globalization. In Globalization and Education. London, UK: Routledge.

Lu, L., Namioka, T., & Yoshikawa, K. (2011). Effects of hydrothermal treatment on characteristics and combustion behaviors of municipal solid wastes. *Applied Energy*, *8*(11), 3659–3664. doi:10.1016/j.apenergy.2011.04.022

Lunder, S., Andrews, D., & Houlihan, J. (2010). *Synthetic estrogen Bisphenol A coats cash register receipts.* Retrieved from http://www.ewg.org/BisphenolA-in-store-receipts

Lundqvist, M., Stigler, J., Elia, G., Lynch, I., Cedervall, T., & Dawson, K. A. (2008). Nanoparticle size and surface properties determine the protein corona with possible implications for biological impacts. *Proceedings of the National Academy of Sciences of the United States of America*, *105*(38), 14265–14270. doi:10.1073/pnas.0805135105 PMID:18809927

Lusher, A., Hollman, P., & Mendoza-Hill, J. (2017). Microplastics in fisheries and aquaculture. *FAO Fisheries and Aquaculture Technical Paper (FAO) eng no. 615.*

Lusher, A. (2015). Microplastics in the marine environment: Distribution, interactions and effects. In M. Bergmann, L. Gutow, & M. Klages (Eds.), *Marine Anthropogenic Litter* (pp. 245–307)., doi:10.1007/978-3-319-16510-3_10

Lusher, A. L., Mchugh, M., & Thompson, R. C. (2013). Occurrence of microplastics in the gastrointestinal tract of pelagic and demersal fish from the English Channel. *Marine Pollution Bulletin*, *67*(1-2), 94–99. doi:10.1016/j.marpolbul.2012.11.028 PMID:23273934

Lyche, J. L. (2011). Phthalates. In R. C. Gupta (Ed.), *Reproductive andDevelopmental Toxicology* (1st ed.; pp. 637–655). Amsterdam: Academic Press. doi:10.1016/B978-0-12-382032-7.10048-7

Macali, A., Semenov, A., Venuti, V., Crupi, V., D'Amico, F., Rossi, B., & Bergami, E. (2018). Episodic records of jellyfish ingestion of plastic items reveal a novel pathway for trophic transference of marine litter. *Scientific Reports*, *8*(1), 6105. doi:10.103841598-018-24427-7 PMID:29666447

Machado, H. M. A. M. M. S., Rodrigues, F. G., Assunc, R. M. N., Soares, H. M., Cangani, A. P., & Cerqueira, D. A. (2010). Chemical recycling of poly (vinyl chloride): Application of partially dehydrochlorinated poly (vinyl chloride) for producing a chemically modified polymer. *Journal of Analytical and Applied Pyrolysis*, *115*, 1474–1479.

Madison, L. L., & Huisman, G. W. (1999). Metabolic engineering of poly (3-hydroxyalkanoates): From DNA to plastic. *Microbiology and Molecular Biology Reviews*, *63*(1), 21–53. PMID:10066830

Maeda, H., Yamagata, Y., Abe, K., Hasegawa, F., Machida, M., Ishioka, R., ... Nakajima, T. (2005). Purification and characterization of a biodegradable plastic-degrading enzyme from Aspergillus oryzae. *Applied Microbiology and Biotechnology*, *67*(6), 778–788. doi:10.100700253-004-1853-6 PMID:15968570

Magliano, D. J., & Lyons, J. G. (2013). Bisphenol A and diabetes, insulin resistance, cardiovascular disease and obesity: Controversy in a (plastic) cup? *The Journal of Clinical Endocrinology and Metabolism*, *98*(2), 502–504. doi:10.1210/jc.2012-3058 PMID:23264398

Magliozzi, R., Nardacci, R., Scarsella, G., Di Carlo, V., & Stefanini, S. (2013). Effects of the plasticiser DEHP on lung of newborn rats: Catalase immunocytochemistry and morphometric analysis. *Histochemistry and Cell Biology*, *120*(1), 41–49. doi:10.100700418-003-0543-2 PMID:12802597

Mahar, A., Malik, R. N., Qadir, A., Ahmed, T., Khan, Z., & Khan, M. A. (2007). Review and Analysis of Current Solid Waste Management Situation. In *Proceedings of the International Conference on Sustainable Solid Waste Management* (pp. 33-41). Chennai: Academic Press. Retrieved from http://citeseerx.ist.psu.edu/viewdoc/download?doi=10.1.1.529.3759&rep=rep1&type=pdf

Maharanaa, T., Negia, Y. S., & Mohanty, B. (2007). Review Article: Recycling of Polystyrene. *Polymer-Plastics Technology and Engineering*, *46*(7), 729–736. doi:10.1080/03602550701273963

Mahar, R. B., Yue, D., Liu, J., Zhang, Y., & Nie, Y. (2009). Biological pretreatment of municipal solid waste prior to landfilling. *Global NEST Journal*, *11*, 510–517.

Mahdiyah, D., & Mukti, B. H. (2013). Isolation of Polyethylene Plastic degrading-Bacteria. *Biosciences International*, *2*, 29–32.

Main, K. M., Mortensen, G. K., Kaleva, M. M., Boisen, K. A., Damgaard, I. N., Chellakooty, M., ... Skakkebaek, N. E. (2006). Human breast milk contamination with phthalates and alterations of endogenous reproductive hormones in infants three months of age. *Environmental Health Perspectives*, *114*(2), 270–276. doi:10.1289/ehp.8075 PMID:16451866

Ma, M., Kondo, T., Ban, S., Umemura, T., Kurahashi, N., Takeda, M., & Kishi, R. (2006). Exposure ofprepubertal female rats to inhaled di (2-ethylhexyl) phthalate affects the onset of puberty andpostpubertal reproductive functions. *Toxicological Sciences*, *93*(1), 164–171. doi:10.1093/toxsci/kfl036 PMID:16763069

Mander, J., & Goldsmith, E. (1996). *The Case Against the Global Economy*. San Francisco, CA: SierraClub Books.

Mandiberg, S. F., & Faure, M. G. (2009). A graduated punishment approach to environmental crimes: Beyond vindication of administrative authority in the United States and Europe. *Colum. J. Envtl. L.*, *34*, 447.

Manikkam, M., Tracey, R., Guerrero-Bosagna, C., & Skinner, M. K. (2013). Plastics derived endocrine disruptors (BPA, DEHP and DBP) induce epigenetic transgenerational inheritance of obesity, reproductive disease and sperm epimutations. *PLoS One*, *8*(1), e55387. doi:10.1371/journal.pone.0055387 PMID:23359474

Mansoor, H. (2018, November 11). *Cabinet approves phase-wise ban on plastic bags across Sindh*. Retrieved from https://www.dawn.com/news/1444812

Mansour, A., & Zarei, M. (2008). A Multi-Period Reverse Logistics Optimization Model for End-Of-Life Vehicles Recovery Based on EU Directive. *International Journal of Computer Integrated Manufacturing*, *21*(7), 764–777. doi:10.1080/09511920701685325

Mantia, P. L. (2002). *Handbook of plastics recycling*. Francesco.

Mantovani, A. (2006). Risk assessment of endocrine disrupters: The role of toxicological studies. *Annals of the New York Academy of Sciences*, *1076*(1), 239–252. doi:10.1196/annals.1371.063 PMID:17119206

Maqbool, F., Mostafalou, S., Bahadar, H., & Abdollahi, M. (2015). Review of endocrine disordersassociated with environmental toxicants and possible involved mechanisms. *Life Sciences*. PMID:26497928

Maragoua, N. C., Makria, A., Lampib, E. N., Thomaidisa, N. S., & Koupparisa, M. A. (2011). Migration of Bisphenol A from polycarbonate baby bottles under real use conditions. *Food Additives and Contaminants*, *25*(3), 373–383. doi:10.1080/02652030701509998 PMID:18311628

Marcel, Y. L., & Noel, S. P. (1970). A plasticizer in lipid extracts of human blood. Chemistry and Physics of Lipids, 4(3), 418–419. doi:10.1016/0009-3084(70)90040-X PubMed doi:10.1016/0009-3084(70)90040-X PMID:5511751

March, J. G., & Cerdà, V. (2015). An innovative arrangement for in-vial membrane-assisted liquid-liquid microextraction: Application to the determination of esters of phthalic acid in alcoholic beverages by gas chromatography-mass spectrometry. *Analytical and Bioanalytical Chemistry*, *407*(14), 4213–4217. doi:10.100700216-015-8646-x PMID:25876533

Marcilla, A., Beltran, M. I., Hernandez, F., & Navarro, R. (2004). HZSM5 and HUSY deactivation during the catalytic pyrolysis of polyethylene. *Applied Catalysis A, General*, *278*(1), 37–43. doi:10.1016/j.apcata.2004.09.023

Marcilla, A., Beltran, M. I., & Navarro, R. (2007). Study of the deactivation process of HZSM5 zeolite during polyethylene pyrolysis. *Applied Catalysis A, General*, *333*(1), 57–66. doi:10.1016/j.apcata.2007.09.004

Marcilla, A., Gómez, A., García, A. N., & Olaya, M. M. (2002). Kinetic study of the catalytic decomposition of the different commercial polyethylenes over an MCM-41 catalyst. *Journal of Analytical and Applied Pyrolysis*, *64*(1), 85–101. doi:10.1016/S0165-2370(01)00174-7

Marcilla, A., Gomez, A., Reyes-Labarta, J. A., Giner, A., & Hernandez, F. (2003). Kinetic study of polypropylene pyrolysis using ZSM-5 and an equilibrium fluid catalytic cracking catalyst. *Journal of Analytical and Applied Pyrolysis*, *68*, 46–48.

Marinova, N., Franckevičius, M., Matulaitienė, I., Devižis, A., Niaura, G., Gulbinas, V., & Delgado, J. L. (2017). Hindered Amine Light Stabilizers Increase the Stability of Methylammonium Lead Iodide Perovskite Against Light and Oxygen. *ChemSusChem*, *10*(19), 3760–3764. doi:10.1002/cssc.201700707 PMID:28762644

Marrack, D., & Meyers, D. (1994). *PP/PE medical syringe recycling system: sharps away. In 87th Annual Meeting and Exhibition.* Air & Waste Manage. Assoc. (Paper No. 94-RP-123B.01)

Marsee, K., Woodruff, T. J., Axelrad, D. A., Calafat, A. M., & Swan, S. H. (2006). Estimated daily phthalate exposures in a population of mothers of male infants exhibiting reduced anogenital distance. *Environmental Health Perspectives*, *114*(6), 805–809. doi:10.1289/ehp.8663 PMID:16759976

Martine, B., Cendrine, D., Fabrice, A., & Marc, C. (2013). Assessment of adult human exposure to phthalate esters in the urban centre of Paris (France). *Bulletin of Environmental Contamination and Toxicology*, *90*(1), 91–96. doi:10.100700128-012-0859-5 PMID:23090363

Martinez, E., Maamaatuaiahutapu, K., & Taillandier, V. (2009). Floating marine debris surface drift: Convergence and accumulation toward the South Pacific subtropical gyre. *Marine Pollution Bulletin*, *58*(9), 1347–1355. doi:10.1016/j.marpolbul.2009.04.022 PMID:19464033

Martins, J., & Sobral, P. (2011). Plastic marine debris on the Portuguese coastline: A matter of size? *Marine Pollution Bulletin*. Retrieved from http://www.sciencedirect.com/science/article/pii/S0025326X1100

Marx, J. L. (1972). Phthalic acid esters – biological impact uncertain. Science, 178(4056), 46–47. doi:10.1126/science.178.4056.46 PubMed doi:10.1126cience.178.4056.46 PMID:5070514

Marx, K., & Engels, F. (1978). *The Marx-Engels Reader* (2nd ed.). New York: W. W. Norton.

Mason, S. A., Kammin, L., Eriksen, M., Aleid, G., Wilson, S., Box, C., ... Riley, A. (2016). Pelagic plastic pollution within the surface waters of Lake Michigan, USA. *Journal of Great Lakes Research*, *42*(4), 753–759. doi:10.1016/j.jglr.2016.05.009

Masood, M., & Barlow, C. Y. (2014). Informal waste sector in Lahore: Role & Motivation. *Second Pakistan Urban Forum.* Retrieved from https://www.researchgate.net/publication/273950122_Informal_waste_sector_in_Lahore_Role_Motivation

Masood, M., & Barlow, C. Y. (2013). Framework for integration of informal waste management sector with the formal sector in Pakistan. *Waste Management & Research*, *31*(10), 93–105. doi:10.1177/0734242X13499811 PMID:23999020

Mastellone, M. L., Perugini, F., Ponte, M., & Arena, U. (2002). Fluidized bed pyrolysis of a recycled polyethylene. *Polymer Degradation & Stability*, *76*(3), 479–487. doi:10.1016/S0141-3910(02)00052-6

Mastral, J. F., Berrueco, C., Gea, M., & Ceamanos, J. (2006). Catalytic degradation of high-density polyethylene over nanocrystalline HZSM-5 zeolite. *Polymer Degradation & Stability*, *91*(12), 3330–3338. doi:10.1016/j.polymdegradstab.2006.06.009

Mastral, J., Esperanza, E., García, P., & Juste, M. (2002). Pyrolysis of high-density polyethylene in a fluidized bed reactor:influence of the temperature and residence time. *Journal of Analytical and Applied Pyrolysis*, *63*(1), 1–15. doi:10.1016/S0165-2370(01)00137-1

Masuno, H., Kidani, T., Sekiya, K., & … . (2002). Bisphenol A in combination with insulin can accelerate the conversion of 3T3-L1 fibroblasts to adipocytes. *Journal of Lipid Research*, *43*(5), 676–684. PMID:11971937

Masuyama, H., Hiramatsu, Y., Kodama, J. I., & Kudo, T. (2003). Expression and potential roles ofpregnane X receptor in endometrial cancer. *The Journal of Clinical Endocrinology and Metabolism, 88*(9), 4446–4454. doi:10.1210/jc.2003-030203 PMID:12970323

Mato, Y., Isobe, T., Takada, H., Kanehiro, H., Ohtake, C., & Kaminuma, T. (2001). Plastic resin pellets as a transport medium for toxic chemicals in the marine environment. *Environmental Science & Technology, 35*(2), 318–324. doi:10.1021/es0010498 PMID:11347604

Matsumoto, A., Kunugita, N., Kitagawa, K., Isse, T., Oyama, T., Foureman, G. L., ... Kawamoto, T. (2003). Bisphenol A levels in human urine. *Environmental Health Perspectives, 111*(1), 101–104. doi:10.1289/ehp.5512 PMID:12515686

Matsumoto, M., Hirata-Koizumi, M., & Ema, M. (2008). Potential adverse effects of phthalic acid esters on human health: A review of recent studies on reproduction. *Regulatory Toxicology and Pharmacology, 50*(1), 37–49. doi:10.1016/j.yrtph.2007.09.004 PMID:17983696

Matsushima, A., Kakuta, Y., Teramoto, T., Koshiba, T., Liu, X., Okada, H., ... Shimohigashi, Y. (2007). Structural evidence for endocrine disruptor Bisphenol A binding to human nuclear receptor ERR gamma. *Journal of Biochemistry, 142*(4), 517–524. doi:10.1093/jb/mvm158 PMID:17761695

Matthews, J. B., Twomey, K., & Zacharewski, T. R. (2001). In vitro and in vivo interactions of Bisphenol A and its metabolite, Bisphenol A glucuronide, with estrogen receptors α and β. *Chemical Research in Toxicology, 14*(2), 149–157. doi:10.1021/tx0001833 PMID:11258963

Mattsson, K., Adolfsson, K., Ekvall, M. T., Borgström, M. T., Linse, S., Hansson, L. A., ... Prinz, C. N. (2016). Translocation of 40 nm diameter nanowires through the intestinal epithelium of Daphnia magna. *Nanotoxicology, 10*(8), 1160–1167. doi:10.1080/17435390.2016.1189615 PMID:27181920

Mattsson, K., Ekvall, M. T., Hansson, L. A., Linse, S., Malmendal, A., & Cedervall, T. (2015). Altered behavior, physiology, and metabolism in fish exposed to polystyrene nanoparticles. *Environmental Science & Technology, 49*(1), 553–561. doi:10.1021/es5053655 PMID:25380515

Mattsson, K., Hansson, L. A., Linse, S., Malmendal, A., & Cedervall, T. (2014). Effect of Nanoparticles in Top Consumers. *Biophysical Journal, 106*(2), 625a. doi:10.1016/j.bpj.2013.11.3454

Mattsson, K., Johnson, E. V., Malmendal, A., Linse, S., Hansson, L. A., & Cedervall, T. (2017). Brain damage and behavioural disorders in fish induced by plastic nanoparticles delivered through the food chain. *Scientific Reports, 7*(1), 11452. doi:10.103841598-017-10813-0 PMID:28904346

Maximenko, N., Hafner, J., & Niiler, P. (2012). Pathways of marine debris derived from trajectories of Lagrangian drifters. *Marine Pollution Bulletin, 65*(1–3), 51–62. doi:10.1016/j.marpolbul.2011.04.016 PMID:21696778

Mayer, A. M., & Staples, R. C. (2002). Laccase new functions for an old enzyme. *Phytochemistry, 60*(6), 561–565. doi:10.1016/S0031-9422(02)00171-1 PMID:12126701

Mazur, S., & Hitchcock, T. (2001). Spontaneous pneumomediastinum, pneumothorax and ecstasy abuse. In *Emergency Medicine* (Vol. 13). CBD Techni. doi:10.1046/j.1442-2026.2001.00190.x

McCauley, S. J., & Bjorndal, K. A. (1999). Conservation implications of dietary dilution from debris ingestion: Sublethal effects in post-hatchling loggerhead sea turtles. *Conservation Biology, 13*(4), 925–929. doi:10.1046/j.1523-1739.1999.98264.x

McChesney, R. (1995). *Telecommunications, Mass Media, and Democracy: The Battle for the Control of U.S. Broadcasting, 1928-1935*. New York: Oxford University Press.

McKay, J. (2017). *A Healthier Planet. Defence Journal, 20(12)*, 41–42. Retrieved from https://search.proquest.com/openview/4905f31a8aacd1a842962bdd2ea2bed3/1?pq-origsite=gscholar&cbl=616545

McKeen, L., W. (2013). 3 Plastics Used in Medical Devices. *Handbook of Polymer Applications in Medicine and Medical Devices, 21*.

McKee, R. H. (2004). Toxicology Research Task G. Phthalate exposure and early thelarche. *Environmental Health Perspectives*, *112*(10), A541–A543. doi:10.1289/ehp.112-a541b PMID:15238295

McKee, R. H., El-Hawari, M., Stoltz, M., Pallas, F., & Lington, A. W. (2002). Absorption, disposition and metabolism of di-isononyl phthalate (DINP) in F-344 rats. *Journal of Applied Toxicology: An International Journal*, *22*(5), 293–302. doi:10.1002/jat.861 PMID:12355558

Mckenna, N. J., Lanz, R. B., & O'malley, B. W. (1999). Nuclear Receptor Coregulators: Cellular and Molecular Biology. *Endocrinology Review*, *20*, 321–344. PMID:10368774

McLaughlin, S. B., & Kszos, L. A. (2005). Development of switchgrass (*Panicum virgatum*) as a bioenergy feedstock in the United States. *Biomass and Bioenergy*, *28*(6), 515–535. doi:10.1016/j.biombioe.2004.05.006

Medina, M. (2010). *Solid wastes, poverty and the environment in developing country cities: Challenges and opportunities*. Helsinki: The United Nations University World Institute for Development Economics Research. Retrieved from https://www.econstor.eu/bitstream/10419/54107/1/63649439X.pdf

Meeker, J.D., Sathyanarayana, S., & Swan, S.H. (2009). Phthalates andother additives in plastics: human exposure and associated healthoutcomes. *Phil. Trans. R. Soc. B, 364*, 2097–2113. doi:10.1098/rstb.2008.0268

Meeker, J. D. (2010). Exposure to environmental endocrine disrupting compounds and men's health. *Maturitas*, *66*(3), 236–241. doi:10.1016/j.maturitas.2010.03.001 PMID:20347536

Meeker, J. D., Calafat, A. M., & Hauser, R. (2007). Di (2-ethylhexyl) phthalate metabolites may alter thyroid hormone levels in men. *Environmental Health Perspectives*, *115*(7), 1029–1034. doi:10.1289/ehp.9852 PMID:17637918

Meeker, J. D., Calafat, A. M., & Hauser, R. (2009). Urinary metabolites of di (2-ethylhexyl) phthalate are associated with decreased steroid hormone levels in adult men. *Journal of Andrology*, *30*(3), 287–297. doi:10.2164/jandrol.108.006403 PMID:19059903

Meeker, J. D., Calafat, A. M., & Hauser, R. (2010). Urinary Bisphenol A concentrations in relation to serum thyroid and reproductive hormone levels in men from an infertility clinic. *Environmental Science & Technology*, *44*(4), 1458–1463. doi:10.1021/es9028292 PMID:20030380

Meeker, J. D., & Ferguson, K. K. (2011). Relationship between urinary phthalate and Bisphenol A concentrations and serum thyroid measures in U. S. adults and adolescents from the National Health and Nutrition Examination Survey (NHANES) 2007-2008. *Environmental Health Perspectives*, *119*(10), 1396–1402. doi:10.1289/ehp.1103582 PMID:21749963

Meeker, J. D., & Ferguson, K. K. (2012). Dioxins and health: including other persistent organic pollutantsand endocrine disruptors. In *Phthalates: human exposure and related health effects*. Hoboken, NJ: Wiley.

Mehala, D., & Venkatesh, S. (2018). A study on bio medical waste disposal in medicare enviro systems in thanjavur. *IJCESR*, *5*(4), 2394–0697.

Mehta, S., Biederman, S., & Shivkumar, S. (1995). Thermal degradation of foamed polystyrene. *Journal of Materials Science*, *30*(11), 2944–2949. doi:10.1007/BF00349667

Meier, E. (2009). *Material Density*. Retrieved December 20, 2018, from A Psimple Psaltery website: http://www.apsimplepsaltery.com/appendices/material_densities/

Melnick, R. L. (2001). Is peroxisome proliferation an obligatory precursor step in the carcinogenicity of di (2-ethylhexyl) phthalate (DEHP)? *Environmental Health Perspectives*, *109*(5), 437–442. doi:10.1289/ehp.01109437 PMID:11401753

Melzer, D., Gates, P., Osborne, N. J., & … ., & Grainger, D. (2012). Urinary Bisphenol A concentration and angiography-defined coronary artery stenosis. *PLoS One*, *7*(8), 43378. doi:10.1371/journal.pone.0043378 PMID:22916252

Melzer, D., Osborne, N. J., Henley, W. E., Cipelli, R., Young, A., Money, C., … Galloway, T. S. (2012). Urinary Bisphenol A concentration and risk of future coronary artery disease in apparently healthy men and women. *Circulation*, *125*(12), 1482–1490. doi:10.1161/CIRCULATIONAHA.111.069153 PMID:22354940

Melzer, D., Rice, N. E., Lewis, C., Henley, W. E., & Galloway, T. S. (2010). Association of urinary Bisphenol A concentration with heart disease: Evidence from NHANES 2003/06. *PLoS One*, *5*(1), 8673. doi:10.1371/journal.pone.0008673 PMID:20084273

Mendez, C. R., Vergaray, G., Vilma, R., Karina, B., & Cardenas, J. (2007). Isolation and characterization of polyethylene-biodegrading mycromycetes. *Revista Peruana de Biología*, *13*(3), 203–205.

Mendiola, J., Stahlhut, R. W., Jørgensen, N., Liu, F., & Swan, S. H. (2011). Shorter anogenital distance predicts poorer semen quality in young men in Rochester, New York. *Environmental Health Perspectives*, *119*(7), 958–963. doi:10.1289/ehp.1103421 PMID:21377950

Mendoza, A. (2018). The Impacts of Plastic Pollution in the Great Lakes. California State University, Sacramento ENVS 190.

Mendum, T., Stoler, E. V., & Warner, J. (2010). *Concentration of Bisphenol A in thermal paper*. Retrieved from http://advancinggreenchemistry.org /?p=1176

Metabolix. (2013a). *Why integrate biopolymers into your conversion process?* Retrieved from http://www.metabolix.com/converters

Metabolix. (2013b). *Crop-based technologies.* Retrieved from http://www.metabolix.com/Products/Crop-based-Technologies

Michalowicz, J. (2014). Bisphenol A--sources, toxicity and biotransformation. Environmental Toxicology and Pharmacology, 37(2), 738–758. doi:10.1016/j.etap.2014.02.003 PubMed doi:10.1016/j.etap.2014.02.003 PMID:24632011

Middleton, J. C., & Tipton, A. J. (1998). Synthetic biodegradable polymers as medical devices. *Med. Plastics Biomater. Mag*, *3*, 30.

Miguel, O., Fernandez-Berridi, M. J., & Iruin, J. J. (1997). Survey on transport properties of liquids, vapors, and gases in biodegradable poly(3-hydroxybutyrate) (PHB). *Journal of Applied Polymer Science, 64*, 1849–1859. DOI: <1849 doi:10.1002/(sici)1097-4628(19970531)64:9

Mihovec-Grdiæ, M., Šmit, Z., Puntariæ, D., & Bošnir, J. (2002). Phthalates in underground waters of the Zagreb area. *Croatian Medical Journal*, *43*(4), 493–497. PMID:12187530

Miller, R. (2005). The landscape for biopolymers in packaging. Miller-Klein Associates report Summary and Full Report.

Miller, K., McAdam, R., & McAdam, M. (2018). A systematic literature review of university technology transfer from a quadruple helix perspective: Toward a research agenda. *R & D Management*, *48*(1), 7–24. doi:10.1111/radm.12228

Milne, B. J., Behie, L. A., & Berruti, F. (1999). Recycling of waste plastics by ultrapyrolysis using an internally circulating fluidized bed reactor. *Journal of Analytical and Applied Pyrolysis*, *51*(1-2), 157–166. doi:10.1016/S0165-2370(99)00014-5

Min, H., & Ko, H.-J. (2008). The Dynamic Design of a Reverse Logistics Network from the Perspective of Third-Party Logistics Service Providers. *International Journal of Production Economics*, *113*(1), 176–192. doi:10.1016/j.ijpe.2007.01.017

Ministry for the Environment. (2006). *Product stewardship case study for end– of– life tyres*. Author.

Ministry for the Environment. (2012). Quantity of solid waste sent to landfill indicator update. *Info*, 654.

Ministry of Environment. (2016). *Forest and Climate Change*. Plastic Waste Management Rules.

Miodovnik, A., Edwards, A., Bellinger, D. C., & Hauser, R. (2014). Developmental neurotoxicity of ortho-phthalate diesters: Review of human and experimental evidence. *Neurotoxicol.*, *41*, 112–122. doi:10.1016/j.neuro.2014.01.007 PMID:24486776

Miodovnik, A., Engel, S. M., Zhu, C., Ye, X., Soorya, L. V., Silva, M. J., ... Wolff, M. S. (2011). Endocrine disruptors and childhood social impairment. *Neurotoxicology*, *32*(2), 261–267. doi:10.1016/j.neuro.2010.12.009 PMID:21182865

Mirenda, P., & Beukelman, D. R. (1987). A Comparison of Speech Synthesis Intelligibility with Listeners from Three Age Groups. *Augmentative and Alternative Communication*, *3*(3), 120–128. doi:10.1080/07434618712331274399

Missiaen, L., Dode, L., Vanoevelen, D., Raeymaekers, L., & Wuytack, F. (2007). Calcium in the Golgi apparatus. *Cell Calcium*, *41*(5), 405–416. doi:10.1016/j.ceca.2006.11.001 PMID:17140658

Miyamoto, K., & Kotake, M. (2006). Estimation of daily Bisphenol A intake of Japanese individuals with emphasis on uncertainty and variability. *Environmental Sciences*, *13*, 15–29. PMID:16685249

Mohamed Nor, N. H., & Obbard, J. P. (2014). Microplastics in Singapore's coastal mangrove ecosystems. *Marine Pollution Bulletin*, *79*(1–2), 278–283. doi:10.1016/j.marpolbul.2013.11.025 PMID:24365455

Mohammed, M., Ozbay, I., Karademir, A., & Isleyen, M. (2017). Pre– treatment and utilization of food waste as energy source by bio– drying process. *Energy Procedia*, *128*, 100–107. doi:10.1016/j.egypro.2017.09.021

Mohan Babu & Mettilda. (2014). Studies on Mechanical, Thermal, and Morphological Properties of Glass Fibre Reinforced Polyoxymethylene Nanocomposite. *Journal of Applied Chemistry*.

Mohan, S. K., & Srivastava, T. (2010). Microbial deterioration and degradation of polymeric materials. *Journal of Biochemical Technology*, *2*, 210–215.

Mohanty, C. R., Mishra, U., & Beuria, P. R. (2014). Municipal solid waste management in Bhubaneswar, India—a review. *Int. J. Latest Trends Eng. Technol*, *3*(3), 303–312.

Mohee, R., Unmar, G. D., Mudhoo, A., & Khadoo, P. (2008). Biodegradability of biodegradable/degradable plastic materials under aerobic and anaerobic conditions. *Waste Management (New York, N.Y.)*, *28*(9), 1624–1629. doi:10.1016/j.wasman.2007.07.003 PMID:17826972

Mok-Lin, E., Ehrlich, S., Williams, P. L., Petrozza, J., Wright, D. L., Calafat, A. M., ... Hauser, R. (2010). Urinary bisphenol A concentrations and ovarian response among women undergoing IVF. *International Journal of Andrology*, *33*(2), 385–393. doi:10.1111/j.1365-2605.2009.01014.x PMID:20002217

Molenaar, E. A., Van Ameijden, E. J., Grobbee, D. E., & Numans, M. E. (2007). Comparison of routine care self-reported and biometrical data on hypertension and diabetes: Results of the Utrecht Health Project. *European Journal of Public Health*, *17*(2), 199–205. doi:10.1093/eurpub/ckl113 PMID:16887835

Moller, L., Leck, F., Og, F., Bo, P., & Larsen, D. H. I. (2012). *Survey of Bisphenol A and Bisphenol A diglycidylether polymer.* The Danish Environmental Protection Agency Strandgade Copenhagen K, Denmark. Retrieved from www.mst.dk/english

Monteith, G. R., McAndrew, D., Faddy, H. M., & Roberts-Thomson, S. J. (2007). Calcium and cancer: Targeting Ca2+ transport. *Nature Reviews. Cancer*, *7*(7), 519–530. doi:10.1038/nrc2171 PMID:17585332

Montuori, P., Jover, E., Morgantini, M., Bayona, J. M., & Triassi, M. (2008). Assessing human exposure to phthalic acid and phthalate esters from mineral water stored in polyethylene terephthalate and glass bottles. *Food Additives and Contaminants*, *25*(4), 511–518. doi:10.1080/02652030701551800 PMID:18348049

Moody, K. (1988). *An Injury to One*. London, UK: Verso.

Moore, C. J. (2008). Synthetic polymers in the marine environment: A rapidly increasing, long-term threat. *Environmental Research*, *108*(2), 131–139. doi:10.1016/j.envres.2008.07.025 PMID:18949831

Moore, C. J., Moore, S. L., Leecaster, M. K., & Weisberg, S. B. (2001). A comparison of plastic and plankton in the North Pacific Central Gyre. *Marine Pollution Bulletin*, *42*(12), 1297–1300. doi:10.1016/S0025-326X(01)00114-X PMID:11827116

Moore, C. J., Moore, S. L., Weisberg, S. B., Lattin, G. L., & Zellers, A. F. (2002). A comparison of neustonic plastic and zooplankton abundance in southern California's coastal waters. *Marine Pollution Bulletin*, *44*(10), 1035–1038. doi:10.1016/S0025-326X(02)00150-9 PMID:12474963

Moore, E., Lyday, S., Roletto, J., Litle, K., Parrish, J. K., Nevins, H., ... Kell, S. (2009). Entanglements of marine mammals and seabirds in central California and the north-west coast of the United States 2001-2005. *Marine Pollution Bulletin*, *58*(7), 1045–1051. doi:10.1016/j.marpolbul.2009.02.006 PMID:19344921

Morales-Suárez-Varela, M. M., Toft, G. V., Jensen, M. S., Ramlau-Hansen, C., Kaerlev, L., Thulstrup, A. M., ... Bonde, J. P. (2011). Parental occupational exposure to endocrine disrupting chemicals and male genital malformations: A study in the Danish National Birth Cohort study. *Environmental Health*, *10*(1), 3. doi:10.1186/1476-069X-10-3 PMID:21235764

Moritz, J. M. (1995). Current legislation governing clinical waste disposal. *The Journal of Hospital Infection*, *30*(supplement), 521–530. doi:10.1016/0195-6701(95)90058-6 PMID:7560993

Moriyama, K., Tagami, T., Akamizu, T., Usui, T., Saijo, M., Kanamoto, N., ... Nakao, K. (2002). Thyroid hormone action is disrupted by Bisphenol A as an antagonist. *The Journal of Clinical Endocrinology and Metabolism*, *87*(11), 5185–5190. doi:10.1210/jc.2002-020209 PMID:12414890

Morrissey, S. (2008).. . *Chemical and Engineering News*.

Mose, T., Mortensen, G. K., Hedegaard, M., & Knudsen, L. E. (2007). Phthalate monoesters in perfusate from a dual placenta perfusion system, the placenta tissue and umbilical cord blood. *Reproductive Toxicology (Elmsford, N.Y.)*, *23*(1), 83–91. doi:10.1016/j.reprotox.2006.08.006 PMID:17049806

Mucha, M., (1976). Thermogravimetric studies on polymethylenes and polyethylenes. *Journal of Polymer Science*, 25-31.

Mu, D., Gao, F., Fan, Z., Shen, H., Peng, H., & Hu, J. (2015). Levels of Phthalate Metabolites in Urine of Pregnant Women and Risk of Clinical Pregnancy Loss. *Environmental Science & Technology*, *49*(17), 10651–10657. doi:10.1021/acs.est.5b02617 PMID:26251123

Muhonja, C. N., Makonde, H., Magoma, G., & Imbuga, M. (2018). Biodegradability of polyethylene by bacteria and fungi from Dandora dumpsite Nairobi-Kenya. *PLoS One*, *13*(7), e0198446. doi:10.1371/journal.pone.0198446 PMID:29979708

Müller, K., Bugnicourt, E., Latorre, M., Jorda, M., Echegoyen Sanz, Y., Lagaron, J. M., ... Schmid, M. (2017). Review on the Processing and Properties of Polymer Nanocomposites and Nanocoatings and Their Applications in the Packaging, Automotive and Solar Energy Fields. *Nanomaterials (Basel, Switzerland)*, *7*(4), 74. doi:10.3390/nano7040074 PMID:28362331

Munguia-Lopez, E. M., Gerardo-Lugo, S., Peralta, E., Bolumen, S., & Soto-Valdez, H. (2005). Migration of Bisphenol A (BISPHENOL A) from can coatings into a fatty-food simulant and tuna fish. *Food Additives and Contaminants*, *22*(9), 892–898. doi:10.1080/02652030500163674 PMID:16192075

Munguia-Lopez, E. M., & Soto-Valtez, H. (2001). Effect of heat processing and storage time on migration of Bisphenol A (BISPHENOL A) and Bisphenol A diglycidyl ether (BADGE) to aqueous food stimulant from Mexican can coatings. *Journal of Agricultural and Food Chemistry*, *49*(8), 3666–3671. doi:10.1021/jf0009044 PMID:11513645

Murakami, K., Ohashi, A., Hori, H., Hibiya, M., Shoji, Y., Kunisaki, M., ... Sugiyama, S. (2007). Accumulation of Bisphenol A in hemodialysis patients. *Blood Purification*, *25*(3), 290–294. doi:10.1159/000104869 PMID:17622711

Murature, D. A., Tang, S. Y., Steinhardt, G., & Dougherty, R. C. (1987). Phthalate esters and semen quality parameters. *Biomedical & Environmental Mass Spectrometry*, *14*(8), 473–477. doi:10.1002/bms.1200140815 PMID:2957007

Murphy, R., & Bartle, I. (2004). *Summary report, biodegradable polymers and sustainability: insight from life cycle assessment*. National Non Food Crops Centre.

Murray, T. J., Maffini, M. V., Ucci, A. A., Sonnenschein, C., & Soto, A. M. (2007). Induction of mammary gland ductal hyperplasias and carcinoma in situ following fetal Bisphenol A exposure. *Reproductive Toxicology (Elmsford, N.Y.)*, *23*(3), 383–390. doi:10.1016/j.reprotox.2006.10.002 PMID:17123778

Musdalslien, M., & Sandberg, P. (2002, April). Energy and HCL recovery from PVC in municipal solid waste incineration. In *PVC 2002: towards a sustainable future Conf. Proc.* London, UK: IOM Communications.

Myers, J. P., vom Saal, F. S., Akingbemi, B. T., Arizono, K., Belcher, S., Colborn, T., . . . Zoeller, R. T. (2009). Why public health agencies cannot depend on good laboratory practices as a criterion for selecting data: The case of bisphenol A. Environmental Health Perspectives, 117(3), 309–315. doi:10.1289/ehp.0800173 PubMed doi:10.1289/ehp.0800173 PMID:19337501

Mylchreest, E., Cattley, R. C., & Foster, P. M. (1998). Male reproductive tract malformations in rats following gestational and lactational exposure to di (n-butyl) phthalate: An antiandrogenic mechanism? *Toxicological Sciences*, *43*(1), 47–60. doi:10.1093/toxsci/43.1.47 PMID:9629619

Mylchreest, E., Sar, M., Cattley, R. C., & Foster, P. M. (1999). Disruption of androgen-regulated male reproductive development by di (n-butyl) phthalate during late gestation in rats is different from flutamide. *Toxicology and Applied Pharmacology*, *156*(2), 81–95. doi:10.1006/taap.1999.8643 PMID:10198273

Mylchreest, E., Wallace, D. G., Cattley, R. C., & Foster, P. M. (2000). Dose-dependent alterations in androgen-regulated male reproductive development in rats exposed to di (n-butyl) phthalate during late gestation. *Toxicological Sciences*, *55*(1), 143–151. doi:10.1093/toxsci/55.1.143 PMID:10788569

Nagorka, R., Conrad, A., Scheller, C., Sussenbach, B., & Moriske, H. J. (2010). Plasticizers and flame retardants in household dust — part 1: Phthalates. Gefahrstoffe — Reinhalt. *Luft*, *70*(3), 70–76.

Nahar, M. S., Liao, C., Kannan, K., & Dolinoy, D. C. (2012). Fetal Liver Bisphenol A Concentrations and Biotransformation Gene Expression Reveal Variable Exposure and Altered Capacity for Metabolism in Humans. *Journal of Biochemical and Molecular Toxicology*, *27*(2), 116–123. doi:10.1002/jbt.21459 PMID:23208979

Nahar, M. S., Soliman, A. S., Colacino, J. A., Calafat, A. M., Battige, K., Hablas, A., ... Rozek, L. S. (2012). Urinary Bisphenol A concentrations in girls from rural and urban Egypt: A pilot study. *Environmental Health, 11*(1), 20. doi:10.1186/1476-069X-11-20 PMID:22472083

Nah, W. H., Park, M. J., & Gye, M. C. (2011). Effects of early prepubertal exposure to Bisphenol A on the onset of puberty, ovarian weights, and estrous cycle in female mice. *Clinical and Experimental Reproductive Medicine*, *38*(2), 75–81. doi:10.5653/cerm.2011.38.2.75 PMID:22384422

Najam, A., & Bari, F. (2017). *Pakistan National Human Development Report 2017.* Islamabad: United Nations Development Programme. Retrieved from http://www.pk.undp.org/content/dam/pakistan/docs/HDR/PK-NHDR.pdf

Nakagawa, Y., & Suzuki, T. (2002). Metabolism of 2-hydroxy-4-methoxybenzophenone in isolated rat hepatocytes and xenoestrogenic effects of its metabolites on MCF-7 human breast cancer cells. *Chemico-Biological Interactions*, *139*(2), 115–128. doi:10.1016/S0009-2797(01)00293-9 PMID:11823001

Nakajima, Y., Goldblum, R. M., & Midoro-Horiuti, T. (2012). Fetal exposure to bisphenol A as a risk factor for the development of childhood asthma: An animal model study. [Excellent animal model of BPA exposure.]. Environmental Health, 11(1), 8. doi:10.1186/1476-069X-11-8 PubMed doi:10.1186/1476-069X-11-8 PMID:22353195

Nam, S., Seo, Y., & Kim, M. (2010). Bisphenol A migration from polycarbonate baby bottle with repeated use. *Chemosphere*, *79*(9), 949–952. doi:10.1016/j.chemosphere.2010.02.049 PMID:20334893

Nanda, S., Sahu, S. S., Abraham, J. (2010). Studies on the biodegradation of natural and synthetic polyethylene by Pseudomonas sp. *Journal of Applied Sciences & Environmental Management,* (2), 57-60.

Nanda, S., Sahu, S., & Abraham, J. (2010). Studies on the biodegradation of natural and synthetic polyethylene by Pseudomonas spp. *Journal of Applied Science & Environmental Management*, *14*(2), 57–60. doi:10.4314/jasem.v14i2.57839

Napper, I. E., & Thompson, R. C. (2016). Release of synthetic microplastic plastic fibres from domestic washing machines: Effects of fabric type and washing conditions. *Marine Pollution Bulletin*, *112*(1-2), 39–45. doi:10.1016/j.marpolbul.2016.09.025 PMID:27686821

Narayan, P. (2001). *Analyzing Plastic Waste Management in India: Case study of Polybags and PET bottles published by IIIEE.* Lund University Sweden.

Narayan, P. (2001). *Analyzing Plastic Waste Management in India: Case study of Polybags and PET bottles.* Lund University.

Narayan, R. (2006a). Biobased and biodegradable polymer materials: rationale, drivers, and technology exemplars. *American Chemical Society Symposium Ser.*, *939*(18), 282. 10.1021/bk-2006-0939.ch018

Narayan, R. (1994). In Y. Doi, & K. Fukuda (Eds.), *Biodegradable plastics and polymers* (p. 261). New York, NY: Elsevier. doi:10.1016/B978-0-444-81708-2.50026-9

Nasser, F., & Lynch, I. (2016). Secreted protein eco-corona mediates uptake and impacts of polystyrene nanoparticles on Daphnia magna. *Journal of Proteomics*, *137*, 45–51. doi:10.1016/j.jprot.2015.09.005 PMID:26376098

Nataraj, S. K., Yang, K. S., & Aminabhabi, T. M. (2012). Polyacrylonitrile-based nanofibers—A state-of-the-art review. *Progress in Polymer Science*, *37*(3), 487–513. doi:10.1016/j.progpolymsci.2011.07.001

National Assembly of Pakistan. (2012, February 28). *The Constitution of the Islamic Republic of Pakistan.* Retrieved from National Assembly of Pakistan: http://na.gov.pk/uploads/documents/1333523681_951.pdf

National Oceanic and Atmospheric Administration. (2012). *How Much Would it Cost to Clean up the Pacific Garbage Patches*. Retrieved August 20, 2016, from Office of Response and Restoration website: http://response.restoration.noaa.gov/about/media/how-much-would-it-cost-clean-pacific-garbage-patches.html

National Research Council. (2008). *Pthalates and cumulative risk assessment the task ahead. Committee on the health risk of pthalates*. National research council.

National Toxicology Program USDOHAHS (2008). *NTP-CERHR Monograph on the Potential Human Reproductive and Developmental Effects of Bisphenol A. 08–5994*. Author.

National Toxicology Program, Center for the Evaluation of Risks to Human Reproduction (NTP-CERHR): Monograph on the Potential Human Reproductive and Developmental Effects of Butyl Benzyl Phthalate (BBP). (2003). NIH Publication No. 03–4487.

National Toxicology Program, Center for the Evaluation of Risks to Human Reproduction. NTP-CERHR Expert Panel Report on Di(2-Ethylhexyl) Phthalate. (2000). Available at: http://cerhr.niehs.nih.gov/news/index.html

National Toxicology Program. (2018). Draft NTP Research Report on the CLARITY-BPA Core Study: A Perinatal and Chronic Extended-Dose-Range Study of Bisphenol A in Rats. Retrieved from https://ntp.niehs.nih.gov/ntp/about_ntp/rrprp/2018/april/rr09peerdraft.pdf

Needham, L. L., Patterson, D. G. Jr, Barr, D. B., Grainger, J., & Calafat, A. M. (2005). Uses of speciation techniques in biomonitoring for assessing human exposure to organic environmental chemi- cals. *Analytical and Bioanalytical Chemistry*, *381*(2), 397–404. doi:10.100700216-004-2975-5 PMID:15616776

Nel, A., Xia, T., Madler, L., Li, N. (2006). *Toxic Potential of Materials at the Nanolevel*. Academic Press.

Nel, A. (2006, February 3). Toxic Potential of Materials at the Nanolevel. *Science*, *311*(5761), 622–627. doi:10.1126cience.1114397

Nelms, S. E., Duncan, E. M., Broderick, A. C., Galloway, T. S., Godfrey, M. H., Hamann, M., ... Godley, B. J. (2016). Plastic and marine turtles: A review and call for research. *ICES Journal of Marine Science*, *73*(2), 165–181. doi:10.1093/icesjms/fsv165

Nerland, I. L., Halsband, C., Allan, I., & Thomas, K. V. (2014). *Microplastics in marine environments: occurrence, distribution and effects (Re.no.6754-2014)*. Oslo: Norwegian Institute for Water Research.

Net, S., Dumoulin, D., El-Osmani, R., Rabodonirina, S., & Ouddane, B. (2014). Case study of PAHs, Me-PAHs, PCBs, phthalates and pesticides contamination in the Somme River water, France. *International Journal of Environmental of Research*, *8*(4), 1159–1170.

Net, S., Rabodonirina, S., Ben Sghaier, R., Dumoulin, D., Chbib, C., Tlili, I., & … . (2015). Distribution of phthalates, pesticides and drug residues in the dissolved, particulate and sedimentary phases from transboundary rivers (France–Belgium). *The Science of the Total Environment*, *521-522*, 152–159. doi:10.1016/j.scitotenv.2015.03.087 PMID:25829293

Net, S., Sempere, R., Delmont, A., Paluselli, A., & Ouddane, B. (2015). Occurrence, fate, behavior and ecotoxicological state of phthalates in different environmental matrices. *Environmental Science & Technology*, *49*(7), 4019–4035. doi:10.1021/es505233b PMID:25730609

Neves, D., Sobral, P., Ferreira, J. L., & Pereira, T. (2015). Ingestion of microplastics by commercial fish off the Portuguese coast. *Marine Pollution Bulletin*, *101*(1), 119–126. doi:10.1016/j.marpolbul.2015.11.008 PMID:26608506

Newbold, R. R., Padilla-Banks, E., Snyder, R. J., Phillips, T. M., Jefferson, W. N. (2007). Developmental exposure to endocrine disruptors and the obesity epidemic. *Reprod Toxicol., 23*. 290–296. doi:10.1016/j.reprotox

Newbold, R. R. (2010). Impact of environmental endocrine disrupting chemicals on the development of obesity. *Hormones (Athens, Greece)*, *9*(3), 206–217. doi:10.14310/horm.2002.1271 PMID:20688618

Newbold, R. R., Padilla-Banks, E., Jefferson, W. N., & Heindel, J. J. (2008). Effects of endocrine disruptors on obesity. *International Journal of Andrology*, *31*(2), 201–208. doi:10.1111/j.1365-2605.2007.00858.x PMID:18315718

News, R. X. (2013, March 5). "Chemically inducible expression of biosynthetic pathways" in patent application approval process. *Life Science Weekly*. Retrieved from http://www.highbeam.com/doc/1G1-323547527.html

Ng, M., Fleming, T., Robinson, M., Thomson, B., Graetz, N., Margono, C., ... Abraham, J. P. (2014). Global, regional, and national prevalence ofoverweight and obesity in children and adults during 1980–2013: A systematic analysis for theGlobal Burden of Disease Study 2013. *Lancet*, *384*(9945), 766–781. doi:10.1016/S0140-6736(14)60460-8 PMID:24880830

Nguyen, A. (2018). *Under the plastic sea, the earth is screaming for help*. Academic Press.

Nie, L., & Wu, H. (2016). Investigation and Analysis of Rural Medical Waste Management. *Journal of Environmental Protection*, *07*(01), 93–98. doi:10.4236/jep.2016.71009

Ni, H.-G., Lu, S.-Y., Mo, T., & Zeng, H. (2016). Brominated flame retardant emissions from the open burning of five plastic wastes and implications for environmental exposure in China. *Environmental Pollution*, *214*, 70–76. doi:10.1016/j.envpol.2016.03.049 PMID:27064612

Niino, T., Ishibashi, T., Itho, T., Sakai, S., Ishiwata, H., Yamada, T., & Onodera, S. (2002). Simultaneous determination of phthalate di-and monoesters in poly (vinylchloride) products and human saliva by gas chromatography–mass spectrometry. *Journal of Chromatography. B, Analytical Technologies in the Biomedical and Life Sciences*, *780*(1), 35–44. doi:10.1016/S1570-0232(02)00413-0 PMID:12383478

Nikbakhsh, E., Eskandarpour, M., & Zegordi, S. H. (2013). Designing a Robust Post-Sales Reverse Logistics Network. *Electrical Engineering and Intelligent Systems*, 313-325.

Nikles, D. E., & Farahat, M. S. (2005). New motivation for the depolymerization products derived from PET waste: A review. *Macromolecular Materials and Engineering*, *290*, 13–30. doi:10.1002/mame.200400186

Nikolaidis, Y. (2012). Reverse Logistics and Quality Management Issues: State-of-the-Art. *Quality Management in Reverse Logistics: A Broad Look on Quality Issues and Their Interaction With Closed-Loop Supply Chains*, 1.

Ning, G., Bi, Y., Wang, T., Xu, M., Xu, Y., Huang, Y., … Wu, Y. (2011). Relationship of urinary Bisphenol A concentration to risk for prevalent type 2 diabetes in Chinese adults: a cross-sectional analysis. *Ann Intern Med.*, *155*(6), 368-374.

Nisar, H., Ejaz, N., Naushad, Z., & Ali, Z. (2008). Impacts of solid waste management in Pakistan: A case study of Rawalpindi city. *WIT Transactions on Ecology and the Environment*, *109*, 685–691. doi:10.2495/WM080701

Nishida, H., & Tokiwa, Y. (1993). Distribution of poly (β-hydroxybutyrate) and poly (ε-caprolactone) aerobic degrading microorganisms in different environments. *Journal of Environmental Polymer Degradation*, *1*(3), 227–233. doi:10.1007/BF01458031

Nishioka, J., Iwahara, C., Kawasaki, M., Yoshizaki, F., Nakayama, H., Takamori, K., . . . Iwabuchi, K. (2012). Di-(2-ethylhexyl) phthalate induces production of inflammatory molecules in human macrophages. Inflammation Research, 61(1), 69–78. doi:10.1007/s00011-011-0390-x PubMed doi:10.100700011-011-0390-x PMID:22005928

Nistor, I., Goseberg, N., & Stolle, J. (2017). Tsunami-Driven Debris Motion and Loads: A Critical Review. *Frontiers in Built Environment*, *3*. doi:10.3389/fbuil.2017.00002

Niu, Y., Zhang, J., Wu, Y., & Shao, B. (2012). Analysis of bisphenol A and alkylphenols in cereals by automated on-line solid-phase extraction and liquid chromatography tandem massspectrometry. *Journal of Agricultural and Food Chemistry*, *60*(24), 6116–6122. doi:10.1021/jf301401k PMID:22646661

Noda, I., Marchessault, R. H., & Terada, M. (1999). *Polymer data handbook*. London: Oxford University Press.

Noorjahan, A., Dhanakumar, S., Mohanraj, R., & Ravichandran, M. (2012). Status of heavy metals distribution in municipal solid waste in Tiruchirappalli City, India. *International Journal of Applied Biology and Pharmaceutical Technology*, *3*(3), 252–258.

North, M. L., Takaro, T. K., Diamond, M. L., & Ellis, A. K. (2014). Effects of phthalates on the development and expression of allergic disease and asthma. Annals of Allergy, Asthma & Immunology, 112(6), 496–502. doi:10.1016/j.anai.2014.03.013 PubMed doi:10.1016/j.anai.2014.03.013 PMID:24726194

North, E. J., & Halden, R. U. (2013). Plastics and environmental health: The road ahead. *Reviews on Environmental Health*, *28*(1), 1–8. doi:10.1515/reveh-2012-0030 PMID:23337043

Northwest Regional Delegation of Public Health. (2005). *Annual Report*. Author.

Nowack, B., & Bucheli, T. D. (2007). Occurrence, behavior and effects of nanoparticles in the environment. *Environmental Pollution*, *150*(1), 5–22. doi:10.1016/j.envpol.2007.06.006 PMID:17658673

NOWPAP MERRAC. (2017). *Understanding of floating marine litter distribution in the NOWPAP region*. MERRAC Technical Report No. 35.

NTP. (1982). Carcinogenesis bioassay of bisphenol A. Natl. Toxicol. Prgram Tech. Rep. 2015, 1–116.

Nwachkwu, S., Obidi, O., & Odocha, C. (2010). Occurrence and recalcitrance of polyethylene bag waste in nigerian soils. *African Journal of Biotechnology*, *9*(37), 6096–6104.

Nwachukwu, S., Obidi, O., & Odocha, C. (2010). Occurrence and recalcitrance of polyethylene bag waste in Nigerian soils. *African Journal of Biotechnology*, *9*, 6096–6104.

O'Brien, E., Bergin, I. L., Dolinoy, D. C., Zaslona, Z., Little, R. J. A., Tao, Y., . . . Mancuso, P. (2014). Perinatal bisphenol A exposure beginning before gestation enhances allergen sensitization, but not pulmonary inflammation, in adult mice. Journal of Developmental Origins of Health and Disease, 5(2), 121–131. doi:10.1017/S204017441400004X PubMed doi:10.1017/S204017441400004X PMID:24847698

O'Brine, T., & Thompson, R. C. (2010). Degradation of plastic carrier bags in the marine environment. *Marine Pollution Bulletin*, *60*(12), 2279–2283. doi:10.1016/j.marpolbul.2010.08.005 PMID:20961585

O'Connor, L. (1994). Improving medical waste disposal. *Mechanical Engineering (New York, N.Y.)*, *116*(5), 56–59.

O'Hanlon, N. J., James, N. A., Masden, E. A., & Bond, A. L. (2017). Seabirds and marine plastic debris in the northeastern Atlantic: A synthesis and recommendations for monitoring and research. *Environmental Pollution*, *231*, 1291–1301. doi:10.1016/j.envpol.2017.08.101 PMID:28917819

O'Toole, G., Kaplan, H. B., & Kolter, R. (2000). Biofilm formation as microbial development. *Annual Review of Microbiology*, *54*(1), 49–79. doi:10.1146/annurev.micro.54.1.49 PMID:11018124

Ochiai, S., ... (2014). CD326(lo)CD103(lo)CD11b(lo) dermal dendritic cells are activated by thymic stromal lymphopoietin during contact sensitization in mice. Journal of Immunology (Baltimore, Md.: 1950), 193(5), 2504–2511. doi:10.4049/jimmunol.1400536 PubMed doi:10.4049/jimmunol.1400536 PMID:25057004

Oeding, V., & Schlegel, H. G. (1973). Beta-ketothiolase from Hydrogenomonas eutropha HI6 and its significance in the regulation of polybeta- hydroxybutyrate metabolism. *The Biochemical Journal*, *134*(1), 239–248. doi:10.1042/bj1340239 PMID:4198758

Office of Technology Assessment (OTA). (1988, October). Issues in medical waste management (Background paper). Washington, DC: U.S. Government Printing Office. (OTA-BP-O-49)

Ogunola, O. S., Onada, O. A., & Falaye, A. E. (2018). Mitigation measures to avert the impacts of plastics and microplasticsin the marine environment (a review). *Environmental Science and Pollution Research International*, *25*(12). doi:10.100711356-018-1499-z PMID:29470754

Oie, L., Hersoug, L. G., & Madsen, J. O. (1997). Residential exposure to plasticizers and its possible role in the pathogenesis of asthma. *Environmental Health Perspectives*, *105*(9), 972–978. doi:10.1289/ehp.97105972 PMID:9374082

Øie, L., Nafstad, P., Botten, G., Magnus, P., & Jaakkola, J. J. (1999). Ventilation in homes and bronchial obstruction in young children. *Epidemiology (Cambridge, Mass.)*, *10*(3), 294–299. doi:10.1097/00001648-199905000-00018 PMID:10230841

Ojo, O. A. (2007). Molecular strategies of microbial adaptation to xenobiotics in natural environment. *Biotechnology and Molecular Biology Review*, *2*(1), 1–13.

Okada, H., Tokunaga, T., Liu, X. H., Takayanagi, S., Matsushima, A., & Shimohigashi, Y. (2008). Direct evidence revealing structural elements essential for the high binding ability of Bisphenol A to human estrogen-related receptor-gamma. *Environmental Health Perspectives*, *116*(1), 32–38. doi:10.1289/ehp.10587 PMID:18197296

Oku, A., Tanaka, S., & Hata, S. (2000). Chemical conversion of poly (carbonate) to bis (hydroxyethyl) ether of bisphenol A. An approach to the chemical recycling of plastic wastes as monomers. *Polymer*, *41*(18), 6749–6753. doi:10.1016/S0032-3861(00)00014-8

Olazar, M., Lopez, G., Amutio, M., Elordi, G., Aguado, R., & Bilbao, J. (2009). Influence of FCC catalyst steaming on HDPE pyrolysis product distribution. *Journal of Analytical and Applied Pyrolysis*, *85*(1-2), 359–365. doi:10.1016/j.jaap.2008.10.016

Olea, N., Pulgar, R., Perez, P., Olea-Serrano, F., Rivas, A., Novillo-Fertrell, A., … Sonnenschein, C. (1996). Estrogenicity of resin-based composites and sealants used in dentistry. *Environ Health Perspect.*, *104*(3), 298-305.

Olea, N., Pulgar, R., P'erez, P., Olea-Serrano, F., Rivas, A., Novillo-Fertrell, A., ... Sonnenschein, C. (1996). Estrogenicity of resinbased composites and sealants used in dentistry. *Environmental Health Perspectives*, *104*(3), 298–305. doi:10.1289/ehp.96104298 PMID:8919768

Oliveira, C. R. D., Bernardes, A. M., & Gerbase, A. E. (2012). Collection and recycling of electronic scrap: A worldwide overview and comparison with the Brazilian situation. *Waste Management.*

Olsén, L., Lampa, E., Birkholz, D. A., Lind, L., & Lind, P. M. (2012). Circulating levels of bisphenol A (BPA) and phthalates in an elderly population in Sweden, based on the Prospective Investigation of the Vasculature in Uppsala Seniors (PIVUS). Ecotoxicology and Environmental Safety, 75(0), 242–248. doi:10.1016/j.ecoenv.2011.09.004 PubMed doi:10.1016/j.ecoenv.2011.09.004 PMID:21955883

Olsen, L., Lind, L., & Lind, P. M. (2012). Associations between circulating levels of Bisphenol A and phthalate metabolites and coronary risk in the elderly. *Ecotoxicol Environ Saf.*, *80*, 179-183.

Onu, P., Vasile, C., Ciocilteu, S., Iojoiu, E., & Darie, H. (1998). Thermal and catalytic decomposition of polyethylene and polypropylene. *Journal of Analytical and Applied Pyrolysis*, *49*(1-2), 145–153. doi:10.1016/S0165-2370(98)00109-0

Onwudilia, J. A., & Williams, P. T. (2016). Catalytic supercritical water gasification of plastics with supported RuO2: A potential solution to hydrocarbonwater pollution problem. *Process Safety and Environmental Protection*, *102*, 140–149. doi:10.1016/j.psep.2016.02.009

Onwudili, J. A., Insura, N., & Williams, P. T. (2009). Composition of products from the pyrolysis of polyethylene and polystyrene in a closed batch reactor: Effects of temperature and residence time. *Journal of Analytical and Applied Pyrolysis*, *86*(2), 293–303. doi:10.1016/j.jaap.2009.07.008

Orós, J., Torrent, A., Calabuig, P., & Déniz, S. (2005). Diseases and causes of mortality among sea turtles stranded in the Canary Islands, Spain (1998-2001). *Diseases of Aquatic Organisms*, *63*(1), 13–24. doi:10.3354/dao063013 PMID:15759796

Ortega, M. A., & Dorrance, A. E. (2011). Microsporogenesis of Rps8/rps8 heterozygous soybean lines. In Euphytica (Vol. 181). doi:10.100710681-011-0422-1

Osz, J., Brelivet, Y., Peluso-Iltis, C., Cura, V., Eiler, S., Ruff, M.,, & .... Moras, D. (2012). Structural basis for a molecular allosteric control mechanism of cofactor binding to nuclear receptors. *Proceedings of the National Academy of Sciences of the United States of America*, *109*(10), 588–594. doi:10.1073/pnas.1118192109 PMID:22203987

Otake, T., Yoshinaga, J., & Yanagisawa, Y. (2001). Analysis of organic esters of plasticizer in indoor air by GC– MS and GC– FPD. *Environmental Science & Technology*, *35*(15), 3099–3102. doi:10.1021/es001914o PMID:11505983

Overington, J. P., Al-Lazikani, B., & Hopkins, A. L. (2006). How many drug targets are there? *Nature Reviews. Drug Discovery*, *5*(12), 993–996. doi:10.1038/nrd2199 PMID:17139284

Owens, B. (2016). *The ghosts of fishers past*. Coastal Science & Societies. Retrieved from www.hakaimagazine.com

Oyedun, A. O., Gebreegziabher, T., Ng, D. K. S., & Hui, C. W. (2014). Mixed-waste pyrolysis of biomass and plastics waste: A modeling approach to reduce energy usage. *Energy*, *75*, 127–135. doi:10.1016/j.energy.2014.05.063

Ozdal, T., & Yesilcubuk, N. S. (2014). Toxicity of Bisphenol A: Effects on health and regulations. *International Scholarly and Scientific Research and Innovation*, *8*(6), 553–557.

Özkır, V., & Başlıgil, H. (2012). Multi-objective optimization of closed-loop supply chains in uncertain environment. *Journal of Cleaner Production*.

Page, B. D., & Lacroix, G. M. (1992). Studies into the transfer and migration of phthalate esters from aluminium foil-paper laminates to butter and margarine. *Food Additives and Contaminants*, *9*(3), 197–212. doi:10.1080/02652039209374064 PMID:1397395

Page, B. D., & Lacroix, G. M. (1995). The occurrence of phthalate ester and di-2-ethylhexyl adipate plasticizers in Canadian packaging and food sampled in 1985–1989: A survey. *Food Additives and Contaminants*, *12*(1), 129–151. doi:10.1080/02652039509374287 PMID:7758627

Pakistan Bureau of Statistics. (2015). *Compendium on Environment Statistics 2015*. Islamabad: Bueau of Statistics, Government of Pakistan. Retrieved from http://www.pbs.gov.pk/sites/default/files//crops_and_climates/compendium_environment/compendium_environment_2015.pdf

Pakistan Bureau of Statistics. (2017). *Provisional Summary Results of 6th Population and Housing Census-2017*. Retrieved from Pakistan Bureau of Statistics, Government of Pakistan: http://www.pbs.gov.pk/content/provisional-summary-results-6th-population-and-housing-census-2017-0

Pałaszewska-Tkacz, A., & Czerczak, S., & Dibutylu, F. (2012). (Di-n-butyl phthalate - inhaled fraction. Occupational exposure limits for phthalates). *Podstawy i Metody Oceny Środ Pracy.*, *73*(3), 37–70.

Panda, A. K., & Singh, R. K. (2011). Catalytic performances of kaoline and silica-alumina in the thermal degradation of polypropylene. *Journal of Fuel Chemistry and Technology*, *39*(3), 198–202. doi:10.1016/S1872-5813(11)60017-0

Panda, A. K., Singh, R. K., & Mishra, D. K. (2010). Thermolysis of waste plastics to liquid fuel: A suitable method for plastic waste management and manufacture of value added products—A world prospective. *Renewable & Sustainable Energy Reviews*, *14*(1), 233–248. doi:10.1016/j.rser.2009.07.005

Pandey, E., Srivastava, K., Gupta, S., Srivastava, S., & Mishra, N. (2016). Some biocompatible materials used in medical practices- A review. *International Journal of Pharmaceutical Sciences and Research.* doi:10.13040/IJPSR.0975-8232.7(7).2748-55

Pandey, A., Ahuja, S., Madan, M., & Asthana, A. K. (2016). Bio-Medical Waste Management in a Tertiary Care Hospital: An Overview. *Journal of Clinical and Diagnostic Research: JCDR*, *10*(11), DC01–DC03. doi:10.7860/JCDR/2016/22595.8822 PMID:28050362

Panepinto, D., Tedesco, V., Brizio, E., & Genon, G. (2015). Environmental performances and energy efficiency for MSW gasification treatment. *Waste and Biomass Valorization*, *6*(1), 123–135. doi:10.100712649-014-9322-7

Pan, G., Hanaoka, T., Yoshimura, M., Zhang, S., Wang, P., Tsukino, H., ... Takahashi, K. (2006). Decreased serum free testosterone in workers exposed to high levels of di-n-butyl phthalate (DBP) and di-2-ethylhexyl phthalate (DEHP): A cross-sectional study in China. *Environmental Health Perspectives*, *114*(11), 1643–1648. doi:10.1289/ehp.9016 PMID:17107847

Pang, X., & Tang, Z. (2010). Polylactic acid (PLA): Research, development and industrialization. *Biotechnology Journal*, *5*(11), 1125–1136. doi:10.1002/biot.201000135 PMID:21058315

Pant, N., Shukla, M., Patel, D. K., Shukla, Y., Mathur, N., Gupta, Y. K., & Saxena, D. K. (2008). Correlation of phthalate exposures with semen quality. *Toxicology and Applied Pharmacology*, *231*(1), 112–116. doi:10.1016/j.taap.2008.04.001 PMID:18513777

Papaconstantinou, A. D., Umbreit, T. H., Fisher, B. R., Goering, P. L., Lappas, N. T., & Brown, K. M. (2000). Bisphenol A-induced increase in uterine weight and alterations in uterine morphology in ovariectomized B6C3F1 mice: role of the estrogen receptor. *Toxicol Sci, 56*, 332–339.

Parcheta, P., & Datta, J. (2017). Environmental impact and industrial development of biorenewable resources for polyurethanes. *Critical Reviews in Environmental Science and Technology*, *47*(20), 1986–2016. doi:10.1080/10643389.2017.1400861

Paris, I., Ruggieri, F., Mazzeo, P., & Carlucci, G. (2003). Simultaneous determination of di (2-ethylhexyl) phthalate and mono (2-ethylhexyl) phthalate in human plasma by high-performance liquid chromatography. *Analytical Letters*, *36*(12), 2649–2658. doi:10.1081/AL-120024639

Park, H. S., & Jeong, J. W. (2001). Recent trends on disposal technologies of medical waste. *J. Korean Solid Wastes Engineering Soc*, *18*(1), 18–27.

Park, H.-J. (2008). Pyrolysis of polypropylene over mesoporous MCM-48 material. *Journal of Physics and Chemistry of Solids*, *69*(5-6), 1125–1128. doi:10.1016/j.jpcs.2007.10.083

Park, J. W., Oh, S. C., Lee, H. P., Kim, H. T., & Yoo, K. O. (2000). Kinetic analysis of thermal decomposition of polymer using a dynamic model. *Korean Journal of Chemical Engineering*, *17*(5), 489–496. doi:10.1007/BF02707154

Park, M. A., Hwang, K. A., Lee, H. R., Yi, B. R., Jeung, E. B., & Choi, K. C. (2012). Cell growth of BG-1 ovarian cancer cells is promoted by di-n-butyl phthalate and hexabromocyclododecane via upregulation of the cyclin D and cyclin-dependent kinase-4 genes. *Molecular Medicine Reports*, *5*(3), 761–766. doi:10.3892/mmr.2011.712 PMID:22179484

Park, S. S., Seo, D. K., Lee, S. H., Yu, T. U., & Hwang, J. (2012). Study on pyrolysis characteristics of refuse plastic fuel using lab-scale tube furnace and thermogravimetric analysis reactor. *Journal of Analytical and Applied Pyrolysis*, *97*, 29–38. doi:10.1016/j.jaap.2012.06.009

Parks, L. G., Ostby, J. S., Lambright, C. R., Abbott, B. D., Klinefelter, G. R., Barlow, N. J., & Gray, L. E. Jr. (2000). The plasticizer diethylhexyl phthalate induces malformations by decreasing fetal testosterone synthesis during sexual differentiation in the male rat. *Toxicological Sciences*, *58*(2), 339–349. doi:10.1093/toxsci/58.2.339 PMID:11099646

Parlikad, A. K., & McFarlane, D. (2009). Strategies for product recovery decisions. *International Journal of Product Lifecycle Management*, *4*(1), 186–206. doi:10.1504/IJPLM.2009.031673

Partk, K. (2016). Nylon (Chemistry, Properties and Uses). *International Journal of Scientific Research*, *5*(9), 349–351.

Partners, C. (2010). *Plastic Products*. Islamabad: State Bank of Pakistan; Retrieved from http://www.sbp.org.pk/departments/ihfd/Sub-Segment%20Booklets/Plastic%20Products.pdf

Passamonti, F. J., & Sedran, U. (2012). Recycling of waste plastics into fuels. LDPE conversion in FCC. *Applied Catalysis B: Environmental*, *125*, 499–506. doi:10.1016/j.apcatb.2012.06.020

Passow, U., De La Rocha, C. L., Fairfield, C., & Schmidt, K. (2014). Aggregation as a function of PCO2and mineral particles. *Limnology and Oceanography*, *59*(2), 532–547. doi:10.4319/lo.2014.59.2.0532

Passow, U., Ziervogel, K., Asper, V., & Diercks, A. (2012). Marine snow formation in the aftermath of the Deepwater Horizon oil spill in the Gulf of Mexico. *Environmental Research Letters*, *7*(3), 1–11. doi:10.1088/1748-9326/7/3/035301

Patel, S., Brehm, E., Gao, L., Rattan, S., Ziv-Gal, A., & Flaws, J. A. (2017). Bisphenol A exposure, ovarian follicle numbers, and female sex steroid hormone levels: Results from a CLARITYBPA study. Endocrinology, 158(6), 1727–1738. doi:10.1210/en.2016-1887 PubMed doi:10.1210/en.2016-1887 PMID:28324068

Pavani & Rajeswari. (2014). Impact of plastics on environmental pollution. *Journal of Chemical and Pharmaceutical Sciences*, 87-93.

Pavani, P., & Raja Rajeswari, T. (2014). Impact of plastics on environmental pollution. *Journal of Chemical and Pharmaceutical Sciences,* 2087-2093.

Pawar. (2016). A Review Article on Acrylic PMMA. *IOSR Journal of Mechanical and Civil Engineering, 13*(2), 1-4.

Pearce, A., Jackson, G., & Cresswell, G. R. (2018). Marine debris pathways across the southern Indian Ocean. *Deep-sea Research. Part II, Topical Studies in Oceanography*. doi:10.1016/j.dsr2.2018.06.009

Peavey, H. S., Donald, R. R., & Gorge, G. (1985). *Environmental Engineering*. Singapore: McGraw– Hill Book Co.

Peciulyte, D. (2002). Microbial colonization and biodeterioration of plasticized polyvinyl chloride plastics. *Ekologija (Lietuvos Mokslu Akademija)*, *4*, 7–15.

Peck, J. D., Sweeney, A. M., Symanski, E., Gardiner, J., Silva, M. J., Calafat, A. M., & Schantz, S. L. (2009). Intra- and inter-individual variability of urinary phthalate metabolite concentrations in Hmong women of reproductive age. *Journal of Exposure Science & Environmental Epidemiology*. doi:10.1038/jes.2009.4 PMID:19223940

Pedà, C., Caccamo, L., Fossi, M. C., Gai, F., Andaloro, F., Genovese, L., ... Maricchiolo, G. (2016). Intestinal alterations in European sea bass Dicentrarchuslabrax (Linnaeus, 1758) exposed to microplastics: Preliminary results. *Environmental Pollution*, *212*, 251–256. doi:10.1016/j.envpol.2016.01.083 PMID:26851981

Peijnenburg, W. J. G. M., Sven, E. J., & Brian, F. (2008). Phthalates. In S. E. Jørgensen & B. D. Fath (Eds.), *Encyclopedia of Ecology*. Oxford, UK: Academic Press. doi:10.1016/B978-008045405-4.00419-5

Peijnenburg, W. J., & Struijs, J. (2006). Occurrence of phthalate esters in the environment of the Netherlands. *Ecotoxicology and Environmental Safety*, *63*(2), 204–215. doi:10.1016/j.ecoenv.2005.07.023 PMID:16168482

Perez, J., Dorada, J. M., & Rubia, T. D. L. (2002). Biodegradation and biological treatments of cellulose, hemicelluloses and lignin: An overview. *International Microbiology*, *5*(2), 53–63. doi:10.100710123-002-0062-3 PMID:12180781

Perrot, J. F., & Subiantoro, A. (2018). Municipal waste management strategy review and waste– to– energy potentials in New Zealand. *Sustainability*, *10*(9), 1–12. doi:10.3390u10093114 PMID:30607262

Petersen, J. H., & Jensen, L. K. (2010). Phthalates and food-contact materials: Enforcing the 2008 European Union plastics legislation. *Food Additives and Contaminants*, *27*(11), 1608–1616. doi:10.1080/19440049.2010.501825 PMID:20737341

Petzold, S., Averbeck, M., Simon, J. C., Lehmann, I., & Polte, T. (2014). Lifetime-dependent effects of bisphenol A on asthma development in an experimental mouse model. PLoS One, 9(6), e100468. doi:10.1371/journal.pone.0100468 PubMed doi:10.1371/journal.pone.0100468 PMID:24950052

Phillip, M. (1996). Clitoral and penile sizes of full term newborns in two different ethnic groups. *Journal of Pediatric Endocrinology & Metabolism*, *9*, 175–179. PMID:8887140

Phillip, M., De, C. B., Pilpel, D., Karplus, M., & Sofer, S. (1996). Clitoral and penile sizes of full term newborns in two different ethnic groups. *Journal of pediatric endocrinology & metabolism. Journal of Pediatric Endocrinology & Metabolism*, *9*(2), 175–179. PMID:8887140

Phua, S. K., Castillo, E., Anderson, J. M., & Hiltner, A. (1987). Biodegradation of polyurethane in vitro. *Journal of Biomedical Materials Research*, *21*(2), 231–246. doi:10.1002/jbm.820210207 PMID:3818683

Pinto, F., Franco, C., Andre, R. N., Miranda, M., Gulyurtlu, I., & Cabrita, I. (2002). Co-gasification study of biomass mixed with plastic wastes. *Fuel*, *3*(81), 291–297. doi:10.1016/S0016-2361(01)00164-8

Pirard, C., Sagot, C., Deville, M., Dubois, N., &Charlier, C. (2012). Urinary levels of Bisphenol A, triclosan and 4-nonylphenol in a general Belgian population. *Environ Int., 48,* 78-83.

Pirolini, A. (2014). *Impact of microplastics/microbeads accumulation on the marine environment.* Retrieved from www.azom.com

Pishvaee, M. S., Kianfar, K., & Karimi, B. (2010). Reverse Logistics Network Design Using Simulated Annealing. *International Journal of Advanced Manufacturing Technology*, *47*(1-4), 269–281. doi:10.100700170-009-2194-5

Plastics Europe. (2008). The compelling facts about Plastics 2007: An analysis of plastics production, demand and recovery for 2007 in Europe. Brussels, Belgium: Plastics Europe.

Plastics Europe. (2015). *Plastics—The Facts 2014/2015 an Analysis of European Plastics Production, Demand and Waste Data. In Plastics Europe* (p. 34). Brussels: Association of Plastic Manufactures.

Plastics in the Marine Environment. (2017). *Annual Review of Marine Science, 9*, 205-229.

PLASTICS. (2012). *History of Plastics.* Retrieved December 1, 2018, from SPI - The Plastics Industry Trade Association website: http://www.plasticsindustry.org/AboutPlastics/content.cfm?ItemNumber=670&navItemNumber=1117

PlasticsEurope. (2013a). *How plastic is made*. Retrieved from http://www.plasticseurope.org/what-is-plastic/how-plastic-is-made.aspx

PlasticsEurope. (2013b). *First estimates suggest around 4% increase in plastics global production from 2010*. Retrieved from http://www.plasticseurope.org/information-centre/press-room-1351/press-releases-2012/first-estimates-suggest-around-4-increase-in-plastics-global-production-from-2010.aspx

Pocar, P., Fiandanese, N., Secchi, C., Berrini, A., Fischer, B., Schmidt, J. S., ... Borromeo, V. (2011). Exposure to di (2-ethyl-hexyl) phthalate (DEHP) in utero and during lactation causeslong-term pituitary-gonadal axis disruption in male and female mouseoffspring. *Endocrinology*, *153*(2), 937–948. doi:10.1210/en.2011-1450 PMID:22147016

Poças, M. F., Oliveira, J. C., Pereira, J. R., & Hogg, T. (2010). Consumer exposure to phthalates from paper packaging: An integrated approach. *Food Additives and Contaminants*, *27*(10), 1451–1459. doi:10.1080/19440049.2010.490790 PMID:20597021

Polyani, K. (1957). *The Great Transformation*. Boston, MA: Beacon Press. (Original work published 1944)

Pometto, A. L., Lee, B., & Johnson, K. E. (1992). Production of an extracellular polyethylene- degrading enzyme(s) by *Streptomyces* species. *Applied and Environmental Microbiology*, *58*(2), 731–733. PMID:1610196

Pometto, A. L., Lee, B., & Johnson, K. E. (1992). Production of an extracellular polyethylene-degrading enzyme(s) by Streptomyces species. *Applied and Environmental Microbiology*, *58*, 731–733. PMID:1610196

Ponsonby, A. L., Dwyer, T., Kemp, A., Cochrane, J., Couper, D., & Carmichael, A. (2003). Synthetic bedding and wheeze in childhood. *Epidemiology (Cambridge, Mass.)*, *14*(1), 37–44. doi:10.1097/00001648-200301000-00012 PMID:12500044

Porte, C., Janer, G., Lorusso, L. C., Ortiz-Zarragoitia, M., Cajaraville, M. P., Fossi, M. C., & Canesi, L. (2006). Endocrine disruptors in marine organisms: Approaches and perspectives. *Comparative Biochemistry and Physiology. Toxicology & Pharmacology: CBP*, *143*(3), 303–315. doi:10.1016/j.cbpc.2006.03.004 PMID:16723279

Powell, J. J., Faria, N., Thomas-McKay, E., & Pele, L. C. (2010). Origin and fate of dietary nanoparticles and microparticles in the gastrointestinal tract. *Journal of Autoimmunity*, *34*(3), 226–233. doi:10.1016/j.jaut.2009.11.006 PMID:20096538

Prakash, B., Veeregowda, B. M., & Krishnappa, G. (2003). Biofilms: A survival strategy of bacteria. *Current Science*, *85*(9), 1299–1307.

Pramila, R., & Ramesh, K. V. (2011). Biodegradation of low density polyethylene (LDPE) by fungi isolated from municipal landfill area. *Journal of Microbiology and Biotechnology Research*, *1*, 131–136.

Premraj, R., & Doble, M. (2005). Biodegradation of polymer. *Indian Journal of Biotechnology*, *4*, 186–193.

Preuss, R., Koch, H. M., & Angerer, J. (2005). Biological monitoring of the five major metabolites of di-(2-ethylhexyl) phthalate (DEHP) in human urine using column-switching liquid chromatography–tandem mass spectrometry. *Journal of Chromatography. B, Analytical Technologies in the Biomedical and Life Sciences*, *816*(1-2), 269–280. doi:10.1016/j.jchromb.2004.11.048 PMID:15664359

Prins, G. S. (2008). Endocrine disruptors and prostate cancer risk. *Endocrine-Related Cancer*, *15*(3), 649–656. doi:10.1677/ERC-08-0043 PMID:18524946

Prins, G. S., Tang, W. Y., Belmonte, J., & Ho, S. M. (2008). Developmental exposure to Bisphenol A increases prostate cancer susceptibility in adult rats: Epigenetic mode of action is implicated. *Fertility and Sterility*, *89*(2), 41. doi:10.1016/j.fertnstert.2007.12.023 PMID:18308059

Priyanka, N., & Archana, T. (2011). Biodegradability of Polythene and Plastic by the Help of Microorganism: A Way for Brighter Future. *Journal of Environmental & Analytical Toxicology*, *1*(02), 111. doi:10.4172/2161-0525.1000111

Priyanka, N., & Archana, T. (2011). Biodegradability of Polythene and Plastic By The Help of Microorganism: A Way for Brighter Future. *Journal of Environmental & Analytical Toxicology*, 1.

Program, N. O., & A. A. M. D. (2014). *Report on the Entanglement of Marine Species in Marine Debris with an Emphasis on Species in the United States*. Silver Spring, MD: Academic Press.

Proshad, R., Kormoker, T., Islam, M. S., Haque, M. A., Rahman, M. M., & Mithu, M. M. (2018). Toxic effects of plastic on human health and environment: A consequences of health risk assessment in Bangladesh. *International Journal of Health*, *6*(1), 1–5. doi:10.14419/ijh.v6i1.8655

Pruss, A., Giroult, E., & Rushbrook, P. (1999). *Safe Management of Wastes from Health-Care Activities*. Geneva, Switzerland: World Health Organization.

Pruter, A. T. (1987). Sources, quantities and distribution of persistent plastics in the marine environment. *Marine Pollution Bulletin*, *18*(6), 305–310. doi:10.1016/S0025-326X(87)80016-4

Psillakis, E., Mantzavinos, D., & Kalogerakis, N. (2004). Monitoring the sonochemical degradation of phthalate esters in water using solid-phase microextraction. *Chemosphere*, *54*(7), 849–857. doi:10.1016/j.chemosphere.2003.09.039 PMID:14637342

Puente, D. L. G., & Sedran, U. (1998). Recycling polystyrene into fuels by means of FCC: Performance of various acidic catalysts. *Applied Catalysis B: Environmental*, *19*(3-4), 305–311. doi:10.1016/S0926-3373(98)00084-8

Puri, N., Kumar, B., & Tyagi, H. (2013). Utilization of recycled wastes as ingredients in concrete mix. *International Journal of Innovative Technology and Exploring Engineering*, *2*(2), 74–78.

Qari, R., & Shaffat, M. (2015). Distribution and Abundance of Marine Debris Along the Coast of Karachi (Arabian Sea), Pakistan. *Pakistan Journal of Scientific and Industrial Research, Series B: Biological Sciences, 58*(2), 98-103. Retrieved from https://www.researchgate.net/profile/Rashida_Qari2/publication/314261050_Distribution_and_Abundance_of_Marine_Debris_Along_the_Coast_of_Karachi_Arabian_Sea_Pakistan/links/58be93c6aca272b9b1805b77/Distribution-and-Abundance-of-Marine-Debris-Along-the-Coast

Qiao, L., Zheng, L., & Cai, D. (2007). Study on the di-n-butyl phthalate and di-2-ethylhexyl phthalate level of girl serum related with precocious puberty in Shanghai. *Wei sheng yanjiu=. Wei Sheng Yen Chiu*, *36*(1), 93–95. PMID:17424861

Qin, Z., & Ji, X. (2010). Logistics Network Design for Product Recovery in Fuzzy Environment. *European Journal of Operational Research*, *202*(2), 479–490. doi:10.1016/j.ejor.2009.05.036

Querol, X., Alastuey, A., López-Soler, A., Plana, F., Andrés, J. M., Juan, R., ... Ruiz, C. R. (1997). A fast method for recycling fly ash: Microwave– assisted zeolite synthesis. *Environmental Science & Technology*, *31*(9), 2527–2533. doi:10.1021/es960937t

Raaman, N., Rajitha, N., Jayshree, A., & Jegadeesh, R. (2012). Biodegradation of plastic by Aspergillus spp. isolated from polythene polluted sites around Chennai. *Journal of Academia and Industrial Research*, *1*, 313–316.

Ragaert, K., Delva, L., & Van Geem, K. (2017). Mechanical and chemical recycling of solid plastic waste. *Waste Management (New York, N.Y.)*, *69*, 24–58. doi:10.1016/j.wasman.2017.07.044 PMID:28823699

Rahman, A. K. M. R. (2009). Jute in South Asia. In *Proceedings of the Symposium on National Fibers* (pp. 19-20). Academic Press.

Rahman, M., & Brazel, C. S. (2004). The plasticizer market: An assessment of traditional plasticizers and research trends to meet new challenges. *Progress in Polymer Science*, *29*(12), 1223–1248. doi:10.1016/j.progpolymsci.2004.10.001

Rai, R., Keshavarz, T., Roether, J. A., Boccaccini, A. R., & Roy, I. (2011). Medium chain length polyhydroxyalkanoates, promising new biomedical medical devices for the future. *Medical devices Science and Engineering: R. Reports*, *72*(3), 29–47. doi:10.1016/j.mser.2010.11.002

Rajesh, P., & Balasubramanian, K. (2014). Phthalate exposure in utero causes epigenetic changes and impairs insulin signalling. *Journal of Endocrinology, 223*(1), 47-66. doi:10.1530/JOE-14-0111

Rajkumar, N., Subramani, T., & Elango, L. (2010). Groundwater contamination due to municipal solid waste disposal-A GIS based study in Erode city. *International Journal of Environmental Sciences, 1*(1), 39.

Raloff, J. (1999). Food for thought: What's coming out of baby's bottle? *Sci. News Online*, *156*, 1–4.

Ramaswamy, V. & Sharma, H. R. (2011). Plastic bags-Threat to environment and cattle health: A retrospective study from Gondar city of Ethiopia. *Environmental Management for Sustainable Development, 2*, 1.

Rashid, S. (2018). *Plastic pollution in the world's oceans is threatening marine life.* Retrieved from News.un.org.

Rashid, R. A., & Frantz, G. C. (1992). MSW incinerator ash as aggregate in concrete and masonry. *Journal of Materials in Civil Engineering*, *4*(4), 353–368. doi:10.1061/(ASCE)0899-1561(1992)4:4(353)

Rathi, S. (2006). Alternative approaches for better municipal solid waste management in Mumbai, India. *Waste Management (New York, N.Y.)*, *26*(10), 1192–1200. doi:10.1016/j.wasman.2005.09.006 PMID:16288861

Rathi, S. (2007). Optimization model for integrated municipal solid waste management in Mumbai, India. *Environment and Development Economics*, *12*(1), 105–121. doi:10.1017/S1355770X0600341X

Raum-Suryan, K. L., Jemison, L. A., & Pitcher, K. W. (2009). Entanglement of Steller sea lions (Eumetopias jubatus) in marine debris: Identifying causes and finding solutions. *Marine Pollution Bulletin*, *58*(10), 1487–1495. doi:10.1016/j.marpolbul.2009.06.004 PMID:19631950

Raynaud, J. (2014). *Valuing Plastics: The Business Case for Measuring, Managing and Disclosing Plastic Use in the Consumer Goods Industry.* UNEP. Retrieved from http://wedocs.unep.org/bitstream/handle/20.500.11822/9238/-Valuing%20plastic%3a%20the%20business%20case%20for%20measuring%2c%20managing%20and%20disclosing%20plastic%20use%20in%20the%20consumer%20goods%20industry-2014Valuing%20plasticsF.pdf?sequence=8&isAl

Rayner, J. L., Wood, C., & Fenton, S. E. (2004). Exposure parameters necessary for delayed puberty and mammary gland development in Long-Evans rats exposed in utero to atrazine. *Toxicology and Applied Pharmacology*, *195*(1), 23–34. doi:10.1016/j.taap.2003.11.005 PMID:14962502

RCO-LIPI. (2018). Kajian Sampah Laut (Marine Debris) dan Dampaknya pada Ekosistem Laut. Jakarta, Indonesia: Author.

Reddy, S. (2018). *Plastic pollution affects sea life throughout the ocean.* Retrieved from www.pewtrust.org

Reddy, B. S., Rozati, R., Reddy, B. V. R., & Raman, N. V. V. S. S. (2006). Association of phthalate esters with endometriosis in Indian women. *BJOG Int J Obstet Gynaecol*, *113*(5), 515–520. doi:10.1111/j.1471-0528.2006.00925.x PMID:16637895

Reddy, C. S. K. (1594). Evolution, site-specific mutagenesis and development of a PHB synthase protein model. *Biochimica et Biophysica Acta*, (1), 178–190.

Reddy, R. M. (2008). Impact of soil composting using municipal solid waste on biodegradation of plastics. *Indian Journal of Biotechnology*, *7*, 235–239.

Reese, A. (2012, September 26). *Eating hot food in plastic containers can lead to serious health problems - Doctor*. Retrieved from https://www.modernghana.com/lifestyle/3733/eating-hot-food-in-plastic-containers-can-lead-to-serious-he.html

Regulation (EC) No 1907/2006 of the European Parliament and of the Council of 18 December 2006 concerning the Registration, Evaluation, Authorisation and Restriction of Chemicals (REACH), establishing a European Chemicals Agency, amending Directive 1999/45/EC and repealing Council Regulation (EEC) No 793/93 and Commission Regulation (EC) No 1488/94 as well as Council Directive 76/769/EEC and Commission Directives 91/155/EEC, 93/67/ EEC, 93/105/EC and 2000/21/EC [displayed 8 May 2017].

Rehm, B.H., Antonio, R.V., Spiekermann, P., Amara, A.A., & Steinb€uchel, A. (2002). *Molecular characterization of the poly(3- hydroxybutyrate) (PHB) synthase from Ralstonia eutropha: in vitro*. Academic Press.

Reischwitz, A., Stoppok, E., & Buchholz, K. (1997). Anaerobic degradation of poly-3-hydroxybutyrate and poly-3-hydroxybutyrate-co-3-hydroxyvalerate. *Biodegradation*, *8*(5), 313–319. doi:10.1023/A:1008203525476 PMID:15765610

Ren, X. (2003). Biodegradable plastics: A solution or a challenge? *Journal of Cleaner Production*, *11*(1), 27–40. doi:10.1016/S0959-6526(02)00020-3

Report, R. A. (2003a). 1,2-benzenedicarboxylic acid, di-C9-11-branched alkyl esters, C10-rich and di-"isodecyl" phthalate (DIDP). Institute for Health and Consumer Protection. *European Chemicals Bureau*, *36*, 234.

Report, R. A. (2003b). 1,2-benzenedicarboxylic acid, di-C8-10-branched alkyl esters, C9-rich and di-"isononyl" phthalate (DINP). Institute for Health and Consumer Protection. *European Chemicals Bureau*, *35*, 290.

Resources for health professionals. (2011). Retrieved from http://www.aoec.org/pehsu/training.html

Restrepo-Flórez, J. M., Bassi, A., & Thompson, M. R. (2014). Microbial degradation and deterioration of polyethylene-a review. *International Biodeterioration & Biodegradation*, *88*, 83–90. doi:10.1016/j.ibiod.2013.12.014

Rezg, R., El-Fazaa, S., Gharbi, N., & Mornagui, B. (2014). Bisphenol A and human chronic diseases: Current evidences, possible mechanisms, and future perspectives. *Environment International*, *64*, 83–90. doi:10.1016/j.envint.2013.12.007 PMID:24382480

Rhie, Y. J., Nam, H. K., Oh, Y. J., Kim, H. S., & Lee, K. H. (2014). Influence of bottle-feeding on serum Bisphenol A levels in infants. *Journal of Korean Medical Science*, *29*(2), 261–264. doi:10.3346/jkms.2014.29.2.261 PMID:24550655

Richiardi, L., Bellocco, R., Adami, H.-O., Torrang, A., Barlow, L., Hakulinen, T., . . . Akre, O. (2004). Testicular Cancer Incidence in Eight Northern European Countries: Secular and Recent Trends. *Cancer Epidemiology, Biomarkers & Prevention, 13*(12), 2157-2166. Retrieved from http://cebp.aacrjournals.org/content/13/12/2157.full-text.pdf

Richter, C. A., Taylor, J. A., Ruhlen, R. L., Welshons, W. V., & vom Saal, F. S. (2007). Estradiol and Bisphenol A stimulate androgen receptor and estrogen receptor gene expression in fetal mouse prostate mesenchyme cells. Environmental Health Perspectives, 115(6), 902–908. doi:10.1289/ehp.9804 PubMed doi:10.1289/ehp.9804 PMID:17589598

Richter, C. A., Birnbaum, L. S., Farabollini, F., Newbold, R. R., Rubin, B. S., Talsness, C. E., ... Vom Saal, F. S. (2007). In vivo effects of Bisphenol A in laboratory rodent studies. *Reproductive Toxicology (Elmsford, N.Y.)*, *24*(2), 199–224. doi:10.1016/j.reprotox.2007.06.004 PMID:17683900

Ritchie Hannah and Roser Max. (2018). *Plastic Pollution*. Avaılable at https://ourworldindata.org/plastic-pollution

Ritter, S. (2011). BPA Is Indispensible For Making Plastics. Chemical and Engineering News, 89. Retrieved from https://pubs.acs.org/cen/coverstory/ 89/8923cover4.html

Ritzer, G. (1996). *The McDonaldization of Society*. Thousand Oaks, CA: Pine Forge Press.

Riu, A., Grimaldi, M., le Maire, A., Bey, G., Phillips, K., Boulahtouf, A., ... Balaguer, P. (2011). Peroxisome proliferator-activated receptor gamma is a target for halogenated analogs of Bisphenol A. *Environmental Health Perspectives*, *119*(9), 1227–1232. doi:10.1289/ehp.1003328 PMID:21561829

Riyad, Ali, & Maqtari. (2014). The Impact of Plastic Bags on the Environment: A field Survey of the City Of Sana'a And The Surrounding Areas, Yemen. *International Journal of Engineering Research and Reviews*, *2*(4), 61–69.

Robertson, R. (1991). *Globalization*. London, UK: Sage.

Robins & Webster. (1999). *Times of the Techno culture*. London, UK: Routledge.

Robinson, L., & Miller, R. (2015). The impact of bisphenol A and phthalates on allergy, asthma, and immune function: A review of latest findings. *Current Environmental Health Reports*, *2*(4), 379–387. doi:10.100740572-015-0066-8 PMID:26337065

Robles-Martínez, F. (2012). Biodrying under greenhouse conditions as pretreatment for horticultural waste. *Journal of Environmental Protection*, *3*(04), 298–303. doi:10.4236/jep.2012.34038

Rochester, J. R., & Bolden, A. L. (2015). Bisphenol S and F: A systematic review and comparison of the hormonal activity of bisphenol A substitutes. Environmental Health Perspectives, 123(7), 643–650. doi:10.1289/ehp.1408989 PubMed doi:10.1289/ehp.1408989 PMID:25775505

Rochman, C. M. (2015). The complex mixture, fate and toxicity of chemicals associated with plastic debris in the marine environment. In Marine Anthropogenic Litter (pp. 117–140). doi:10.1007/978-3-319-16510-3_5

Rochman, C. M., Hoh, E., Kurobe, T., & Teh, S. J. (2013). Ingested plastic transfers hazardous chemicals to fish and induces hepatic stress. *Scientific Reports*, *3*(1), 3263. doi:10.1038rep03263 PMID:24263561

Rochman, C. M., Tahir, A., Williams, S. L., Baxa, D. V., Lam, R., Miller, J. T., ... Teh, S. J. (2015). Anthropogenic debris in seafood: Plastic debris and fibers from textiles in fish and bivalves sold for human consumption. *Scientific Reports*, *5*(1), 14340. doi:10.1038rep14340 PMID:26399762

Rodríguez, B., Bécares, J., Rodríguez, A., & Arcos, J. M. (2013). Incidence of entanglements with marine debris by northern gannets (Morus bassanus) in the non-breeding grounds. *Marine Pollution Bulletin*, *75*(1–2), 259–263. doi:10.1016/j.marpolbul.2013.07.003 PMID:23932474

Rogers, D. S., Melamed, B., & Lembke, R. S. (2012). Modeling and Analysis of Reverse Logistics. *Journal of Business Logistics*, *33*(2), 107–117. doi:10.1111/j.0000-0000.2012.01043.x

Rohrmann, S., Nelson, W. G., Rifai, N., Brown, T. R., Dobs, A., Kanarek, N., ... Platz, E. A. (2007). Serum estrogen, but not testosterone, levels differ between black and white men in a nationally representative sample of Americans. *The Journal of Clinical Endocrinology and Metabolism*, *92*(7), 2519–2525. doi:10.1210/jc.2007-0028 PMID:17456570

Ronn, M., Lind, L., Örberg, J., Kullberg, J., Söderberg, S., Larsson, A., ... Lind, P. M. (2014). Bishenol A is related to circulating levels of adiponectin, leptin and ghrelin, but not to fat mass or fat distribution in humans. *Chemosphere*, *112*, 42–48. doi:10.1016/j.chemosphere.2014.03.042 PMID:25048886

Rosenfeld, C. S. (2015). Bisphenol A and phthalate endocrine disruption of parental and social behaviors. Frontiers in Neuroscience, 9, 57. doi:10.3389/fnins.2015.00057 PubMed doi:10.3389/fnins.2015.00057 PMID:25784850

Rosevelt, C., Los Huertos, M., Garza, C., & Nevins, H. M. (2013a). Marine debris in central California: Quantifying type and abundance of beach litter in Monterey Bay, CA. In Marine Pollution Bulletin (Vol. 71). doi:10.1016/j.marpolbul.2013.01.015

Routledge, E. J., White, R., Parker, M. G., & Sumpter, J. P. (2000). Differential effects of xenoestrogens on coactivator recruitment by estrogen receptor (ER) α and ER β. *The Journal of Biological Chemistry*, *275*(46), 35986–35993. doi:10.1074/jbc.M006777200 PMID:10964929

Rowdhwal, S. S., & Chen, J. (2018). Toxic Effects of Di-2-ethylhexyl Phthalate: An Overview. *BioMed Research International*. doi:10.1155/2018/1750368

Rowsell, V. F., Tangney, P., Hunt, C., & Voulvoulis, N. (2010). Estimating levels of micro pollutants in municipal waste water. *Water, Air, and Soil Pollution*, *206*(1–4), 357–368. doi:10.100711270-009-0112-y

Royal Commission on Environmental Pollution. (1984). *10th Report tackling pollution—experience and prospects*. London: HMSO.

Rozati, R., Reddy, P. P., Reddanna, P. A., & Mujtaba, R. (2002). Role of environmental estrogens in the deterioration of male factor fertility. *Fertility and Sterility*, *78*(6), 1187–1194. doi:10.1016/S0015-0282(02)04389-3 PMID:12477510

Rubin, B. S. (2011). Bisphenol A: an endocrine disruptor with widespread exposure and multiple effects. *Journal of Steroid Biochemistry and Molecular Biology, 127,* 27–34. doi:10.1016/j.jsbmb.2011.05.002

Rubin, B. S., & Soto, A. M. (2009). Bisphenol A: Perinatal exposure and body weight. *Mol Cell Endocrinol, 304*(1-2), 55–62. doi:10.1016/j.mce.2009.02.023

Rubin, B. S., Murray, M. K., Damassa, D. A., King, J. C., & Soto, A. M. (2001). Perinatal exposure to low doses of Bisphenol A affects body weight, patterns of estrous cyclicity, and plasma LH levels. *Environmental Health Perspectives*, *109*(7), 675–680. doi:10.1289/ehp.01109675 PMID:11485865

Rudel, R. A., Gray, J. M., Engel, C. L., Rawsthorne, T. W., Dodson, R. E., Ackerman, J. M., . . . Brody, J. G. (2011). Food packaging and bisphenol A and bis(2-ethyhexyl) phthalate exposure: Findings from a dietary intervention. Environmental Health Perspectives, 119(7), 914–920. doi:10.1289/ehp.1003170 PubMed doi:10.1289/ehp.1003170 PMID:21450549

Rudel, R., Camann, D., Spengler, J. D., Barr, D., & Brody, J. G. (2003, March). Household exposure to phthalates, pesticides, alkylphenols, pbdes, and other endocrine active compounds. In Toxicological Sciences (Vol. 72, pp. 184-184). Oxford Univ Press.

Rudel, R.A., Dodson, R.E., Newton, E., Zota, A.R., & Brody, J.G. (2008). Correlations between urinary phthalate metabolites and phthalates, estrogenic compounds 4-butyl phenol and o-phenyl phenol, and some pesticides in home indoor air and house dust. *Epidemiology, 19*, S332.

Rudel, R. A., Camann, D. E., Spengler, J. D., Korn, L. R., & Brody, J. G. (2003). Phthalates, alkylphenols, pesticides, polybrominated diphenyl ethers, and other endocrinedisrupting compounds in indoor air and dust. *Environmental Science & Technology*, *37*(20), 4543–4553. doi:10.1021/es0264596 PMID:14594359

Ruj, B., Pandey, V., Jash, P., & Srivastava, V. K. (2015). Sorting of plastic waste for effective recycling. *Int. Journal of Applied Sciences and Engineering Research*, *4*(4). doi:10.6088/ijaser.04058

Rummel, C. D., Jahnke, A., Gorokhova, E., Kühnel, D., & Schmitt-Jansen, M. (2017). Impacts of biofilm formation on the fate and potential effects of microplastic in the aquatic environment. *Environmental Science & Technology Letters*, *4*(7), 258–267. doi:10.1021/acs.estlett.7b00164

Ryan, P. G. (2015). A brief history of marine litter research. In Marine Anthropogenic Litter (pp. 1–25). doi:10.1007/978-3-319-16510-3_1

Ryan, P.G., Moore, C.J., Franeker, J.A., & Moloney, C.L. (2009). Monitoring the abundanceof plastic debris in the marine environment. *Philos Trans R Soc Lond BBiol Sci B, 364*, 1999-2012.

Ryan, P. G. (2018). Entanglement of birds in plastics and other synthetic materials. *Marine Pollution Bulletin, 135*, 159–164. doi:10.1016/j.marpolbul.2018.06.057 PMID:30301025

Ryan, P. G., Moore, C. J., van Franeker, J. A., & Moloney, C. L. (2009). Monitoring the abundance of plastic debris in the marine environment. *Philosophical Transactions of the Royal Society of London. Series B, Biological Sciences, 364*(1526), 1999–2012. doi:10.1098/rstb.2008.0207 PMID:19528052

Ryan, P. G., & Rice, N. (1996). The Free Shopping Bag Debate: Costs and Attitudes. *South African Journal of Science, 92*(4), 163–164.

Rykowska, I., & Wasiak, W. (2006). Properties, threats and methods of analysis of Bisphenol A and its derivatives. *Acta Chromatographica, 16*, 7–27.

Ryu, C., Sharifi, V. N., & Swithenbank, J. (2007). Waste pyrolysis and generation of storable char. *International Journal of Energy Research, 31*(2), 177–191. doi:10.1002/er.1241

Saal, F. S., Akingbemi, B. T., Belcher, S. M., Birnbaum, L. S., Crain, D. A., Eriksen, M., & ... . (2007). Chapel Hill bisphenol A expert panel consensus statement: Integration of mechanisms, effects in animals and potential to impact human health at current levels of exposure. *Reproductive Toxicology (Elmsford, N.Y.), 24*(2), 131–138. doi:10.1016/j.reprotox.2007.07.005 PMID:17768031

Sabanayagam, C., Teppala, S., & Shankar, A. (2013). Relationship between urinary Bisphenol A levels and prediabetes among subjects free of diabetes. *Acta Diabetologica, 50*(4), 625–631. doi:10.100700592-013-0472-z PMID:23636267

Sachin, S. S., & Mishra, R. L. (2013). Screening and identification of soil fungi with potential of plastic degrading ability. *Indian Journal of Applied Research, 3*(11), 34–36.

Sadef, Y., Nizami, A. S., Batool, S. A., Chaudary, M. N., Ouda, O. K., Asam, Z. Z., ... Demirbas, A. (2016). Waste-to-energy and recycling value for developing integrated solid waste management plan in Lahore. *Energy Sources. Part B, Economics, Planning, and Policy, 11*(7), 569–579. doi:10.1080/15567249.2015.1052595

Sadri, S. S., & Thompson, R. C. (2014). On the quantity and composition of floating plastic debris entering and leaving the Tamar Estuary, Southwest England. *Marine Pollution Bulletin, 81*(1), 55–60. doi:10.1016/j.marpolbul.2014.02.020 PMID:24613232

Safety4sea. (2018). *How plastic affects marine life.* Retrieved from Safety4sea.com

Sahajwalla, V., & Gaikwad, V. (2018). The present and future of e-waste plastics recycling. *Current Opinion in Green and Sustainable Chemistry, 13*, 102–107. doi:10.1016/j.cogsc.2018.06.006

Sajiki, J., Miyamoto, F., Fukata, H., Mori, C., Yonekubo, J., & Hayakawa, K. (2007). Bisphenol A (BISPHENOL A) and its source in foods in Japanese markets. *Food Additives and Contaminants, 24*(1), 103–112. doi:10.1080/02652030600936383 PMID:17164221

Sakurai, K., Kawazuma, M., Adachi, T., Harigaya, T., Saito, Y., Hashimoto, N., & Mori, C. (2004). Bisphenol A affects glucose transport in mouse 3T3-F442A adipocytes. *British Journal of Pharmacology, 141*(2), 209–214. doi:10.1038j.bjp.0705520 PMID:14707028

Salazar-Martinez, E., Romano-Riquer, P., Yanez-Marquez, E., Longnecker, M. P., & Hernandez-Avila, M. (2004). Anogenital distance in human male and female newborns: A descriptive, cross-sectional study. *Environmental Health*, *3*(1), 8. doi:10.1186/1476-069X-3-8 PMID:15363098

Salehi, A., Gustafsson, J., Quesada, I., & Nadal, A. (2012). Rapid insulinotropic action of low doses of Bisphenol-A on mouse and human islets of langerhans: Role of estrogen receptor β. *PLoS One*, *7*(2), 31109. doi:10.1371/journal.pone.0031109 PMID:22347437

Saliba, M., Matsui, T., Seo, J. Y., Domanski, K., Correa-Baena, J. P., Nazeeruddin, M. K., ... Grätzel, M. (2016). Cesium-containing triple cation perovskite solar cells: Improved stability, reproducibility and high efficiency. *Energy & Environmental Science*, *9*(6), 1989–1997. doi:10.1039/C5EE03874J PMID:27478500

Salkin, I. F., & Krisiunas, E. (1998). Alternatives to medical waste incinerators. *Journal of Solid Waste Technology Management*, *25*(1), 9–13.

Sannigrahi, A. K., & Chakrabortty, S. (2002). Beneficial management of organic wastes by vermi composting. *Indian Journal of Environmental Protection*, *22*, 405–408.

Sargis, R. M., Johnson, D. N., Choudhury, R. A., & Brady, M. J. (2010). Environmental endocrine disruptors promote adipogenesis in the 3T3- L1 cell line through glucocorticoid receptor activation. *Obesity (Silver Spring, Md.)*, *18*(7), 1283–1288. doi:10.1038/oby.2009.419 PMID:19927138

Sarigiannis, D. A. (2017). Assessing the impact of hazardous waste on children's health: The exposome paradigm. *Environmental Research*, *158*, 531–541. doi:10.1016/j.envres.2017.06.031 PMID:28711809

Sarkis, J., Helm, M. M., & Hervani, A. A. (2010). Reverse Logistics and Social Sustainability. *Corporate Social Responsibility and Environmental Management*, *17*(6), 337–354. doi:10.1002/csr.220

Sasikumar, P., Kannan, G., & Haq, A. N. (2010). A Multi-Echelon Reverse Logistics Network Design for Product Recovery - Case of Truck Tire Remanufacturing. *International Journal of Advanced Manufacturing Technology*, *49*(9-12), 1223–1234. doi:10.100700170-009-2470-4

Sasse, F., & Emig, G. (1998). Chemical recycling of polymer materials. *Chemical Engineering & Technology*, *21*(10), 777–789. doi:10.1002/(SICI)1521-4125(199810)21:10<777::AID-CEAT777>3.0.CO;2-L

Satapathy, S. (2017). An analysis of barriers for plastic recycling in the Indian plastic industry. *Benchmarking: An International Journal*, *24*(2), 415–430. doi:10.1108/BIJ-11-2014-0103

Sathya, R., Ushadevi, T., & Panneerselvam, A. (2012). Plastic degrading actinomycetes isolated from mangrove sediments. *International Journal of Current Research, 4*(10), 1–3.

Sathyanarayana, S. (2008) Baby care products: possible sources of infant phthalate exposure. *Pediatrics, 121*.

Sathyanarayana, S. (2008). Phthalates and children's health. *Current Problems in Pediatric and Adolescent Health Care*, *38*(2), 34–49. doi:10.1016/j.cppeds.2007.11.001 PMID:18237855

Sathyanarayana, S., Karr, C. J., Lozano, P., Brown, E., Calafat, A. M., Liu, F., & Swan, S. H. (2008). Baby care products: Possible sources of infant phthalate exposure. *Pediatrics*, *121*(2), e260–e268. doi:10.1542/peds.2006-3766 PMID:18245401

Savaskan, R. C., & van Wassenhove, L. N. (2006). Reverse Channel Design: The Case of Competing Retailers. *Management Science*, *52*(1), 1–14. doi:10.1287/mnsc.1050.0454

Saxena, S., Srivastava, R. K., & Samaddar, A. B. (2010). Sustainable Waste Management Issues in India. *IUP Journal of Soil & Water Sciences, 3*(1).

Schecter, A., Lorber, M., Guo, Y., Wu, Q., Yun, S. H., Kannan, K., ... Colacino, J. A. (2013). Phthalate concentrations and dietary exposure from food purchased in New York State. *Environmental Health Perspectives*, *121*(4), 473–479. doi:10.1289/ehp.1206367 PMID:23461894

Scheirs, J., & Kaminsky, W. (2006). *Feedstock Recycling and Pyrolysis of Waste Plastics. In Converting Waste Plastics into Diesel and Other Fuels*. Wiley – VCH. doi:10.1002/0470021543

Schink, B., Janssen, P. H., & Frings, J. (1992). Microbial degradation of natural and of new synthetic polymers. *FEMS Microbiology Reviews*, *103*(2/4), 311–316. doi:10.1111/j.1574-6968.1992.tb05852.x PMID:1476775

Schmidt, C., Krauth, T., & Wagner, S. (2017). Export of Plastic Debris by Rivers into the Sea. *Environmental Science & Technology*, *51*(21), 12246–12253. doi:10.1021/acs.est.7b02368 PMID:29019247

Schneider, J. E., Brozek, J. M., & Keen-Rhinehart, E. (2014). Our stolen figures: the interface of sexualdifferentiation, endocrine disruptors, maternal programming, and energy balance. *Hormones and Behavior, 66*(1), 104-119.

Schnurr, R. E., Alboiu, V., Chaudhary, M., Corbett, R. A., Quanz, M. E., Sankar, K., ... Walker, T. R. (2018). Reducing marine pollution from single-use plastics (SUPs): A review. *Marine Pollution Bulletin*, *137*, 157–171. doi:10.1016/j.marpolbul.2018.10.001 PMID:30503422

Schonfelder, G., Wittfoht, W., Hopp, H., Talsness, C. E., Paul, M., & Chahoud, I. (2002). Parent bisphenol A accumulation in the human maternal-fetal-placental unit. *Environmental Health Perspectives*, *110*(11), 703–707. doi:10.1289/ehp.021100703 PMID:12417499

Schreiber, A., Fu, F., Yang, O., Wan, E., Gu, E., & Le Blanc, Y. (2011). Increasing Selectivity and Confidence in Detection When Analyzing Phthalates by LC–MS/MS. *AB Sciex (AN 3690411–01)*.

Schug, T. T., Heindel, J. J., Camacho, L., Delclos, K. B., Howard, P., Johnson, A. F., . . . Bucher, J. R. (2013). A new approach to synergize academic and guideline-compliant research: The CLARITY-BPA research program. Reproductive Toxicology (Elmsford, N.Y.), 40, 35–40. doi:10.1016/j.reprotox.2013.05.010 PubMed doi:10.1016/j.reprotox.2013.05.010 PMID:23747832

Schuler, K. (2008). *Smart Plastics Guide: Healthier Food Uses of Plastics*. Minneapolis, MN: Academic Press.

Science for Environment Policy. (2011). *Plastic Waste: Ecological and HumanHealth Impacts*. In-depth Reports.

Scott, G. (2000). 'Green' polymers. *Polymer Degradation & Stability*, *68*(1), 1–7. doi:10.1016/S0141-3910(99)00182-2

Scott, G. (2007). Plastic packaging and coastal pollution. *The International Journal of Environmental Studies*, *3*(4), 35–39.

Seachrist, D. D., Bonk, K. W., Ho, S.-M., Prins, G. S., Soto, A. M., & Keri, R. A. (2016). A review of the carcinogenic potential of bisphenol A. *Reproductive Toxicology (Elmsford, N.Y.)*, *59*, 167–182. doi:10.1016/j.reprotox.2015.09.006 PMID:26493093

Seltenrich, N. (2015). New Link in the Food Chain? Marine Plastic Pollution and Seafood Safety. *Environmental Health Perspectives, 123*(2), A34-A41.

Selvin, E., Feinleib, M., Zhang, L., Rohrmann, S., Rifai, N., Nelson, W. G., ... Platz, E. A. (2007). Androgens and diabetes in men results from the Third National Health and Nutrition Examination Survey (NHANES III). *Diabetes Care*, *30*(2), 234–238. doi:10.2337/dc06-1579 PMID:17259487

Senate of Pakistan. (1997). *Act,1997.* Retrieved from ELAW: https://www.elaw.org/system/files/Law-PEPA-1997.pdf

Senatore, P. J. (1994). Medical waste disposal alternatives: selection and implementation. In *87th Annual Meeting and Exhibition.* Air & Waste Manage. Assoc. (Paper No. 94-RP123B.03)

Seneviratne, G., Tennakoon, N. S., Weerasekara, M. L. M. A. W., & Nandasena, K. A. (2006). Polyethylene biodegradation by a developed *Penicillium–Bacillus* biofilm. *Current Science*, *90*, 20–22.

Senior, P. J., Beech, G. A., Ritchie, G. A. F., & Dawes, E. A. (1972). The role of oxygen limitation in the formation of poly-b-hydroxybutyrate during batch and continuous culture of Azobacter beijerinckii. *The Biochemical Journal*, *128*(5), 1193–1201. doi:10.1042/bj1281193 PMID:4643700

Senior, P. J., & Dawes, E. A. (1973). The regulation of poly-beta-hydroxybutyrate metabolism in Azotobacter beirjerinckii. *The Biochemical Journal*, *134*(1), 225–238. doi:10.1042/bj1340225 PMID:4723225

Seo, Y.-H., Lee, K.-H., & Shin, D.-H. (2003). Investigation of catalytic degradation of high-density polyethylene by hydrocarbon group type analysis. *Journal of Analytical and Applied Pyrolysis*, *70*(2), 383–398. doi:10.1016/S0165-2370(02)00186-9

Seretoudi, G., Bikiaris, D., & Panayiotou, C. (2002). Synthesis, characterization and biodegradability of poly (ethylene succinate)/poly (ε-caprolactone) block copolymers. *Polymers*, *43*(20), 5405–5415. doi:10.1016/S0032-3861(02)00433-0

Serrano, D. P., Aguado, J., Escola, J. M., Rodriguez, J. M., Morselli, L., & Orsi, R. (2003). Thermal and catalytic cracking of a LDPE-EVA copolymer mixture. *Journal of Analytical and Applied Pyrolysis*, *68–69*, 481–494. doi:10.1016/S0165-2370(03)00037-8

Shaffer, C. B., Carpenter, C. P., & Smyth Jr., H. F. (1945). Acute and subacute toxicity of di (2- ethylhexyl) phthalate with note upon its metabolism. The Journal of Industrial Hygiene and Toxicology, 27(5), 130–135.

Shafiei, S. R., Melville, B. W., Beskhyroun, S., & Shamseldin, A. Y. (2014). Preliminary investigation of the tsunami-borne debris impact on structures: a new method for impact force measurement. *Hydraulic Structures and Society - Engineering Challenges and Extremes*, 1–9. doi:10.14264/uql.2014.44

Shah, P. (2001). *The Plastic Devil: Ecological Menace*. Academic Press.

Shah, A. A., Hasan, F., Akhter, J. I., Hameed, A., & Ahmed, S. (2008a). Degradation of polyurethane by novel bacterial consortium isolated from soil. *Annals of Microbiology*, *58*(3), 381–386. doi:10.1007/BF03175532

Shah, A. A., Hasan, F., Akhter, J., Hameed, A., & Ahmed, S. (2009). Isolation of *Fusarium* sp. AF4 from sewage sludge, with the ability to adhere the surface of polyethylene. *African Journal of Microbiological Research*, *3*, 658–663.

Shah, A. A., Hasan, F., Hameed, A., & Ahmed, S. (2008). Biological degradation of plastics: A comprehensive review. *Biotechnology Advances*, *26*(3), 246–265. doi:10.1016/j.biotechadv.2007.12.005 PMID:18337047

Shaikh, H., Memon, N., Bhanger, M. I., & Nizamani, S. M. (2014). GC/MS Based Non-target Screening of Organic Contaminants in River Indus and its Tributaries in Sindh (Pakistan). *Pakistan Journal of Analytical & Environmental Chemistry, 15*(1), 24. Retrieved from http://pjaec.pk/index.php/pjaec/article/view/210

Shaikh, H., Anis, A., Poulose, A. M., Alam, M., A-Otaibi, M. N., Alam, M. A., & Al-Zahrani, S. M. (2016). Studies on High Density Polyethylene Reinforced with Phosphate Ore Particles: Thermal, Rheological, Mechanical and Morphological Properties. *J of Polymer Plastic Technology and Engineering*, *55*(17), 1831–1841. doi:10.1080/03602559.2016.1171875

Shamsuddin, I. M., Jafar, J. A., Shawai, A. S. A., Yusuf, S., Lateefah, M., & Aminu, I. (2017). Bioplastics as Better Alternative to Petroplastics and Their Role in National Sustainability: A Review. *Advances in Bioscience and Bioengineering*, *5*(4), 63–70. doi:10.11648/j.abb.20170504.13

Shang, J., Chai, M., & Zhu, Y. (2003). Photocatalytic degradation of polystyrene plastic under fluorescent light. *Environmental Science & Technology*, *37*(19), 4494–4499. doi:10.1021/es0209464 PMID:14572106

Shankar, A., & Teppala, S. (2011). Relationship between urinary Bisphenol A levels and diabetes mellitus. *The Journal of Clinical Endocrinology and Metabolism*, *96*(12), 3822–3826. doi:10.1210/jc.2011-1682 PMID:21956417

Shankar, A., & Teppala, S. (2012). Urinary Bisphenol A and hypertension in a multiethnic sample of US adults. *Journal of Environmental and Public Health*, *2012*, 481–641. doi:10.1155/2012/481641 PMID:22363351

Shankar, A., Teppala, S., & Sabanayagam, C. (2012). Bisphenol A and peripheral arterial disease: Results from the NHANES. *Environmental Health Perspectives*, *120*(9), 1297–1300. doi:10.1289/ehp.1104114 PMID:22645278

Shanle, E. K., & Xu, W. (2010). *Endocrine disrupting chemicals targeting estrogen receptor signaling*. Academic Press.

Shan, X. Y., Xi, B., Cheng, H., Hou, D. Q., Wang, Y., & Mi, J. (2010). Prevalence and behavioral risk factors of overweight and obesity among children aged 2–18 in Beijing, China. *International Journal of Pediatric Obesity; IJPO*, *5*(5), 383–389. doi:10.3109/17477160903572001 PMID:20233154

Shao, B., Han, H., Li, D., Ma, Y., Tu, X., & Wu, Y. (2007). Analysis ofalkylphenol and bisphenol A in meat by accelerated solvent extraction and liquid chromatography with tandem massspectrometry. *Food Chemistry*, *105*(3), 1236–1241. doi:10.1016/j.foodchem.2007.02.040

Sharma, A., & Sharma, A. (2004). Degradation assessment of low density polythene (LDPE) and polythene (PP) by an indigenous isolate of *Pseudomonas stutzeri*. *Journal of Scientific and Industrial Research (New Delhi, India)*, *63*, 293–296.

Sharma, S., & Chatterjee, S. (2017). Microplastic pollution, a threat to marine ecosystem and human health: A short review. *Environmental Science and Pollution Research International*, *24*(27), 21530–21547. doi:10.100711356-017-9910-8 PMID:28815367

Sharpe, R. M. (2001). Hormones and testis development and the possible adverse effects of environmental chemicals. *Toxicology Letters*, *120*(1-3), 221–232. doi:10.1016/S0378-4274(01)00298-3 PMID:11323180

Sharpe, R. M., & Drake, A. J. (2013). Obesogens and obesity—An alternative view? *Obesity (Silver Spring, Md.)*, *21*(6), 1081–1083. doi:10.1002/oby.20373 PMID:23512350

Sharpe, R. M., & Irvine, D. S. (2004). How strong is the evidence of a link between environmental chemicals and adverse effects on human reproductive health? *BMJ (Clinical Research Ed.)*, *328*(7437), 447–451. doi:10.1136/bmj.328.7437.447 PMID:14976101

Sharpe, R. M., & Skakkebaek, N. E. (1993). Are oestrogens involved in falling sperm counts and disorders of the male reproductive tract? *Lancet*, *341*(8857), 1392–1396. doi:10.1016/0140-6736(93)90953-E PMID:8098802

Sharpe, R. M., & Skakkebaek, N. E. (2008). Testicular dysgenesis syndrome: Mechanstic insights and potential new downstream effects. *Fertility and Sterility*, *89*(2), 33–38. doi:10.1016/j.fertnstert.2007.12.026 PMID:18308057

Shea, K. M. (2003). Pediatric exposure and potential toxicity of phthalate plasticizers. *Pediatrics*, *111*(6), 1467–1474. doi:10.1542/peds.111.6.1467 PMID:12777573

Sheavly, S. B., & Register, K. M. (2007). Marine debris & plastics: Environmental concerns, sources, impacts and solutions. *Journal of Polymers and the Environment*, *15*(4), 301–305. doi:10.100710924-007-0074-3

Sheikh, I. A. (2016). Stereoselectivity and the potential endocrine disrupting activity of di-(2-ethylhexyl) phthalate (DEHP) against human progesterone receptor: A computational perspective. *Journal of Applied Toxicology*, *36*(5), 741–747. doi:10.1002/jat.3302 PMID:26879776

Shelby, M. D. (2008). *NTP-CERHR Monograph on the Potential Human Reproductive and Developmental Effects of Bisphenol-A. National Toxicology Program, US Department of Health and Human Services. Center for the Evaluation of Risks to Human Reproduction*. Washington, DC: CERHR-NTP.

Shemwell, B. E., & Levendis, Y. A. (2000). Particulates generated from combustion of polymers. *JAPCA J Air Waste Ma*, 27, *50*(1), 94–102.

Sheng, Z. G., Tang, Y., Liu, Y. X., Yuan, Y., Zhao, B. Q., Chao, X. J., & Zhu, B. Z. (2012). Low concentrations of bisphenol a suppressthyroid hormone receptor transcription through anongenomic mechanism. *Toxicology and Applied Pharmacology*, *259*(1), 133–142. doi:10.1016/j.taap.2011.12.018 PMID:22227104

Shenk, D. (1997). *Data Smog: Surviving the Information Glut*. New York: HarperCollins.

Sheriff, K. M., Gunasekaran, A., & Nachiappan, S. (2012). Reverse logistics network design: A review on strategic perspective. *International Journal of Logistics Systems and Management*, *12*(2), 171–194. doi:10.1504/IJLSM.2012.047220

Sheriff, K. M., Subramanian, N., Rahman, S., & Jayaram, J. (2017). Integrated optimization model and methodology for plastics recycling: Indian empirical evidence. *Journal of Cleaner Production*, *153*, 707–717. doi:10.1016/j.jclepro.2016.07.137

Shigeno, T., Katakuse, M., Fujita, T., Mukoyama, Y., & Watanabe, H. (2009). Phthalate ester-induced thymic stromal lymphopoietin mediates allergic dermatitis in mice. Immunology, 128(1Suppl), e849–e857. doi:10.1111/j.1365-2567.2009.03094.x PubMed doi:10.1111/j.1365-2567.2009.03094.x PMID:19740346

Shimao. (2001). Biodegradation of plastics. *Current Opinion in Biotechnology, 12,* 242–247.

Shimao, M. (2001). Biodegradation of plastics. *Current Opinion in Biotechnology*, *12*(3), 242–247. doi:10.1016/S0958-1669(00)00206-8 PMID:11404101

Shin, I. S., Lee, M.-Y., Cho, E.-S., Choi, E., Son, H.-Y., & Lee, K.-Y. (2014). Effects of maternal exposure to di(2-ethylhexyl)phthalate (DEHP) during pregnancy on susceptibility to neonatal asthma. Toxicology and Applied Pharmacology, 274(3), 402–407. doi:10.1016/j.taap.2013.12.009 PubMed doi:10.1016/j.taap.2013.12.009 PMID:24370437

Shin, S.-M., Yoshioka, T., & Okuwaki, A. (1998). Dehydrochlorination behavior of flexible PVC pellets in NaOH solutions at elevated temperature. *Journal of Applied Polymer Science*, *67*(13), 2171–2177. doi:10.1002/(SICI)1097-4628(19980328)67:13<2171::AID-APP7>3.0.CO;2-B

Shiri, N. D., Kajava, P. V., Ranjan, H. V., Pais, N. L., & Naik, V. M. (2015). Processing of Waste Plastics into Building Materials Using a Plastic Extruder and Compression Testing of Plastic Bricks. *Journal of Mechanical Engineering and Automation.*, *5*(3B), 39–42. doi:10.5923/c.jmea.201502.08

Shivley, J. M. (2006). Preface. In J. M. Shivley (Ed.), *Inclusions in Prokaryotes*. Berlin: Springer-Verlag. doi:10.1007/3-540-33774-1

Shneider, B., Schena, J., Truog, R., Jacobson, M., & Kevy, S. (1989). Exposure to di (2-ethylhexyl) phthalate in infants receiving extracorporeal membrane oxygenation. *The New England Journal of Medicine*, *320*(23), 1563–1563. doi:10.1056/NEJM198906083202322 PMID:2725593

Shulman, J. D., Coughlan, A. T., & Savaskan, R. C. (2010). Optimal Reverse Channel Structure for Consumer Product Returns. *Marketing Science*, *29*(6), 1071–1085. doi:10.1287/mksc.1100.0578

Siddiqi, M. A., Laessig, R. H., & Reed, K. D. (2003). Polybrominated Diphenyl Ethers (PBDEs): New Pollutants-Old Diseases. *Clinical Medicine & Research*, *1*(4), 281–290. doi:10.3121/cmr.1.4.281 PMID:15931321

Siddique, R. (2010). Utilization of municipal solid waste (MSW) ash in cement and mortar. *Resources, Conservation and Recycling*, *54*(12), 1037–1047. doi:10.1016/j.resconrec.2010.05.002

Siddiqui, M. N., Achilias, D. S., Redhwi, H. H., Bikiaris, D. N., Katsogiannis, K.-A. G., & Karayannidis, G. P. (2010). Hydrolytic Depolymerization of PET in a Microwave Reactor. *Macromolecular Materials and Engineering*, *295*(6), 575–584. doi:10.1002/mame.201000050

Sifniades, S., Levy, A., & Hendrix, J. (1999a). *Process for depolymerizing nylon-containing waste to form caprolactam.* U.S. Patent 5,932,724.

Sifniades, S., Levy, A., & Hendrix, J. (1999b). *Process for depolymerizing nylon-containing whole carpet to form caprolactam.* U.S. Patent 5,929,234.

Sigler, M. (2014). The effects of plastic pollution on aquatic wildlife: Current situations and future solutions. *Water, Air, and Soil Pollution*, *225*(11), 2184. doi:10.100711270-014-2184-6

Silva, M. J., Reidy, J. A., Herbert, A. R., Preau, J. L., Needham, L. L., & Calafat, A. M. (2004). Detection of phthalate metabolites in human amniotic fluid. *Bulletin of Environmental Contamination and Toxicology, 72*(6), 1226-1231.

Silva, M. J. (2007). Quantification of 22 phthalate metabolites in human urine. *Journal of Chromatography. A, 860*, 106–112. PMID:17997365

Silva, M. J., Barr, D. B., Reidy, J. A., Kato, K., Malek, N. A., Hodge, C. C., ... Brock, J. W. (2003). Glucuronidation patterns of common urinary and serum monoester phthalate metabolites. *Archives of Toxicology*, *77*(10), 561–567. doi:10.100700204-003-0486-3 PMID:14574443

Silva, M. J., Barr, D. B., Reidy, J. A., Malek, N. A., Hodge, C. C., Caudill, S. P., ... Calafat, A. M. (2004). Urinary levels of seven phthalate metabolites in the U.S. population from the National Health and Nutrition Examination Survey (NHANES) 1999–2000. *Environmental Health Perspectives*, *112*(3), 331–338. doi:10.1289/ehp.6723 PMID:14998749

Silva, M. J., Kato, K., Gray, E. L., Wolf, C., Needham, L. L., & Calafat, A. M. (2005). Urinary metabolites of di-n-octyl phthalate in rats. *Toxicology*, *210*(2-3), 123–133. doi:10.1016/j.tox.2005.01.012 PMID:15840426

Silva, M. J., Malek, N. A., Hodge, C. C., Reidy, J. A., Kato, K., Barr, D. B., ... Brock, J. W. (2003). Improved quantitative detection of 11 urinary phthalate metabolites in humans using liquid chromatography–atmospheric pressure chemical ionization tandem mass spectrometry. *Journal of Chromatography. B, Analytical Technologies in the Biomedical and Life Sciences*, *789*(2), 393–404. doi:10.1016/S1570-0232(03)00164-8 PMID:12742130

Silva, M. J., Samandar, E., Preau, J. L. Jr, Reidy, J. A., Needham, L. L., & Calafat, A. M. (2007). Quantification of 22 phthalate metabolites in human urine. *Journal of Chromatography. B, Analytical Technologies in the Biomedical and Life Sciences*, *860*(1), 106–112. doi:10.1016/j.jchromb.2007.10.023 PMID:17997365

Silva, M. J., Slakman, A. R., Reidy, J. A., Preau, J. L. Jr, Herbert, A. R., Samandar, E., ... Calafat, A. M. (2004). Analysis of human urine for fifteen phthalate metabolites using automated solid-phase extraction. *Journal of Chromatography. B, Analytical Technologies in the Biomedical and Life Sciences*, *805*(1), 161–167. doi:10.1016/j.jchromb.2004.02.038 PMID:15113553

Silver, M. K., O'Neill, M. S., Sowers, M. R., & Park, S. K. (2011). Urinary Bisphenol A and type-2 diabetes in U.S. adults: data from NHANES 2003–2008. *PlOS 1, 6*, 26868.

Simmons, C. (2005). *It's in the Bag: An Estimate of the Effect of CO2 Emissions of the Irish Plastic Bag Tax.* Academic Press.

Singh, A. (2018). *Plastic waste burning at Yamuna Biodiversity Park.* Academic Press.

Singhal, R., Singhal, C., & Upadhyayula, S. (2010). Thermal catalytic degradation of polyethylene over silicoaluminophosphate molecular sieves- A thermogravimetric study. *Journal of Analytical and Applied Pyrolysis*, *89*(2), 313–317. doi:10.1016/j.jaap.2010.09.007

Singh, B., & Sharma, N. (2008). Mechanistic implications of plastic degradation. *Polymer Degradation & Stability*, *93*(3), 561–584. doi:10.1016/j.polymdegradstab.2007.11.008

Singh, J., & Gupta, K. (2014). Screening and Identification of Low density Polyethylene (LDPE) Degrading Soil Fungi Isolated from Polythene Polluted Sites around Gwalior city (MP). *International Journal of Current Microbiology and Applied Sciences*, *3*, 443–448.

Singh, N., Hui, D., Singh, R., Ahuja, I. P. S., Feo, L., & Fraternali, F. (2017). Recycling of plastic solid waste: A state of art review and future applications. *Composites. Part B, Engineering*, *115*, 409–422. doi:10.1016/j.compositesb.2016.09.013

Singh, P., & Sharma, V. P. (2016). Integrated Plastic Waste Management: Environmental and Improved Health Approaches. *Procedia Environmental Sciences*, *35*, 692–700. doi:10.1016/j.proenv.2016.07.068

Singh, S., & Shoei-Lung, L. S. (2011). Phthalates: Toxicogenomics and inferred human diseases. *Genomics*, *97*(3), 148–157. doi:10.1016/j.ygeno.2010.11.008 PMID:21156202

Singh, S., & Shoei-Lung, L. S. (2012). Bisphenol A and phthalates exhibit similar toxicogenomics and health effects. *Gene*, *494*(1), 85–91. doi:10.1016/j.gene.2011.11.035 PMID:22173104

Sivan, A. (2011). New perspectives in plastic biodegradation. *Current Opinion in Biotechnology*, *22*(3), 422–426. doi:10.1016/j.copbio.2011.01.013 PMID:21356588

Sivan, A., Szanto, M., & Pavlov, V. (2006). Biofilm development of the polyethylenedegrading bacterium *Rhodococcus ruber. Applied Microbiology and Biotechnology*, *72*(2), 346–352. doi:10.100700253-005-0259-4 PMID:16534612

Sklair, L. (2001). *The Transnational Capitalist Class*. Cambridge, UK: Blackwell.

Slapak, M. J. P., Kasteren, J. M. N., & Drinkenburg, B. A. A. H. (1999). Hydrothermal recycling of PVC in a bubbling fluidized bed reactor: The influence of bed material and temperature. *Polymers for Advanced Technologies*, *10*(10), 596–602. doi:10.1002/(SICI)1099-1581(199910)10:10<596::AID-PAT913>3.0.CO;2-J

Slouka, M. (1995). *War of the Worlds*. New York: Harper and Row.

Smith, S. D. A. (2012). Marine debris: A proximate threat to marine sustainability in Bootless Bay, Papua New Guinea. *Marine Pollution Bulletin*, *64*(9), 1880–1883. doi:10.1016/j.marpolbul.2012.06.013 PMID:22770700

Smolders, K., & Baeyens, J. (2004). Thermal degradation of PMMA in fluidized beds. *Waste Management (New York, N.Y.)*, *24*(8), 849–857. doi:10.1016/j.wasman.2004.06.002 PMID:15381237

Snell, K. D., & Peoples, O. P. (2009). PHA Bioplastic: A valueadded coproduct for biomass biorefineries. *Biofuels, Bioproducts & Biorefining*, *3*(4), 456–467. doi:10.1002/bbb.161

Soeborg, T., Frederiksen, H., & Andersson, A. M. (2012). Cumulative risk assessment of phthalate exposure of Danish children and adolescents using the hazard index approach. *International Journal of Andrology*, *35*(3), 245–252. doi:10.1111/j.1365-2605.2011.01240.x PMID:22320716

Sohail, M. S., & Sohal, A. S. (2003). The Use of Third Party Logistics Services: A Malaysian Perspective. *Technovation*, *23*(5), 401–408. doi:10.1016/S0166-4972(02)00003-2

Sohoni, P., & Sumpter, J. P. (1998). Several environmental estrogens are also anti-androgens. *The Journal of Endocrinology*, *158*(3), 327–339. doi:10.1677/joe.0.1580327 PMID:9846162

Soja, E. (1989). *Postmodern Geographies*. London, UK: Verso.

Somleva, M. N., Snell, K. D., Beaulieu, J. J., Peoples, O. P., Garrison, B. R., & Patterson, N. A. (2008). Production of polyhydroxybutyrate in switchgrass, a value-added co-product in an important lignocellulosic biomass crop. *Plant Biotechnology Journal*, *6*(7), 663–678. doi:10.1111/j.1467-7652.2008.00350.x PMID:18498309

Somm, E., Schwitzgebel, V. M., Toulotte, A., Cederroth, C. R., Combescure, C., Nef, S., ... Hüppi, P. S. (2009). Perinatal exposure to Bisphenol A alters early adipogenesis in the rat. *Environmental Health Perspectives*, *117*(10), 1549–1555. doi:10.1289/ehp.11342 PMID:20019905

Song, J. H., Murphy, R. J., Narayan, R., & Davies, G. B. H. (2009). Biodegradable and compostable alternatives to conventional plastics. *Philosophical Transactions of the Royal Society of London. Series B, Biological Sciences*, *364*(1526), 2127–2139. doi:10.1098/rstb.2008.0289 PMID:19528060

Song, S. S., Hein, S., & Steinbuchel, A. (1999). Production of poly(4- hydroxybutyric acid) by fed-batch cultures of recombinant strains of Escherichia coli. *Biotechnology Letters*, *21*(3), 193–197. doi:10.1023/A:1005451810844

Song, Y., Hauser, R., Hu, F. B., Franke, A. A., Liu, S., & Sun, Q. (2014). Urinary concentrations ofbisphenol A and phthalate metabolites and weight change: A prospective investigation in USwomen. *International Journal of Obesity*, *38*(12), 1532–1537. doi:10.1038/ijo.2014.63 PMID:24722546

Sonoda, E., Sasaki, M. S., Morrison, C., Yamaguchi-Iwai, Y., Takata, M., & Takeda, S. (1999). Sister chromatid exchanges are mediated by homologous recombination in vertebrate cells. *Molecular and Cellular Biology*, *19*(7), 5166–5169. doi:10.1128/MCB.19.7.5166 PMID:10373565

Soriano, S., Alonso-Magdalena, P., García-Arévalo, M., Novials, A., Muhammed, S. J., Stahlhut, R. W., ... Swan, S. H. (2009). Bisphenol A data in NHANES suggest longer than expected half-life, substantial nonfood exposure, or both. *Environmental Health Perspectives*, *117*(5), 784–789. doi:10.1289/ehp.0800376 PMID:19479022

Soto, A. M., & Sonnenschein, C. (2010). Environmental causes of cancer: Endocrine disruptors as carcinogens. *Nature Reviews. Endocrinology*, (6): 364–371. PMID:20498677

Soto, A. M., & Sonnenschein, C. (2010). Environmental causes of cancer: Endocrine disruptors as carcinogens. *Nature Reviews. Endocrinology*, *6*(7), 363–370. doi:10.1038/nrendo.2010.87 PMID:20498677

Souza, W. R. D. (2013). *Microbial degradation of lignocellulosic biomass*. West Palm Beach, FL: InTech.

Sowmya, H., Ramalingappa, M. K., & Thippeswamy, B. (2014). Biodegradation of Polyethylene by Bacillus cereus. *Advances in Polymer Science and Technology. International Journal (Toronto, Ont.)*, *4*, 28–32.

Specht, I. O., Bonde, J. P., Toft, G., Lindh, C. H., Jönsson, B. A., & Jørgensen, K. T. (2015). Serum phthalate levels and time to pregnancy in couples from Greenland, Poland and Ukraine. *PLoS One*, *10*(3), e0120070. doi:10.1371/journal.pone.0120070 PMID:25786246

Spivey, A. (2003). Plastic Bags – Prolific Problems. *Environmental Health Perspectives, 111*(4), A208.

Srivastava, S. K. (2007). Green Supply-Chain Management: A State-Of-The-Art Literature Review. *International Journal of Management Reviews*, *9*(1), 53–80. doi:10.1111/j.1468-2370.2007.00202.x

Srivastava, S. K., & Srivastava, R. K. (2006). Managing Product Returns for Reverse Logistics. *International Journal of Physical Distribution & Logistics Management*, *36*(7), 524–546. doi:10.1108/09600030610684962

Srivastava, S. P., Srivastava, S., Saxena, D. K., Chandra, S. V., & Seth, P. K. (1990). Testicular effects of di-n-butyl phthalate (DBP): Biochemical and histopathological alterations. *Archives of Toxicology*, *64*(2), 148–152. doi:10.1007/BF01974401 PMID:2350234

Stahel, W. R. (2016, March 23). The circular economy. *Nature International Weekly Journal of Science*, *531*, 435–438. doi:10.1038/531435a PMID:27008952

Stahlhut, R. W., Van Wijngaarden, E., Dye, T. D., Cook, S., & Swan, S. H. (2007). Concentrations of urinary phthalate metabolites are associated with increased waist circumference and insulin resistance in adult U.S. males. *Environmental Health Perspectives*, *115*(5), 876–882. doi:10.1289/ehp.9882 PMID:17589594

Staples, C. A., Peterson, D. R., Parkerton, T. F., & Adams, W. J. (1997). The environmental fate of phthalate esters: A literature review. *Chemosphere*, *35*(4), 667–749. doi:10.1016/S0045-6535(97)00195-1

Steer, M., Cole, M., Thompson, R. C., & Lindeque, P. K. (2017). Microplastic ingestion in fish larvae in the western English Channel. *Environmental Pollution*, *226*, 250–259. doi:10.1016/j.envpol.2017.03.062 PMID:28408185

Steger, M. (2002). *Globalism: The New Market Ideology*. Lanham, MD: Rowman and Littlefield.

Stelfox, M., Hudgins, J., & Sweet, M. (2016). A review of ghost gear entanglement amongst marine mammals, reptiles and elasmobranchs. *Marine Pollution Bulletin*, *111*(1–2), 6–17. doi:10.1016/j.marpolbul.2016.06.034 PMID:27345709

Sterling, W. J., Walline, K. S., & McCoy, B. J. (2001). Experimental study of polystyrene thermolysis to moderate conversion. *Polymer Degradation & Stability*, *73*(1), 75–82. doi:10.1016/S0141-3910(01)00069-6

Sticklen, M. (2008). Plant genetic engineering for biofuel production: Towards affordable cellulosic ethanol. *Nature Reviews. Genetics*, *9*(6), 433–443. doi:10.1038/nrg2336 PMID:18487988

Stiglitz, J. E. (2002). *Globalization and Its Discontents*. New York: Norton.

Stoll, C. (1995). *Silicon Snake Oil: Second Thoughts on the Information Highway*. New York: Doubleday.

Street, M. E., Angelini, S., Bernasconi, S., Burgio, E., Cassio, A., & Catellani, C., … Amarri, S. (2018). Current Knowledge on Endocrine Disrupting Chemicals (EDCs) from Animal Biology to Humans, from Pregnancy to Adulthood: Highlights from a National Italian Meeting. *International Journal of Molecular Sciences*, *19*(6), 1647. doi:10.3390/ijms19061647

Strong, A. B. (2006). *Plastics: materials and processing* (3rd ed.). Upper Saddle River, NJ: Pearson Prentice Hall.

Sudesh, K., Abe, H., & Doi, Y. (2000). Synthesis, structure and properties of polyhydroxyalkanoates: Biological polyesters. *Progress in Polymer Science*, *25*(10), 1503–1555. doi:10.1016/S0079-6700(00)00035-6

Sudhire, V., Muraleedharan, V. R., &Srinivasan, G. (1996). Integrated solid waste management in urban India: a critical operational research framework. *Journal of Socio-Economic Planning Science, 30*, 163–181.

Sugii, T. (2008). *Plastic Bag Reduction*. Policies to Reduce Environmental Impact.

Sugni, M., Calcaterra, E., & Adani, F. (2005). Biostabilization–biodrying of municipal solid waste by inverting air– flow. *Bioresource Technology*, *96*(12), 1331–1337. doi:10.1016/j.biortech.2004.11.016 PMID:15792579

Sui, Y., Ai, N., Park, S. H., Rios-Pilier, J., Perkins, J. T., Welsh, W. J., & Zhou, C. (2012). Bisphenol A and its analogues activate human pregnane X receptor. *Environmental Health Perspective, 120,* 399–405. doi:.1104426 doi:10.1289/ehp

Suleman, Khan, Gull, Aleem, Shafiq, & Jamil. (2014). *A Comprehensive Short Review on Polyurethane Foam*. Academic Press.

Sun, Q., Cornelis, M. C., Townsend, M. K., Tobias, D. K., Eliassen, A. H., Franke, A. A., ... Hu, F. B. (2014). Association of urinary concentrations of Bisphenol A and phthalate metabolites with risk of type 2 diabetes: A prospective investigation in the Nurses' Health Study (NHS) and NHSII cohorts. *Environmental Health Perspectives*, *122*(6), 616–623. doi:10.1289/ehp.1307201 PMID:24633239

Sun, Y., Tao, F. B., Su, P. Y., Mai, J. C., Shi, H. J., Han, Y.-T., ... Liu, J. (2012). National estimates of the pubertal milestones among urban and rural Chinese girls. *The Journal of Adolescent Health*, *51*(3), 279–284. doi:10.1016/j.jadohealth.2011.12.019 PMID:22921139

Sun, Y., Zhang, Q., Hou, J., Wang, P., & Sundell, J. (2017). Exposure of phthalates in residential buildings and its health effects. *Procedia Engineering*, *205*, 1901–1904. doi:10.1016/j.proeng.2017.10.286

Supreme Court of Pakistan. (1994). *Zia v. WAPDA, PLD 1994 Supreme Court 693*. Islamabad: Supreme Court of Pakistan. Retrieved from https://www.elaw.org/pk.shehla.zia.1994

Suresh, B., Maruthamuthu, S., Palanisamy, N., Ragunathan, R., Pandiyaraj, K. N., & Muralidharan, V. S. (2011). Investigation on biodegradability of polyethylene by Bacillus cereus strain Ma-Su isolated from compost soil. *International Research Journal of Microbiology*, *2*, 292–302.

Suriyamongkol, P., Weselake, R., Narine, S., Moloney, M., & Shah, S. (2007). Biotechnological approaches for the production of polyhydroxyalkanoates in microorganisms and plants—A review. *Biotechnology Advances*, *25*(2), 148–175. doi:10.1016/j.biotechadv.2006.11.007 PMID:17222526

Sussarellu, R., Suquet, M., Thomas, Y., Lambert, C., Fabioux, C., Pernet, M. E. J., … Huvet, A. (2016). Oyster reproduction is affected by exposure to polystyrene microplastics. *Proceedings of the National Academy of Sciences*, *113*(9), 2430–2435. 10.1073/pnas.1519019113

Suyama, K., Masafumi, K., Masamitsu, S., & Hiroyuki, Y. (2010). Chemical recycling of networked polystyrene derivatives using subcritical water in the presence of an aminoalchocol. *Polymer Degradation & Stability*, *95*(9), 1588–1592. doi:10.1016/j.polymdegradstab.2010.05.034

Suzuki, T., Yaguchi, K., Suzuki, S., & Suga, T. (2001). Monitoring of phthalic acid monoesters in river water by solid-phase extraction and GC-MS determination. *Environmental Science & Technology*, *35*(18), 3757–3763. doi:10.1021/es001860i PMID:11783656

Suzuki, Y., Yoshinaga, J., Mizumoto, Y., Serizawa, S., & Shiraishi, H. (2012). Foetal exposure tophthalate esters and anogenital distance in male newborns. *International Journal of Andrology*, *35*(3), 236–244. doi:10.1111/j.1365-2605.2011.01190.x PMID:21696396

Svensson, K., Hernández-Ramírez, R. U., Burguete-García, A., Cebrián, M. E., Calafat, A. M., Needham, L., ... López-Carrillo, L. (2011). Phthalate exposure associated with self-reported diabetes among Mexican women. *Environmental Research*, *111*(6), 792–796. doi:10.1016/j.envres.2011.05.015 PMID:21696718

Swan, S. H. (2008). Environmental phthalate exposure in relation to reproductive outcomes and other health endpoints in humans. *Environmental Research, 108*, 177–184. doi:10.1016/j.envres.2008.08.007

Swan, S. H. (2008). Environmental phthalate exposure in relation to reproductive outcomes and other health endpoints in humans. *Environmental Research*, *108*(2), 177–184. doi:10.1016/j.envres.2008.08.007 PMID:18949837

Swan, S. H., Elkin, E. P., & Fenster, L. (2000). The question of declining sperm density revisited: An analysis of 101 studies published 1934-1996. *Environmental Health Perspectives*, *108*(10), 961–966. doi:10.1289/ehp.00108961 PMID:11049816

Swan, S. H., Main, K. M., Liu, F., Stewart, S. L., Kruse, R. L., Calafat, A. M., ... Teague, J. L. (2005). Decrease in anogenital distance among male infants with prenatal phthalate exposure. *Environmental Health Perspectives*, *113*(8), 1056–1061. doi:10.1289/ehp.8100 PMID:16079079

Swan, S., Liu, F., Hines, M., Kruse, R. L., Wang, C., Redmon, J. B., ... Weiss, B. (2010). Prenatal phthalate exposure and reduced masculine play in boys. *International Journal of Andrology*, *33*(2), 259–269. doi:10.1111/j.1365-2605.2009.01019.x PMID:19919614

Swift, G. (1993). Directions for environmentally biodegradable polymer research. *Accounts of Chemical Research*, *26*(3), 105–110. doi:10.1021/ar00027a005

Syed, S. (2006). Solid and liquid waste management. *Emirates J. Eng. Res*, *11*(2), 19–36.

Takatori, S., Kitagawa, Y., Kitagawa, M., Nakazawa, H., & Hori, S. (2004). Determination of di (2-ethylhexyl) phthalate and mono (2-ethylhexyl) phthalate in human serum using liquid chromatography-tandem mass spectrometry. *Journal of Chromatography. B, Analytical Technologies in the Biomedical and Life Sciences*, *804*(2), 397–401. doi:10.1016/j.jchromb.2004.01.056 PMID:15081935

Takayanagi, S., Tokunaga, T., Liu, X., Okada, H., Matsushima, A., & Shimohigashi, Y. (2006). Endocrine disruptor Bisphenol A strongly binds to human estrogen-related receptor gamma (ERRgamma) with high constitutive activity. *Toxicology Letters*, *167*(2), 95–105. doi:10.1016/j.toxlet.2006.08.012 PMID:17049190

Takeshita, A., Inagaki, K., Igarashi-Migitaka, J., Ozawa, Y., & Koibuchi, N. (2006). Th endocrinedisrupting chemical, diethylhexyl phthalate, activates MDR1 gene expression in human colon cancer LS174T cells. *The Journal of Endocrinology*, *190*(3), 897–902. doi:10.1677/joe.1.06664 PMID:17003290

Takeuchi, T., Tsutsumi, O., Ikezuki, Y., Takai, Y., & Taketani, Y. (2004). Positive relationship between androgen and the endocrine disruptor, bisphenol A, in normal women and women with ovarian dysfunction. *Endocrine Journal*, *51*(2), 165–169. doi:10.1507/endocrj.51.165 PMID:15118266

Takeuchi, T., Tsutsumi, O., Nakamura, N., Ikezuki, Y., Takai, Y., Yano, T., & Taketani, Y. (2004). Gender difference in serum Bisphenol A levels may be caused by liver UDP glucuronosyl transferase activity in rats. *Biochemical and Biophysical Research Communications*, *325*(2), 549–554. doi:10.1016/j.bbrc.2004.10.073 PMID:15530427

Talsness, C. E., Andrade, A. J., Kuriyama, S. N., Taylor, J. A., & Vom Saal, F. S. (2009). Components of plastic: Experimental studies in animals and relevance for human health. *Philosophical Transactions of the Royal Society of London. Series B, Biological Sciences*, *364*(1526), 2079–2096. doi:10.1098/rstb.2008.0281 PMID:19528057

Talvitie, J., Heinonen, M., Pääkkönen, J. P., Vahtera, E., Mikola, A., Setälä, O., & Vahala, R. (2015). Do wastewater treatment plants act as a potential point source of microplastics? Preliminary study in the coastal Gulf of Finland, Baltic Sea. *Water Science and Technology*. PMID:26524440

Talvitie, J., Mikola, A., Setälä, O., Heinonen, M., & Koistinen, A. (2017). How well is microlitter purified from wastewater?–A detailed study on the stepwise removal of microlitter in a tertiary level wastewater treatment plant. *Water Research*, *109*, 164–172. doi:10.1016/j.watres.2016.11.046 PMID:27883921

Tammemagi, H. Y. (1999). *The Waste Crisis: Landfills Incinerators and the Searchfor a Sustainable Future*. Oxford University Press.

Tang-Peronard, J. L., Andersen, H. R., Jensen, T. K., & Heitmann, B. L. (2011). Endocrine disrupting chemicals and obesity development in humans: A review. *Obesity Reviews*, *12*(8), 622–636. doi:10.1111/j.1467-789X.2011.00871.x PMID:21457182

Tang, W. Y., Morey, L. M., Cheung, Y. Y., Birch, L., Prins, G. S., & Ho, S. M. (2010). Neonatal exposure to estradiol/bisphenol A alters promoter methylation and expression of *Nsbp1* and *Hpcal1* genes and transcriptional programs of Dnmt3a/b and Mbd2/4 in the rat prostate gland throughout life. *Endocrinology*, *153*(1), 42–55. doi:10.1210/en.2011-1308 PMID:22109888

Tarantino, G., Valentino, R., Di Somma, C., D'Esposito, V., Passaretti, F., Pizza, G., & .... (2012). Bisphenol A in Polycystic Ovary Syndrome and its Association with Liver-Spleen Axis. *Horumon To Rinsho*, *78*(3), 447–453. doi:10.1111/j.1365-2265.2012.04500.x PMID:22805002

Taskeen, A., & Naeem, I. (2009). Bisphenol A Toxicity in Milk: A Review. *Nature and Science, 7*(8), 83-85. Retrieved from http://www.sciencepub.net/nature/0708/10_0981_Bisphenol_ns0708.pdf

Taskeen, A. (2012). *Qualitative and Quantitative Analysis of Bisphenol-A in Foods and Beverages Stored in Plastic Containers and Wraps in Pakistan.* Lahore: Department of Chemistry, Lahore College for Women University. Retrieved from http://prr.hec.gov.pk/jspui/bitstream/123456789/504/1/1734S.pdf

Taylor, J. A., Vom Saal, F. S., Welshons, W. V., Drury, B., Rottinghaus, G., Hunt, P. A., ... VandeVoort, C. A. (2010). Similarity of bisphenol A pharmacokinetics in rhesus monkeys and mice: Relevance for human exposure. *Environmental Health Perspectives*, *119*(4), 422–430. doi:10.1289/ehp.1002514 PMID:20855240

Taylor, M. L., Gwinnett, C., Robinson, L. F., & Woodall, L. C. (2016). Plastic microfibre ingestion by deep-sea organisms. *Scientific Reports*, *6*(1), 33997. doi:10.1038rep33997 PMID:27687574

Tchobanoglous, Theisen, & Vigil. (n.d.). *Integrated Solid Waste Management.* McGraw Hill.

Teitelbaum, S. L., Britton, J. A., Calafat, A. M., Ye, X., Silva, M. J., Reidy, J. A., ... Wolff, M. S. (2008). Temporal variability in urinary concentrations of phthalate metabolites, phytoestrogens and phenols among minority children in the United States. *Environmental Research*, *106*(2), 257–269. doi:10.1016/j.envres.2007.09.010 PMID:17976571

Teitelbaum, S. L., Mervish, N., Moshier, E. L., Vangeepuram, N., Galvez, M. P., Calafat, A. M., ... Wolff, M. S. (2012). Associations between phthalate metabolite urinaryconcentrations and body size measures in New York City children. *Environmental Research*, *112*, 186–193. doi:10.1016/j.envres.2011.12.006 PMID:22222007

Tekman, M. B., Krumpen, T., & Bergmann, M. (2017). Marine litter on deep Arctic seafloor continues to increase and spreads to the North at the HAUSGARTEN observatory. *Deep-sea Research. Part I, Oceanographic Research Papers*, *120*, 88–99. doi:10.1016/j.dsr.2016.12.011

ten Brink, P., Schweitzer, J.-P., Watkins, E., Janssens, C., De Smet, M., Leslie, H., & Galgani, F. (2018). Circular economy measures to keep plastics and their value in the economy, avoid waste and reduce marine litter. *Economics*. Retrieved from https://archimer.ifremer.fr/doc/00419/53002/53950.pdf

Teppala, S., Madhavan, S., & Shankar, A. (2012). Bisphenol A and metabolic syndrome: Results from NHANES. *International Journal of Endocrinology*, (5): 98–180. PMID:23251154

Tepper, L. B. (1973). Phthalic acid esters – An overview. Environmental Health Perspectives, 3, 179–182. PubMed PMID:4704568

Testa, C., Nuti, F., Hayek, J., De Felice, C., Chelli, M., Rovero, P., ... Papini, A. M. (2012). Di-(2-ethylhexyl) phthalate and autism spectrum disorders. *ASN Neuro*, *4*(4), AN20120015. doi:10.1042/AN20120015 PMID:22537663

Teuten, E. L., Saquing, J. M., Knappe, D. R. U., Barlaz, M. A., Jonsson, S., Bjo¨rn, A., . . . Ochi, D. (2009). Transport and release of chemicals from plastics to the environment and to wildlife. Philos. Trans. R. Soc. B Biol. Sci., 364, 2027–2045. PubMed PMID:19528054

Teuten, E. L., Saquing, J. M., Knappe, D. R., Barlaz, M. A., Jonsson, S., Bjorn, A., … Ochi, D. (2009). Transport and release of chemicals from plastics to the environment and to wildlife. *Philosophical Transactions of the Royal Society B: Biological Sciences, 364*(1526), 2027–2045. doi:10.1098/rstb.2008.0284

Teuten, E. L., Saquing, J. M., Knappe, D. R. U., Barlaz, M. A., Jonsson, S., Björn, A., ... Takada, H. (2009). Transport and release of chemicals from plastics to the environment and to wildlife. *Philosophical Transactions of the Royal Society of London. Series B, Biological Sciences*, *364*(1526), 2027–2045. doi:10.1098/rstb.2008.0284 PMID:19528054

Thayer, K. A., Heindel, J. J., Bucher, J. R., & Gallo, M. A. (2012). Role of environmental chemicals in diabetes and obesity: A national toxicology program workshop review. *Environmental Health Perspectives*, *120*(6), 779–789. doi:10.1289/ehp.1104597 PMID:22296744

The Ministry of Environment and Forests. (2011). *Plastic Waste (Management and Handling)*. Author.

The News International. (2016, August 21). *Packaging industry enjoys 15 percent annual growth*. Retrieved from https://www.thenews.com.pk/print/143977-Packaging-industry-enjoys-15-percent-annual-growth

The ocean plastic pollution challenge: Towards solutions in the UK. (n.d.). Grantham Institute.

The World Bank. (2018a). *Solid Waste Management*. Washington DC: The World Bank. Retrieved from http://www.worldbank.org/en/topic/urbandevelopment/brief/solid-waste-management

The World Bank. (2018b). *Urban population (% of total)*. Retrieved from The World Bank Group: https://data.worldbank.org/indicator/SP.URB.TOTL.IN.ZS

Thiel, M., Luna-Jorquera, G., Álvarez-Varas, R., Gallardo, C., Hinojosa, I. A., Luna, N., ... Portflitt-Toro, M. (2018). Impacts of Marine Plastic Pollution From Continental Coasts to Subtropical Gyres—Fish, Seabirds, and Other Vertebrates in the SE Pacific. *Frontiers in Marine Science, 5*(238).

Thompson, R. C. (2017). *Future of the Sea: Plastic Pollution*. Foresight, Government Office for Science.

Thompson, C. J., Ross, S. M., Hensley, J., Liu, K., Heinze, S. C., Young, S. S., & Gaido, K. W. (2005). Differential steroidogenic gene expression in the fetal adrenal gland versus the testis and rapid and dynamic response of the fetal testis to di(n-butyl) phthalate. *Biology of Reproduction*, *73*(5), 908–917. doi:10.1095/biolreprod.105.042382 PMID:15987825

Thompson, R. C. (2015). Microplastics in the marine environment: Sources, consequences and solutions. In *Marine anthropogenic litter* (pp. 185–200). Cham: Springer. doi:10.1007/978-3-319-16510-3_7

Thompson, R. C., Moore, C. J., Saal, F. S. V., & Swan, S. H. (2009). Plastics, the environment and human health: Current consensus and future trends. *Philosophical Transactions of the Royal Society of London. Series B, Biological Sciences*, *364*(1526), 2153–2166. doi:10.1098/rstb.2009.0053 PMID:19528062

Thompson, R. C., Olson, Y., Mitchell, R. P., Davis, A., Rowland, S. J., John, A. W. G., ... Russell, A. E. (2004). Lost at Sea: Where Is All the Plastic? *Science*, *304*(5672), 838. doi:10.1126cience.1094559 PMID:15131299

Thomson, B. M., & Grounds, P. R. (2005). Grounds, Bisphenol A in canned foods in New Zealand: An exposure assessment. *Food Additives and Contaminants*, *22*(1), 65–72. doi:10.1080/02652030400027920 PMID:15895613

Thornton, J., Lewis, J., Lebrun, C. M., & Licskai, C. J. (2012). Clinical characteristics of women with menstrual-linked asthma. Respiratory Medicine, 106(9), 1236–1243. doi:10.1016/j.rmed.2012.05.003 PubMed doi:10.1016/j.rmed.2012.05.003 PMID:22703945

Though, R. (2007). Plastic Shopping Bags: Environmental Impacts and Policy Options. New Zealand: Victoria University of Wellington.

Thurston, S. W., Mendiola, J., Bellamy, A. R., Levine, H., Wang, C., Sparks, A., ... Swan, S. H. (2016). Phthalate exposure and semen quality in fertile US men. *Andrology*, *4*(4), 632–638. doi:10.1111/andr.12124 PMID:26601918

Thushari, G. G. N., Senevirathna, J. D. M., Yakupitiyage, A., & Chavanich, S. (2017). Effects of microplastics on sessile invertebrates in the eastern coast of Thailand: An approach to coastal zone conservation. *Marine Pollution Bulletin*, *124*(1), 349–355. doi:10.1016/j.marpolbul.2017.06.010 PMID:28760587

Tian, X., Takamoto, M., & Sugane, K. (2003). Bisphenol A promotes IL-4 production by Th2 cells. International Archives of Allergy and Immunology, 132(3), 240–247. doi:10.1159/000074305 PubMed doi:10.1159/000074305 PMID:14646385

Tian, X., Zhang, X., Liu, W., Zheng, J., Ruan, C., & Cui, P. (2006). Preparation and Properties of Poly (ethylene terephthalate)/Silica Nanocomposites. *Journal of Macromolecular Science, Part B: Physics*, *45*(4), 507–513. doi:10.1080/00222340600769782

Tibbetts, J. H. (2015). Managing Marine Plastic Pollution: Policy Initiatives to Address Wayward Waste. *Environmental Health Perspectives, 123*(4), A90-A93.

Tickner, J. (2011). Phthalates and Their Alternatives: Health and Environmental Concerns. Lowell Center for Sustainable Production. Retrieved from https://www.uml.edu/docs/Phthalate%20and%20their%20 Alternatives_tcm18-229903.pdf

Tokiwa, Y., Calabia, B., Ugwu, C., & Aiba, S. (2009). Review: Biodegradability of Plastics. *International Journal of Molecular Sciences*, *10*(9), 3722–3742. doi:10.3390/ijms10093722 PMID:19865515

Tom, A. P., Haridas, A., & Pawels, R. (2016). Biodrying process efficiency: – significance of reactor matrix height. *Procedia Technology*, *25*, 130–137. doi:10.1016/j.protcy.2016.08.240

Tongamp, W., Kano, J., Zhang, Q., & Saito, F. (2008). Simultaneous treatment of PVC and oyster-shell wastes by mechanochemical means. *Waste Management (New York, N.Y.)*, *28*(3), 484–488. doi:10.1016/j.wasman.2007.01.022 PMID:17475466

Topçu, E. N., Tonay, A. M., Dede, A., Öztürk, A. A., & Öztürk, B. (2013). Origin and abundance of marine litter along sandy beaches of the Turkish Western Black Sea Coast. *Marine Environmental Research*, *85*, 21–28. doi:10.1016/j.marenvres.2012.12.006 PMID:23290790

Touati-Moungla, N., & Jost, V. (2012). Combinatorial optimization for electric vehicles management. *Journal of Energy and Power Engineering*, *6*(5), 738–743.

Toxics Link. (2014). *Report: Plastics and The Environment.* Assessing The Impact of The Complete Ban on Plastic Carry Bag.

Tran, T. T. H., & Luc, T. T. H. (2018). Reverse Logistics in Plastic Supply Chain: The Current Practice in Vietnam. In Nachhaltige Impulse für Produktion und Logistikmanagement (pp. 219-233). Springer Gabler.

Tranfo, G., Papaleo, B., Caporossi, L., Capanna, S., De Rosa, M., Pigini, D., ... Paci, E. (2013). Urinary metabolite concentrations of phthalate metabolites in Central Italy healthyvolunteers determined by a validated HPLC/MS/MS analytical method. *International Journal of Hygiene and Environmental Health*, *216*(4), 481–485. doi:10.1016/j.ijheh.2012.11.003 PMID:23270838

Trasande, L., Attina, T. M., & Blustein, J. (2012). Association between urinary Bisphenol A concentration and obesity prevalence in children and adolescents. *JAMA, 308,* 1113–1121. doi:10.1001/2012.jama.11461

Trasande, L., Attina, T. M., Sathyanarayana, S., Spanier, A. J., & Blustein, J. (2013b). Race/ethnicity specific associations of urinary phthalates with childhood body mass in a nationally representative sample. *Environmental Health Perspectives*, *121*(4), 501–506. doi:10.1289/ehp.1205526 PMID:23428635

Trasande, L., Sathyanarayana, S., Messito, M. J., Gross, R. S., Attina, T. M., & Mendelsohn, A. L. (2013). Phthalates and the diets of US children and adolescents. *Environmental Research*, *126*, 84–90. doi:10.1016/j.envres.2013.07.007 PMID:24041780

Trasande, L., Spanier, A. J., Sathyanarayana, S., Attina, T. M., & Blustein, J. (2013a). Urinary phthalates and increased insulin resistance in adolescents. *Pediatrics*, *132*(3), e646–e655. doi:10.1542/peds.2012-4022 PMID:23958772

Tseng, M., Hoang, K. C., Yang, M. K., Yang, S. F., & Chu, W. S. (2007). Polyester-degrading thermophilic actinomycetes isolated from different environment in Taiwan. *Biodegradation*, *18*(5), 579–583. doi:10.100710532-006-9089-z PMID:17653512

Turner, J. T. (2015). Zooplankton fecal pellets, marine snow, phytodetritus and the ocean's biological pump. *Progress in Oceanography*, *130*, 205–248. doi:10.1016/j.pocean.2014.08.005

Two Oceans Aquarium. (2018). *The plastic problem: How does plastic pollution affect wildlife.* Retrieved from www.aquarium.co.za

Tyl, R. W., Myers, C. B., Marr, M. C., Fail, P. A., Seely, J. C., Brine, D. R., ... Butala, J. H. (2004). Reproductive toxicity evaluation of dietary butyl benzyl phthalate (BBP) in rats. *Reproductive Toxicology (Elmsford, N.Y.)*, *18*(2), 241–264. doi:10.1016/j.reprotox.2003.10.006 PMID:15019722

U.S. Department of Energy. (2013a). *How fossil fuels were formed.* Retrieved from http://www.fe.doe.gov/education/energylessons/coal/gen_howformed.html

U.S. Department of Energy. (2013b). *Total petroleum consumption (thousand barrels per day).* Retrieved from http://www.eia.gov/cfapps/ipdbproject/iedindex3.cfm?tid=5&pid=5&aid=2&cid=regions&syid=1980&eyid=2010&unit=TBPD

U.S. Environmental Protection Agency. (2003). Framework for Cumulative Risk Assessment. U.S. Environmental Protection Agency, Office of Research and Development, National Center for Environmental Assessment, Washington Office, Washington, DC. EPA/600/P-02/001F.

U.S. Environmental Protection Agency. (2007). Concepts, Methods, and Data Sources for Cumulative Health Risk Assessment of Multiple Chemicals, Exposures and Effects: A Resource Document (Final Report). U.S. Environmental Protection Agency, Washington, DC. EPA/600/R-06/013F.

Udyawer, V., Read, M. A., Hamann, M., Simpfendorfer, C. A., & Heupel, M. R. (2013). First record of sea snake (*Hydrophis elegans*, Hydrophiinae) entrapped in marine debris. *Marine Pollution Bulletin*, *73*(1), 336–338. doi:10.1016/j.marpolbul.2013.06.023 PMID:23809333

Uemichi, Y., Makino, Y., & Kanazuka, T. (1989). Degradation of polypropylene to aromatic hydrocarbons over Pt- and Fe- containing activated carbon. *Journal of Analytical and Applied Pyrolysis*, *16*(3), 229–238. doi:10.1016/0165-2370(89)80027-0

Uemura, Y., Liu, T.-Y., Narita, Y., Suzuki, M., & Matsushita, S. (2008). 17 Beta-estradiol (E2) plus tumor necrosis factor-alpha induces a distorted maturation of human monocyte-derived dendritic cells and promotes their capacity to initiate T-helper 2 responses. Human Immunology, 69(3), 149–157. doi:10.1016/j.humimm.2008.01.017 PubMed doi:10.1016/j.humimm.2008.01.017 PMID:18396206

Uhrin, A. V., Matthews, T. R., & Lewis, C. (2014). Lobster Trap Debris in the Florida Keys National Marine Sanctuary: Distribution, Abundance, Density, and Patterns of Accumulation. *Marine and Coastal Fisheries*, *6*(1), 20–32. doi:10.1080/19425120.2013.852638

Ukei, H., Hirose, T., Horikawa, S., Takai, Y., Taka, M., Azuma, N., & Ueno, A. (2000). Catalytic degradation of polystyrene into styrene and design of recyclable polystyrene with dispersed catalysts. *Catalysis Today*, *62*(1), 67–75. doi:10.1016/S0920-5861(00)00409-0

Ulutan, S. (1998). A recycling assessment of PVC bottles by means of heat impact evaluation on its reprocessing. *Journal of Applied Polymer Science*, *69*(5), 865–869. doi:10.1002/(SICI)1097-4628(19980801)69:5<865::AID-APP4>3.0.CO;2-K

Umer, M., & Abid, M. (2017). Economic Practices in Plastic Industry from Raw Material to Waste in Pakistan: A Case Study. *Asian Journal of Water, Environment and Pollution, 14*(2), 81-90. Retrieved from https://content.iospress.com/articles/asian-journal-of-water-environment-and-pollution/ajw170018

Underkofler, L. A. (1958). Production of microbial enzymes and their applications. *Applied Microbiology*, *6*, 212–221. PMID:13534309

UNEP & FAO. (2009). *Abandoned, lost or otherwise discarded fishing gear*. FAO Fisheries and Aquaculture Technical Paper No. 523, UNEP Regional Seas Reports and Studies No. 185. Available at: http://www.fao.org/docrep/011/i0620e/i0620e00.htm

UNEP. (2011). *NEP Year book 2011: Emerging Issues in Our Global Environment*. Retrieved from http://wedocs.unep.org/bitstream/handle/20.500.11822/17716/UNEP_Year_Book_Emerging_Issues_in_our_Global.pdf?sequence=1&isAllowed=y

UNEP. (2013). Retrieved from http://www.unep.org/Documents.Multilingual/Default.asp?

UNEP. (2015). *Biodegradable Plastics and Marine Litter.Misconceptions, concerns and impacts on marine environments*. UNEP.

United States Census Bureau. (2018, December 28). *Current Population*. Retrieved from https://www.census.gov/popclock/print.php?component=counter

United States Environmental Protection Agency (USEPA). (n.d.). *Phthalates action plan summary*. Retrieved from http://www.epa.gov/oppt/existingchemicals/pubs/ actionplans/phthalates.html

United States Environmental Protection Agency. (2010). *Waste and cleanup risk assessment*. Retrieved from http://www.epa.gov/oswer/riskassessment/glossary.htm

United States Environmental Protection Agency. (2013). *Types of crude oil*. Retrieved from http://www2.epa.gov/emergency-response/types-crude-oil

United States Government Accountability Office. (1979). Operations of the National Cancer Institute's Carcinogenesis Programs, HRD-79-51. Retrieved from http://www.gao.gov/products/HRD-79-51

Upreti, M. C., & Srivastava, R. B. (2003). A potential Aspergillus species for biodegradation of polymeric materials. *Current Science*, *84*(11), 1399–1402.

Upson, K., Sathyanarayana, S., De Roos, A. J., Thompson, M. L., Scholes, D., Dills, R., & Holt, V. L. (2013). Phthalates and risk of endometriosis. *Environmental Research*, *126*, 91–97. doi:10.1016/j.envres.2013.07.003 PMID:23890968

Urban, R. M., Jacobs, J. J., Tomlinson, M. J., Gavrilovic, J., Black, J., & Peoc'H, M. (2000, April). Dissemination of wear particles to the liver, spleen, and abdominal lymph nodes of patients with hip or knee replacement. *J. Bone. Joint. Surg.*, *82*(4), 457–457. doi:10.2106/00004623-200004000-00002 PMID:10761937

Uren-Webster, T. M., Lewis, C., Filby, A. L., Paull, G. C., & Santos, E. M. (2010). Mechanisms of toxicity of di (2-ethylhexyl) phthalate on the reproductive health of male zebra fish. *AquaticToxicology*, *99*(3), 360–369. PMID:20561692

US Department of Health and Human Services Centers for Disease Control and Prevention. (2013). *Fourth national report on human exposure to environmental chemicals*. Atlanta, GA: Author.

US Environmental Protection Agency (2012). Phthalates Action Plan, Revised 03/14/2012.

US Environmental Protection Agency. (1999). *Introduction to Water Policy Standards*. Washington, DC: Office of Water.

US EPA. (2002). *Municipal Solid Waste in the United States: 2000 Facts and Figures (EPA-530-R-02-001)*. US Environmental Protection Agency.

US FDA. (2000). *Contaminates: Action Levels for Poisonous or Deleterious Substances in Human Food and Animal Feed*. Author.

US FDA. (2003). *Labeling & Nutrition: Interim Procedures for Qualified Health Claims in the Labeling of Conventional Human Food and Human Dietary Supplements*. Author.

Usha, R., Sangeetha, T., & Palaniswamy, M. (2011). Screening of Polyethylene degrading microorganisms from garbage soil. *Libyan Agricultural Research Center Journal International*, *2*, 200–204.

Usha, R., Sangeetha, T., & Palaniswamy, M. (2011). Screening of Polyethylene Degrading Microorganisms from Garbage Soil. *Libyan Agriculture Research Center Journal International*, *2*, 200–204.

Valles, E. G., Laughter, A. R., & Dunn, C. S. (2003). Role of the perox- isome proliferator-activated receptor alpha in responses to diisononyl phthalate. *Toxicology*, *191*(2–3), 211–225. doi:10.1016/S0300-483X(03)00260-9 PMID:12965124

Van Cauwenberghe, L., Claessens, M., Vandegehuchte, M., & Janssen, C. R. (2014). XXII International Pigment Cell Conference (IPCC) "Bringing Colors to Life: Advances in Pigment Cell Research and Translation into Clinical Practice" Organised by the Asian Society for Pigment Cell Research (ASPCR), in partnership with the Dermatological. In *Pigment Cell & Melanoma Research* (Vol. 27). 10.1111/pcmr.12292

Van Cauwenberghe, L., Claessens, M., Vandegehuchte, M. B., & Janssen, C. R. (2015). Microplastics are taken up by mussels (Mytilus edulis) and lugworms (Arenicola marina) living in natural habitats. *Environmental Pollution*, *199*, 10–17. doi:10.1016/j.envpol.2015.01.008 PMID:25617854

Van Cauwenberghe, L., Claessens, M., Vandegehuchte, M. B., Mees, J., & Janssen, C. R. (2013). Assessment of marine debris on the Belgian Continental Shelf. *Marine Pollution Bulletin*, *73*(1), 161–169. doi:10.1016/j.marpolbul.2013.05.026 PMID:23790460

Van Cauwenberghe, L., & Janssen, C. R. (2014). Microplastics in bivalves cultured for human consumption. *Environmental Pollution*, *193*, 65–70. doi:10.1016/j.envpol.2014.06.010 PMID:25005888

Van Cauwenberghe, L., Vanreusel, A., Mees, J., & Janssen, C. R. (2013). Microplastic pollution in deep-sea sediments. *Environmental Pollution*, *182*, 495–499. doi:10.1016/j.envpol.2013.08.013 PMID:24035457

van den Oever, Molenveld, van der Zee, & Bos. (2017). *Report No. 1722*. Wageningen Food & Biobased Research.

Van Sebille, E., Spathi, C., & Gilbert, A. (2016). The ocean plastic pollution challenge: Towards solutions in the UK. *Grant. Brief. Pap*, *19*, 1–16.

Van Tongeren, M., Nieuwenhuijsen, M. J., Gardiner, K., Armstrong, B., Vrijheid, M., Dolk, H., & Botting, B. (2002). A job–exposure matrix for potential endocrine-disrupting chemicals developed for a study into the association between maternal occupational exposure and hypospadias. *The Annals of Occupational Hygiene*, *46*(5), 465–477. PMID:12176761

van Veilen, J. B., & Poirier, Y. (2008). Production of renewable polymers from crop plants. *The Plant Journal*, *54*(4), 684–701. doi:10.1111/j.1365-313X.2008.03431.x PMID:18476872

Vandenberg, L. N., Chahoud, I., Heindel, J. J., Padmanabhan, V., Paumgartten, F. J. R., & Schoenfelder, G. (2010). Urinary, circulating, and tissue biomonitoring studies indicate widespread exposure to bisphenol A. Environmental Health Perspectives, 118(8), 1055–1070. doi:10.1289/ehp.0901716 PubMed doi:10.1289/ehp.0901716 PMID:20338858

Vandenberg, L. N., Colborn, T., Hayes, T. B., Heindel, J. J., Jacobs, D. R., Jr., Lee, D.-H., . . . Myers, J. P. (2012). Hormones and endocrinedisrupting chemicals: Low-dose effects and nonmonotonic dose responses. Endocrine Reviews, 33(3), 1–378. doi:10.1210/er.2011-1050 PubMed doi:10.1210/er.2011-1050 PMID:22419778

Vandenberg, L. N., Colborn, T., Hayes, T. B., Heindel, J. J., Jacobs, D. R., Jr., Lee, D.-H., . . . Zoeller, R. T. (2013). Regulatory decisions on endocrine disrupting chemicals should be based on the principles of endocrinology. Reproductive Toxicology (Elmsford, N.Y.), 38, 1–15. doi:10.1016/j.reprotox.2013.02.002 PubMed doi:10.1016/j.reprotox.2013.02.002 PMID:23411111

Vandenberg, L. N., Hauser, R., Marcus, M., Olea, N., & Welshons, W. V. (2007). Human exposure to bisphenol A (BPA). *Reproductive Toxicology (Elmsford, N.Y.)*, *24*(2), 139–177. doi:10.1016/j.reprotox.2007.07.010 PMID:17825522

Vandenberg, L. N., Maffini, M. V., Sonnenschein, C., Rubin, B. S., & Soto, A. M. (2009). Bisphenol-A and the great divide: A review of controversies in the field of endocrine disruption. *Endocrine Reviews*, *30*(1), 75–95. doi:10.1210/er.2008-0021 PMID:19074586

Van, G. R., Serrano, D. P., Aguado, J., García, R., & Rojo, C. (2001). Thermal and catalytic Cracking of polyethylene under mild conditions. *Journal of Analytical and Applied Pyrolysis*, *58*, 127–142.

Varotto, L., Domeneghetti, S., Rosani, U., Manfrin, C., Cajaraville, M. P., Raccanelli, S., ... Venier, P. (2013). DNA Damage and Transcriptional Changes in the Gills of Mytilus galloprovincialis Exposed to Nanomolar Doses of Combined Metal Salts (Cd, Cu, Hg). *PLoS One*, *8*(1), e54602. doi:10.1371/journal.pone.0054602 PMID:23355883

Vélez-Rubio, G. M., Estrades, A., Fallabrino, A., & Tomás, J. (2013). Marine turtle threats in Uruguayan waters: Insights from 12 years of stranding data. *Marine Biology*, *160*(11), 2797–2811. doi:10.100700227-013-2272-y

Velis, C. (2017). Waste pickers in Global South: Informal recycling sector in a circular economy era. *Waste Management & Research*, 35(4), 329-331

Velis, C. A., Longhurst, P. J., Drew, G. H., Smith, R., & Pollard, S. J. (2009). Biodrying for mechanical–biological treatment of wastes: A review of process science and engineering. *Bioresource Technology*, *100*(11), 2747–2761. doi:10.1016/j.biortech.2008.12.026 PMID:19216072

Vendel, A. L., Bessa, F., Alves, V. E. N., Amorim, A. L. A., Patrício, J., & Palma, A. R. T. (2017). Widespread microplastic ingestion by fish assemblages in tropical estuaries subjected to anthropogenic pressures. *Marine Pollution Bulletin*, *117*(1-2), 448–455. doi:10.1016/j.marpolbul.2017.01.081 PMID:28214011

Venkatesh, S., & Kukreti, I. (2018). *India's plastic consumption increases at over 10 percent year-on-year*. Down to Earth.

Ventrice, P., Ventrice, D., Russo, E., & De Sarro, G. (2013). Phthalates: European regulation, chemistry, pharmacokinetic and related toxicity. *Environmental Toxicology and Pharmacology*, *36*(1), 88–96. doi:10.1016/j.etap.2013.03.014 PMID:23603460

Vergara, S. E., & Tchobanoglous, G. (2012). Municipal Solid Waste and the Environment: A Global Perspective. *Annual Review of Environment and Resources*, *37*(1), 277–309. doi:10.1146/annurev-environ-050511-122532

Verma, R., Vinoda, K. S., Papireddy, M., & Gowda, A. N. (2016). Toxic Polluntants from Plasti Waste - A Review. *Procedia Environmental Sciences*, *35*, 701–708. doi:10.1016/j.proenv.2016.07.069

Vert, M. (2011). Not any new functional polymer can be for medicine: What about artificial biopolymers? *Macromolecular Bioscience*, *11*(12), 1653–1661. doi:10.1002/mabi.201100224 PMID:22052691

Vigiak, O., Ribolzi, O., Pierret, A., Sengtaheuanghoung, O., & Valentin, C. (2008). Trapping Efficiencies of Cultivated and Natural Riparian Vegetation of Northern Laos. *Journal of Environment Quality*, 889. doi:10.2134/jeq2007.0251

Vijayalakshmi, Mekala, Yoganand, & Pandiyaraj. (2011). Studies on Modification of Surface Properties in Polycarbonate (PC) Film Induced by DC Glow Discharge Plasma. *International Journal of Polymer Science*, 1-7.

Vikelsøe, J., Thomsen, M., & Carlsen, L. (2002). Phthalates and nonylphenols in profiles of differently dressed soils. *The Science of the Total Environment*, *296*(1-3), 105–116. doi:10.1016/S0048-9697(02)00063-3 PMID:12398330

Vilaplana, F., Ribes-Greus, A., & Karlsson, S. (2006). Degradation of recycled high-impact polystyrene: Simulation by reprocessing and thermooxidation. *Polymer Degradation & Stability*, *91*(9), 2163–2170. doi:10.1016/j.polymdegradstab.2006.01.007

Villalobos, M., Olea, N., Brontons, J. A., Olea-Serrano, M. F., & Pedraza, V. (1995). The E-screen assay: A comparison of different MCF7 cell stocks. *Environmental Health Perspectives*, *103*(9), 844–850. doi:10.1289/ehp.95103844 PMID:7498097

Vinas, R., Jeng, Y. J., & Watson, C. S. (2012). Non-genomic effects of xenoestrogen mixtures. *International Journal of Environmental Research and Public Health*, *9*(8), 2694–2714. doi:10.3390/ijerph9082694 PMID:23066391

Vince, J., & Hardesty, B. D. (2017). Plastic pollution challenges in marine and coastal environments: From local to global governance. *Restoration Ecology*, *25*(1), 123–128. doi:10.1111/rec.12388

Virilio, P. (1998). The Virilio Reader. Malden, MA: Blackwell Publishers.

Vishwakarma, S. K., Pandey, P., & Gupta, N. K. (2017). Characterization of ABS Material: A Review. *Journal of Research in Mechanical Engineering*, *3*(5), 13–16.

Vogel, S. A. (2009). The politics of plastics: The making and unmaking of bisphenol A 'safety'. American Journal of Public Health, 99(S3), S559–S566. doi:10.2105/AJPH.2008.159228 PubMed doi:10.2105/AJPH.2008.159228 PMID:19890158

Volkel, W., Colnot, T., Csanady, G. A., Filser, J. G., & Dekant, W. (2002). Metabolism and kinetics of Bisphenol A in humans at low doses following oral administration. *Chemical Research in Toxicology*, *15*(10), 1281–1287. doi:10.1021/tx025548t PMID:12387626

Volke-Sepulveda, T., Saucedo-Castaneda, G., Gutierrez-Rojas, M., Manzur, A., & Favela-Torres, E. (2002). Thermally treated low density polyethylene biodegradation by *Penicillium pinophilum* and *Aspergillus niger*. *Journal of Applied Polymer Science*, *83*(2), 305–314. doi:10.1002/app.2245

Vom Saal, F. S. (2018). Commentary: FDA Statement on BPA's Safety Is Premature. Environ. Heal. News. Retrieved from https://www.ehn.org/ fda-flawed-statement-science-bpa-2542621453.html

Vom Saal, F. S., & Hughes, C. (2005). an extensive new literature concerning low-dose effecs of bisphenol A shows the need for a newrisk assessment. *Environmental Health Perspectives*, *113*(8), 926–933. doi:10.1289/ehp.7713 PMID:16079060

Vom Saal, F. S., Nagel, S. C., Coe, B. L., Angle, B. M., & Taylor, J. A. (2012). The estrogenic endocrine disrupting chemical Bisphenol A (BISPHENOL A) and obesity. *Molecular and Cellular Endocrinology*, *354*(1-2), 74–84. doi:10.1016/j.mce.2012.01.001 PMID:22249005

Von Moos, N., Burkhardt-Holm, P., & Köhler, A. (2012). Uptake and effects of microplastics on cells and tissue of the blue mussel Mytilus edulis L. after an experimental exposure. *Environmental Science & Technology*, *46*(20), 11327–11335. doi:10.1021/es302332w PMID:22963286

Vroman, I., & Tighzert, L. (2009). Biodegradable Polymers. *Materials (Basel)*, *2*(2), 307–344. doi:10.3390/ma2020307

Výnos Ministerstva Pôdohospodárstva Slovenskej republiky a Ministerstva Zdravotníctva Slovenskej republiky z 15. marca 2004 No. 608/3/2004 - 100, ktorým sa vydáva hlava Potravinového Kódexu Slovenskej republiky upravujúca kontaminanty v potravinách [Slovak decree of the Ministry of Agriculture of the Slovak Republic and the Slovak Ministry of Health of 15 March 2004 No. 608/3/2004 - 100, issuing the chapter Slovak Republic Foodstuffs Code governing contaminants in food, in Slovak]. Ministerstva Pôdohospodárstva Slovenskej republiky 2004.

Wabnitz, C., & Nichols, W. J. (2010). Editorial: Plastic Pollution: An Ocean Emergency. *Marine Turtle Newsletter*, *20*(129), 1–4. Retrieved from http://search.proquest.com/docview/924334169?accountid=27795

Wackett, L. P., & Hershberger, C. D. (2001). *Biocatalysis and Biodegradation; Microbial Transformation of Organic Compounds*. Washington, DC: ASM Press.

Wada, K., Sakamoto, H., Nishikawa, K., Sakuma, S., Nakajima, A., Fujimoto, Y., & Kamisaki, Y. (2007). Lifestyle-related diseases of the digestive system: Endocrine disruptors stimulate lipid accumulation in target cells related to metabolic syndrome. *Journal of Pharmacological Sciences*, *105*(2), 133–137. doi:10.1254/jphs.FM0070034 PMID:17928741

Wadge, A., & Hutton, M. (1986). The uptake of cadmium, lead and selenium by barley and cabbage grown on soils amended with refuse incinerator fly ash. *Plant and Soil*, *96*(3), 407–412. doi:10.1007/BF02375144

Wagner, M., & Oehlmann, J. (2009). Endocrine disruptors in bottledmineral water: total estrogenic burden and migration from plasticbottles. *Environ. Sci. Pollut. Res*, *16*, 278–286. -009-0107-7 doi:10.100711356

Wagner, M., Scherer, C., Alvarez-Muñoz, D., Brennholt, N., Bourrain, X., Buchinger, S., ... Reifferscheid, G. (2014). Microplastics in freshwater ecosystems: What we know and what we need to know. *Environmental Sciences Europe*, *26*(1), 1–9. doi:10.118612302-014-0012-7 PMID:28936382

Wagner, T. P. (2012). Examining the concept of convenient collection: An application to extended producer responsibility and product stewardship frameworks. *Waste Management (New York, N.Y.)*, *33*(3), 499–507. doi:10.1016/j.wasman.2012.06.015 PMID:22818910

Walvoord, E. C. (2010). The Timing of Puberty: Is it changing? Does it matter? *The Journal of Adolescent Health*, *47*(5), 433–439. doi:10.1016/j.jadohealth.2010.05.018 PMID:20970077

Wang, H. X., Zhou, Y., Tang, C. X., Wu, J. G., Chen, Y., & Jiang, Q. W. (2012). Association between Bisphenol A exposure and body mass index in Chinese school children: A cross sectional study. *Environmental Health*, *11*(1), 79. doi:10.1186/1476-069X-11-79 PMID:23083070

Wang, H., Zhou, Y., Tang, C., He, Y., Wu, J., Chen, Y., & Jiang, Q. (2013). Urinary phthalate metabolites are associated with body mass index and waist circumference in Chinese schoolchildren. *PLoS One*, *8*(2), e56800. doi:10.1371/journal.pone.0056800 PMID:23437242

Wang, I. J., Karmaus, W. J., Chen, S. L., Holloway, J. W., & Ewart, S. (2015). Effects of phthalate exposure on asthma may be mediated through alterations in DNA methylation. *Clinical Epigenetics*, *7*(1), 1. doi:10.118613148-015-0060-x PMID:25960783

Wang, J. G., & Bakken, L. R. (1998). Screening of soil bacteria for polybeta- hydroxybutyric acid production and its role in the survival of starvation. *Microbial Ecology*, *35*(1), 94–101. doi:10.1007002489900063 PMID:9459662

Wang, J., Li, X., Zhang, Q., Xiong, J., & Li, H. (2015). Determination of phthalate esters in Chinese spirits using isotope dilution gaschromatography with tandem mass spectrometry. *Journal of Separation Science*, *38*(10), 1700–1710. doi:10.1002/jssc.201401001 PMID:25755215

Wang, S. F., & Grosssman, S. J. (1987). Plastic materials for insulating applications. *Journal of Chemical Education*, *64*(1), 39–44. doi:10.1021/ed064p39

Wang, T., Li, M., Chen, B., Xu, M., Xu, Y., Huang, Y., ... Ning, G. (2012). Urinary Bisphenol A (BISPHENOL A) Concentration Associates with Obesity and Insulin Resistance. *The Journal of Clinical Endocrinology and Metabolism*, *97*(2), E223–E227. doi:10.1210/jc.2011-1989 PMID:22090277

Wang, T., Lu, J., Xu, M., Xu, Y., Li, M., Liu, Y., ... Ning, G. (2013). Urinary bisphenol Aconcentration and thyroid function in Chinese adults. *Epidemiology (Cambridge, Mass.)*, *24*(2), 295–302. doi:10.1097/EDE.0b013e318280e02f PMID:23337242

Wang, X., Tao, W., Xu, Y., Feng, J., & Wang, F. (2014). Indoor phthalate concentration and exposure in residential and office buildings in Xi'an, China. *Atmospheric Environment*, *87*, 146–152. doi:10.1016/j.atmosenv.2014.01.018

Wang, Y., & Lobstein, T. (2006). Worldwide trends in childhood overweight and obesity. *International Journal of Pediatric Obesity; IJPO*, *1*(1), 11–25. doi:10.1080/17477160600586747 PMID:17902211

Ward, P. G., Goff, M., Donner, M., Kaminsky, W., & O'Connor, K. E. (2006). A two-stepchemo-biotechnological conversion of polystyrene to a biodegradable thermoplastic. *Environmental Science & Technology*, *40*(7), 2433–2437. doi:10.1021/es0517668 PMID:16649270

Warkentin, I. G., Sodhi, N. S., Espie, R. H. M., & Poole, A. F. (2005). Merlin (Falco columbarius). *The Birds of North America Online*. doi:10.2173/bna.44

Warner, M., Eskenazi, B., Mocarelli, P., Gerthoux, P. M., Samuels, S., Needham, L., ... Brambilla, P. (2002). Serum dioxin concentrations and breast cancer risk in the Seveso Women's Health Study. *Environmental Health Perspectives*, *110*(7), 625–628. doi:10.1289/ehp.02110625 PMID:12117637

Waste Prevention Association. (2003). *Medical Waste Treatment Technologies-Alternatives to Incineration.* Available from http://www.otzo.most.org.pl/en/docs/med_tech.pdf

Watanabe, M., Yasuaki, M., Takashi, M., Hiroshi, I., Toshiyuki, M., & Katsuhiko, H. (2009). Chemical recycling of polycarbonate in high-pressurehigh-temperature steam at 573 K. *Polymer Degradation & Stability*, *94*(12), 2157–2162. doi:10.1016/j.polymdegradstab.2009.09.010

Waterman, P. (1992). *Internationallabour Communication by Computer: The Fifth International?* Working.

Watson, J. L. (Ed.). (1997). *Golden Arches East: McDonald's in East Asia*. Palo Alto, CA: Stanford University Press.

Watters, D. L., Yoklavich, M. M., Love, M. S., & Schroeder, D. M. (2010). Assessing marine debris in deep seafloor habitats off California. *Marine Pollution Bulletin*, *60*(1), 131–138. doi:10.1016/j.marpolbul.2009.08.019 PMID:19751942

Webb, H. K., Arnott, J., Crawford, R. J., & Ivanova, E. P. (2013). Plastic Degradation and Its Environmental Implications with Special Reference to Poly (ethylene terephthalate). *Polymers*, *5*(1), 1–18. doi:10.3390/polym5010001

Webb, H. K., Crawford, R. J., Sawabe, T., & Ivanova, E. P. (2009). Poly(ethylene terephthalate) Polymer Surfaces as a Substrate for Bacterial Attachment and Biofilm Formation. *Microbes and Environments*, *24*(1), 39–42. doi:10.1264/jsme2.ME08538 PMID:21566352

Webb, J. S., Nixon, M., Eastwood, I. M., Greenhalgh, M., Robson, G. D., & Handley, P. S. (2000). Fungal colonization and biodeterioration of plasticized polyvinyl chloride. *Applied and Environmental Microbiology*, *66*(8), 3194–3200. doi:10.1128/AEM.66.8.3194-3200.2000 PMID:10919769

Webster, F. (1995). Theories of the Information Society. London, UK: Routledge. doi:10.4324/9780203991367

Wegner, A., Besseling, E., Foekema, E. M., Kamermans, P., & Koelmans, A. A. (2012). Effects of nanopolystyrene on the feeding behavior of the blue mussel (Mytilus edulis L.). *Environmental Toxicology and Chemistry*, *31*(11), 2490–2497. doi:10.1002/etc.1984 PMID:22893562

Wei, J., Zhao, J., & Sun, X. (2012). Reverse channel decisions for a fuzzy closed-loop supply chain. *Applied Mathematical Modelling*.

Weinstein, J. E., Crocker, B. K., & Gray, A. D. (2016). From macroplastic to microplastic: Degradation of high-density polyethylene, polypropylene, and polystyrene in a salt marsh habitat. *Environmental Toxicology and Chemistry*, *35*(7), 1632–1640. doi:10.1002/etc.3432 PMID:26992845

Weiss, T., & Angerer, J. (2002). Simultaneous determination of various aromatic amines and metabolites of aromatic nitro compounds in urine for low level exposure using gas chromatography–mass spectrometry. *Journal of Chromatography. B, Analytical Technologies in the Biomedical and Life Sciences*, *778*(1-2), 179–192. doi:10.1016/S0378-4347(01)00542-4 PMID:12376125

Welden, N. A., Abylkhani, B., & Howarth, L. M. (2018). The effects of trophic transfer and environmental factors on microplastic uptake by plaice, Pleuronectes plastessa, and spider crab, Maja squinado. *Environmental Pollution*, *239*, 351–358. doi:10.1016/j.envpol.2018.03.110 PMID:29674213

Wellisch, M., Jungmeier, G., Karbowski, A., Patel, M.K., & Rogulska, M. (2010). Biorefinery systems – potential contributors to sustainable innovation. *Biofuels, Bioproducts & Biorefining*, *4*(3), 275-286. Doi:10.1002/bbb.217

Welsh, M., Saunders, P. T., Fisken, M., Scott, H. M., Hutchison, G. R., Smith, L. B., & Sharpe, R. M. (2008). Identification in rats of a programming window for reproductive tract masculinization, disruption of which leads to hypospadias and cryptorchidism. *The Journal of Clinical Investigation*, *118*(4), 1479–1490. doi:10.1172/JCI34241 PMID:18340380

Welshons, W. V., Nagel, S. C., & vom Saal, F. S. (2006). Saal FSv. Large effects from small exposures. III. Endocrine mechanisms mediating effects of bisphenol A at levels of human exposure. Endocrinology, 147(6), s56–s69. doi:10.1210/en.2005-1159 PubMed doi:10.1210/en.2005-1159 PMID:16690810

Welshons, W. V., Nagel, S. C., Thayer, K. A., Judy, B. M., & Vom Saal, F. S. (1999). Low-dose bioactivity of xenoestrogens in animals: Fetal exposure to low doses of methoxychlor and other xenoestrogens increases adult prostate size in mice. *Toxicology and Industrial Health*, *15*(1), 12–25. doi:10.1191/074823399678846745 PMID:10188188

Welshons, W. V., Thayer, K. A., Judy, B. M., Taylor, J. A., Curran, E. M., & Vom Saal, F. S. (2003). large effects from small exposures. I. Mechanisms for endocrine-disrupting chemicals with estrogenic activity. *Environmental Health Perspectives*, *111*(8), 994–1006. doi:10.1289/ehp.5494 PMID:12826473

Weng, Y. I., Hsu, P. Y., Liyanarachchi, S., Liu, J., Deatherage, D. E., Huang, Y.-W., ... Cheng, A.-L. (2010). Epigenetic influences of low-dose Bisphenol A in primary human breast epithelial cells. *Toxicology and Applied Pharmacology*, *248*(2), 111–121. doi:10.1016/j.taap.2010.07.014 PMID:20678512

Westerhout, R. W. J., Waanders, J., Kuipers, J. A. M., & Swaaij, W. P. M. (1997). Kinetics of the low-temperature pyrolysis of polyethene, polypropene, and polystyrene modeling, experimental determination, and comparison with literature models and data. *Industrial & Engineering Chemistry Research*, *36*(6), 1955–1964. doi:10.1021/ie960501m

Wetherill, Y. B., Akingbemi, B. T., Kanno, J., McLachlan, J. A., Nadal, A., Sonnenschein, C., ... Belcher, S. M. (2007). In vitro molecular mechanisms of Bisphenol A action. *Reproductive Toxicology (Elmsford, N.Y.), 24*(2), 178–198. doi:10.1016/j.reprotox.2007.05.010 PMID:17628395

WHO. (2003). Retrieved from http://www.who.int/water_sanitation_health/dwq/chemicals/di2ethylhexyphthalate.pdf

Whyatt, R. M., Perzanowski, M. S., Just, A. C., Rundle, A. G., Donohue, K. M., Calafat, A. M., . . . Miller, R. L. (2014). Asthma in inner-city children at 5-11 years of age and prenatal exposure to phthalates: The Columbia Center for Children's Environmental Health Cohort. Environmental Health Perspectives, 122(10), 1141–1146. doi:10.1289/ehp.1307670 PubMed doi:10.1289/ehp.1307670 PMID:25230320

Wiedinmyer, C., Yokelson, R. J., & Gullett, B. K. (2014). Global Emissions of Trace Gases, Particulate Matter, and Hazardous Air Pollutants from Open Burning of Domestic Waste. *Environmental Science & Technology, 48*(16), 9523–9530. doi:10.1021/es502250z PMID:25019173

Wiewel, B. V., & Lamoree, M. (2016). Geotextile composition, application and ecotoxicology—A review. *Journal of Hazardous Materials, 317*, 640–655. doi:10.1016/j.jhazmat.2016.04.060 PMID:27283344

Willhite, C. C., Ball, G. L., & McLellan, C. J. (2008). Derivation of a bisphenol A oral reference dose (RfD) and drinking-water equivalent concentration. *Journal of Toxicology and Environmental Health, 11*(2), 69–146. doi:10.1080/10937400701724303 PMID:18188738

Williams, P.T., & Williams, E.A. (1998). Recycling plastic waste by pyrolysis. *Journal of the Energy Institute, 71*, 81-93.

Williams, E. S., Panko, J., & Paustenbach, D. J. (2008). The European Union's REACH regulation: A review of its history and requirements. *Critical Reviews in Toxicology, 39*(7), 553–575. doi:10.1080/10408440903036056 PMID:19650717

Williams, G. (2012). Aromatase up-regulation, insulin and raised intracellular oestrogens in men, induce adiposity, metabolic syndrome and prostate disease, via aberrant ER-α and GPER signalling. *Molecular and Cellular Endocrinology, 351*(2), 269–278. doi:10.1016/j.mce.2011.12.017 PMID:22233684

Williams, G. P. (2010). The role of oestrogen in the pathogenesis of obesity, type 2 diabetes, breast cancer and prostate disease. *European Journal of Cancer Prevention, 19*(4), 256–271. doi:10.1097/CEJ.0b013e328338f7d2 PMID:20535861

Williamson, D. H., & Wilkinson, J. F. (1958). The isolation and estimation of the poly-beta-hydroxybutyrate inclusions of Bacillus species. *Journal of General Microbiology, 19*(1), 198–209. doi:10.1099/00221287-19-1-198 PMID:13575768

Williamson, L. J. (2003). It's Not My Bag, Baby! *Onearth, 25*(2), 32–34.

Wilson, A. S. (1995). *Plasticizers. Principles and practices*. Cambridge, MA: The Institute of Materials.

Wilson, D. C., Araba, A. O., Chinwah, K., & Cheeseman, C. R. (2009). Building recycling rates through the informal sector. *Waste Management (New York, N.Y.), 29*(2), 629–635. doi:10.1016/j.wasman.2008.06.016 PMID:18701272

Wilson, D. C., Costas, V., & Cheeseman, C. (2006). Role of informal sector recycling in waste management in developing countries. *Habitat International, 30*(4), 797–808. doi:10.1016/j.habitatint.2005.09.005

Wilson, N. K., Chuang, J. C., Morgan, M. K., Lordo, R. A., & Sheldon, L. S. (2007). An observational study of the potential exposures of preschool children to pentachlorophenol, bisphenol-A, and nonylphenol at home and daycare. *Environmental Research, 103*(1), 9–20. doi:10.1016/j.envres.2006.04.006 PMID:16750524

Wilson, R. (1995). Nature and Young Children. *Young Children, 50*(6), 4–11.

Wilson, V. S., Blystone, C. R., Hotchkiss, A. K., Rider, C. V., & Gray, L. E. (2008). Diverse mechanisms of anti-androgen action: Impact on male rat reproductive tractdevelopment. *International Journal of Andrology*, *31*(2), 178–187. doi:10.1111/j.1365-2605.2007.00861.x PMID:18315717

Wilson, V. S., Lambright, C., Furr, J., Ostby, J., Wood, C., Held, G., & Gray, L. E. Jr. (2004). Phthalate ester-induced gubernacular lesions are associated with reduced insl3 gene expression in the fetal rat testis. *Toxicology Letters*, *146*(3), 207–215. doi:10.1016/j.toxlet.2003.09.012 PMID:14687758

Windfeld, E. S., & Brooks, M. S. (2015). Medical Waste Management – A Review. *Journal of Environmental Management*, *163*, 98–108. doi:10.1016/j.jenvman.2015.08.013 PMID:26301686

Wirth, J. J., Rossano, M. G., Potter, R., Puscheck, E., Daly, D. C., Paneth, N., ... Diamond, M. P. (2008). A pilot study associating urinary concentrations of phthalate metabolites and semen quality. *Systems Biology in Reproductive Medicine*, *54*(3), 143–154. doi:10.1080/19396360802055921 PMID:18570050

Wittassek, M., & Angerer, J. (2008). Phthalates: Metabolism and exposure. *International Journal of Andrology*, *31*(2), 131–138. doi:10.1111/j.1365-2605.2007.00837.x PMID:18070048

Wittassek, M., Angerer, J., Kolossa-Gehring, M., Schäfer, S. D., Klockenbusch, W., Dobler, L., ... Wiesmüller, G. A. (2009). Fetal exposure to phthalates–a pilot study. *International Journal of Hygiene and Environmental Health*, *212*(5), 492–498. doi:10.1016/j.ijheh.2009.04.001 PMID:19423389

Wittassek, M., Koch, H. M., Angerer, J., & Brüning, T. (2011). Assessing exposure to phthalates–the human biomonitoring approach. *Molecular Nutrition & Food Research*, *55*(1), 7–31. doi:10.1002/mnfr.201000121 PMID:20564479

Wittassek, M., Wiesmüller, G. A., Koch, H. M., Eckard, R., Dobler, L., Müller, J., ... Schlüter, C. (2007). Internal phthalate exposure over the last two decades–a retrospective humanbiomonitoring study. *International Journal of Hygiene and Environmental Health*, *210*(3), 319–333. doi:10.1016/j.ijheh.2007.01.037 PMID:17400024

Witt, U., Einig, T., Yamamoto, M., Kleeberg, I., Deckwer, W. D., & Müller, R. J. (2001). Biodegradation of aliphatic–aromatic copolyesters: Evaluation of the final biodegradability and ecotoxicological impact of degradation intermediates. *Chemosphere*, *44*(2), 289–299. doi:10.1016/S0045-6535(00)00162-4 PMID:11444312

Wojanowski, R., Verter, V., & Boyaci, T. (2007). Retail-Collection Network Design under Deposit-Refund. *Computers & Operations Research*, *34*(2), 324–345. doi:10.1016/j.cor.2005.03.003

Wolf, C., Lambright, C., Mann, P., Price, M., Cooper, R. L., Ostby, J., & Gray, L. E. Jr. (1999). Administration of potentially antiandrogenic pesticides (procymidone, linuron, iprodione, chlozolinate, p, p′-DDE, and ketoconazole) and toxic substances (dibutyl-and diethylhexyl phthalate, PCB 169, and ethane dimethanesulphonate) during sexual differentiation produces diverse profiles of reproductive malformations in the male rat. *Toxicology and Industrial Health*, *15*(1-2), 94–118. doi:10.1177/074823379901500109 PMID:10188194

Wolfer, S., Sander, H., & Gogoll, F. (2012). *Reverse Logistics for Waste Electrical and Electronic Equipment (WEEE) in China*. Academic Press.

Wolff, M. S., Engel, S. M., Berkowitz, G. S., Ye, X., Silva, M. J., Zhu, C., ... Calafat, A. M. (2008). Prenatal phenol and phthalate exposures and birth outcomes. *Environmental Health Perspectives*, *116*(8), 1092–1097. doi:10.1289/ehp.11007 PMID:18709157

Woodall, L. C., Robinson, L. F., Rogers, A. D., Narayanaswamy, B. E., & Paterson, G. L. J. (2015). Deep-sea litter: A comparison of seamounts, banks and a ridge in the Atlantic and Indian Oceans reveals both environmental and anthropogenic factors impact accumulation and composition. *Frontiers of Materials Science*, *2*. doi:10.3389/fmars.2015.00003

Woods, L., & Bakshi, B. R. (2014). Reusable vs. disposable cups revisited: Guidance in life cycle comparisons addressing scenario, model, and parameter uncertainties for the US consumer. *The International Journal of Life Cycle Assessment*, *19*(4), 931–940. doi:10.100711367-013-0697-7

Woodward, B. L., Winn, J. P., Moore, M. J., & Peterson, M. L. (2006). Experimental modeling of large whale entanglement injuries. *Marine Mammal Science*, *22*(2), 299–310. doi:10.1111/j.1748-7692.2006.00020.x

Woo, O. S., Ayala, N., & Broadbelt, L. J. (2000). Mechanistic interpretation of base-catalyzed depolymerization of polystyrene. *Catalysis Today*, *55*(1-2), 161–171. doi:10.1016/S0920-5861(99)00235-7

World Health Organization (WHO). (2017). *Guidelines for Drinking-Water Quality*. WHO.

Worm, B., Barbier, E. B., Beaumont, N., Duffy, J. E., Folke, C., Halpern, B. S., ... Watson, R. (2006). Impacts of biodiversity loss on ocean ecosystem services. *Science*, *314*(5800), 787–790. doi:10.1126cience.1132294 PMID:17082450

Wormuth, M., Scheringer, M., Vollenweider, M., & Hungerbuhler, K. (2006). What are the sources of exposure to eight frequently used phthalic acid esters in Europeans. Risk Analysis, 26(3), 803–824. doi:10.1111/j.1539-6924.2006.00770.x PubMed doi:10.1111/j.1539-6924.2006.00770.x PMID:16834635

Wozniak, A. L., Bulayeva, N. N., & Watson, C. S. (2005). Xenoestrogens at picomolar to nanomolar concentrations trigger membrane estrogen receptor-alphamediated Ca2+ fluxes and prolactin release in GH3/B6 pituitary tumor cells. *Environmental Health Perspectives*, *113*(4), 431–439. doi:10.1289/ehp.7505 PMID:15811834

WRAP. (2009). *Biopolymer packaging in UK grocery market*. Banbury, UK: WRAP.

Wright, S. L., Thompson, R. C., & Galloway, T. S. (2013). The physical impacts of microplastics on marine organisms: A review. *Environmental Pollution*, *178*, 483–492. doi:10.1016/j.envpol.2013.02.031 PMID:23545014

Wrya, M., Joseph, R. C., & Paul, D. E. (2018). Using Solar Thermal Collectors for Plastic Recycling in Additive Manufacturing. *UKH Journal of Science and Engineering*.

Wu, B., Wang, D., Chai, X., Takahashi, F., & Shimaoka, T. (2016). Characterization of chlorine and heavy metals for the potential recycling of bottom ash from municipal solid waste incinerators as cement additives. *Frontiers of Environmental Science & Engineering*, *10*(4), 1–8. doi:10.100711783-016-0847-9

Wu, M. T., Wu, C. F., Chen, B. H., Chen, E. K., Chen, Y. L., Shiea, J., ... Wu, J. R. (2013). Intake of phthalate-tainted foods alters thyroid functions in Taiwanese children. *PLoS One*, *8*(1), e55005. doi:10.1371/journal.pone.0055005 PMID:23383031

Wu, S., Zhu, J., Li, Y., Lin, T., Gan, L., Yuan, X., ... Wei, G. (2010). Dynamic effect of di-2- (ethylhexyl) phthalate on testicular toxicity: Epigenetic changes and their impact on gene expression. *International Journal of Toxicology*, *29*(2), 193–200. doi:10.1177/1091581809355488 PMID:20335514

Wu, Y.-H., Zhou, Q., Zhao, T., Deng, M.-L., Zhang, J., & Wang, Y.-Z. (2009). Poly (ethylene glycol) enhanced dehydrochlorination of poly (vinyl chloride). *Journal of Hazardous Materials*, *163*(2-3), 1408–1411. doi:10.1016/j.jhazmat.2008.07.047 PMID:18723284

Wyszkowska, J., & Wyszkowski, M. (2002). Effect of cadmium and magnesium on microbiological activity in soil. *Polish Journal of Environmental Studies*, *11*(5), 585–591.

Wyszkowski, M., & Sivitskaya, V. (2012). Changes in the content of organic carbon and available forms of macronutrients in soil under the influence of soil contamination with fuel oil and application of different substances. *Journal of Elementology*, *17*(1), 139–148.

Wyszkowski, M., & Wyszkowska, J. (2009). The effect of contamination with cadmium on spring barley (Hordeum vulgare L.) and its relationship with the enzymatic activity of soil. *Fresenius Environmental Bulletin*, *18*(7), 1046–1053.

Xiao, G., Ni, M.-J., Chi, Y., Jin, B.-S., Xiao, R., Zhong, Z.-P., & Huang, Y.-J. (2009). Gasification characteristics of MSW and an ANN prediction model. *Waste Management (New York, N.Y.)*, *29*(1), 240–244. doi:10.1016/j.wasman.2008.02.022 PMID:18420400

Xia, T., Kovochich, M., Liong, M., Zink, J. I., & Nel, A. E. (2008). Cationic polystyrene nanosphere toxicity depends on cell-specific endocytic and mitochondrial injury pathways. *ACS Nano*, *2*(1), 85–96. doi:10.1021/nn700256c PMID:19206551

Xie & Qi. (2011). *Environmental impacts from PET packaging waste management using Life Cycle Assessment: A case study in China. International Symposium.*

Xie, C., Liu, F., Yu, S., Xie, F., Li, L., Zhang, S., & Yang, J. (2008). Catalytic cracking of polypropylene into liquid hydrocarbons over Zr and Mo modified MCM-41 mesoporous molecular sieve. *Catalysis Communications*, *10*(1), 79–82. doi:10.1016/j.catcom.2008.08.001

Xie, Z., Ebinghaus, R., Temme, C., Lohmann, R., Caba, A., & Ruck, W. (2007). Occurrence and air– sea exchange of phthalates in the Arctic. *Environmental Science & Technology*, *41*(13), 4555–4560. doi:10.1021/es0630240 PMID:17695896

Xue, Y., Wang, C., Hu, Z., Zhou, Y., Liu, G., Hou, H., ... Li, J. (2018). Thermal treatment on sewage sludge by electromagnetic induction heating: Methodology and drying characterization. *Waste Management (New York, N.Y.)*, *78*, 917–928. doi:10.1016/j.wasman.2018.07.009

Xu, X., Tan, L., Himi, T., Sadamatsu, M., Tsutsumi, S., Akaike, M., & Kato, N. (2011). Changed preference for sweet taste in adulthood induced by perinatal exposure to Bisphenol A—A probable link to overweight and obesity. *Neurotoxicology and Teratology*, *33*(4), 458–463. doi:10.1016/j.ntt.2011.06.002 PMID:21704699

Yamada-Onodera, K., Mukumoto, H., Katsuyaya, Y., Saiganji, A., & Tani, Y. (2001). Degradation of polyethylene by a fungus *Penicillium simplicissimum* YK. *Polymer Degradation & Stability*, *72*(2), 323–327. doi:10.1016/S0141-3910(01)00027-1

Yamaguchi, A., Ishibashi, H., Kohra, S., Arizono, K., & Tominaga, N. (2005). Short-term effects of endocrine-disrupting chemicals on the expression of estrogen-responsive genes in male medaka (Oryzias latipes*). Aquatic Toxicology (Amsterdam, Netherlands)*, *72*(3), 239–249. doi:10.1016/j.aquatox.2004.12.011 PMID:15820104

Yamamoto, T., Isaka, K., Sato, H., Matsukura, Y., & Ishida, H. (2000). Gasification and smelting system using oxygen blowing for municipal waste. *ISIJ International*, *40*(3), 260–265. doi:10.2355/isijinternational.40.260

Yang, G. C., & Yang, T. Y. (1998). Synthesis of zeolites from municipal incinerator fly ash. *Journal of Hazardous Materials*, *62*(1), 75–89. doi:10.1016/S0304-3894(98)00163-0

Yang, M., Kim, S. Y., Chang, S. S., Lee, I. S., & Kawamoto, T. (2006). Urinary concentrations of bisphenol A in relation to biomarkers of sensitivity and effect and endocrine-related health effects. *Environmental and Molecular Mutagenesis*, *47*(8), 571–578. doi:10.1002/em.20230 PMID:16795089

Yarsley, V. E., & Couzens, E. G. (1945). *Plastics*. Middlesex, UK: Penguin Books Limited.

Yawson, R. M. (2009). *The Ecological System of Innovation: A New Architectural Framework for a Functional Evidence-Based Platform for Science and Innovation Policy*. doi:10.2139srn.1417676

Yin, X., Zhang, J., & Wang, X. (2004a). *Sequential injection analysis system for the determination of arsenic by hydride generation atomic absorption spectrometry*. doi:10.1017/CBO9781107415324.004

Yokota, H., Iwano, H., Endo, M., Kobayashi, T., Inoue, H., Ikushiro, S., & Yuasa, A. (1999). Glucuronidation of the environmental oestrogen Bisphenol A by an isoform of UDP-glucuronosyl transferase, UGT2B1, in the rat liver. *The Biochemical Journal*, *340*(2), 405–409. doi:10.1042/bj3400405 PMID:10333482

Yonekubo, J., Hayakawa, K., & Sajiki, J. (2008). Concentrations of bisphenol A, bisphenol A diglycidyl ether, and their derivatives in canned foods in Japanese markets. *Journal of Agricultural and Food Chemistry*, *56*(6), 2041–2047. doi:10.1021/jf073106n PMID:18284199

Yoon, O. S. (2001). Disposal measures and problems of medical waste. *Journal of Korean Solid Wastes Engineering Soc*, *18*(1), 1–12.

Yoshida, S., Hiraga, K., Takehana, T., Taniguchi, I., Yamaji, H., Maeda, Y., ... Oda, K. (2016). A bacterium that degrades and assimilates polyethylene terephthalate. *Science*, *351*(6278), 1196–1199. doi:10.1126cience.aad6359 PMID:26965627

Yoshida, T., Horie, M., Hoshino, Y., Nakazawa, H., Horie, M., & Nakazawa, H. (2001). Determination of bisphenol A in canned vegetables and fruitby high performance liquid chromatography. *Food Additives and Contaminants*, *18*(1), 69–75. doi:10.1080/026520301446412 PMID:11212549

Yoshioka, T., Furukawa, K., Sato, T., & Okuwaki, A. (1998). Chemical recycling of flexible PVC by oxygen oxidation in NaOH solutions at elevated temperatures. *Journal of Applied Polymer Science*, *70*(1), 129–135. doi:10.1002/(SICI)1097-4628(19981003)70:1<129::AID-APP13>3.0.CO;2-2

Yuan, B. L., Li, X. Z., & Graham, N. (2008). Aqueous oxidation of dimethyl phthalate in a Fe (VI)-TiO2-UV reaction system. *Water Research*, *42*(6-7), 1413–1420. doi:10.1016/j.watres.2007.10.010 PMID:17977571

Zacharewski, T. R., Meek, M. D., Clemons, J. H., Wu, Z. F., Fielden, M. R., & Matthews, J. B. (1998). Examination of the in vitro and in vitro estrogenic activities of eight commercial phthalate esters. *Toxicological Sciences*, *46*(2), 282–293. PMID:10048131

Zalasiewicz, J., Waters, C. N., Ivar do Sul, J. A., Corcoran, P. L., Barnosky, A. D., Cearreta, A., ... Yonan, Y. (2016). The geological cycle of plastics and their use as a stratigraphic indicator of the Anthropocene. *Anthropocene*, *13*, 4–17. doi:10.1016/j.ancene.2016.01.002

Zalko D, Jacques C, Duplan H, Bruel S, Perdu E. (2011). Viable skin efficiently absorbs and metabolizes Bisphenol A. *Chemosphere, 82,* 424–430. doi.: PMID. 21030062 doi:10.1016/j.chemosphere.2010.09.058

Zaman, T. (2010). *The Prevalence and Environmental Impact of Single Use Plastic Products*. Academic Press.

Zare Jeddi, M., Eshaghi Gorji, M., Rietjens, I., Louisse, J., Bruinen de Bruin, Y., & Liska, R. (2018). Biomonitoring and subsequent risk assessment of combined exposure to phthalates in Iranian children and adolescents. *International Journal of Environmental Research and Public Health*, *15*(11), 2336. doi:10.3390/ijerph15112336 PMID:30360526

Zeeshan, M. F., Al Ibad, A., Aziz, A., Subhani, A., Shah, A., & Khan, T. (2018). Practice and enforcement of national Hospital Waste Management 2005 rules in Pakistan. *Eastern Mediterranean Health Journal, 24*(5), 443+. doi:10.26719/2018.24.5.443

Zettler, E. R., Mincer, T. J., & Amaral-Zettler, L. A. (2013). Life in the "plastisphere": Microbial communities on plastic marine debris. *Environmental Science & Technology*, *47*(13), 7137–7146. doi:10.1021/es401288x PMID:23745679

Zhang, D. Q., He, P. J., Yu, L. Z., & Shao, L. M. (2009). Effect of inoculation time on the bio– drying performance of combined hydrolytic–aerobic process. *Bioresource Technology*, *100*(3), 1087–1093. doi:10.1016/j.biortech.2008.07.059 PMID:18835776

Zhang, H., Obias, V., Gonyer, K., & Dennis, D. (1994). Production of polyhydroxyalkanoates in sucrose-utilizing recombinant Escherichia coli and Klebsiella strains. *Applied and Environmental Microbiology*, *60*, 1198–1205. PMID:8017916

Zhang, K., Su, J., Xiong, X., Wu, X., Wu, C., & Liu, J. (2016). Microplastic pollution of lakeshore sediments from remote lakes in Tibet plateau, China. *Environmental Pollution*, *219*, 450–455. doi:10.1016/j.envpol.2016.05.048 PMID:27238763

Zhang, Y. H. (2006). Phthalate exposure and human semen quality in Shanghai: a cross-sectional study. *Biomedical and Environmental Sciences*, *19*, 205–209. PMID:16944777

Zhang, Y., Meng, X., Chen, L., Li, D., Zhao, L., Zhao, Y., ... Shi, H. (2014). Age and sex-specific relationships between phthalate exposures and obesity in Chinese children at puberty. *PLoS One*, *9*(8), e104852. doi:10.1371/journal.pone.0104852 PMID:25121758

Zhang, Z., Alomirah, H., Cho, H. S., Li, Y. F., Liao, C., Minh, T. B., ... Kannan, K. (2011). Urinary Bisphenol A concentrations and their implications for human exposure in several Asian countries. *Environmental Science & Technology*, *1*(45), 7044–7050. doi:10.1021/es200976k PMID:21732633

Zhang, Z., Hirose, T., Nishio, S., Morioka, Y., Azuma, N., Ueno, A., ... Okada, M. (1995). Chemical recycling of waste polystyrene into styrene over solid acids and bases. *Industrial & Engineering Chemistry Research*, *34*(12), 4514–4519. doi:10.1021/ie00039a044

Zhao, W., Hasegawa, S., Fujita, J., Yoshii, F., Sasaki, T., Makuuchi, K., ... Nishimoto, S. (1996). Effects of zeolites on the pyrolysis polypropylene. *Polymer Degradation & Stability*, *53*(1), 129–135. doi:10.1016/0141-3910(96)00080-8

Zhou, R., Zhang, Z., Zhu, Y., Chen, L., Sokabe, M., & Chen, L. (2009). Deficits in development of synaptic plasticity in rat dorsal striatum following prenatal and neonatal exposure to lowdose Bisphenol A. *Neuroscience*, *159*(1), 161–171. doi:10.1016/j.neuroscience.2008.12.028 PMID:19162132

Zhu, D., Asnani, P. U., Zurbrugg, C., Anapolsky, S., & Mani, S. K. (2007). *Improving municipal solid waste management in India: A sourcebook for policymakers and practitioners*. The World Bank. doi:10.1596/978-0-8213-7361-3

Zimmerman-Downs, J. M., Shuman, D., Stull, S. C., & Ratzlaff, R. E. (2010). Bisphenol A blood and saliva levels prior to and after dental sealant placement in adults. *Journal of Dental Hygiene*, *84*(3), 145–150. PMID:20579427

Ziółkowska, A., & Wyszkowski, M. (2010). Toxicity of petroleum s ubstances to microorganisms and plants. *Ecological Chemistry and Engineering. S*, *17*(1), 73–82.

Zion Research Analysis. (2016). *Plastics: Complex systems problem*. Academic Press.

Zoeller, R. T., Bansal, R., & Parris, C. (2005). Bisphenol A- an environmental contaminant that acts as a thyroid hormone receptor antagonist in vitro, increases serum thyroxine, and alters RC3/neurogranin expression in the developing rat brain. *The Journal of Endocrinology*, *146*(2), 607–612. doi:10.1210/en.2004-1018 PMID:15498886

Zota, A. R., Calafat, A. M., & Woodruff, T. J. (2014). Temporal trends in phthalate exposures: Findings from the National Health and Nutrition Examination Survey, 2001–2010. *Environmental Health Perspectives*, *122*(3), 235–241. doi:10.1289/ehp.1306681 PMID:24425099

Zota, A. R., Phillips, C. A., & Mitro, S. D. (2016). *Recent Fast Food Consumption and Bisphenol A andPhthalates Exposures among the US Population in NHANES, 2003–2010*. Environmental HealthPerspective.

Zuberi, M. J., & Ali, S. F. (2015). Greenhouse effect reduction by recovering energy from waste landfills in Pakistan. *Renewable & Sustainable Energy Reviews*, *44*, 117–131. doi:10.1016/j.rser.2014.12.028

Zubris, K. A. V., & Richards, B. K. (2005). Synthetic fibers as an indicator of land application of sludge. *Environmental Pollution*, *138*(2), 201–211. doi:10.1016/j.envpol.2005.04.013 PMID:15967553

About the Contributors

Khursheed Ahmad Wani is Lecturer in the Department of Environmental Science, Government Degree College Bijbehara, J&K. Dr. Wani served at ITM University Gwalior as Assistant Professor in the Department of Environmental Science from 2011 to 2017. He has completed his M. Sc. and Ph. D. in Environmental Science from Jiwaji University, Gwalior, Madhya Pradesh. He has also qualified Jammu and Kashmir State Level Eligibility Test (JKSET). His areas of interest include Environmental management, Environmental Impact Assessment and Occupational Health. He has published research papers in various national and international journals and is the author of three books on Environmental Science. He is a member of several national and international organizations and is in the editorial board of various journals. He has organized different programmes on Environmental Awareness and has completed research project sponsored by Madhya Pradesh Council of Science and Technology, Bhopal, India. Dr. Wani has organized various national and international conferences/seminars/workshops as well.

S. M. Zuber is presently working as Sr. Assistant Professor in Government Degree College Bijbehara, Kashmir, India. Dr. Zuber has more than 15 papers to his credit published in Journals of national and international repute.

* * *

Toqeer Ahmed is currently working as Assistant Professor at Centre for Climate Research and Development (CCRD), COMSATS University Islamabad. Since his education, he has worked at responsible positions in several different Government departments and R & D organizations. He has completed several national as well as international projects in collaboration with the University of Edinburgh, UK, UNDP, IISD, SDC Islamabad, national NGOs and Government departments. He has more than 35 peer reviewed research publications in the field of food and water quality assessment, wastewater treatment, climate impacts on health and Nano-biotechnology. Dr. Ahmed has lectured and presented Research Papers in both national and international conferences. He has organized different seminars, training workshops, conferences on water quality, water management and environmental issues. He introduced the concept of Smart Water Metering (SWM) in Pakistan. He is currently working on Environmental Issues, Climate Change Impacts on Health, Water Management and Environmental Nanotechnology.

Md Ali is presently An Associate professor at Centre of Research for Development (CORD), University of Kashmir.

Zainab Kalimuddin Ali is currently working as a lecturer of Zoology at Wahed College of Science, Amravati. Maharashtra. She has completed her Masters in Zoology from Sant Gadge Baba Amravati University. She has also completed Advance Diploma in Cosmetology from Shri Shivaji Science College, Amravati besides having the DNYS from Akhil Bhartiya Prakritik Chikitsa Parishad, New Delhi. She is the gold medal awardee in the subject chemistry and microbiology in BSC. She is also the recipient of certificate and memento given by Afroz jahan Memorial e-trust for outstanding success in education.

Attiya Baddar has completed post-graduation in Education (M. Ed) from the Department of Education, University of Kashmir Srinagar. She has qualified State Eligibility Test (JKSET) and is presently pursuing Doctorate in the Postgraduate Department of Education, University of Kashmir.

Irfan Ashraf Badroo is a research scholar in the Department of Zoology, Sant Gadge Baba Amravati University, Amravati Maharashtra. The area of research is toxicology. He has qualified Graduate Aptitude test in Engineering (GATE) organized by Indian Institute of Technology Bombay. He has also qualified Jammu and Kashmir State level Eligibility Test (JKSET). He has also been declared successful and qualified Joint CSIR-UGC test for Junior Research Fellowship and Eligibility for Lectureship. His area of interest include biochemistry, aquaculture, biodiversity cytotoxity and genotoxicity. He has publication in national and international journals and is a co-author of a book chapter. He has also been an organizing member of National conference. He has won best paper presentation awards in both international and national conferences. He has also actively participated and attended various workshops.

Suriya Ashraf Badroo is currently working as a lecturer at Muslim Education Trust, Sopore, Jammu and Kashmir. She has completed her Masters in Zoology from Barkatuallah University, Madhya Pradesh. She has also completed B.Ed. from University of Kashmir, Jammu and Kashmir.

Yahya Bakhtiyar obtained his M. Sc. (Zoology) in 2002 from Aligarh Muslim University, Aligarh, and was awarded Ph.D. in Zoology with Ichthyology / Fish and Fisheries specialization from University of Jammu in 2008. He worked as a Lecturer in Zoology, School Education Department before joining Department of Zoology, University of Kashmir, as Assistant Professor in 2013. He has worked as Junior Research Fellow and Senior Research Fellow in DST (J&K Govt.) project entitled "Nutritional Requirements of Certain Fresh Water Prawns of Local Commercial Importance and Development of Low-Cost Formula Feeds" for 3 years and has also worked as Senior Research Fellow in another DST (GOI) funded Project entitled "Demonstration of Mono and polyculture of Macrobrachium rosenbergii and Indian major carps in Jammu" for 1 year. Dr. Yahya Bakhtiyar has a Post-Graduate teaching experience of 05 years and research experience of more than 07 years in the field of Zoology. His major research highlights include Nutritional requirements of freshwater prawn of Jammu region; Development of low-cost formula feeds for Macrobrachium dayanum; Food preferences of Macrobrachium dayanum (Henderson) and Labeo rohita (Hamilton); Nutritional status and culture of food organisms; Mono and polyculture of Macrobrachium rosenbergii and Indian major carps; Proximate composition of various Fish, prawns and natural and artificial food ingredients. It's worth to mention that Dr. Bakhtiyar is the Top rank holder in the State in 10+2 Zoology Lecturer (School Education) list conducted by Jammu and Kashmir Public service Commission in the year 2008. He has published 27 research papers in reputed

National and International Journals in the field of Fish and Fisheries. Moreover, he has participated in 30 International/National Conferences/Regional conferences besides attending the number of workshops as well. He is a life member of various societies including Indian Science Congress Association, Inland Fisheries Society of India, Indian Fisheries Association, Indian Academy of Environmental Biology etc. Presently his focus of research is Fish Biology especially the impact of exotic carps on local fish fauna and water ecosystem.

Monika Bhadauria is an Associate Professor, Toxicology and Pharmacology Laboratory, Department of Zoology, Guru Ghasidas Vishwavidyalaya.

Sajood Bhat is a research Scholar at Department of chemistry Govt of S.G.S. P.G.(Autom) College Sidhi Madhy Pradesh.

Rayees Ahmad Bhat is a research scholar at Centre of Research for Chemical Sciences, Govt Model Science College, Jiwaji University, Gwalior.

Trinath Biswal has done their PhD at Utkal University, Bhubaneswer in the broad area of complex catalyses polymerization and co-polymerization. Their research area is polymer biocomposite and environmental science. They have published about 20 research papers in national and international Journal along with three books.

Muhammad Reza Cordova is a researcher work on the topic of marine pollution, marine ecology and biology, ecotoxicology and environmental stress. He worked more than ten years in marine pollution project including heavy metal and marine plastic pollution, particularly in distribution, occurrence, and toxicology of marine debris and microplastic, in Indonesian Seas. He already published scientific publications correlated to marine pollution and get a grant from research grants, scholarships, and travel awards. Reza has experience as a lecturer in undergraduate level at three universities in Indonesia and as industrial experience as an environmental impact assessment consultant.

Ashaq Ahmad Dar is a Research Scholar pursuing his Ph. D. from Department of Ecology and Environmental Science, Pondicherry University, Puducherry. He had published a number of papers and also attended a lot of international and national conferences. Moreover, he had qualified JRF-NET, ASRB-NET and JK-SET.

Ankita Dhillon obtained her M.Sc. and Ph.D. degree in 2013 and 2017, respectively from Banasthali Vidyapith, Rajasthan, India. Her Ph.D. supervisor was Dr. Dinesh Kumar, School of Chemical Sciences, Central University of Gujarat, Gandhinagar, India. Presently, she has been working as an Assistant Professor at Department of Chemistry, Banasthali Vidyapith since 2017. She has published more than a dozen papers in various journals of international repute. She has authored eight book chapters in different books published by various publishers of international repute. She has presented her work in several national and international conferences. She has received three young scientist awards for best paper presentation in international conferences. Her research interest includes the development of water purification technology.

Prachi Dixit is presently working as Junior Research Fellow in MPCST funded project in Dept. of Environmental Science, ITM University, Gwalior, Madhya Pradesh. Participated in 06 National/International conferences/seminars. Actively engaged in research activities and presently enrolled for Ph. D in ITM University, Gwalior, Madhya Pradesh. Published 1 research paper in National journal of repute. The broad areas of interest are Biotechnology, Environmental Science and Microbiology.

Hamid Iqbal has completed his post graduation from Aligarh Muslim University, Aligarh and completed his Ph.D. in Botany in the year 2010. He is presently serving as Assistant Professor, College of Applied Biotechnology, Ministry of Higher Education, Sur- Sultanante of Oman. He was a Postdoctoral Fellow - Department of Biological Sciences, Faculty of Agriculture, Science and Technology, North-West University, Mafikeng Campus, South Africa. from Feb, 2012 to Aug 2014. He has published about 12 papers in national and international journal with high impact factor. Has received many awards in the form of NRF Free standing Post-Doctoral Fellowship 2013 Ref No: SFP12090312175, Grant No. 85210 Dated 19th March 2013. Post-Doctoral Fellowship, North West University, South Africa 2012. UGC Research Fellowship, University Grants Commission (U.G.C.), New Delhi, India 2007- 2010. Dr. Mohd. Farooq Memorial Scholarship for the session 2005-06 for Merit in MSc.

Ashiq Hussain Khanday is a research scholar in the Department of Botany, Sant Gadge Baba Amravati University, Amravati Maharashtra. The area of research is Genetic Divergence phylogenetic analysis. He has qualified Graduate Aptitude test in Engineering (GATE). He has qualified twice Joint CSIR-UGC test for Eligibility for Lectureship. His area of interest include genetic divergence, phylogenetic analysis, biodiversity and bioinformatics. He has various publications in international and national journals and is a co-author of a book chapter. He has also actively participated and attended various workshops.

D. Kumar is Professor at Centre of Research for Chemical Sciences, Govt Model Science College, Jiwaji University, Gwalior.

Dinesh Kumar is an academician and researcher of international recognition in School of Chemical Sciences at the Central University of Gujarat, Gandhinagar. He has joined as an Associate Professor in the School of Chemical Sciences at the Central University of Gujarat, Gandhinagar in 2017. Prior to the Central University of Gujarat, Gandhinagar, he taught at the Banasthali University, Rajasthan as an Assistant Professor of Chemistry from 2007 to 2011, and as an Associate Professor of Chemistry from 2011 to 2017. Dr. Kumar has obtained his master and Ph.D. degrees in Chemistry from the Department of Chemistry, University of Rajasthan, Jaipur. Dr. Kumar has received many national awards and fellowships like young scientist awards, excellent speaker, a young researcher award in National and International conferences, CSIR-HRDG fellowship, Departmental Scholarship od Department of Chemistry and University Fellowship of the University of Rajasthan. He has been invited as a speaker in a workshop in Trieste, The World Academy of Sciences (TWAS), Italy. His research interest focuses on the development of capped nanoparticles, core-shell, metal oxide-based nanoadsorbent and nanosensors for the removal and sensing of health hazardous inorganic toxicants like fluoride and heavy metal ions from aqueous media. To boot, his research interests also focus on the synthesis of supramolecular metal complexes, metal chelates and searching for their biological effectiveness. He has authored more than ninety publications in journals of international repute, one book, and more than four dozen book chapters. He has been delivered more than fifteen invited lectures and over than 40 oral and poster presentations in national and international conferences and symposia.

Hendrik Lamsali is an associate professor in Universiti Utara Malaysia, under the College of Business. He is a faculty member of UUM School of Technology Management and Logistics. His research area includes operations management, reverse logistics, green supply chains, decisions science/operations research. Currently he is also the director of the Student Affairs Department.

Javid Manzoor is a PhD student in the Department of Environmental Science (IGAEERE), Jiwaji University, Gwalior, Madhya Pradesh, India. He has obtained his Master's degree from the same university. He has two years of teaching experience. He is an awardee of University Research Scholarship. He is a permanent member of people for animal. His areas of interest include environmental pollution, occupational health and biomedical waste management. He has published research papers and book chapters in various national and international journals with impact factor.

Sajad Hussain Mir is presently working as Lecturer in zoology in the Department of Education, Govt. of Jammu and Kashmir, India. He has completed M. Sc. (Zoology), M. Phil and Ph. D from the Postgraduate Department of Zoology, University of Kashmir. He has worked extensively on "Experimental Diabetology". He has contributed more than 25 research papers in reputed national and international journals and has authored two books. He has completed a project in the Department of School Education entitled, "Study of role and functioning of village education committee in management of schools and participation of community in school affairs" under Sarva Shiksha Abhiyan. He is a member of editorial board of many international journals and is actively involved in promotion of science learning by presenting Live Tele-Classes besides, working as a reviewer of many international journals.

Rafiya Munvar is Research Scholar at School of Studies in Environmental Science Jiwaji University, Gwalior India. she has published various research papers in reputed journals and her area of research is nanotechnology and toxicology.

Sapna Nehra received her M.Sc. degree in 2014 from Banasthali Vidyapith, Rajasthan, India. Since July 2015, she has been pursuing her research work under the supervision of Dr. Dinesh Kumar, School of Chemical Sciences, Central University of Gujarat, Gandhinagar. She has published four papers and book publishers of international repute, respectively. She has presented her work in several national and international conferences. Her research interests include the development of smart materials for water purification.

Sapna Raghav was awarded her master's degree (Chemistry) in 2014 from Banasthali Vidyapith, Rajasthan, India. Since April 2016, she has been pursuing her research work under the supervision of Dr. Dinesh Kumar, School of Chemical Sciences, Central University of Gujarat, Gandhinagar. She has published seven papers and four book chapters in various journals and book publishers of international repute, respectively. She has presented her work in several national and international conferences. Her research interests include the development of water purification technology.

Kajal S. Rathore is working at Department of Department of Biotechnology, Govt. KRG (Autonomous) PG College, Gwalior, India. She also worked as Post Doctoral Fellow at the G. B. Pant University of Agriculture and Technology, Pantnagar, India. Following a guest faculty at Department of Botany, Bareilly College, Bareilly. She received her doctoral degree in Botany, from MJP Rohilkhand University, Bareilly, India and had studied post graduation in Industrial Biotechnology from Ch. Charan Singh University, Meerut, India. Dr. Rathore is the author of over 40 peer-reviewed publications in national and international journals and edited two books on bioremediation and neutraceuticals (IGI Global Publisher, USA). She also holds membership of many professional bodies and is awarded as fellow of Indian Botanical Society. Her research specifically focuses on rhizosphere biology, plant biochemistry and environmental biotechnology. She is life member of various national as well as international scientific bodies/societies in the field of plant and environmental biotechnology.

Pushkar Singh Rawat is currently pursuing PhD in the Department of Biochemistry, University of Lucknow, Lucknow. He has completed his M.Sc in Biochemistry from the Department of Biochemistry, University of Lucknow, Lucknow. He has University Gold Medalist in Graduation. He has qualified Uttarakhand State Eligibility Test (USET), Himachal Pradesh State Eligibility Test (HPSET) & Chhattisgarh State Eligibility Test (CGSET). He has also selected for the prestigious ICMR SRF fellowship. His areas of expertise are Biochemical toxicology and Clinical Biochemistry. He has more than 5 years research experience. He likes to write on several emerging research contents.

Summia Rehman is a PhD student in the Department of Botany, University of Kashmir, Srinagar, J&K India.

Manoj Sharma born on 1st September 1977, obtained his B. Pharm from Barkatullah University, Bhopal in 1999 and M. Pharm (Pharmacology) from Rajiv Gandhi University of Health Sciences, Bangalore, Karnataka in March 2003. After Qualifying Junior Research Fellowship (JRF) Examination of DRDO, New Delhi in 2004, He joined as JRF in the Laboratory of Dr. R. Vijayaraghavan Head, Division of Pharmacology and Toxicology, Defence Research and Development Establishment (DRDE), Gwalior (MP) Followed by Senior Research Fellow (SRF) by in 2006 to pursue his Doctoral Work. He was awarded his PhD from Jiwaji University, Gwalior in April 2009. He is presently working as an Associate Professor in Pharmacology and Toxicology Department, School of Studies in Pharmaceutical Sciences, Jiwaji University Gwalior-India. His area of Specialization is Development of Cytoprotective agent against alkylating anticancer agents and Drug Discovery & Development and Nerve agent Toxicity. He has published several research papers in Journal of National and International repute. He received Jewel of India Award in 2014 and Best paper award in 2009 at DRDE Award Ceremony, Gwalior, India. He has authored / co-authored of four books and also applied for one patent. He has completed one project as Principal investigator funded by DRDE, Gwalior and also completed 08 projects as team member during fellowship period. He has supervised 02 Phd thesis & 20 M.Pharm student`s dissertations. He has Honour of Fellow of International Science Congress Association (FISCA). He has been nominated as "CPCSEA Nominee" by Ministry of Environment and Forest, Govt. of India in 2014. He has also been nominated as Young Pharmacologist Fellow from Central Region by Indian Pharmacological Society (IPS).

Neha Sharma is working as Assistant Professor in Amity Institute of Biotechnology, Amity University Madhya Pradesh, Gwalior. She has more than 10 years experience of teaching and research. She has participated in more than forty National/International conferences/seminars. She is actively engaged in research activities and members of reputed scientific societies. She has published 17 research papers and 03 book chapters in National and International journal of repute. The broad areas of her interest are Microbiology and Biotechnology. She got ;Young Biotechnologist Award 2019; "Young Scientist Award 2018" and "Junior Scientist of the year 2015" by different scientific bodies.

Shalini Singh is a Research Scholar pursuing PhD from the Department of Biochemistry, University of Lucknow, Lucknow. She has qualified GATE and ASRB NET examination. She has also University Gold Medalist and selected for the prestigious DST INSPIRE fellowship. She is a passionate researcher in the area of Molecular biology, Microbiology and Enzymology. She has published various book chapters and research papers in many national and international journals. She also presented her research findings in national and international conferences.

Shivom Singh is working as Assistant Professor, Department of Environmental Science, ITM University, Gwalior, India. He also worked as Postdoctoral Fellow at the Department of Biological Science, G. B. Pant University of Agriculture and Technology, Pantnagar (UK). Dr. Shivom Singh received two Ph.D. degrees first in Botany from MJP Rohilkhand University, Bareilly and second in Environmental Sciences from Gurukul Kangri University, Haridwar. His postgraduate degree is from the Gurukul Kangri University, Haridwar, India. He is a Fellow of Action for Sustainable, Efficacious Development and Awareness (FASEA) and fellow of Indian Botanical Society. Dr. Singh research on Environmental monitoring of different aspects of pollutions and their biological managements and rhizosphere biology. His current work is aimed on biofertilizer and biopesticides. He has written two edited books (IGI Global Publisher, USA) and more than forty research and review articles in reputed national and international journals. He is life member of various national as well as international scientific bodies/societies in the field of bryology, plant science, and environmental science.

Hassaan Sipra is working as Scientific Officer at Centre for Climate Research and Development, COMSATS University Islamabad. His work focuses on water conservation, climate impacts and air pollution. Previously, he has served at Lahore Waste Management Company and Asian Development Bank. He has a Master's in Environmental Management from Yale School of Forestry & Environmental Studies and a Bachelor's in Economics and Environmental Science from Westminster College MO.

Irfan Rashid Sofi has done his M.Sc. in Environmental Science from HNB Gharwal University Dehradun, Uttarakhand and M.Phil. from Jiwaji University Gwalior and is pursuing PhD from School of Studies in Environmental Science Jiwaji University Gwalior M.P. India. He has published research papers and various book chapters in national and international journals.

Ruchi Srivastava is a research scholar in Jiwaji University Gwalior, Madhya Pradesh.

Vaishali Tomar is currently working in the capacity of Formulation Scientist in New York, USA and is leading the complete formulation department for a prestigious organization. Dr. Tomar is also an active member of editor board of International Journal of Nanotechnology in Medicine and Engineering

(Bio Core) and Open Access Journal of Chemistry (Sryahwa Publications). Dr. Tomar is also a reviewer for many prestigious journals, viz: Chemistry Central Journal, Journal of Fluorine Chemistry etc. She has good publication track in very prestigious journal like Microchemical Journal and have published quality papers in the field of Nanotechnology. She has awarded with Young Scientist Award in 2011 by Indian Council of Chemists and in 2013 by Current Research in Engineering Sciences and Technology. Dr. Tomar holds a doctorate degree from Banasthali University, where her research circled mostly around nanotechnology space. Dr. Tomar and her husband have a wonderful daughter, age four. She enjoys meeting people and explore places.

Index

L

M

N

O

P

R

S

T

U

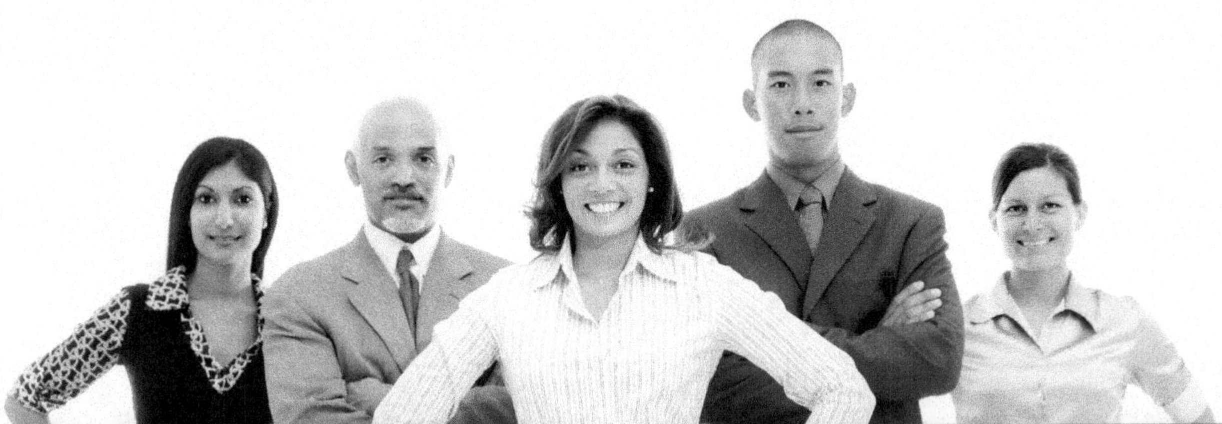

www.ingramcontent.com/pod-product-compliance
Lightning Source LLC
LaVergne TN
LVHW080618300926
849162LV00005B/1197